Multidisciplinary Management of
Gastrointestinal Cancers

Multidisciplinary Management of
Gastrointestinal
Cancers

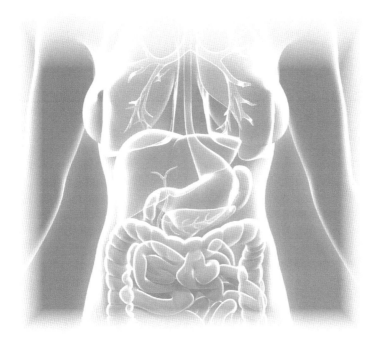

Edited by

Weijing SUN
University of Pittsburgh, USA

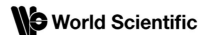 **World Scientific**

NEW JERSEY · LONDON · SINGAPORE · BEIJING · SHANGHAI · HONG KONG · TAIPEI · CHENNAI · TOKYO

Published by

World Scientific Publishing Co. Pte. Ltd.

5 Toh Tuck Link, Singapore 596224

USA office: 27 Warren Street, Suite 401-402, Hackensack, NJ 07601

UK office: 57 Shelton Street, Covent Garden, London WC2H 9HE

Library of Congress Cataloging-in-Publication Data

Names: Sun, Weijing, editor.

Title: Multidisciplinary management of gastrointestinal cancers / [edited by] Weijing Sun.

Description: New Jersey : World Scientific, 2016. | Includes bibliographical references and index.

Identifiers: LCCN 2016007773 | ISBN 9789814651868 (hardback : alk. paper)

Subjects: | MESH: Digestive System Neoplasms--therapy | Digestive System
  Neoplasms--diagnosis

Classification: LCC RC280.D5 | NLM WI 149 | DDC 616.99/433--dc23

LC record available at http://lccn.loc.gov/2016007773

British Library Cataloguing-in-Publication Data

A catalogue record for this book is available from the British Library.

Typeset by Stallion Press

Email: enquiries@stallionpress.com

Printed in Singapore

Contents

Preface

About a quarter of all diagnosed malignancies originate from the gastrointestinal (GI) system, which in nature demands multidisciplinary management because of the complexity of heterogeneity in etiology, great variations in molecular biology/genetic characteristics, involvement of multiple organs and their distinctive functions, and the tremendous differences in treatment options and outcomes for each different disease.

With the expeditious advancement in molecular biology/genetic profile analyses (such as next generation DNA sequencing [NGS], circulating tumor cells [CTCs], cell-free DNA [cfDNA] from liquid biopsy samples, and TCGA programs) and technology (e.g. robotic surgery), as well as recent discoveries of new therapeutic agents (e.g. target-oriented agents, tyrosine kinase inhibitors [TKIs], and immune checkpoint inhibitors), multidisciplinary management for GI cancers is required to achieve the best outcome for both the individual cancer patient (personalized medicine/precision medicine) and the general society (preventive medicine).

With the principles given above, this book is designed to provide up-to-date, evidence-based information and knowledge on the multidisciplinary management of the major malignancies in the GI system, including etiology analysis, genetic and hereditary evaluation, critical diagnostic procedures/processes, new surgical and technology advantages, the role of radiation therapy, and novel systemic agents' development and application in clinical practice. The book also covers the significant issues of quality of life and supportive care of GI cancer patients. We hope this book may facilitate oncology practitioners, including those in all sub-specialty areas, to view and manage GI cancers with multidisciplinary perspective in their daily practice.

Weijing Sun, MD, FACP
Professor of Medicine
University of Pittsburgh Medical Center
Pittsburgh, PA

List of Contributors

Mark Agulnik, MD, FRCPC
Associate Professor of Medicine
Director, Hematology/Oncology Fellowship Training Program
Division of Hematology/Oncology
Robert H. Lurie Comprehensive Cancer Center
Northwestern University Feinberg School of Medicine
Chicago, IL

Nathan Bahary, MD, PhD
Associate Professor of Medicine
Department of Medicine
Division of Hematology/Oncology
University of Pittsburgh Cancer Institute
Pittsburgh, PA

Brian C. Baumann MD
Resident, Class of 2017
Department of Radiation Oncology
Hospital of the University of Pennsylvania
Perelman Center for Advanced Medicine
Philadelphia, PA

Edgar Ben-Josef, MD
Professor of Radiation Oncology
Department of Radiation Oncology
Hospital of the University of Pennsylvania
Perelman Center for Advanced Medicine
Philadelphia, PA

Randall E. Brand, MD
Professor of Medicine
Division of Gastroenterology, Hepatology & Nutrition
University of Pittsburgh Medical Center
Pittsburgh, PA

Edward Chu, MD
Professor of Medicine and Pharmacology & Chemical Biology
Chief, Division of Hematology-Oncology
Deputy Director, University of Pittsburgh Cancer Institute
University of Pittsburgh School of Medicine
Pittsburgh, PA

Mauro Cives, MD
Department of GI Oncology
H. Lee Moffitt Cancer Center and Research Institute
Tampa, FL

Tong Dai, MD, PhD
Assistant Professor of Medicine
Division of Hematology and Medical Oncology
GI Oncology Program
Weill Cornell Medical College, Cornell University
New York, NY

Neha J. Darrah, MD
Supportive Medicine Physician
Division of General Internal Medicine
Cedars-Sinai Medical Center
Los Angeles, CA

Beth Dudley, MS, MPH, CGC
Licensed Genetic Counselor
University of Pittsburgh Medical Center
Pittsburgh, PA

Jennifer Eads, MD
Assistant Professor of Medicine
Division of Hematology and Oncology
University Hospitals Seidman Cancer Center
Case Comprehensive Cancer Center
Case Western Reserve University
Cleveland, OH

Alyssa D. Fajardo, MD
Assistant Professor of Surgery
Department of Surgery
Division of Colorectal Surgery
Indiana University School of Medicine
Indianapolis, IN

Kenneth E. Fasanella, MD
Assistant Professor of Medicine
Program Director, Gastroenterology Fellowship
Division of Gastroenterology, Hepatology and Nutrition
University of Pittsburgh
Pittsburgh, PA

Theofanis Floros, MD
Athens Naval & Veterans' Hospital
Athens, Greece
University of Pittsburgh Cancer Institute
Pittsburgh, PA

David A. Geller, MD
Richard L. Simmons Professor of Surgery
Chief, Division of Hepatobiliary and Pancreatic Surgery
Director, UPMC Liver Cancer Center
University of Pittsburgh
Pittsburgh, PA

Bruce J. Giantonio, MD
Associate Professor of Medicine
The Abramson Cancer Center
The University of Pennsylvania
Philadelphia, PA

Michael K. Gibson, MD, PhD, FACP
Associate Professor of Medicine
Medical Director, Head and Neck Team
Medical Director, Clinical Trials Unit
Division of Hematology and Oncology
University Hospitals Seidman Cancer Center
Case Comprehensive Cancer Center
Case Western Reserve University
Cleveland, OH

Gaurav Goel, MD
Assistant Professor of Medicine
Division of Medical Oncology
University of Kentucky Markey Cancer Center
Lexington, KY

Yoon-Koo Kang, MD, PhD
Professor of Internal Medicine
Department of Oncology
Asan Medical Center
University of Ulsan College of Medicine
Seoul, Republic of Korea

Jonathan C. King, MD
Assistant Professor of Surgery
Surgical Oncology and General Surgery
Department of Surgery
David Geffen School of Medicine at UCLA
Los Angeles, CA

James J. Lee, MD, PhD
Assistant Professor of Medicine
Division of Hematology/Oncology
University of Pittsburgh School of Medicine
Pittsburgh, PA

James D. Luketich, MD
Henry T. Bahnson Professor of Cardiothoracic Surgery
Chair, Department of Cardiothoracic Surgery
Chief, Division of Thoracic and Foregut Surgery
Director, Thoracic Surgical Oncology
Director, UPMC Esophageal and Lung Surgery Institute
Director, Mark Ravitch/Leon C. Hirsch Center for Minimally Invasive Surgery
Co-Director, Surgical Oncology Services
University of Pittsburgh Cancer Institute
Pittsburgh, PA

Aju Mathew, MD
Assistant Professor
Department of Medicine
Division of Medical Oncology
Markey Cancer Center
University of Kentucky
Lexington, KY

Kevin McGrath, MD
Professor of Medicine
Director, Endoscopic Ultrasound
Division of Gastroenterology, Hepatology and Nutrition
University of Pittsburgh
Pittsburgh, PA

Jennifer Miller, MD
Postdoctoral Fellow
Division of Gastrointestinal (GI) Surgical Oncology
University of Pittsburgh
Pittsburgh, PA

Christina A. Minami, MD
General Surgery Resident
Department of Surgery
Northwestern University
Chicago, IL

Nisha A. Mohindra, MD
Assistant Professor of Medicine
Division of Hematology/Oncology
Northwestern University Feinberg School of Medicine
Chicago, IL

Michael A. Morse, MD
Professor of Medicine
Professor in the Department of Surgery
Duke Cancer Institute
Durham, NC

Caroline Novak, MD
Resident (Graduated)
Department of Medicine
Northwestern University
Chicago, IL

Mark H. O'Hara, MD
Assistant Professor of Medicine
The Abramson Cancer Center
The University of Pennsylvania
Philadelphia, PA

Bert H. O'Neil, MD
Professor of Medicine
Director of the Gastrointestinal Cancer Research Program
Division of Hematology Oncology Department of Medicine
Indiana University
Indianapolis, IN

Sook Ryun Park, MD, PhD
Associate Professor of Internal Medicine
Department of Oncology
Asan Medical Center
University of Ulsan College of Medicine
Seoul, Republic of Korea

Anuj Patel, MD
Instructor in Medicine, Harvard Medical School
Dana-Farber Cancer Institute
Boston, MA

Arjun Pennathur, MD, FACS
Associate Professor of Cardiothoracic Surgery
Sampson Family Endowed Chair in Thoracic Surgical Oncology
University of Pittsburgh School of Medicine
Pittsburgh, PA

James F. Pingpank, Jr., MD, FACS
Associate Professor of Medicine
Division of Surgical Oncology
Department of Surgery, University of Pittsburgh Medical Center
Pittsburgh, PA

Manuel Villa Sanchez, MD
Assistant Professor of Cardiothoracic Surgery
Department of Cardiothoracic Surgery
University of Pittsburgh
Pittsburgh, PA

Savreet Sarkaria, MD
Clinical Associate Professor of Medicine
Division of Gastroenterology, Hepatology and Nutrition
University of Pittsburgh Medical Center
Pittsburgh, PA

Bhavin C. Shah, MD
Fellow — Surgical Oncology (Graduated)
Division of Surgical Oncology
Department of Surgery, University of Pittsburgh Medical Center
Pittsburgh, PA

Manish A. Shah, MD
Bartlett Family Associate Professor of Gastrointestinal Oncology
Director, Gastrointestinal Oncology Program
Co-Director, Center for Advanced Digestive Care
Sandra and Edward Meyer Cancer Center at Weill Cornell Medicine
New York, NY

Safi Shahda, MD
Assistant Professor of Clinical Medicine
Indiana University School of Medicine
Indiana University Health Simon Cancer Center
Indianapolis, IN

Evan S. Siegelman, MD
Associate Professor of Radiology
Perelman School of Medicine
University of Pennsylvania
Philadelphia, PA

Jonathan Strosberg, MD
Associate Professor
Section Head, Neuroendocrine Tumor Program
Chair, GI Research Committee
Chair, Scientific Review Committee
Moffitt Cancer Center
Tampa, FL

Weijing Sun, MD, FACP
Professor of Medicine
Division of Hematology/Oncology
University of Pittsburgh Medical Center and University of Pittsburgh
Pittsburgh, PA

Ursina R. Teitelbaum, MD
Associate Professor of Clinical Medicine
Division of Hematology/Oncology
University of Pennsylvania Perelman Center for Advanced Medicine
Philadelphia, PA

Andrew Z. Wang, MD
Associate Professor
Director of Clinical and Translational Research
Department of Radiation Oncology
Lineberger Comprehensive Cancer Center
University of North Carolina at Chapel Hill School of Medicine
Chapel Hill, NC

Jeffrey D. Wayne, MD
Professor of Surgery
Division of Surgical Oncology
Northwestern University
Chicago, IL

Valaree Williams, MS, RD, CSO, LDN
Clinical Dietitian
University of Colorado Health
Aurora, Colorado

Benjamin L. Yam, MD
Senior Resident — Radiation Oncology
Hospital of the University of Pennsylvania
Philadelphia, PA

Herbert J. Zeh III, MD
Associate Professor of Surgery
Chief, Division of Gastrointestinal (GI) Surgical Oncology
Co-Director, UPMC Pancreatic Cancer Center and
Co-Director, GI Oncology Program
University of Pittsburgh
Pittsburgh, PA

Amer H. Zureikat, MD
Assistant Professor of Surgery
Division of Gastrointestinal (GI) Surgical Oncology
Co-Director, UPMC Pancreatic Cancer Center
University of Pittsburgh
Pittsburgh, PA

Chapter 1

The Role of Hereditary and Environmental Factors in Gastrointestinal Cancers

Beth Dudley, Savreet Sarkaria and Randall E. Brand

1 Introduction

One major approach to reduce gastrointestinal (GI) cancer mortality is through the implementation of prevention and/or early detection strategies. However, with the exception of colon cancer, it is not feasible to screen the general population in the United States for GI malignancies due to their low incidence. Currently, early detection strategies for other GI malignancies focus on those subsets of the population in whom the risk for a cancer is substantially greater than the general population. Recognition of environmental and hereditary factors that predispose to a GI malignancy is necessary for the successful development and application of prevention and surveillance approaches.

Risk factors can be divided into modifiable and non-modifiable factors. Most modifiable risk factors are environmental, behavioral, or diet-related, while non-modifiable risk factors include heredity, age, gender, and medical conditions, especially those associated with inflammation. This chapter reviews our current knowledge regarding hereditary and environmental risk factors for the following GI malignancies: esophageal, gastric, biliary, small bowel, pancreas, and colorectal.

2 Colon Cancer

Colorectal cancer is the second leading cause of cancer death in the United States with an estimated 132,700 new cases of colorectal cancer diagnosed and 49,700 deaths from this disease in 2015.[1]

2.1 *Non-genetic risk factors*

Age and medical conditions such as personal history of colon cancer or inflammatory bowel disease are associated with an increased risk for colon cancer.[1] The following modifiable risk factors are also associated with increased risk: cigarette smoking, alcohol consumption, physical inactivity, a low-fiber, high-fat diet, and obesity.[2]

Individuals who have a family history of colorectal cancer have an increased risk for the disease, presumably as the result of both genetic and shared environmental risk factors. A meta-analysis of familial colorectal risk estimated the relative risks shown in Table 1.[3]

Although colon cancer diagnoses in first-degree relatives have the most impact on risk, affected second- and third-degree relatives can also increase risk to some extent, especially if there are multiple affected family members or if there are affected first-degree relatives as well.[4]

2.2 *Genetic risk factors*

Up to 10% of colorectal cancer is presumed to be due to a genetic cause. There are a number of different hereditary cancer syndromes that are associated with an increased risk for colon cancer. Recently, there have been other genes identified that modify colon cancer risk, probably to a smaller degree than the genes associated with previously described syndromes. Refer to Table 2 for details regarding the genetic basis and associated cancer risks for these inherited predispositions.

2.2.1 *Lynch syndrome*

Lynch syndrome is the most common hereditary predisposition to colon cancer and accounts for approximately 3% of all colon cancer diagnoses.[5,6] The most significant

Table 1   Risk for colorectal cancer based on family history.

Family History of Colorectal Cancer	Relative Risk
One first-degree relative	2.25
More than first-degree relative	4.25
First-degree relative diagnosed before 45	3.87

Table 2 Hereditary syndromes and susceptibility genes associated with colorectal cancer.

Syndrome	Gene(s)	Colon Cancer Risk	Other Cancers	Other Cancer Risks
Lynch syndrome	*MLH1*	15–70%	Uterine	15–60%
	MSH2	Second colon	Stomach	5–8%
	MSH6	cancer	Ovarian	7%
	PMS2	62% at 30 years	Urinary tract	6%
	EPCAM		Small bowel	4%
			Pancreas	4%
			Brain	2%
Familial adenomatous polyposis (FAP)	*APC*	~100%	Small bowel	4–12%
			Pancreas	2%
			Thyroid	2%
			Brain	1%
			Hepatoblastoma	1.6%
Attenuated familial adenomatous polyposis (AFAP)	*APC*	Up to 70%	Same as FAP	
MUTYH-associated neoplasia (MAN)	*MUTYH*	28-fold	Small bowel	4%
			Breast	Possible
			Ovarian	two-fold
			Bladder	increase
Juvenile polyposis syndrome (JPS)	*SMAD4*	39–68%	Stomach	Up to 21%
	BMPR1A		Small bowel, pancreas	Unknown, but reported
Peutz–Jeghers syndrome (PJS)	*STK11*	39%	Breast	45%
			Stomach	29%
			Small bowel	13%
			Pancreas	36%
			Lung	15%
Cowden syndrome	*PTEN*	4–14%	Breast	Up to 85%
			Thyroid	Up to 35%
			Uterine	Up to 28%
			Kidney	10–57%
			Melanoma	2–9%
Hereditary diffuse gastric cancer (HDGC)	*CDH1*	Unknown, but reported	Gastric (diffuse)	56–70%
			Breast (lobular)	42%
Serrated polyposis syndrome (SPS)	*Unknown*	Unknown	None	

(*Continued*)

Table 2   (*Continued*)

Syndrome	Gene(s)	Colon Cancer Risk	Other Cancers	Other Cancer Risks
Newly identified genes	*ATM*	2.5-fold	Breast	17%
			Pancreas	2.41-fold
	AXIN2	Unknown	None	
	CHEK2 (*c.407T>C mutation*)	1.5- to two-fold	Breast Prostate	1.5-fold Unknown
	GREM1	Unknown	None	
	POLE/ POLD1	Unknown	Uterine Brain	Unknown Unknown

risks are for colon and endometrial cancer; as is the case with colon cancer, Lynch syndrome accounts for up to 3% of all endometrial cancer diagnoses.[7] Lynch syndrome also confers modestly increased risks for a number of other cancers. Recent studies have suggested the possibility of an increased risk for breast and prostate cancers,[8] although the data is somewhat conflicting. Some families also have sebaceous neoplasms of the skin and have historically been considered to have Muir–Torre syndrome, although we now know the molecular basis is the same as Lynch syndrome.[9]

Lynch syndrome is caused by mutations in four mismatch repair (*MMR*) genes[9–11] and by deletions of the 3' end of *EPCAM*, a gene located immediately upstream of *MSH2*.[12] A clinical diagnosis of Lynch syndrome can be established using the Amsterdam criteria:[13]

- Three or more family members diagnosed with cancer of the colon, endometrium, small bowel, renal pelvis, or ureter, one of whom is a first degree relative of the other two
- Cancer diagnoses across at least two generations of the family
- At least one diagnosis before age 50

These criteria are stringent and may detect as few as 39% of families with a mismatch repair gene mutation.[14]

In an attempt to capture more families with Lynch syndrome, the Bethesda guidelines were developed.[15] These guidelines were designed to determine when microsatellite instability testing should be performed on a tumor:

- An individual with colorectal cancer diagnosed before age 50

- An individual with multiple HNPCC-related cancers* diagnosed at any age
- An individual with colorectal cancer that has histological features of MSI^ diagnosed before age 60
- An individual with colorectal cancer who has a first degree relative with an HNPCC-related cancer* diagnosed before age 50
- An individual with colorectal cancer who has two or more first- or second-degree relatives diagnosed with an HNPCC-related cancer* at any age

The Bethesda guidelines also fail to identify about one quarter of families with a mismatch repair gene mutation,[14] so universal screening of all colon[16] and endometrial[17] cancers for Lynch syndrome has been proposed.

Information about impaired mismatch repair gene function can be gained by evaluating the presence of microsatellite instability (MSI) testing in a tumor.[18] The majority of colorectal and endometrial cancers associated with Lynch syndrome demonstrate microsatellite instability,[19,20] whereas only 10–15% of sporadic colorectal cancers[21] and 20–25% of sporadic endometrial cancers[22] do; in sporadic cases, *MLH1* transcription has been silenced in the tumor as the result of somatic promoter hypermethylation.[23,24]

Immunohistochemistry (IHC) studies can also provide information about Lynch syndrome since tumors related to Lynch syndrome are likely to demonstrate loss of mismatch repair protein expression.[25] The pattern of loss observed can provide information about which gene is not functioning properly; see Figure 1 for a guide to interpreting *MMR* IHC results.

If a tumor demonstrates loss of MLH1 and PMS2 protein expression, additional studies can be performed to differentiate between somatic promoter

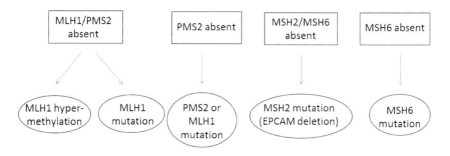

Figure 1   Mismatch repair IHC interpretation.

---

*Colorectal, endometrial, stomach, ovarian, pancreas, ureter and renal pelvis, biliary tract, brain, small bowel, and sebaceous neoplasms/keratocanthomas.
^Tumor-infiltrating lymphocytes, Crohn's-like lymphocytic reaction, mucinous/signet ring differentiation, or medullary growth pattern.

hypermethylation and a germline mutation. For both colon and endometrial tumors, molecular tumor studies can identify the presence or absence of hyper-methylation. For colon tumors, identification of the *BRAF* (V600E) mutation can be used as a surrogate since this mutation is identified in 50–70% of colon tumors that have *MLH1* promoter hypermethylation and is not observed in tumors without hypermethylation.[26]

Several recent studies have demonstrated that in some cases, loss of *MMR* function in a tumor is the result of biallelic somatic mutations.[27] In this case, an individual does not have Lynch syndrome. The studies published to date suggest that 50–70% of individuals who have loss of *MMR* expression identified in their tumor but do not have an identified germline mutation in the corresponding gene(s) have biallelic somatic mutations.

A rare childhood cancer syndrome, called biallelic mismatch repair deficiency, results when an individual carries inherited mutations in both copies of a *MMR* gene.[28] These individuals develop brain tumors, hematologic malignancies, and GI cancers at very young ages and also have features of neurofibromatosis type I.

2.2.2 *Familial adenomatous polyposis (FAP)*

Classic FAP is a hereditary condition that is characterized by hundreds to thousands of adenomas in the colon that begin to develop during adolescence. A clinical diag-nosis of FAP is established if an individual has at least 100 colon adenomas. The majority of individuals with FAP (~90%) have a mutation identified in the tumor suppressor gene *APC*.[29] *APC* mutations are inherited in an autosomal dominant manner, but up to one-third of individuals with FAP have a *de novo* mutation.

To a lesser degree, individuals with FAP may also develop polyps in the stomach and small intestine, particularly in the duodenum and the periampullary region. The polyps in the stomach are usually fundic gland polyps and therefore have a low risk of becoming cancerous; as a result, the risk for gastric cancer in individuals with FAP is not dramatically increased. The polyps in the small intestine are typically adenomas.

There are several benign findings that are associated with FAP; these include desmoid tumors, osteomas, lipomas, fibromas, dental abnormalities (extra or miss-ing teeth), and CHRPE (congenital hypertrophy of the retinal epithelium). Historically, the term 'Gardner syndrome' was used for a family with FAP that also has some of these benign findings.

2.2.3 *Attenuated familial adenomatous polyposis (AFAP)*

Attenuated FAP is a milder form of FAP. Most individuals with AFAP develop between 20 and 100 adenomas beginning in early-mid adulthood. Upper GI polyps

may also develop. The genetic basis of AFAP is heterogeneous and not fully elucidated. A recent study suggested that only approximately 10% of individuals with an
AFAP phenotype have identified *APC* mutations.[30] This study also suggested that
approximately 7% of these individuals have mutations identified in the *MUTYH*
gene (see section below). This indicates that the majority of individuals with AFAP
have no identified genetic basis for their polyp burden.

2.2.4 *MUTYH-associated neoplasia (MAN)*

Biallelic *MUTYH* mutations, resulting in an autosomal recessively inherited predisposition to colon polyps, were originally reported in siblings with an attenuated
adenomatous polyposis phenotype; the resulting condition was referred to as
MYH-associated polyposis.[31] Since then, it has become evident that while most
individuals with biallelic *MUTYH* mutations have between 20 and 100 colon adenomas, the clinical presentation of this disease can be widely variable, with some
individuals having colon cancer in the absence of multiple polyps and some individuals having florid polyposis.[32] Several studies indicate that approximately 3% of
individuals diagnosed with colorectal cancer before age 50 carried biallelic *MYH*
mutations.[33] Individuals with multiple serrated polyps have also been found to have
biallelic *MUTYH* mutations. Given the phenotypic variability that can result from
biallelic *MUTYH* mutations, it has been proposed that the associated condition be
referred to as MUTYH-associated neoplasia (MAN) rather than MUTYH-
associated polyposis.[24]

2.2.5 *Juvenile polyposis syndrome (JPS)*

Individuals with JPS develop multiple juvenile polyps. For many individuals with
JPS, polyps are most likely to develop in the colon; the pathology can be variable,
with tubular adenomas, sessile serrated adenomas, and hyperplastic polyps being
present in addition to juvenile polyps. Individuals with JPS may also have polyps
in the stomach (usually hyperplastic) and throughout the small bowel (juvenile,
hyperplastic, and adenomatous). They often begin to develop polyps in childhood.
The clinical presentation can be widely variable with respect to polyp number and
distribution.[35] A clinical diagnosis of JPS is established when an individual meets
one of the following criteria:[36]

- More than five juvenile polyps in the colon
- Multiple juvenile polyps throughout the GI tract
- Any number of juvenile polyps with a family history of juvenile polyps

Approximately 50–60% of individuals with JPS have a mutation in either *SMAD4* or *BMPR1A*, both of which are inherited in an autosomal dominant fashion.[35] Approximately 25% of individuals with JPS have no reported family history of the condition. Mutations in *SMAD4* tend to be associated with a more severe phenotype, with a higher incidence of adenomas and carcinomas, and are strongly correlated with upper GI polyposis.[35] Some individuals with *SMAD4* mutations have both JPS and hereditary hemorrhagic telangiectasia (HHT), a syndrome characterized by arteriovenous malformations and mucocutaneous telangiectasia.[37] Recently, thoracic aortic aneurysms have also been reported in individuals with *SMAD4* mutations.[38]

2.2.6 *Peutz–Jeghers syndrome (PJS)*

PJS is characterized by hamartomatous GI polyps and mucocutaneous hyperpigmentation.[39] The polyps associated with PJS are characteristic of the syndrome and are called Peutz–Jeghers (PJ) polyps; they are most common in the small bowel, but can also occur in the stomach and colon. Many individuals with PJS begin to develop polyps in childhood and the presenting symptom can be intussusception. Other types of polyps, including adenomas, are also observed in association with PJS. The mucocutaneous hyperpigmentation associated with PJS usually presents as dark blue or brown freckles on the lips and fingers, inside the mouth, and around the eyes, nostrils, and anus. Hyperpigmentation usually appears by age five, but often fades in puberty or adulthood.[40]

A clinical diagnosis of PJS can be made if any of the following criteria are met:[41]

- Two or more histologically confirmed PJ polyps
- Any number of PJ polyps and characteristic mucocutaneous hyperpigmentation
- Any number of PJ polyps in an individual with a family history of PJS
- Characteristic mucocutaneous hyperpigmentation in an individual with a family history of PJS

Approximately 94% of individuals with a clinical diagnosis of PJS have a mutation identified in the *STK11* gene.[42] Mutations in this gene are inherited in an autosomal dominant fashion, although as many as 45% of individuals with PJS are the first person in their family to have the diagnosis. Individuals with PJS have significantly increased risks for a number of cancers.[43] Reproductive system tumors, including sex cord ovarian tumors with annular tubules (SCTAT) and adenoma malignum of the cervix in women and Sertoli cell tumors of the testes in males, are also associated with PJS.

2.2.7 *Cowden syndrome*

Cowden syndrome is associated with a number of benign and malignant tumors. It is caused by mutations in the tumor suppressor gene *PTEN*, which are inherited in an autosomal dominant fashion.[44] Up to 80% of individuals with an operational diagnosis[45] of Cowden syndrome have an identifiable mutation.[46]

Refer to Table 2 for a summary of the malignant tumors associated with Cowden syndrome.[47] The benign findings associated with Cowden syndrome can be observed in a number of different body systems.[48] The hallmark features of Cowden syndrome are Lhermitte–Duclos disease (LDD) and mucocutaneous growths, including trichilemmomas, papillomatosis papules on the face and inside the mouth, acral keratoses, and lipomas. Fibrocystic breast disease, uterine fibroids, and benign thyroid disease (nodules, adenomas, and goiter) are common in Cowden syndrome. Arterial vascular malformations and hemangiomas are also reported with increased frequency in individuals with Cowden syndrome. Although not tumor-related, most individuals with Cowden syndrome (at least 80%) also have macrocephaly.

Most, if not all, individuals with Cowden syndrome have some type of GI involvement.[49] Polyps are the most common GI finding in Cowden syndrome and can be observed in the stomach, small bowel, and colon. Hyperplastic polyps seem to be the most frequently observed type of polyp, although hamartomas, juvenile polyps, ganglioneuromas, and adenomas are also observed. Glycogenic acanthosis is also reported in individuals with Cowden syndrome.

2.2.8 *Hereditary diffuse gastric cancer (HDGC)*

HDGC is discussed in more detail in the gastric cancer section of this chapter. There are reports of signet-ring cell colon cancer in individuals with *CDH1* mutations,[50] although no risk has been published for colon cancer.

2.2.9 *Serrated polyposis syndrome (SPS)*

Serrated polyposis syndrome, formerly known as hyperplastic polyposis syndrome, is characterized by the presence of multiple hyperplastic polyps or serrated adenomas in the colon. The polyps associated with SPS should not be confused with common sporadic rectal hyperplastic polyps, as the former tend to be larger, more numerous, and associated with risk for malignancy.

Although we suspect a genetic susceptibility to polyp development in individuals with SPS, at least in some cases, we have not identified a causative gene to date.

Currently, the diagnosis of SPS is established solely through the World Health Organization's proposed clinical diagnosis, when one of the following criteria is met:[51]

- At least five serrated polyps to the right of the sigmoid colon, of which two are greater than 1 cm
- Any number of serrated polyps occurring to the right of the sigmoid colon in an individual who has a first degree relative with serrated polyposis syndrome
- More than 20 serrated polyps throughout the colon

Individuals with serrated polyposis syndrome have a tendency to develop numerous hyperplastic polyps and serrated adenomas at a rapid pace.[52] It has also been demonstrated that no individuals developed upper GI polyps. The risk for colon cancer has not been well defined, but is increased; one recent study reported a risk of 7% after five years of surveillance and found that this risk is directly correlated with number of polyps.[53] A recent publication demonstrated that individuals with SPS do not appear to have an increased risk for extracolonic cancers.[54]

Although no genetic cause has been identified for SPS, an individual's diagnosis of the condition does have implications for family members. Approximately 32% of first-degree relatives were also given the diagnosis of SPS during screening colonoscopy[55] and the relative risk for colon cancer in first-degree relatives of individuals with SPS is 5.4.[56]

2.2.10 *Other genes*

Mutations in a number of genes, including *ATM*,[57] *AXIN2*,[58] *CHEK2*,[59] *GREM1*,[60] and *POLE/POLD1*,[61] have been recently described in association with an increased risk for colon polyps and colon cancer. Mutations in *ATM* and *CHEK2* are not rare, but seem to be associated with a modest increase in risk. Mutations in the other genes seem to individually account for a very small proportion of hereditary colon cancer and are not well defined.

3 Esophageal Cancer

Esophageal cancer is the eighth most common cancer worldwide with a five-year survival rate of less than 15%, thus ranking sixth among all cancers in mortality. Although the incidence of squamous cell carcinoma is decreasing in the United States, the incidence of esophageal adenocarcinoma continues to rise at dramatic rates.[62] There are significant geographic variations in the incidence of esophageal cancers worldwide.[63]

3.1 *Adenocarcinoma*

Esophageal adenocarcinoma (EAC) has increased in incidence by more than seven-fold in the United States in the past several decades.[64] This is likely due at least in part to an increased incidence of Barrett's esophagus (BE) and gastroesophageal reflux disease (GERD). Increased rates of obesity and lower incidence of *H. pylori* infection may also play a major role.

BE is considered a precursor to and the greatest risk factor for EAC. Among patients who have BE, the risk of developing EAC is increased 30–40-fold above that of the general population. The risk of developing EAC in patients with BE is proportional to the extent and grade of dysplasia. The annual incidence of progression to EAC is 0.12% to 0.38% per year for nondysplastic lesions.[64] This risk, however, rises dramatically to 6% per year in patients with high-grade dysplasia.[65]

Rates of adenocarcinoma of the esophagus are higher in smokers compared to nonsmokers and increase with higher pack year histories.[66] The rates are increased even further in smokers with BE. While the risk is reduced after smoking cessation, it does not return to the level of never-smokers.[66] Obesity has also been linked to adenocarcinomas of the esophagus and gastric cardia. There is accumulating data that central obesity, rather than body mass index (BMI), is associated with both BE and EAC.[67] Unlike squamous cell carcinoma (SCC), discussed below, studies have found no association between alcohol consumption and the development of EAC.[68]

Having a family history of EAC increases the risk for the disease and approximately 7% of EAC is considered familial.[69] Some data suggests that individuals who have one first-degree relative with EAC have a two-fold higher risk than the general population, while having more than one affected first-degree relative increases the risk threefold.[70] A significant proportion of this increased risk has traditionally been attributed to shared lifestyle risk factors, although several genes have recently been identified in association with BE/EAC, including *MSR1*, *ASCC1*, and *CTHRC1*.[71] The role of these genes in EAC development is not clear, although it may be related to the inflammatory process.

3.2 *Squamous cell carcinoma*

The incidence of SCC of the esophagus varies considerably by geographic region. The role of various risk factors also varies in different parts of the world. Chronic irritation of the esophagus appears to have a role in the process of carcinogenesis. To that effect, causative "modifiable" factors are thought to be history of smoking,[72] alcohol consumption,[72] and diet.[73,74]

Tylosis is a rare autosomal dominant disorder caused by mutations in the *RHBDF2* gene, characterized by hyperkeratosis of the palms of the hands and soles of feet and a life-time risk as high as 40% for developing esophageal SCC.[75] Plummer–Vinson syndrome (PVS) is the triad of iron deficiency anemia, dysphagia, and cervical esophageal webs; its cause is unknown.[76] Patients with PVS have a higher life-time rate of SCC of 10%.

The risk of esophageal SCC is increased by 16- to 28-fold in patients with achalasia.[77] Caustic injuries such as lye ingestion have been associated with higher incidence of SCC.[78] Conditions that cause gastric atrophy, such as atrophic gastritis, are associated with a two-fold increase in risk of esophageal SCC.[79] Several studies have found an association between a history of SCC of the head and neck, lung, or esophagus and synchronous or metachronous SCC of the esophagus.[80] It is unclear if this reflects common risk factors or independent mechanisms.

4 Gastric Cancer

The lifetime risk of developing gastric cancer in the United States is 0.9%.[81] It is estimated in 2015 that 24,590 individuals will be diagnosed and 10,720 individuals will die from this cancer.[1] Gastric cancer is associated with a variety of genetic and environmental risk factors. The role of environmental influences is supported by the fact that emigrants from high-incidence to low-incidence countries often experience a decrease in risk of developing gastric cancer.[82]

4.1 *Non-genetic risk factors*

4.1.1 *Medical*

H. pylori infection has been associated with approximately a six-fold increase in the risk of adenocarcinomas distal to the gastric cardia and likely accounts for greater than 75% of distal gastric cancers.[83] The purposed mechanism of carcinogenesis is inflammation of the mucosa triggered by *H. pylori* infection which results in atrophy and intestinal metaplasia. Despite this clear association, less than 1% of individuals infected with *H. pylori* will develop gastric cancer.

Gastric atrophy (e.g. atrophic gastritis) increases the risk of gastric cancer by 3 to 18 times that of the general population.[79] Similarly, pernicious anemia is associated with a two- to six-fold excess risk of developing gastric cancer.[84] Patients with blood group A have a 20% increased rate of developing gastric cancer. It is not known if this association is due to the blood group antigens themselves or the effects of closely associated genes.[85] Ménétrier's disease is also a possible risk factor for gastric cancer, with risk estimates varying from 2 to 15%.[86]

The relative risk of developing gastric cancer after gastric surgery is 1.5–3.0, with the risk increasing over time and is greatest approximately 15–20 years after surgery. This risk is greater in patients who have undergone Billroth II in comparison to Billroth I surgery.[87] While the mechanism is not known, regurgitation of bile and pancreatic juices into the stomach has been postulated as having a causative role.

4.1.2 *Lifestyle*

Tobacco use,[88] dietary risk factors,[89] obesity,[90] and occupational exposures[91] have also been linked to gastric cancer. Various demographic factors such as socioeconomic status also seem to play a role in the development of the disease. More than 70% of gastric cancers occur in developing countries. Although there is a higher prevalence of *H. pylori* in these areas, poor hygiene is another key factor[63] and likely accounts for the increased risk of distal gastric cancer in areas of lower socioeconomic status. On the other hand, higher socioeconomic status has been associated with an increased risk of proximal gastric cancers and parallels the demographic and pathological features of Barrett's-associated esophageal adenocarcinoma.[92]

4.2 *Genetic risk factors*

Up to 3% of gastric cancers are hereditary.[93] Hereditary diffuse gastric cancer (HDGC) is a familial form of gastric cancer with an autosomal dominant pattern of inheritance primarily associated with diffuse gastric cancer and lobular breast cancer.[94] A clinical diagnosis of HDGC is established if a family has:[95]

- At least two documented cases of diffuse gastric cancer in first- or second-degree relatives, with one diagnosis before 50
- At least three documented cases of diffuse gastric cancer in first- or second-degree relatives, regardless of age

Approximately 30–50% of individuals with a clinical diagnosis of HDGC carry a mutation in the *CDH1* gene, which encodes for the E-cadherin protein.[96] The criteria for *CDH1* testing are somewhat broader than the clinical diagnostic criteria.[97]

Several other genetic syndromes are associated with intestinal-type gastric cancer, including Lynch syndrome, FAP, PJS, and JPS, all of which are discussed in more detail in the colon cancer section of this chapter.

5 Pancreatic Cancer

Pancreatic cancer has now become the third leading cause of cancer death in the United States, with ~49,000 new cases of pancreatic cancer estimated to be diagnosed in 2015.[1] Ninety-six percent of cases are adenocarcinomas (PDAC). Five-year survival rates remain dismal at 6% despite our increased knowledge of the molecular biology of this disease.[98,99]

5.1 *Non-genetic risk factors*

Cigarette smoking is the most reproducible modifiable risk factor, doubling one's risk as compared to nonsmokers.[100] It has been estimated that up to 20% of PDAC cases can be attributed to smoking.[1] Obesity has been associated with increased risk for PDAC, with a meta-analysis demonstrating an increase in relative risk for PDAC with each 5 kg/m^2 increase in BMI.[101] Diet also plays a factor, with studies demonstrating increased meat consumption associated with PDAC risk. *H. pylori* infection, prior cholecystectomy or gastrectomy, and pipe or cigar smoking also increase PDAC risk. Data is inconclusive regarding alcohol and caffeine intake. Non-modifiable risk factors for PDAC include age, with 70% of patients diagnosed at older than 65, African-American ethnicity, Ashkenazi-Jewish descent and areas in the world with higher socioeconomic development.[102]

Medical conditions such as chronic pancreatitis (CP) and diabetes mellitus (DM) are associated with increased risks for PDAC. There is a wide variation in reported PDAC incidence in CP patients, ranging from 2- to 19-fold.[103–105] A recent meta-analysis found a relative risk of 5.8 (2.1–15.9) for pancreatic cancer after two years of the chronic pancreatitis diagnosis.[106] In this same study, it was shown that over a 20-year period, ~5% of all patients with chronic pancreatitis will be diagnosed with PDAC. The association between diabetes and PDAC is difficult to determine since there is strong evidence to support that PDAC can cause DM. It has been reported that up to 80% of PDAC patients will have DM or impaired fasting glucose levels at the time of diagnosis.[107] However, long-standing type 1 and 2 DM have both been shown to be associated with an approximately two-fold risk for PDAC development.[108,109]

5.2 *Genetic risk factors*

It has been estimated that up to 10% of PDAC cases have a hereditary component. Some individuals have well-described cancer predisposing syndromes such as hereditary breast ovarian cancer (HBOC),[110,111] familial atypical multiple mole melanoma (FAMMM),[112] Lynch syndrome,[113] PJS,[43] FAP,[114]

Li–Fraumeni syndrome[115] and hereditary pancreatitis.[116] With the exception of hereditary pancreatitis, all of these syndromes are associated with an increased risk for developing pancreatic cancer, but are more strongly associated with other cancers.

Monoallelic mutations in genes associated with rare autosomal recessive conditions have recently been identified as an etiology for some cases of hereditary pancreatic cancer as well. These genes include *ATM*,[57,117] which is associated with ataxia-telangiectasia, and *PALB2*,[118] which is associated with Fanconi's anemia. To date, a mutation in *PALLD*, a gene that encodes for the palladin protein, has been

Table 3 Hereditary syndromes and susceptibility genes associated with pancreatic adenocarcinoma.

Syndrome	Gene(s)	Relative Risk of PC	Other Cancers	Other Cancer Risks
Familial atypical multiple mole melanoma (FAMMM)	*CDKN2A*	13- to 39-fold	Melanoma	58–92%
Hereditary breast ovarian cancer (HBOC)	*BRCA1* *BRCA2*	Two-fold 3- to 9-fold	Breast Ovary	50–87% 27–44%
Familial adenomatous polyposis (FAP)	*APC*	Five-fold	Colon	70–100%
Lynch syndrome	*MLH1, MSH2 MSH6, PMS2, EPCAM*	9- to 11-fold	Colon Endometrial	15–70% 15–60%
Peutz–Jeghers syndrome (PJS)	*STK11/LKB1*	Up to 132-fold	GI Breast	15–40% 45%
Li–Fraumeni syndrome	*TP53*	7.3-fold	Sarcomas Breast Brain Adrenocortical	61- to 107-fold 6.4-fold 35-fold Not calculated
Hereditary pancreatitis	*PRSS1*	53-fold	None	—
Cystic fibrosis	*CFTR*	2.6-fold	None	—
Newly identified genes	*ATM*	Three-fold	Breast Colon	17% 2.5-fold
	PALB2	Unknown	Breast	35%

Table 4   Relative risk of pancreatic cancer by blood type.

Blood Type	Relative Risk of Pancreatic Adenocarcinoma
O	1.0
A	1.38 (relative to type O)
B	1.53 (relative to type O)
AB	1.47 (relative to type O)

described in a single large kindreds (Family X) followed at the University of Washington,[119] but has not been identified in other families. The relative risks for developing PC and commonly associated extra-pancreatic cancers with inherited mutations are shown in Table 3.

Familial pancreatic cancer (FPC) is defined as families with two or more first-degree relatives with pancreatic adenocarcinoma that do not meet criteria for any of the known pancreatic cancer-associated hereditary syndromes listed in Table 3.[120] Studies have demonstrated that family members in FPC kindreds are at an increased risk for pancreatic cancer development. An FPC family member with one or two first-degree relatives has a 4- to 7-fold increased risk for developing pancreatic cancer, respectively, while those individuals with three or more first-degree relatives have a 17- to 32-fold risk.[120]

The recognition of modest differences for PDAC development based on blood type has been observed; see Table 4 for odds ratios.[121]

6   Cholangiocarcinoma

Cholangiocarcinoma accounts for approximately 3% of all gastrointestinal malignancies and carries an incidence of two cases per 100,000 in the United States.[122]

6.1   *Non-genetic risk factors*

Primary sclerosing cholangitis (PSC) is an inflammatory condition of the bile ducts and accounts for 30% of cases of cholangiocarcinoma with a lifetime risk of 10–15%.[123] Choledochal cysts are more common in Asian populations and are associated with the development of cholangiocarcinoma with rates ranging from 10 to 30%.[124]

Parasitic infections are more commonly associated with the development of cholangiocarcinoma in areas of Asia where infection with liver flukes consumed in under-cooked fish result in adult worms inhabiting the bile ducts.[125] This causes chronic inflammation and possibly malignant transformation of the biliary epithelium. Hepatolithiasis, also known as chronic intrahepatic stone disease or recurrent pyogenic cholangitis, is a strong risk factor for cholangiocarcinoma; between 4 and 11% of patients with chronic hepatolithiasis develop intrahepatic cholangiocarcinoma.[126] While the cause of hepatolithiasis is not known, it is thought that these stones are likely secondary to chronic inflammation from bacteria or parasitic infections, congenital duct abnormalities or perhaps dietary influences.

Exposure to the radiologic contrast agent Thorotrast is a strong risk factor for developing cholangiocarcinoma. Patients typically develop cancer 30–35 years after exposure.[127] Increased rates of cholangiocarcinoma have been detected in patients with hepatitis C, hepatitis B, and chronic liver disease of nonviral causes to varying degrees in different parts of the world.[128] The associations between cholangiocarcinoma and diabetes, obesity, and tobacco use are less clear, but these factors may increase risk.[129]

6.2 *Genetic risk factors*

Lynch syndrome carries a 2–7% risk of developing cholangiocarcinoma.[130] Biliary papillomatosis is a rare genetic disorder characterized by multiple adenomatous polyps in the bile ducts; patients have up to an 80% risk of developing cholangiocarcinoma.[131]

7 Gallbladder Cancer

Gallbladder adenocarcinomas are uncommon in the United States with fewer than 5,000 cases diagnosed each year.[132] In contrast, rates are high in areas of South America and Asia which share a high prevalence of gallstones or *Salmonella* infection.[133] Gallstones are the most well-established risk factor and are present in 70–90% of patients with gallbladder cancer, although the incidence of developing gallbladder cancer in patients with cholelithiasis is only 0.5–3%.[134] The incidence of developing gallbladder cancer is 2–15% in patients with porcelain gallbladder.[135] Adenomas are considered to have a neoplastic potential, but they account for less than 5% of all gallbladder polyps.[136] The most useful predictor of malignancy in a gallbladder polyp is size of the polyp, with larger polyps being more likely to be malignant. Other risk factors for gallbladder cancer include anomalous pancreatico-biliary junction,[137] *Salmonella* exposure,[138] tobacco use,[128] and obesity.[128]

8 Small Intestine Cancers

Cancers of the small intestine are rare and represent only 3% of all GI tract malignancies and 0.5% of all cancers in the United States, with approximately 9,000 new cases diagnosed each year.[139] Most small intestinal adenocarcinomas arise from adenomas and occur either in the setting of a hereditary cancer syndrome or chronic inflammation. Individuals with Lynch syndrome, FAP, and PJS have an increased risk for small bowel cancer; see the colon cancer section for more details. Similar to other sites in the GI tract, chronic inflammation appears to play a role in the etiology of some small bowel adenocarcinomas. This is supported by the fact that inflammatory conditions of the small intestine such as Crohn's disease[140] and celiac disease[141] are associated with higher rates of adenocarcinoma in the small intestine. A few modifiable risk factors, including smoking, alcohol consumption, and diet, have also been associated with small bowel adenocarcinomas.[142]

References

1. American Cancer Society, Cancer Facts & Figures 2015. Atlanta: American Cancer Society; 2015.
2. Durko L, Malecka-Panas E. Lifestyle modifications and colorectal cancer. *Curr Colorectal Cancer Rep* 2014;**10**(1):45–54.
3. Johns LE, Houlston RS. A systematic review and meta-analysis of familial colorectal cancer risk. *Am J Gastroenterol* 2001;**96**(10):2992–3003.
4. Taylor DP, *et al.* Population-based family history-specific risks for colorectal cancer: A constellation approach. *Gastroenterology* 2010;**138**(3):877–885.
5. Hampel H, *et al.* Screening for the Lynch syndrome (hereditary nonpolyposis colorectal cancer). *N Engl J Med* 2005;**352**(18):1851–1860.
6. Hampel H, *et al.* Feasibility of screening for Lynch syndrome among patients with colorectal cancer. *J Clin Oncol* 2008;**26**(35):5783–5788.
7. Hampel H, *et al.* Comment on: Screening for Lynch syndrome (hereditary nonpolyposis colorectal cancer) among endometrial cancer patients. *Cancer Res* 2007;**67**(19):9603.
8. Win AK, *et al.* Risks of primary extracolonic cancers following colorectal cancer in Lynch syndrome. *Natl Cancer Inst* 2012;**104**(18):1363–1372.
9. Nystrom-Lahti M, *et al.* Mismatch repair genes on chromosomes 2p and 3p account for a major share of hereditary nonpolyposis colorectal cancer families evaluable by linkage. *Am J Hum Genet* 1994;**55**(4):659–665.
10. Miyaki M, *et al.* Germline mutation of *MSH6* as the cause of hereditary nonpolyposis colorectal cancer. *Nat Genet* 1997;**17**(3)271–272.
11. Nakagawa H, *et al.* Mismatch repair gene *PMS2*: Disease-causing germline mutations are frequent in patients whose tumors stain negative for PMS2 protein, but paralogous genes obscure mutation detected and interpretation. *Cancer Res* 2004;**64**(14):4721–4727.

12. Ligtenberg MJ, *et al.* Heritable somatic methylation and inactivation of *MSH2* in families with Lynch syndrome due to deletion of the 3' exons of *TACSTD1*. *Nat Genet* 2009;**41**(1):112–117.

13. Vasen HF, *et al.* New clinical criteria for hereditary nonpolyposis colorectal cancer (HNPCC, Lynch syndrome) proposed by the International Collaborative Group on HNPCC. *Gastroenterology* 1999;**116**(6):1453–1456.

14. Hampel H, *et al.* Feasibility of screening for Lynch syndrome among patients with colorectal cancer. *J Clin Oncol* 2008;**26**(35):5783–5788.

15. Umar A, *et al.* Revised Bethesda guidelines for hereditary nonpolyposis colorectal cancer (Lynch syndrome) and microsatellite instability. *J Natl Cancer Inst* 2004;**96**(4):261–268.

16. EGAPP Working Group, Recommendations from the EGAPP Working Group: Genetic testing strategies in newly diagnosed individuals with colorectal cancer aimed at reducing morbidity and mortality from Lynch syndrome in relatives. *Genet Med* 2009;**11**(1):35–41.

17. Hampel H, *et al.* Screening for Lynch syndrome (hereditary nonpolyposis colorectal cancer) among endometrial cancer patients. *Cancer Res* 2006;**66**(15):7810–7817.

18. Zhang L. Immunohistochemistry versus microsatellite instability testing for screening colorectal cancer patients at risk for hereditary nonpolyposis colorectal cancer syndrome: Part II. The utility of microsatellite instability testing. *J Mol Diagn* 2008;**10**(4):301–307.

19. Thibodeau SN, *et al.* Microsatellite instability in cancer of the proximal colon. *Science* 1993;**260**(5 109):816–819.

20. Risinger JI, *et al.* Genetic instability of microsatellites in endometrial carcinoma. *Cancer Res* 1993;**53**(21):5100–5103.

21. Ionov Y, *et al.* Ubiquitous somatic mutations in simple repeated sequences reveal a new mechanism for colonic carcinogenesis. *Nature* 1993;**363**(6429):558–561.

22. Burks RT, *et al.* Microsatellite instability in endometrial carcinoma. *Oncogene* 1994;**9**(4):1163–1166.

23. Cunningham JM, *et al.* Hypermethylation of the *hMLH1* promoter in colon cancer with microsatellite instability. *Cancer Res* 1998;**58**(15):3455–3460.

24. Simpkins SB. *MLH1* promoter methylation and gene silencing is the primary cause of microsatellite instability in sporadic endometrial cancers. *Hum Mol Genet* 1999;**8**(4):661–666.

25. Shia J. Immunohistochemistry versus microsatellite instability testing for screening colorectal cancer patients at risk for hereditary nonpolyposis colorectal cancer syndrome: Part I. The utility of immunohistochemistry. *J Mol Diagn* 2008;**10**(4):293–300.

26. Deng G, *et al.* *BRAF* mutation is frequently present in sporadic colorectal cancer with methylated *MLH1*, but not in hereditary nonpolyposis colorectal cancer. *Clin Cancer Res* 2004;**10**(1):191–195.

27. Haraldsdottir S, *et al.* Colon and endometrial cancers with mismatch repair deficiency can arise from somatic, rather than germline, mutations. *Gastroenterology* 2014;**147**(6):1308–1316.

28. Durno CA, *et al.* Oncologic surveillance for subjects with biallelic mismatch repair gene mutations: 10 year follow-up of a kindred. *Pediatr Blood Cancer* 2012;**59**(4):652–656.

29. Nishisho I, *et al.* Mutations of chromosome 5q21 genes in FAP and colorectal cancer patients. *Science* 1991;**253**(5020):665–669.

30. Grover S, *et al.* Prevalence and phenotypes of *APC* and *MUTYH* mutations in patients with multiple colorectal adenomas. *JAMA* 2012;**308**(5):485–492.

31. Al-Tassan N, *et al.* Inherited variants of MYH associated with somatic G:C◊T: A mutations in colorectal tumors. *Nat Genet* 2002;**30**(2):227–232.

32. Wang L, *et al. MYH* mutations in patients with attenuated and classic polyposis and with young-onset colorectal cancer without polyps. *Gastroenterology* 2004;**127**(1):9–16.

33. Giraldez MD, *et al. MSH6* and *MUTYH* deficiency is a frequent event in early-onset colorectal cancer. *Clin Cancer Res* 2010;**16**(22):5402–5413.

34. Church J, *et al.* Understanding MYH-associated neoplasia. *Dis Colon Rectum* 2012;**55**(3):359–362.

35. Brosens LAA, *et al.* Juvenile polyposis syndrome. *World J Gastroenterol* 2011;**17**(44):4839–4844.

36. Jass JR, *et al.* Juvenile polyposis — a precancerous condition. *Histopathology* 1988;**13**(6):619–630.

37. Schwenter F, *et al.* Juvenile polyposis, hereditary hemorrhagic telangiectasia, and early onset colorectal cancer in patients with *SMAD4* mutation. *J Gastroenterol* 2012;**47**(7):795–804.

38. Teekakirikul P, *et al.* Thoracic aortic disease in two patients with juvenile polyposis syndrome and SMAD4 mutations. *Am J Med Genet Part A* 2013;**161A**(1):185–191.

39. Bruwer A, *et al.* Surface pigmentation and generalized intestinal polyposis (Peutz–Jeghers syndrome). *Proc Staff Meet Mayo Clin* 1954;**29**(6):168–171.

40. Beggs AD, *et al.* Peutz–Jeghers syndrome: A systematic review and recommendations for management. *Gut* 2010;**59**(7):975–986.

41. Tomlinson IP, Houlston RS. Peutz–Jeghers syndrome. *J Med Genet* 1997;**34**(12):1007–1011.

42. Aretz S, *et al.* High proportion of large genomic deletions in Peutz–Jeghers syndrome. *Hum Mutat* 2005;**26**(6):513–519.

43. Giardiello FM, *et al.* Very high cancer risk in familial Peutz–Jeghers syndrome. *Gastroenterology* 2000;**119**(6):1447–1453.

44. Nelen MR, *et al.* Localization of the gene for Cowden disease to chromosome 10q22-23. *Nat Genet* 1996;**13**(1):114–116.

45. Pilarski R, Eng C. Will the real Cowden syndrome please stand up (again)? Expanding mutational and clinical spectra of the *PTEN* hamartoma tumour syndrome. *J Med Genet* 2004;**41**(5):323–326.

46. Marsh DJ, *et al.* Mutation spectrum and genotype-phenotype analyses in Cowden disease and Bannayan–Zonana syndrome, two hamartoma syndromes with germline *PTEN* mutation. *Hum Mol Genet* 1998;**7**(3):507–515.

47. Min-Han T, *et al.* Lifetime cancer risks in individuals with germline *PTEN* mutations. *Clin Cancer Res* 2012;**18**(2):400–407.

48. Pilarski R. Cowden syndrome: A critical review of the clinical literature. *J Genet Couns* 2009;**18**(1):13–27.

49. Heald B, *et al.* Frequent gastrointestinal polyps and colorectal adenocarcinomas in a prospective series of *PTEN* mutation carriers. *Gastroenterology* 2010;**139**(6): 1927–1933.

50. Richards FM, *et al.* Germline E-cadherin gene (*CDH1*) mutations predispose to familial gastric cancer and colorectal cancer. *Hum Mol Genet* 1999;**8**(4):607–610.

51. Snover DC, *et al.* Serrated polyps of the colon and rectum and serrated ("hyperplastic") polyposis. In: Bosman ST, *et al.* eds. WHO Classification of tumours of the digestive system. Berlin: Springer-Verlag, 2010, pp. 160–165.

52. Edelstein DL, *et al.* Serrated polyposis: Rapid and relentless development of colorectal neoplasia. *Gut* 2013;**62**(3):404–408.

53. Boparai KS, *et al.* Increased colorectal cancer risk during follow-up in patients with hyperplastic polyposis syndrome: A multicentre cohort study. *Gut* 2010;**59**(8):1094–1100.

54. Hazewinkel Y, *et al.* Extracolonic cancer risk in patients with serrated polyposis syndrome and their first-degree relatives. *Fam Cancer* 2013;**12**(4):669–673.

55. Oquinena S, *et al.* Serrated polyposis: Prospective study of first-degree relatives. *Eur J Gastroenterol Hepatol* 2013;**25**(1):28–32.

56. Boparai KS, *et al.* Increased colorectal cancer risk in first-degree relatives of patients with hyperplastic polyposis syndrome. *Gut* 2010;**59**(9):1222–1225.

57. Thompson D, *et al.* Cancer risks and mortality in heterozygous *ATM* mutation carriers. *J Natl Cancer Inst* 2005;**97**(11):813–822.

58. Lammi L, *et al.* Mutations in *AXIN2* cause familial tooth agenesis and predispose to colorectal cancer. *Am J Hum Genet* 2004;**74**(5):1043–1050.

59. Liu C, *et al.* The *CHEK2* I157T variant and colorectal cancer susceptibility: A systematic review and meta-analysis. *Asian Pac J Cancer Prev* 2012;**13**(5):2051–2055.

60. Jaeger E, *et al.* Hereditary mixed polyposis syndrome is caused by a 40-kb upstream duplication that leads to increased and ectopic expression of the BMP antagonist GREM1. *Nat Genet* 2012;**44**(6):699–703.

61. Palles C, *et al.* Germline mutations affecting the proofreading domains of *POLE* and *POLD1* predispose to colorectal adenomas and carcinomas. *Nat Genet* 2013;**45**(2):136–144.

62. Pohl H, *et al.* Esophageal adenocarcinoma incidence: Are we reaching the peak? *Cancer Epidemiol Biomarkers Prev* 2010;**19**(6):1468–1470.

63. Jemal A, *et al.* Global cancer statistics. *CA Cancer J Clin* 2011;**61**(2): 69–90.

64. Desai TK, *et al.* The incidence of oesophageal adenocarcinoma in non-dysplastic Barrett's oesophagus: A meta-analysis. *Gut* 2012;**61**(7):970–976.

65. Spechler SJ. Barrett esophagus and risk of esophageal cancer: A clinical review. *JAMA* 2013;**310**(6):627–636.

66. Cook MB, *et al*. Cigarette smoking and adenocarcinomas of the esophagus and esophagogastric junction: A pooled analysis from the international BEACON consortium. *J Natl Cancer Inst* 2010;**102**(17):1344–1353.
67. Chang P, Friedenberg F. Obesity and GERD. *Gastroenterol Clin North Am* 2014;**43**(1):161–173.
68. Thrift AP, *et al*. Alcohol and the risk of Barrett's esophagus: A pooled analysis from the International BEACON Consortium. *Am J Gastroenterol* 2014;**109**(10): 1586–1594.
69. Chak A, *et al*. Familiality in Barrett's esophagus, adenocarcinoma of the esophagus, and adenocarcinoma of the gastroesophageal junction. *Cancer Epidemiol Biomarkers Prev* 2006;**15**(9):1668–1673.
70. Wu M, *et al*. Does family history of cancer modify the effects of lifestyle risk factors on esophageal cancer? A population-based case-control study in China. *Int J Cancer* 2011;**128**(9):2147–2157.
71. Orloff M, *et al*. Germline mutations in *MSR1*, *ASCC1*, and *CTHRC1* in patients with Barrett esophagus and esophageal adenocarcinoma. *JAMA* 2011;**306**(4):410–419.
72. Castellsague X, *et al*. Independent and joint effects of tobacco smoking and alcohol drinking on the risk of esophageal cancer in men and women. *Int J Cancer* 1999;**82**(5):657–664.
73. Navarro Silvera SA, *et al*. Diet and lifestyle factors and risk of subtypes of esophageal and gastric cancers: Classification tree analysis. *Ann Epidemiol* 2014;**24**(1):50–57.
74. Tang L, *et al*. High temperature of food and beverage intake increases the risk of oesophageal cancer in Xinjiang, China. *Asian Pac J Cancer Prev* 2013;**14**(9):5085–5088.
75. Iwaya T, *et al*. Tylosis esophageal cancer locus on chromosome 17q25.1 is commonly deleted in sporadic human esophageal cancer. *Gastroenterology* 1998;**114**(6): 1206–1210.
76. Novacek G. Plummer–Vinson syndrome. *Orphanet J Rare Dis* 2006;**1**:36.
77. Leeuwenburgh I, *et al*. Long-term esophageal cancer risk in patients with primary achalasia: A prospective study. *Am J Gastroenterol* 2010;**105**(10):2144–2149.
78. Appelqvist P, Salmo M. Lye corrosion carcinoma of the esophagus: A review of 63 cases. *Cancer* 1980;**45**(10):2655–2658.
79. Islami F, *et al*. Gastric atrophy and risk of oesophageal cancer and gastric cardia adenocarcinoma — a systematic review and meta-analysis. *Ann Oncol* 2011;**22**(4):754–760.
80. Erkal HS, *et al*. Synchronous and metachronous squamous cell carcinomas of the head and neck mucosal sites. *J Clin Oncol* 2001;**19**(5):1358–1362.
81. National Cancer Institute. SEER Cancer Statistics Factsheets: Stomach Cancer, 2013.
82. Haenszel W, Kurihara M. Studies of Japanese migrants: Mortality from cancer and other diseases among Japanese in the United States. *J Natl Cancer Inst* 1968;**40**(1):43–68.
83. Uemura N, *et al*. *Helicobacter pylori* infection and the development of gastric cancer. *N Engl J Med* 2001;**345**(11):784–789.
84. Hsing AW, *et al*. Pernicious anemia and subsequent cancer. A population-based cohort study. *Cancer* 1993;**71**(3):745–750.
85. Edgren G, *et al*. Risk of gastric cancer and peptic ulcers in relation to ABO blood type: A cohort study. *Am J Epidemiol* 2010;**172**(11):1280–1285.

86. Fieber SS, Rickert RR, Hyperplastic gastropathy. Analysis of 50 selected cases from 1955–1980. *Am J Gastroenterol* 1981;**76**(4):321–329.

87. Tersmette AC, *et al.* Meta-analysis of the risk of gastric stump cancer: Detection of high risk patient subsets for stomach cancer after remote partial gastrectomy for benign conditions. *Cancer Res* 1990;**50**(20):6486–6489.

88. Ladeiras-Lopes R, *et al.* Smoking and gastric cancer: systematic review and meta-analysis of cohort studies. *Cancer Causes Control* 2008;**19**(7):689–701.

89. Lazarevic K, *et al.* Dietary factors and gastric cancer risk: Hospital based case control study. *J Buon* 2010;**15**(1):89–93.

90. Turati F, *et al.* A meta-analysis of body mass index and esophageal and gastric cardia adenocarcinoma. *Ann Oncol* 2013;**24**(3):609–617.

91. Ekstrom AM, *et al.* Occupational exposures and risk of gastric cancer in a population-based case-control study. *Cancer Res* 1999;**59**(23):5932–5937.

92. Powell J, McConke, CC. Increasing incidence of adenocarcinoma of the gastric cardia and adjacent sites. *Br J Cancer* 1990;**62**(3):440–443.

93. McLean MH, El-Omar EM. Genetics of gastric cancer. *Nat Rev Gastroenterol Hepatol* 2014;**11**(11):664–674.

94. Hansford S, *et al.* Hereditary diffuse gastric cancer: *CDH1* mutations and beyond. *JAMA Oncol* 2015;**1**(1):23–32.

95. Caldas C, *et al.* Familial gastric cancer: Overview and guidelines for management. *J Med Genet* 1999;**36**(12):873–880.

96. Guilford P, *et al.* E-cadherin mutations in familial gastric cancer. *Nature* 1998;**392**(6674):402–405.

97. Fitzgerald RC, *et al.* Hereditary diffuse gastric cancer: Updated consensus guidelines for clinical management and directions for future research. *J Med Genet* 2010;**47**(7):436–444.

98. Yachida S, *et al.* Distant metastasis occurs late during the evolution of pancreatic cancer. *Nature* 2010;**467**(7319):1114–1117.

99. Zamboni G, *et al.* Precancerous lesions of the pancreas. *Best Pract Res Clin Gastroenterol* 2013;**27**(2):299–322.

100. Iodice S, *et al.* Tobacco and the risk of pancreatic cancer: A review and meta-analysis. *Langenbecks Arch Surg* 2008;**393**(4):535–545.

101. Larsson SC, *et al.* Body mass index and pancreatic cancer risk: A meta-analysis of prospective studies. *Int J Cancer* 2007;**120**(9):1993–1998.

102. Veedu JS, *et al.* Epidemiology of gastrointestinal cancers #5: Dissecting the epidemiology of pancreatic adenocarcinoma. *Pract Gastro* 2015;**39**(1):12–29.

103. Lowenfels AB, *et al.* Pancreatitis and the risk of pancreatic cancer. International Pancreatitis Study Group. *N Engl J Med* 1993;**328**(20):1433–1437.

104. Bansal P, Sonnenberg A. Pancreatitis is a risk factor for pancreatic cancer. *Gastroenterology* 1995;**109**(1):247–251.

105. Malka D, *et al.* Risk of pancreatic adenocarcinoma in chronic pancreatitis. *Gut* 2002;**51**(6):849–852.

106. Raimondi S, *et al.* Pancreatic cancer in chronic pancreatitis: Aetiology, incidence, and early detection. *Best Pract Res Clin Gastroenterol* 2010;**24**(3):349–358.

107. Li D. Diabetes and pancreatic cancer. *Mol Carcinog* 2012;**51**(1):64–74.
108. Stevens RJ, *et al.* Pancreatic cancer in type 1 and young-onset diabetes: Systemic review and meta-analysis. *Br J Cancer* 2007;**96**(3):507–509.
109. Huxley R, *et al.* Type-II diabetes and pancreatic cancer: A meta-analysis of 36 studies. *Br J Cancer* 2005;**92**(11):2076–2083.
110. Thompson D, *et al.* Cancer Incidence in *BRCA1* mutation carriers. *J Natl Cancer Inst* 2002;**94**(18):1358–1365.
111. Breast Cancer Linkage Consortium, Cancer risks in *BRCA2* mutation carriers. *J Natl Cancer Inst* 1999;**91**(15):1310–1316.
112. Goldstein AM, *et al.* Increased risk of pancreatic cancer in melanoma-prone kindreds with p16INK4 mutations. *N Engl J Med* 1995;**333**(15):970–974.
113. Kastrinos F, *et al.* Risk of pancreatic cancer in families with Lynch syndrome. *JAMA* 2009;**302**(16):1790–1795.
114. Giardiello FM, *et al.* Increased risk of thyroid and pancreatic carcinoma in familial adenomatous polyposis. *Gut* 1993;**34**(10):1394–1396.
115. Ruijs MW, *et al.* *TP53* germline mutation testing in 180 families suspected of Li–Fraumeni syndrome: Mutation detection rate and relative frequency of cancers in different familial phenotypes. *J Med Genet* 2010;**47**(6):421–428.
116. Lowenfels AB, *et al.* Hereditary pancreatitis and the risk of pancreatic cancer. International Hereditary Pancreatitis Study Group. *J Natl Cancer Inst* 1997;**89**(6):442–446.
117. Roberts NJ, *et al.* *ATM* mutations in patients with hereditary pancreatic cancer. *Cancer Discov* 2012;**2**(1):41–46.
118. Jones S, *et al.* Exomic sequencing identified *PALB2* as a pancreatic cancer susceptibility gene. *Science* 2009;**324**(5924):217.
119. Pogue-Geile KL, *et al.* Palladin mutation causes familial pancreatic cancer and suggests a new cancer mechanism. *PLoS Med* 2006;**3**(12):e516.
120. Klein AP, *et al.* Prospective risk of pancreatic cancer in familial pancreatic cancer kindreds. *Cancer Res* 2004;**64**(7):2634–2638.
121. Wolpin BM, *et al.* Pancreatic cancer risk and ABO blood group alleles: Results from the pancreatic cancer cohort consortium. *Cancer Res* 2010;**70**(3):1015–1023.
122. Vauthey JN, Blumgart LH. Recent advances in the management of cholangiocarcinomas. *Semin Liver Dis* 1994;**14**(2):109–114.
123. Claessen MM, *et al.* High lifetime risk of cancer in primary sclerosing cholangitis. *J Hepatol* 2009;**50**(1):158–164.
124. Soreide K, Soreide JA. Bile duct cyst as precursor to biliary tract cancer. *Ann Surg Oncol* 2007;**14**(3):1200–1211.
125. Watanapa P, Watanapa WB. Liver fluke-associated cholangiocarcinoma. *Br J Surg* 2002;**89**(8):962–970.
126. Lee CC, *et al.* What is the impact of coexistence of hepatolithiasis on cholangiocarcinoma. *J Gastroenterol Hepatol* 2002;**17**(9):1015–1020.
127. Lipshutz GS, *et al.* Thorotrast-induced liver neoplasia: A collective review. *J Am Coll Surg* 2002;**195**(5):713–718.

128. Shaib Y, El-Serag HB. The epidemiology of cholangiocarcinoma. *Semin Liv Dis* 2004;**24**(2):115–125.

129. Grainge MJ, *et al*. The antecedents of biliary cancer: A primary case-control study in the United Kingdom. *Br J Cancer* 2009;**100**(1):178–180.

130. Watson P, *et al*. The risk of extra-colonic, extra-endometrial cancer in the Lynch syndrome. *Int J Cancer* 2008;**123**(2):444–449.

131. Lee SS, *et al*. Clinicopathologic review of 58 patients with biliary papillomatosis. *Cancer* 2004;**100**(4):783–793.

132. Carriaga MT, Henson DE. Liver, gallbladder, extrahepatic bile ducts, and pancreas. *Cancer* 1995;**75**(1 Suppl.):171–190.

133. Randi G, *et al*. Gallbladder cancer worldwide: Geographical distribution and risk factors. *Int J Cancer* 2006;**118**(7):1591–1602.

134. Maringhini A, *et al*. Gallstones, gallbladder cancer, and other gastrointestinal malignancies. An epidemiologic study in Rochester, Minnesota. *Ann Intern Med* 1987;**107**(1):30–35.

135. Kan ZS, *et al*. Reassessing the need for prophylactic surgery in patients with porcelain gallbladder: Case series and systematic review of the literature. *Arch Surg* 2011;**146**(10):1143–1147.

136. Farinon AM, *et al*. "Adenomatous polyps of the gallbladder" adenomas of the gallbladder. *HPB Surg* 1991;**3**(4):251–258.

137. Elnemr A, *et al*. Anomalous pancreatobiliary ductal junction without bile duct dilatation in gallbladder cancer. *Hepatogastroenterology* 2001;**48**(38):382–386.

138. Nagaraja V, Eslick GD. Systematic review with meta-analysis: The relationship between chronic *Salmonella typhi* carrier status and gallbladder cancer. *Aliment Pharmacol Ther* 2014;**39**(8):745–750.

139. Weiss NS, Yang CP. Incidence of histologic types of cancer of the small intestine. *J Natl Cancer Inst* 1987;**78**(4):653–656.

140. Canavan C, *et al*. Meta-analysis: Colorectal and small bowel cancer risk in patients with Crohn's disease. *Aliment Pharmacol Ther* 2006;**23**(8):1097–1104.

141. Green PH, Jabri B. Celiac disease and other precursors to small-bowel malignancy. *Gastroenterol Clin North Am* 2002;**31**(2):625–639.

142. Bennett CM, *et al*. Lifestyle factors and small intestine adenocarcinoma risk: A systematic review and meta-analysis. *Cancer Epidemiol* 2015 [Epub ahead of print]

Chapter 2

Immunotherapy in Gastrointestinal Malignancies

Michael A. Morse

Recent reports of efficacy of immune therapies in solid tumors other than melanoma and renal cell carcinoma have raised enthusiasm for testing immunotherapy in gastrointestinal (GI) malignancies. Strategies under development include antibodies and related molecules that mediate cellular cytotoxicity, vaccines intended to activate tumor-specific T cell and antibody responses, adoptive transfer of natural killer (NK) cells, tumor infiltrating lymphocytes, and chimeric antigen receptor T cells, and immunomodulatory drugs such as checkpoint blocking antibodies. Thus far, benefit has been modest although insights from these studies have provided new directions for testing. We will review the current status of the various immunotherapy approaches undergoing testing in GI malignances.

1 Introduction

As evident in its proclamation as the "breakthrough of the year 2013" by *Science*,[1] immunotherapy is enthusiastically being promoted for malignancies beyond the traditional targets of melanoma and renal cell carcinoma. An understanding of the determinants of a successful anti-tumor immune response is continuing to evolve;[2] however, a balance of immunostimulatory and immunoinhibitory cellular subsets, cytokines, and surface-expressed molecules is clearly critical. These components may occasionally assemble in a pattern typical of the response to acute viral infections leading to tumor rejection or may create a pattern more typical of chronic

27

inflammation that favors immune evasion, angiogenesis and tumor growth.[3] A fundamental requirement for immune rejection of tumor is the presence of immune effectors (cytolytic T cells [CTLs], helper T cells [Th], and NK cells) and antibodies to recognize and mediate destruction of tumor cells. Implicit in this fundamental requirement are differences between malignant cells and normal tissue that allow recognition by immune effectors. Previous concepts of self and non-self antigens are being replaced by a nuanced view that suggests immunogenicity of tumor cells relates to the rapid appearance of adequate quantities of antigens significantly different from those normally encountered by the receptors of the host's immune cells.[4] While the innate cellular arm of the immune system (NK cells, macrophages, neutrophils) recognizes aberrant molecular patterns including loss of HLA molecules, the adaptive cellular arm (CTL, Th) recognizes tumor antigens, unique or inappropriately expressed molecules that are the product of genetic instability and epigenetic changes of tumor cells. Interestingly, the tumor types with the greatest mutation rate are those which have demonstrated the most prominent efficacy for immunotherapy.[5] Tumor antigens targeted by CTL are expressed at the tumor cell surface as short (usually nine amino acid long) peptide sequences bound within MHC class I molecules where they can be recognized by activated T cells with the appropriate cognate receptor, resulting in tumor destruction by either granzyme delivery or Fas/Fas-ligand interactions, both of which trigger apoptotic pathways.

Because only activated T cells are capable of specific tumor recognition and killing, a critical event is activation of a sufficient number of tumor-antigen-specific T cells, a process that relies on co-operation of the innate and adaptive immune systems through type I interferons.[6] The initial death of some tumor cells and the associated inflammatory environment result in recruitment of dendritic cells (DCs) which take up antigens in their environment and process and present these antigens as small peptides within MHC class I and II molecules to CD8+ and CD4+ T cells respectively with receptors capable of recognizing the antigens (often called signal 1). The different subtypes of dendritic cells appear at first to affect tumor immunity in contrasting ways, plasmacytoid DCs are sometimes reported to be immunosuppressive and myeloid-derived DCs are associated with activation of antigen-specific immune responses, but in fact they may cooperate through interferon production by plasmacytoid DCs.[7] Subsequently, costimulatory molecules (CD80 and CD86) on myeloid-derived DCs engage CD28 on T cells providing "signal 2" for T cell activation and proliferation.[8] Other costimulatory pair interactions such as ICOS-L/ICOS, CD70/CD27, OX40L/OX40 and 4-1BBL/4-1BB also may amplify T cell responses.[9] The lack of costimulatory molecule expression on most tumor cells is one explanation for their inability to activate T cells directly. Following delivery of signal 2, further activation and proliferation of T cells occurs in response to local cytokine secretion, IL-2 from CD4+ T helper (Th1) cells, and IL-12 from dendritic cells in response to engagement of their CD40 by CD40L expressed by CD4+ T cells. Activated T cells, responding to chemokines emanating from the tumor environment[10] and recruited by high endothelial venules[11] are capable of trafficking to tumors and mediating cytolysis.

Because T cell activation could also result in autoimmunity, a number of controls throughout the T cell life cycle exist but may also be usurped by tumors to inhibit anti-tumor immune responses. The most avid auto-reactive T cells are deleted in the thymus; however, T cell activation and function are also controlled at "check points." At the site of activation, T cells upregulate CTLA4[12] which preferentially competes for CD28 and delivers inactivating signals to the T cell. In peripheral tissues, PD-1 expressed by activated T cells in response to inter-feron-gamma engages tissue expressed PD-L1 resulting in T cell "exhaustion." Other T cell inhibitory combinations described include HVEM/BTLA, TIM-3/Galectin-9, and MHC class II/LAG3.[13] These inhibitory pathways are usurped or activated by tumors to prevent T cell mediated destruction. Further, other cells in the tumor milieu such as CD4+CD25+FOXP3+ regulatory T cells (Treg) inhibit effector T cells by cell-cell contact or through the secretion of cytokines, such as interleukin-10 or TGF-β.[14] Monocytic myeloid-derived suppressor cells (MDSC) suppress antigen-specific T cells mainly through nitric oxide.[15] TH17 cells[16] and tumor associated macrophages[17] inhibit dendritic cell and T cell function by immunomodulatory (Th2) cytokine production (such as IL-10). The rare popula-tion NKT cells, lymphocytes that express NK markers but also a T cell receptor which recognizes only the lipid and glycolipid-binding molecule CD1d, are of two subsets that have opposite immunoregulatory functions related to their inter-action with Treg.[18] Metabolic enzymes and their products such as the tryptophan catabolizing enzyme, indoleamine 2,3-dioxygenase (IDO) and its product kynure-nine, have also been implicated in tumor-induced immunosuppression (reviewed in Ref. 19). IDO is upregulated by loss of the tumor suppressor Bin-1 in tumor cells and by interferons produced in the tumor microenvironment. As originally described, depletion of tryptophan on which T cells are dependent leads to impaired T cell activation. IDO activity also suppresses NK cells, and leads to enhanced Treg and MDSC levels or function. More recently, a more complex view of its immunosuppressive effects has included a role in inflammation and angiogenesis. In addition to Th2 cytokines (IL-4, IL-5, IL-6, IL-10 and IL-13), other cytokines in the tumor environment inhibit the host immune response. TGF-β, initially an inhibitor of tumor proliferation, subsequently promotes angiogenesis and immune evasion.

Opportunities to interact with or modulate the host response to tumor underpin the immunotherapies in development. Cytokines such as IL-2, IL-12, and interferon alpha nonspecifically activate immune effectors. Cancer vaccines deliver tumor antigens in a form that allows their uptake by *in situ* DC which can then cross-present the antigen to T cells with the appropriate receptor. Vaccines may consist of whole autologous or allogeneic tumor cells, genes modified to enhance immunogenicity or processed to generate lysates. Specific tumor antigens have been delivered as peptide epitopes, full length protein or fragments of tumor antigens, glycoproteins or carbohydrates, idiotype, genetic material (within plasmids, viral vectors, mRNA, bacterial or yeast vectors), or with DC and DC/tumor fusions. Adoptive transfer of antigen-specific T cells such as chimeric antigen-receptor CAR-T or tumor infiltrating lymphocytes (TILs) provides a large number of antigen-specific T cells which are expected to traffic to tumors. Delivery of antibodies or bispecific molecules permits engagement of tumors by NK cells (ADCC) or T cells. For example, cetuximab is able to mediate ADCC although this has not been conclusive in humans. Although the most recent strategies to counter tumor-induced suppression of T cells have focused on checkpoint inhibitors, including blocking antibodies against PD-1 and PD-L1, biologics that target the other inhibitory pathways are also being rapidly developed.

The remainder of this chapter will describe the immune basis for targeting each of the GI malignancies and review the immunotherapies that have been or are being tested. Because there are numerous recent reviews for some gastrointestinal malignancies, we will reference those and not exhaustively catalogue each study performed, but will highlight the challenges and promising areas. Data predominantly from clinical studies will be emphasized. A few additional points should be considered when surveying data across studies. The definition of response/progression has varied and the standard definitions may not be appropriate for immunotherapy studies. While Response Evaluation Criteria in Solid Tumors (RECIST ver 1.1) is the standard for most oncology studies currently, immune-related Response Criteria (ir-RC) were developed[20] to account for the possibility that immune responses may be delayed and progression may occur before clinical benefit is observed or the immune response to tumor may give the appearance of progression, so called pseudo-progression. Another consideration is whether expression of the target antigen is required for enrollment and if so, how the expression is identified. For example, tumor antigens may be assessed at the protein level by immunohistochemistry or at the gene expression level by polymerase chain reaction. It is also possible to identify peptides residing in MHC molecules though this is primarily used for antigen discovery currently.[21] Definition of T cell and antibody responses also varies considerably across studies depending on the assay used. The

ELISPOT assay, in which the number of T cells secreting cytokine in response to test antigen is quantified, has been the most frequently used to detect antigen-specific immune responses, but newer assays including sequencing of T cell receptors to detect oligoclonality may provide more refined characterization of the immune response. ELISA is typically used to measure antibody responses, but assays testing the function of the induced antibodies may provide additional insights about the immune response induced by immunization. Most studies analyze peripheral blood T cell responses but it is more likely that the immune cells infiltrate and elaborated cytokines at the site of tumor would provide more robust information about immunogenicity of the vaccine; however, this is logistically more challenging to achieve.

2 Colorectal Cancer Immunotherapy

2.1 *The immune response to colorectal cancer*

Extensive evaluation of colorectal cancer (CRC)[22] has identified infiltration of the tumor with lymphocytes (TILs), particularly prominent in those with microsatellite instability (MSI).[23] Increased TIL, both cytolytic and memory, are associated with improved survival for early stage colon cancer,[24,25] a concept under development as an "Immunoscore".[26] The relationship of granzyme B expression with improved outcome is indicated by the greater invasiveness of CRCs with low granzyme levels.[27] NK cell density in the tumor stroma is also associated with improved prognosis in patients with stage III CRC.[28] Although low in frequency, NKT cells are also associated with improved prognosis of CRC.[29] Surprisingly, Treg, although often associated with poor prognosis in other malignancies, have generally been associated with a good or neutral prognosis in colorectal cancer as reported in two recent meta-analyses.[30,31] Ladoire has suggested that this paradox can be explained by the role of Treg in controlling the pro-inflammatory/protumorigenic Th17 cells responding to the constant bacterial assault on the large intestine.[32]

The role of other immune cell subtypes has been somewhat inconclusive. While one would expect DC infiltration to be associated with improved outcome, this is an inconsistent finding possibly related to their specific intratumoral location.[33,34] Depending on their subtype, tumor-associated macrophages (TAMs) have been reported to confer better or worse tumor control. For example, a worse outcome has been associated with TAM that secrete pro-angiogenic molecules.[35] An increased frequency of peripheral blood and tumor MDSC were identified in patients with colorectal cancer and correlated with stage and metastasis. Further relevance of MDSC for immunotherapy is the observation that immune responses to a MUC-1 vaccine were attenuated in patients with high peripheral blood MDSC levels.[36]

The cytokine patterns expressed within CRCs are prognostic. Th1 cytokines (IL-2, IFN-γ, IL-12), providers of effector T cell help, have generally been associated with improved prognosis[37] while Th2 cytokines (IL-4, IL-5, IL-6, IL-10 and IL-13), modulators of effector T cell function, have had an inconsistent impact,[37] although some (such as IL-10) are more consistently associated with a higher relapse rate.[38] Similarly, Th17 cytokines (IL-17, IL-6 and IL-8)[39] and TGF-β[40] are associated with poorer prognosis. Other molecules in the colorectal tumor environment have an immunomodulatory role. Elevated expression of IDO was associated with poorer survival[41] while low plasma levels of its product, the tryptophan metabolite L-kynurenine were associated with increased survival.[42]

Regarding markers of immune suppression or immune escape, PD-L1 expression has been quite variable and has somewhat of a paradoxical association with outcome. In CRC, PD-L1 expression by tumor was inversely correlated with CD8+ T cells and intratumoral PD-1+ T cells were associated with advanced tumor stage and poorer prognosis;[43] however, Taube[44] found only one out of eight CRC specimens with PD-L1 expression using a cutoff for positivity of >5% of cells with cell surface expression using the monoclonal antibody 5H1. Surprisingly, the immune infiltrates expressed PD-L1 expression in 4/8 specimens. Droesser[45] however observed PD-L1 expression in 37% of mismatch repair (MMR)-proficient and in 29% of MMR-deficient CRC. Among MMR-proficient CRC, PD-L1 expression was associated with improved survival independent of other established prognostic factors. As expected, PD-L1 expression was associated with IFN-γ gene expression and infiltration by CD8+ lymphocytes suggesting that the PD-L1 expression in this scenario is a marker for CTL infiltration rather than a cause of immune suppression.

CRC has well established antigen targets including CEA,[46] MUC-1, β-HCG, EpCAM, p53, gastrin, 5T4, survivin, SART3, and NY-ESO-1, all of which have been found to be immunogenic when used as part of vaccines. The hypermutation rate in MSI-H tumors (particularly frame shift mutations) may generate a large number of neoantigens that can be targeted by the T cell response to tumor vaccines. Indeed, the immune response against peptides derived from frame shift mutations in MSI tumors is more frequent than the response against more well-established antigens such as CEA and MUC1.[47] Recurrence-free survival was most impacted among patients with MSI-high cancer following immunization with a tumor vaccine.[48] One challenge is that MHC molecules are downregulated in 72% of colorectal cancer.[49] In this study there was a positive correlation with CD8+ T cell infiltration suggesting that the down regulation of MHC served as a protective mechanism against CTL.

2.2 Immune therapies for CRC

2.2.1 Non-specific immune activation

There is no current established role for non-specific immune stimulation in colorectal cancer. Previously levamisole was combined with fluorouracil for the adjuvant treatment of CRC[50] and was suggested to work through immune activation, although it was not clear that this was involved in its mechanism of action against colon cancer[51] and it has been supplanted by folinic acid for modulation of fluorouracil. There have been occasional studies reporting cytokine combinations that enhance CTL responses and clinical outcome in colorectal cancer. For example, when GM-CSF and low-dose IL-2 were combined with chemotherapy, there was an increased frequency of tumor antigen-specific CTL and a reduction in Treg.[52] The combination of subcutaneous IL-2 and melatonin resulted in higher one year survival compared with best supportive care in patients with refractory CRC.[53] However, in larger studies interferon alone[54] and combined with fluorouracil[55] did not have benefit in the adjuvant setting; nor was the stimulatory adjuvant Bacillus Calmette-Guerin (BCG) associated with improvements in relapse-free survival in the adjuvant setting.[56,57] Interestingly, and as has been observed with other immunotherapies, despite the lack of improvement in relapse free survival, overall survival was improved in those patients who received BCG. The variable results with non-specific immune stimulants have resulted in more focus on antigen-specific immune activators.

2.2.2 Cancer vaccines for CRC

Vaccines for CRC have been summarized in a meta-analysis of data from phase I/II studies of tumor cell, peptide, viral vector, and dendritic cell-based strategies. This analysis concluded there was immunogenicity (59% humoral response rate, 44% cellular response rate), but minimal clinical activity as judged by the response rate of <1%.[58] Although some have concluded from the low response rate that CRC vaccines have little efficacy, there are a number of potential criticisms of this conclusion. Few vaccine studies in any malignancy have reported tumor regression, likely due to the extended time required to develop a clinically relevant expansion of tumor antigen-specific immune effectors during which tumors will have progressed; however, delayed evidence of tumor control and overall survival benefit has been observed in the absence of tumor regression in CRC and other malignancies. Marshall and colleagues[59] reported that 12 of 23 patients who progressed after two vaccinations achieved stable disease at 4 months. As many of the early phase studies have been summarized, the remainder of this section will focus on a discussion of newer studies and important issues raised by them.

The first issue is whether there is a preferred vaccine strategy. In the aforementioned meta-analysis, no single strategy was clearly superior, although there may be differences in the rate of humoral versus cellular responses with different strategies. Some have suggested that tumor cell vaccines have the advantage of providing a wide array of tumor antigens, mutated and non-mutated, and indeed have demonstrated clinical benefit;[60,61] however, autologous CRC vaccines are cumbersome to produce and have a high degree of variability in the administered product. More recent attempts have used allogeneic tumor cells[62] but clinical experience remains limited because of the small numbers of patients treated in these studies. Further, it is possible that immunosuppressive molecules such as TGF-β could be released by these tumors which may be countered by attempting to suppress production of these molecules.[63] Others have favored the use of individual peptides, peptide pools,[64] or proteins to allow a more focused induction of immune responses which can also be readily measured using assays that quantify antigen-specific T cell frequencies. Tumor antigen-encoding viral vectors[65] or oncolytic viruses such as Newcastle Disease Virus[66] injected into tumors or used to infect autologous tumor which then serves as a vaccine, because of the additional immunogenicity provided by the viral constituents, is also under development. Unfortunately, there have been few comparative studies. We randomized patients with resected metastases of CRC to receive autologous dendritic cells mixed with a poxvirus construct encoding CEA and MUC1 called PANVAC-V,F or the PANVAC-V,F poxvirus plus *in situ* GM-CSF.[67] There was no difference in progression free or overall survival between the two vaccine strategies; however, there was a higher rate of CEA-specific T cell response using the dendritic cells.

Many have suggested that the typical scenario in which vaccines have been tested, advanced disease, is destined to fail because of a weakened immune response and insufficient survival time to allow the immune response to achieve clinical efficacy. This is supported by reports of clinical benefit in vaccine studies for earlier stage disease. For example, a meta-analysis of studies in which patients with resected stage II and III CRC received active specific immunotherapy (ASI) with autologous tumor vaccines reported a significantly improved disease-free and overall survival.[68] Others have argued the ability of the vaccine to induce an immune response should be the relevant criterion, rather than the stage of the disease. Many studies have concluded that the immune response often correlates with survival. While some have argued that this correlation merely means that healthier patients destined to live longer also achieve more robust immune responses, this has been refuted by others who point out that immune responses against control, non-tumor antigens are not correlated with clinical outcome. When

Marshall and colleagues administered poxvector vaccines encoding CEA,[69] patients with higher T cell responses by ELISPOT assay had greater clinical response, but Flu-specific immune responses were not correlated with any trend towards clinical response. The association of outcome with immune response is not limited to T cell responses. In a randomized phase II study of CTP37-DT in metastatic colorectal cancer, patients who developed anti-β-HCG antibodies had improved overall survival (45 weeks vs. 25 weeks; $p = 0.0002$) compared to patients who did not.[70]

If as most data suggests, vaccination is unlikely to cause tumor regressions, then therapeutic vaccines will likely need to be combined with immune or targeted therapy. Fortunately, this appears to be feasible. When ALVAC-CEA, a nonreplicating canarypox vector encoding CEA and the B7.1 (CD80) costimulatory molecule, was combined with chemotherapy, overall immunologic and clinical responses were similar across all groups.[71] Similarly, 62% of patients developed antibody responses against G17DT, a gastrin-17/diphtheria fusion when it was administered concurrently with irinotecan and immune responders had a longer survival.[72] When TroVax, a modified vaccinia virus Ankara (MVA) encoding 5T4, a human oncofetal protein with elevated expression in CRC, was administered with fluorouracil and oxaliplatin, a majority of patients developed a humoral response to 5T4 and 41% of patients with metastatic disease had disease stabilization.[73]

Other important insights about vaccination against CRC have included demonstration of enhanced immunogenicity by co-delivery of tumor antigen and costimulatory molecules such as B7-1 (CD80), ICAM-1 (CD54), and LFA-3 (CD58) (using a three-gene construct called TRICOM). Using poxvectors encoding CEA and the TRICOM costimulatory molecules, Marshall reported a trend towards enhanced CEA-specific immune response and an increase in progression-free survival with the prime-boost strategy and the further addition of GM-CSF at the injection site.[59]

Among the explanations for impaired immune responses to vaccines for CRCs includes the presence of Treg and for viral vectors, neutralizing antibody and strategies to evade these challenges may be necessary. We demonstrated that AVX701, a novel CEA-expressing alphaviral-based vaccine with tropism for dendritic cells, was immunogenic over multiple immunizations despite neutralizing antiviral antibodies and elevated Tregs in the advanced cancer patients studied.[74] We also tested a novel Ad5 [E1-E2b-] adenoviral vector encoding CEA and demonstrated that it could increase the frequency of CEA-specific T cells despite the development of anti-adenoviral neutralizing antibody.[75] Because of the potentially better efficacy in patients with no evidence of disease, we are now testing AVX701 in the adjuvant setting for stage III colorectal cancer following standard chemotherapy (NCT01890213) (see Table 1). The role of heterologous prime-boost immunizations, sequentially using two different vectors to deliver

Table 1 Open clinical trials of immunotherapy for gastrointestinal malignancies.

Number	Title	Immunotherapy
Anal Cancer		
NCT01585428	A Phase II Study of Lymphodepletion Followed by Autologous Tumor-Infiltrating Lymphocytes and High-Dose Aldesleukin for Human Papillomavirus-Associated Cancers	TIL
NCT01923116	Therapeutic Vaccination Against Human Papillomavirus Type 16 for the Treatment of Anal Intraepithelial Neoplasia in HIV+ Men	SLP-HPV-01 (Synthetic long E6/E7 peptide)
NCT01653249	A Phase I Clinical Trial of an HPV Therapeutic Vaccine	Vaccine consisting of four HPV-16 E6 peptides in combination with Candin®
HCC		
NCT01995227	An Individualized Anti-Cancer Vaccine Study in Patients With HCC	AlloVax(TM): a personalized anti-cancer vaccine combining Chaperone Rich Cell Lysate (CRCL) as a source of tumor antigen prepared from patient's tumor and AlloStim(TM), allogeneic Th1 memory cell with CD3/CD28-coated microbeads attached
NCT01923233	*In Situ* Therapeutic Cancer Vaccine for Refractory Liver Cancer	Radiofrequency ablation followed by intratumoral, and IV AlloStim(TM)
NCT01749865	CIK Treatment for HCC Patient Underwent Radical Resection	Cytokine-Induced Killer Cells
NCT01974661	Phase I Safety Study of Dendritic Cell *Vaccine* to Treat Patients With *Hepatocellular Carcinoma*	COMBIG-DC
Pancreatic Cancer		
NCT01836432	A Phase III Study of Chemotherapy with or without Algenpantucel-L (HyperAcute®-Pancreas) Immunotherapy in Subjects With Borderline Resectable or Locally Advanced Unresectable Pancreatic Cancer	Algenpantucel-L (HyperAcute®-Pancreas) allogeneic tumor cell

(Continued)

Table 1   (*Continued*)

Number	Title	Immunotherapy
NCT01903083	Phase I Trial of Chemoimmunotherapy and Hypofractionated Radiation Therapy for Borderline Resectable and Locally Advanced Pancreatic Adenocarcinoma.	Tadalafil (phopshodiesterase 5) inhibitor
NCT01959672	A Phase II Study of Neoadjuvant Chemotherapy with and without Immunotherapy to CA125 (Oregovomab) Followed by Hypofractionated Stereotactic Radiotherapy and Concurrent HIV Protease Inhibitor Nelfinavir in Patients with Locally Advanced Pancreatic Cancer	oregovomab
NCT00727441	A Randomized Three-arm Neoadjuvant and Adjuvant Feasibility and Toxicity Study of a GM-CSF Secreting Allogeneic Pancreatic Cancer Vaccine Administered Either Alone or in Combination with Either a Single Intravenous Dose or Daily Metronomic Oral Doses of Cyclophosphamide for the Treatment of Patients with Surgically Resected Adenocarcinoma of the Pancreas	GVAX
NCT01313416	A Pilot Study to Test the Feasibility of the Combination of Gemcitabine and Anti-PD1 Monoclonal Antibody (CT-011) in the Treatment of Resected Pancreatic Cancer	Anti-PD1 Monoclonal Antibody (CT-011)
NCT01896869	A Phase II, Multicenter Study of FOLFIRINOX Followed by Ipilimumab in Combination with Allogeneic GM-CSF Transfected Pancreatic Tumor Vaccine (GVAX) in the Treatment of Metastatic Pancreatic Cancer	Ipilimumab plus GVAX (PANC 6.03 pcDNA-1/GM-Neo and PANC 10.05 pcDNA-1/ GM-Neo; Allogeneic GM-CSF- Transduced Pancreatic Tumor Cell Vaccine)
NCT01595321	Pilot Study Evaluating an Allogeneic GM-CSF-Transduced Pancreatic Tumor Cell Vaccine (GVAX) and Low Dose Cyclophosphamide Integrated With Fractionated Stereotactic Body Radiation Therapy (SBRT) and FOLFIRINOX Chemotherapy in Patients with Resected Adenocarcinoma of the Pancreas	GVAX (PANC 6.03 pcDNA-1/ GM-Neo and PANC 10.05 pcDNA-1/GM-Neo; Allogeneic GM-CSF-Transduced Pancreatic Tumor Cell Vaccine)

(Continued)

Table 1   (*Continued*)

Number	Title	Immunotherapy
NCT01088789	A Safety and Feasibility Trial of Boost Vaccinations of a Lethally Irradiated, Allogeneic Pancreatic Tumor Cell Vaccine Transfected with the GM-CSF Gene	GVAX (PANC 6.03 pcDNA-1/GM-Neo and PANC 10.05 pcDNA-1/GM-Neo; Allogeneic GM-CSF-Transduced Pancreatic Tumor Cell Vaccine)
NCT02004262	A Phase 2B, Randomized, Controlled, Multicenter, Open-Label Study of the Efficacy and Immune Response of GVAX Pancreas Vaccine (with Cyclophosphamide) and CRS 207 Compared to Chemotherapy or to CRS-207 Alone in Adults with Previously-Treated Metastatic Pancreatic Adenocarcinoma	GVAX (PANC 6.03 pcDNA-1/GM-Neo and PANC 10.05 pcDNA-1/GM-Neo; Allogeneic GM-CSF-Transduced Pancreatic Tumor Cell Vaccine) plus CRS-207 (listeria-mesothelin vaccine)
NCT01420874	Treatment of Advanced Colorectal or Pancreatic Cancer with Anti-CD3 x Anti-EGFR-Armed Activated T Cells (Phase Ib)	EGFR2Bi-specific antibody armed activated autologous T cells
NCT01583686	Phase I/II Study of Metastatic Cancer Using Lymphodepleting Conditioning Followed by Infusion of Anti-mesothelin Gene Engineered Lymphocytes	Anti-mesothelin CAR engineered PBL
NCT01781520	Study of S-1 Plus DC-CIK for Patients with Unresectable Locally Advanced Pancreatic Cancer	Cultured autologous peripheral blood mononuclear cells
NCT01473940	Ipilimumab and Gemcitabine for Advanced Pancreas Cancer: A Phase Ib Study	Ipilimumab
NCT02077881	A Phase I/II Study of Indoximod in Combination with Gemcitabine and Nab-Paclitaxel in Patients with Metastatic Adenocarcinoma of the Pancreas	Indoximod (IDO inhibitor)
NCT02154646	A Phase 1b Study of LY2157299 in Combination with Gemcitabine in Patients with Advanced or Metastatic Unresectable Pancreatic Cancer	LY2157299 (small molecule inhibitor of the TGF-β receptor type 1 kinase)

Colorectal Cancer

Number	Title	Immunotherapy
NCT01348256	Randomized Phase II Study with Dendritic Cell Immunotherapy in Patients with Resected Hepatic Metastasis of Colorectal Carcinoma	Autologous dendritic cells loaded with autologous tumor antigens

(*Continued*)

Table 1 (*Continued*)

Number	Title	Immunotherapy
NCT01890213	A Pilot Study of Active Immunotherapy With CEA(6D) VRP Vaccine (AVX701) in Patients with Stage III Colorectal Cancer	Alphaviral vector encoding CEA
NCT02176746	A Phase I/II Study of Active *Immunotherapy* with Cancer Stem Cells Vaccine for *Colorectal* Cancer (CSC)	Cancer stem cell loaded DCs
NCT01929499	Efficacy of Adjuvant Cytokine-induced Killer Cells in Colon Cancer (CIKCC)	Cytokine-induced killer cells
NCT01885702	Dendritic Cell Vaccination in Patients with Lynch Syndrome or Colorectal Cancer with MSI	Frameshift-derived neoantigen-loaded DC
NCT01952730	A Pilot Safety Study of Vaccination with Autologous, Lethally Irradiated Colorectal Cancer Cells Engineered by Adenoviral Mediated Gene Transfer to Secrete Human Granulocyte-Macrophage Stimulating Factor	Autologous GVAX
NCT01462513	L-BLP25 in Patients with *Colorectal* Carcinoma After Curative Resection of Hepatic Metastases (LICC)	L-BLP25
NCT01309126	A Phase 3 Open-Label, Randomized, Multicenter Study of Imprime PGG® in Combination With Cetuximab (Erbitux®) in Subjects With Recurrent or Progressive KRAS Wild Type Colorectal Cancer	Imprime PGG + cetuximab

Gastroesophageal

Number	Title	Immunotherapy
NCT01227772	A Phase I/IIa Study of OTSGC-A24 Vaccine in Advanced Gastric Cancer	OTSGC-A24: HLA A24 binding peptide cocktail targeting FOXM1, DEPDC1, KIF20A, URLC10 and VEGFR1
NCT02215837	Randomized, Controlled, Multicenter Study of Autologous Tumor Lysate-pulsed Dendritic and Cytokine-induced Killer Cells (Ag-D-CIK) Combined With Chemotherapy for Gastric Cancer.	Dendritic cells and cytokine induced killer cells

(*Continued*)

Table 1   (*Continued*)

Number	Title	Immunotherapy
NCT02030561	Phase I/II Study of Expanded, Activated Autologous Natural Killer Cell Infusions With Trastuzumab for Patients with HER2+ Breast and Gastric Cancer	NK cells and trastuzumab
NCT01783951	The purpose of this study is to evaluate the antitumor effect and safety of clinical effectiveness S-1 plus dendritic cell activated Cytokine induced killer treatment (DC-CIK) for advanced gastric cancer.	Dendritic cell activated cytokine induced killer cells
NCT01143545	Allogeneic Tumor Cell Vaccine with Metronomic Oral Cyclophosphamide and Celecoxib as Adjuvant Therapy for Lung and Esophageal Cancers, Thymic Neoplasms, Thoracic Sarcomas, and Malignant Pleural Mesotheliomas	K526-GM vaccine
NCT01258868	Epigenetically-Modified Autologous Tumor Cell Vaccines With ISCOMATRIX(TM) Adjuvant and Oral Celecoxib in Patients Undergoing Resection of Lung and Esophageal Cancers, Thymic Neoplasms, Thoracic Sarcomas, and Malignant Pleural Mesotheliomas	Autologous Tumor cell vaccine
NCT02054104	Adjuvant Tumor Lysate Vaccine and Iscomatrix with or without Metronomic Oral Cyclophosphamide and Celecoxib in Patients with Malignancies Involving Lungs, Esophagus, Pleura, or Mediastinum	H1299 Lysate Vaccine
NCT01928394	A Phase I/II, Open-label Study of Nivolumab Monotherapy or Nivolumab Combined with Ipilimumab in Subjects with Advanced or Metastatic Solid Tumors (Gastric subgroup)	Anti-PD-1 and Ant-CTLA4
NCT01772004	Phase I, Open-label, Multiple-ascending Dose Trial to Investigate the Safety, Tolerability, Pharmacokinetics, Biological and Clinical Activity of MSB0010718C in Subjects with Metastatic or Locally Advanced Solid Tumors and Expansion to Selected Indications	Anti-PD-L1

(*Continued*)

Table 1   (*Continued*)

Number	Title	Immunotherapy
NCT01375842	A Phase I, Open Label, Dose Escalation Study of the Safety and Pharmacokinetics of MPDL3280A Administered Intravenously as a Single Agent to Patients with Locally Advanced or Metastatic Solid Tumors or Hematologic Malignancies	Anti-PD-L1
NCT02340975	A Phase 1b/2 Study of MEDI4736 With Tremelimumab, MEDI4736 or Tremelimumab Monotherapy in Gastric or GEJ Adenocarcinoma	Anti-PD-L1
Various		
NCT01928394	A Phase I/II, Open-label Study of Nivolumab Monotherapy or Nivolumab Combined with Ipilimumab in Subjects with Advanced or Metastatic Solid Tumors	Nivolumab (anti-PD-1 Ab) and ipilimumab (anti-CTLA4 antibody)
NCT01174121	A Phase II Study Using Short-Term Cultured, CD8+-Enriched Autologous Tumor-infiltrating Lymphocytes Following a Lymphocyte Depleting Regimen in Metastatic Digestive Tract Cancers	Combination of TIL and aldesleukin
NCT01868490	The Adoptive *Immunotherapy* for Solid Tumors Using Modified Autologous Cytokine-induced Killer Cells	Cytokine-induced killer (CIK) cells
NCT01522820	Vaccine Therapy with or without Sirolimus in Treating Patients With NY-ESO-1 Expressing Solid Tumors	DEC-205-NY-ESO-1 fusion protein vaccine
NCT01801852	Autologous Natural Killer T Cells Infusion for the Treatment of Cancer	Autologous natural killer T (NKT) cells
NCT00553683	Cyclophosphamide, Radiation Therapy, and Poly ICLC in Treating Patients with Unresectable, Recurrent, Primary, or Metastatic Liver Cancer	Poly ICLC

(*Continued*)

Table 1   (*Continued*)

Number	Title	Immunotherapy
NCT01526473	A Phase I Study To Evaluate the Antitumor Activity and Safety of DUKE-002-VRP(HUHER2-ECD+TM), an Alphaviral Vector Encoding the HER2 Extracellular Domain and Transmembrane Region, in Patient with Locally Advanced or Metastatic Human Epidermal Growth Factor Receptor 2-Positive (HER2+) Cancers Including Breast Cancer	Alphavirus encoding HER2
NCT02133079	Immunotherapy of Tumor with Autologous Tumor Derived Heat Shock Protein gp96	Autologous tumor derived heat shock protein gp96
NCT01284231	A Study to Evaluate the Safety and Tolerability of MEDI-565 in Adults with Gastrointestinal Adenocarcinomas	MEDI-565 (Bispecific T cell engaging molecule)

the same antigen avoids the neutralizing or excessive response to the single vector while enhancing immune responses to the antigen was studied by Marshall and colleagues[69] who reported that one vaccinia encoding CEA followed by three boosts of fowlpox encoding CEA was superior to the reverse order in the generation of CEA-specific T cell responses. Theoretically, any heterologous combination of vaccines (e.g. plasmids,[65] peptides, DCs, bacterial vectors) could serve as a component of a prime-boost strategy. Because the number of permutations of prime-boost strategies is large, it is unlikely that they can be directly compared in human clinical trials and rather data from preclinical models, safety, convenience and other pragmatic issues (plasmids are cheaper to manufacture than viral vectors for example) will likely guide these combination strategies in the future.

In summary, currently, there is no lead CRC vaccine. Those that have had suggestion of benefit in later phase trials (such as the autologous tumor cell vaccines[60,61] or Newcastle disease virus in a subgroup)[66] have been challenging to develop further due to regulatory concerns. Some that have progressed to late phase II or III such as the idiotype vaccines (CeaVac[76] and Onyvax-105[77,78]) and 17-1a glycoprotein (SCV106)[79] did not reach their study endpoints and/or have had their development discontinued. Newer vaccine designs based on optimized viral vectors, heterologous prime boost strategies, targeting more relevant antigens, and intended to avoid host inhibitory or immunosuppressive responses or combined with newer immunomodulatory strategies await more advanced testing.

2.2.3 *Adoptive transfer of T cells, CAR-T cells, BiTE and antibodies mediating ADCC*

There are few studies of TIL or CAR-T for CRC.[80] In a study of patients with stage II to IV CRC,[81] CD4+ T cells were obtained from sentinel lymph nodes, expanded *in vitro* with autologous tumor extract and administered with little associated toxicity. Of the nine patients with metastatic disease, four experienced complete regressions CRC. This impressive result clearly requires follow-up studies. Caution regarding possible toxicity of T cell therapy is suggested by a study where three of three patients who received autologous T cells engineered with high-avidity CEA-specific T cell receptors experienced severe transient inflammatory colitis, although they all had a decline in CEA level.[82] In a single patient with CRC receiving CAR-T cells specific for HER2, cytokine storm led to the patient's death.[83] Ongoing studies are included in the table. BiTE molecules, bispecific antibody like molecules which can simultaneously bind a surface expressed tumor antigen and CD3 on T cells are capable of connecting cytotoxic T cells to a cancer cell, independently of T cell receptor specificity or peptide antigen presentation. We have previously shown that CEA-BiTE (Medi-565) mediates killing of CEA-expressing, human CRC *in vitro*.[84] Early phase testing of this molecule is ongoing, but BiTE has demonstrated activity in hematologic malignancies. The concept of monoclonal antibodies to induce ADCC has been tested in a late phase study with edrecolomab which did not reach its endpoint,[85] but newer antibodies optimized for binding to Fcγ receptors or targeted against potentially more relevant antigens are in development (Table 1).

2.2.4 *Checkpoint blockade*

There is limited data from studies testing checkpoint blockade in colorectal cancer. In a phase II study of the anti-CTLA4 Ab tremelimumab, a partial response was documented in only one out of 47 patients with colorectal cancer.[86] One potential criticism of this study is that patients were not allowed to continue on the study drug beyond first progression to determine if they might be late responders. In a phase I trial of the anti-PD-1 antibody nivolumab, one of 14 patients with metastatic colorectal cancer had a complete response,[87] but no response was observed in another phase I study of 19 patients.[88] One possible explanation was the low level of PD-L1, identified in only one of seven colorectal cancers analyzed, and a possible biomarker for sensitivity to anti-PD-1 antibodies. Finally, in a phase I study of the anti-PD-L1 antibody BMS-936559, there was no response among 18 CRC patients.[89] Another anti-PD-L1 antibody (MPDL3280A) is currently being tested with chemotherapy in colorectal cancer and nivolumab is being studied in MSI-H metastatic colorectal cancers (Table 1; see section 9 for newer data).

3 Pancreatic Cancer Immunotherapy

3.1 *The immune response to pancreatic cancer*

Pancreatic cancer has a prominent stromal component that prominently alters the host response to the malignancy and with relevance to the immune response, favors an immune evasive response.[90] This is supported by studies such as that of Ino and colleagues[91] who reported that shorter survival was associated with higher levels of M2 TAM, neutrophils, and the ratio of Tregs to CD4+ T cells. Conversely, longer survival was associated with higher levels of cells associated with immune attack (tumor-infiltrating CD4+ and CD8+ lymphocytes, and M1 TAM). Others have identified increasing levels of Treg as pancreatic adenocarcinoma progresses.[92] The stroma may also serve as a physical barrier to efficient immune cell infiltration.

3.2 *Tumor antigens in pancreatic cancer*

Pancreatic cancers share many tumor antigens for which endogenous T cell responses may be identified including MAGE-A3, p53, CEA, human telomerase reverse transcriptase (hTERT), Wilms tumor (WT)-1, and vascular endothelial growth factor receptor (VEGFR)2.[93] The mutations of Kras present opportunities for immune targeting as Kras is critical for driving tumor proliferation; however, as Kras is an early mutation, there may also be the possibility of tolerance to these antigens. One of the antigens of particular interest has been mesothelin, expressed by the majority of pancreatic cancers, minimally expressed by normal peritoneum and pleural tissues,[94] and to which patients with pancreatic adenocarcinoma harbor antigen-specific T cells.[95]

3.3 *Vaccines for pancreatic cancer*

Vaccine therapy for pancreatic cancer has been recently reviewed[96] and tumor vaccines, the leading candidates being GVAX and Algenpantucel-L, are among those undergoing advanced phase testing. The Johns Hopkins group has performed a series of studies with GVAX, a combination of two allogeneic human pancreatic cancer cell lines, engineered to express GM-CSF, testing its effects in patients with either resected pancreatic adenocarcinoma or metastatic disease.[97,98] GM-CSF, likely due to its role as a dendritic cell growth and maturation fact, had been previously demonstrated to be the most effective cytokine for inducing immune responses to the vaccine and enhancing tumor free survival in mouse models. Although as a tumor vaccine, there are a number of potential antigenic targets, recent studies have identified a high rate of mesothelin-specific immune responses leading to efforts to clone mesothelin into other vaccine platforms such as the ΔactA/ΔinlB strain of live-attenuated *L. monocytogenes* (CRS-207). These studies also demonstrated that higher avidity mesothelin-specific T cell responses which correlated with survival could be induced by the GVAX after pre-administration of cyclophosphamide, used to deplete regulatory T cells. Importantly, this vaccine strategy was demonstrated to modify the tumor environment from non-immunogenic to immunogenic as suggested by the formation of intratumoral tertiary lymphoid aggregates following vaccination. Gene expression profiling of these aggregates demonstrated that a suppressed Treg pathway was associated with improved survival, but again illustrated complexities in our understanding of the role of Th17 because an enhanced Th17 pathway was also associated with improved outcome.[99] This promising line of research led to a recent randomized phase II study of patients with previously treated metastatic pancreatic cancer in which the prime-boost strategy of cyclophosphamide/GVAX followed by CRS-207 improved median overall survival compared with GVAX alone (6 months vs. 3.4 months).[100] The design of this study raises the question of whether the GVAX actually has a role; therefore, a phase IIb study is currently enrolling patients with previously treated metastatic pancreatic cancer to cyclophosphamide/GVAX/CRS207 or CRS207 alone or physician choice of chemotherapy.

Algenpantucel-L (also known as hyperacute-pancreatic cancer vaccine) which consists of two irradiated, live, human allogeneic pancreatic cancer cell lines modified to express murine α-1,3-galactosyltransferase, generates highly immunogenic α-galactosylated epitopes onto the tumor cell surface proteins. Because humans usually have IgG that recognize this epitope, the vaccine is rapidly attacked releasing antigen for cross presentation by DC. In a highly promising phase II study, Algenpantucel-L was administered with adjuvant gemcitabine and chemoradiotherapy following surgical resection for pancreatic cancer.[101] The 12-month disease-free survival was 62%, and the 12-month overall survival was 86%, impressive results that have led to a fully enrolled phase III clinical study testing this approach. A study of Algenpantucel-L with chemoradiotherapy for locally advanced pancreatic cancer is also ongoing (Table 1).

Similar to the experiments in colon cancer, there have been hints of activity for peptide vaccines, but no compelling late phase data. A study testing immunization with a modified CEA peptide mixed with GM-CSF in the adjuvant montanide supported the concept of dose–immunologic response as patients with advanced pancreatic cancer receiving the vaccine with CEA peptide at 1mg had the highest rate of CEA-specific immune response by ELISPOT assay compared with lower doses of peptide.[102] Small studies of vaccination with mutated Kras peptides have demonstrated feasibility and immunogenicity that was associated with survival benefit, but studies were not designed to demonstrate definitive clinical efficacy.[103] Similarly, only small studies have been performed with survivin peptide vaccine, but again immunogenicity was demonstrated.[104] Because of the importance of telomerase in preserving the telomeres of chromosomes during multiple rounds of replication, it has been suggested that a vaccine against telomerase may target resistant, persistent, and proliferating tumor cells. Immunization with G1001 (TeloVAC), a human telomerase reverse transcriptase catalytic subunit (hTERT) class II 16 amino acid peptide induced CD4+ and CD8+ T cell clones that could recognize hTERT. GV1001 demonstrated promising phase II data in which pancreatic cancer patients with an immune response survived longer.[105] However, GV1001 failed to improve outcome in two phase III studies in patients with nonresectable pancreatic ductal adenocarcinoma (PDA), the first testing GV1001 monotherapy (followed by combination with gemcitabine in progressors) versus gemcitabine alone[106] and the second combined simultaneously or sequentially with gemcitabine/capecitabine versus gemcitabine/capecitabine.[107] An attempt to identify biomarkers of activity of GV1001 yielded the hypothesis that eotaxin levels may predict overall survival in patients receiving concurrent vaccine and chemotherapy.[108] The significance of this finding remains to be demonstrated as eotaxin (CCL11), a chemotactic factor for eosinophils, has been more typically associated with allergic responses rather than immunity to tumors.

In addition to peptide vaccine studies intended to activate T cells, protein based vaccines have also been tested with the intention of activating antibody responses. Because pancreatic cancers depend on autocrine and paracrine cytokine and growth factor secretion, inducing antibodies that target growth factors may lead to a growth inhibitory effect. In a double-blinded, placebo-controlled clinical trial of previously treated advanced pancreatic cancer patients, the administration of G17DT, a fragment of gastrin which can serve as a growth factor for GI malignancies, fused to diphtheria toxin to enhance immunogenicity, increased survival in a re-analysis of the data excluding protocol violators.[109] Longer survival was documented for patients developing anti-G17DT responses compared with nonresponders.

Viral, yeast, and bacterial vectors have all been employed as immunotherapy for pancreatic cancer. Unfortunately, a phase III, randomized clinical trial comparing PANVAC-V/F to physician choice chemotherapy in second line pancreatic cancer failed to meet its survival endpoints (J. Marshall, personal communication). The GlobeImmune yeast vector containing mutated Kras has also been tested in combination with gemcitabine in a phase IIb study demonstrating a 2.6 month improvement in median overall survival in patients who had undergone pancreaticoduodenectomy and had positive microscopic margins (17.2 vs. 14.6 months).[110] As described above, the ΔactA/ΔinlB strain of live-attenuated *Listeria monocytogenes* (*Lm*) variant into which mesothelin has been cloned was (*Lm* Δ*actA*/Δ*inlB*/hMesothelin) developed as a single agent or prime boost partner with GVAX,[100] demonstrating clinical benefit in a phase II study. *Lm* is taken up by macrophages and other phagocytes in the liver resulting in an inflammatory response, activation of NK cells and responses of T cells against the encoded antigen.

Due to the complexity of generating dendritic cells, studies in pancreatic cancer have been limited. In a retrospective review of 138 patients treated with a DC based therapy,[111] six month survival was 72.2% and nine month survival was 50.4%, which were similar to survivals for chemotherapy treated patients in the current era. In a study of patients with refractory pancreatic cancer, a DC vaccine plus lymphokine-activated killer (LAK) cells in combination with gemcitabine and/ or S-1 enhanced survival compared with the DC vaccine in combination with chemotherapy but no LAK cells.[112] Survival correlated with decreased regulatory T cells on therapy. Therefore, the role of DCs in both of these studies is unclear, but warrants further evaluation.

3.4 *Adoptive immunotherapy for pancreatic cancer*

There is limited data with TILs and CAR-T for pancreatic cancer, although a mesothelin-specific CAR-T has been developed.[113] Because the chimeric antigen receptor is a foreign antigen, allergic reactions and other undesirable immune responses may be limitations as with other CAR-T.[114,115] A different cell-based strategy is to activate macrophages to degrade the tumor stroma which is otherwise a major barrier to therapy of pancreatic cancer. Beatty reported that a CD40 agonistic antibody activated macrophages which rapidly infiltrated tumors and destroyed their stroma.[116] A phase I study utilizing this approach along with gemcitabine[117] demonstrated uniform decreases in FDG-PET of the primary tumor but heterogeneity of metastatic lesions. Unfortunately, this approach does not seem to lead to induction of T cell responses but does depend on a Th1 environment within the tumor.[118]

3.5 *Checkpoint blockade*

The immunosuppressive pancreatic tumor environment would seem ideal for testing checkpoint blockade. Unfortunately, ipilimumab as a single agent had minimal activity in a phase II trial in locally advanced and metastatic pancreatic cancer. However, one patient did have a delayed, but substantial, response of the primary and hepatic metastases.[119] More promising data was reported when ipilimumab was combined with GVAX in locally advanced or metastatic pancreatic cancer.[120] In this randomized study, among patients receiving ipilimumab plus GVAX, 3 out of 15 had prolonged disease stabilization and 7 out of 15 experienced CA19-9 declines, whereas among patients receiving only ipilimumab, 2 out of 15 had brief disease stabilization and none had CA19-9 declines. Survival also favored the combination therapy. Studies with PD-1 and anti-PD-L1 are ongoing (Table 1).

4 Hepatocellular Carcinoma Immunotherapy

4.1 *The immune response to hepatocellular carcinoma*

The host immune response to hepatocellular carcinoma (HCC) is both pro-tumorigenic and tumor-inhibitory.[121] It is well established that HCC develops in the setting of chronic inflammation. While the release of reactive oxygen species in this environment generates mutations through DNA damage, inflammation also alters and impairs anti-tumor immune response. Further, although an "inflammatory environment" is associated with an improved outcome,[122,123] particularly if associated with infiltration of HCC by TILS with activated signaling pathways,[124] an immunosuppressive environment generally predominates (as has been recently reviewed in Ref. 125). The underlying cause of the cirrhosis and HCC may impact immunity as functional defects in peripheral blood DCs have been identified in patients with hepatitis B and C.[126] Indeed, the diseased liver may contribute to imbalances in immune response due to alteration in the numbers of myeloid DC which decline in diseased livers accompanied by an increase in plasmacytoid DC.[127] Increased Treg levels have been found in the peripheral blood and among tumor infiltrating lymphocytes of HCC patients[128–130] where they are associated with a reduction in CD8+ T cells,[131] more advanced disease and worse survival.[132] Studies have been fairly consistent in their identification of Treg as poor prognostic factors in HCC as reported in recent meta-analyses.[133,134] In addition to their role in suppressing CD8+ T cells, Treg in liver tumors are associated with reduced number and function of peripheral and intratumoral CD56(dim)CD16+ NK subsets in patients with HCC.[31] These studies would suggest that depletion of Treg could be useful in management of HCC; however, there is likely more complexity to this issue. Greten[135] reported that depletion of Tregs, as could be achieved with cyclophosphamide, allowed detection of AFP-specific T cell responses among peripheral blood mononuclear cells *in vitro*. In contrast, Flecken[136] noted that depletion of Treg *in vitro* resulted in enhanced proliferation but not function of tumor antigen-specific T cells suggesting Treg depletion alone may be insufficient. Monocytic myeloid derived suppressor cells identified in patients with HCC[137] were reported to suppress antigen specific T cells and NK cells.[138] Increased Th17 cells and secreted cytokines (IL-17 and IL-23) in the peripheral blood of HCC patients where they are associated with worse outcome.[139,140] Further, IL-17 recruits neutrophils to HCC where they are associated with enhanced angiogenesis.[141] PD-L1 expression has been identified in HCC but a novel role was identified by Kuang who reported peritumoral monocyte-expressed PD-L1 could suppress T cell responses.[142] PD-1 expression is greater on intratumoral T cells than peripheral blood of HCC patients suggesting PD-1 blockade may provide benefit, but in this study, blockade of PD-1/PD-L1 during T cell stimulation in vitro increased the frequency but not the function of "exhausted" T cells of HCC patients.[143] It should also be noted that standard therapies for HCC may have immunomodulatory effects. For example, sorafenib treated tumor associated macrophages had enhanced IL-12 secretion;[144] further, sorafenib may suppress Treg.[145–147]

4.2 *Tumor antigens*

Spontaneous and vaccine induced immune responses against NY-ESO-1, MAGE, SSX, and AFP have been identified in HCC patients;[143,148–150] however, there is no dominant response to a particular antigen as suggested by Flecken[136] who non-specifically expanded T cells from peripheral blood and tumor tissue and detected CD8+ T cells specific for AFP, glypican-3, MAGE-A1 and NY-ESO-1 without a predominance of any specificity.

4.3 *Review of immune therapies for hepatocellular carcinoma*

Vaccines have mainly been tested in phase I/II studies for HCC with small numbers of subjects. Examples have included peptide vaccines against glipican-3 (reviewed in Ref. 151) and telomerase,[152] and DC loaded with AFP peptides,[153] autologous tumor cells,[154] HepG2 lysates[155] or administered intratumorally.[156] In general, these studies have demonstrated immunogenicity, suggestions tumor responses, and improved clinical outcome. As with other malignancies, there is wide variation in inter-patient responses to the immunizations, suggested by a two patient study with detailed immune analysis.[157] The subjects received a plasmid encoding AFP as a prime and then adenoviral vector encoding AFP as a boost. One patient experienced only activation of adenoviral vector specific T cells. The other patient activated AFP-specific T cells but only minimal adenoviral vector-specific T cells. The positive response was hypothesized to be related to their lower MDSC, greater activation of NK cells at baseline, and serum type I cytokine response. This raises the question of whether an immune biomarker could predict responses to the vaccine.

Adoptive immunotherapy with LAK cells, TILs, and ex vivo IL-2 or IL-2/CD3 stimulated PBMC have been reported to improve survival or reduce recurrence in resected HCC or HCC treated with transcatheter chemoembolization or radiofrequency ablation in phase II or non-randomized studies. The details of these studies have been recently reviewed.[158] A potential benefit of this approach may also be some degree of hepatitis infection control.[159]

There is little data on checkpoint blockade, but one study did administer the anti-CTLA4 antibody tremelimumab to patients with chronic HCV and HCC.[160] In addition to a decrease in viral load and anti-HCV immune responses, the tremelimumab was associated with an HCC time to progression of 6.48 months, a partial response rate of 17.6% and disease control rate of 76.4%. Ongoing studies of immunotherapy for HCC are listed in Table 1.

5 Immunotherapy for Biliary Cancers

5.1 *The immune response to biliary malignancies*

In the limited study of the immune response to biliary malignancies, a similar pattern, as has been reported for other liver tumors, has emerged. Goeppert demonstrated that T cells were the most prevalent inflammatory cell type in biliary tract cancers.[161] During the biliary intraepithelial neoplasia to primary carcinoma to metastasis sequence, evidence of adaptive immunity declined while evidence of innate immunity increased. Tumor infiltrating CD4+, CD8+, and Foxp3+ T lymphocytes were associated with a significantly longer overall survival but only in extrahepatic cholangiocarcinoma and gallbladder cancer, not intrahepatic cholangiocarcinoma. It was noticed that in cholangiocarcinoma, CD8+ T cells were more numerous in the tumor than interface of tumor and normal liver, but CD4+ cells exhibited the opposite pattern. CD56+ NK and CD20+ B cells were infrequent in either location.[162] The high levels of M2 macrophages was found in intrahepatic cholangiocarcinoma positively correlated with angiogenesis, Treg frequency, and worse disease-free survival.[163] It appears that cytokines/chemokines produced by the cholangiocarcinoma were responsible for the M2 polarization through activation of STAT3 as evidenced by suppressed IL-10 production by the macrophages when exposed to STAT3 siRNA. It is considered that the number of mature (CD83+) DC at the invasive margin of cholangiocarcinoma correlated with the number of CD8-positive or CD4-positive T cells in the tumor and was associated with a lower rate of lymph node metastasis and a better clinical outcome.[164] Among mechanisms for resistance to immune responses is the upregulation of FAS-L on cholangiocarcinoma and downregulation of FAS rendering the tumor cells less sensitive to killing and more capable of inhibiting T cells.[165] The PD-1/PD-L1 axis has been studied to a limited extent, but as in other malignancies, PD-L1 expression was inversely correlated with stage of disease and intratumoral CD8+ T cells which were found to be apoptotic, suggesting suppression of effector immunity by tumor expressed PD-L1.[166]

5.2 *Tumor antigens*

Twenty-two to twenty-nine percent intrahepatic cholangiocarcinomas express cancer testis antigens such as MAGE-A1, MAGE-A3/4 and NY-ESO-1 and the half cases express at least one of the antigens suggesting they may be potential targets for cancer vaccines.[167] The mucin molecules, predominantly MUC1 and MUC5AC are expressed in slightly less than half of the cases.[168] If mutations, fusions, or amplifications generating neoantigens or overexpression of proteins are also potentially targetable, then a number of molecular abnormalities that have been identified in cholangiocarcinoma (such as ARID1A, IDH1/2, TP53, FGFR2, KRAS, and others) could represent potential targets.[169] The Rosenberg group at NCI identified type I CD4+ T helper cells recognizing a mutation in erbb2 interacting protein (ERBB2IP) expressed by the cancer within the patient's TILS. On two occasions, adoptive transfer of TILS enriched for mutation-specific polyfunctional Th1 cells resulted in disease regression.[170]

5.3 *Immunotherapy for biliary malignancies*

As has been the case with other malignancies, vaccine studies have been single arm and/or phase I. Aruga and colleagues tested two different peptide cocktails. In the first study,[171] nine patients with advanced, refractory biliary tract malignancy received escalating doses of HLA-A*2402–restricted epitope peptides derived from lymphocyte antigen 6 complex locus K (LY6K), TTK protein kinase, insulin-like growth factor-II mRNA-binding protein 3 (IMP-3), and DEP domain containing 1 (DEPDC1). The vaccine was well tolerated with no grade 3 or 4 adverse events and was immunogenic (ELISPOT detected immune responses to at least one antigen in seven of nine patients and the response increased with increasing doses). Some degree of epitope dominance was suggested by the observation that the anti-LY6K and DEPDC1 responses exceeded those to TTK or IMP3.The immune response (injection site reaction or T cell response) was associated with longer survival. In the second study,[172] nine patients with advanced, refractory biliary tract malignancies, received HLA-A*2402-restricted peptides derived from cell division cycle associated 1 (CDCA1), cadherin 3 (CDH3) and kinesin family member 20A (KIF20A) subcutaneously. As before, the peptide combination was well tolerated and ELISPOT detected T cell responses in five of nine patients. Injection site reaction was associated with longer overall survival. In an attempt to enhance immunogenicity, dendritic cell vaccines have also been utilized in biliary malignancies. Autologous tumor lysate pulsed dendritic cells plus *ex vivo* activated T cell transfer was tested in patients with resected intrahepatic cholangiocarcinoma. The median progression-free survival (PFS) and overall survival (OS) were 18.3 and 31.9 months in the vaccinated patients compared with 7.7 and 17.4 months in the (non-randomized) control unvaccinated group.[173] An injection site skin reaction to the vaccine was associated with a longer PFS and OS. Patients with advanced biliary tract cancers were immunized with dendritic cells loaded with WT1 and MUC-1 peptides in a different study.[174] Median survival was related to improved nutritional status, reaction to the vaccine (fever), low baseline C-reactive protein, and use of chemotherapy. While all are small studies, taken in aggregate they suggest that patients with biliary malignancies are capable of mounting an immune response to tumor antigens and the immune response is associated with outcome, but patients with better clinical status and less advanced disease may benefit more as has been suggested for other malignancies. Ongoing studies continue to test similar strategies (see Table 1).

6 Immunotherapy for Gastroesophageal Malignancies

6.1 *The immune response to esophagogastric cancers and targeted tumor antigens*

Both gastric and esophageal cancers develop in the setting of inflammation[175,176] suggesting positive and negative roles for immune cells in the tumor environment of these malignancies. Studies reported that a high Th1/Th2 cytokine ratio is associated with improved disease free survival while high Th17 and MDSC are associated with worse outcome.[177] Intratumoral DCs, memory T cells, B cells, and NK cells were associated with improved outcome. An analysis of the peripheral blood immune cell population from patients with advanced gastric and GE junction adenocarcinomas noted that while the frequency and activation status of total T and NK cells were similar between the cancer patients and healthy volunteers, there were fewer CD4+ T cells, fewer B cells, increased MDSC subpopulations, and an increased frequency of activated Treg in the cancer patients.[178] At the site of the tumor, Treg has been associated with a worse prognosis in one meta-analyses of gastric cancer, but not a second.[30,31]

Potential tumor antigen targets in gastric cancer and esophageal adenocarcinoma are similar to those found in other gastrointestinal malignancies and include p53, HER2, cancer testis antigens such as MAGE-1,-2,-3, and NY-ESO-1.[179,180] Esophageal squamous cell carcinoma has also been noted to express cancer testis antigens.[180]

6.2 *Immunotherapy strategies for gastroesophageal cancer*

Vaccine studies in gastroesophageal malignancies have included peptide and dendritic cell vaccines. In a study for patients with advanced gastric cancer, DCs loaded with HER2/neu-derived peptides induced tumor-specific T cell responses and clinical responses were reported in two out of nine patients.[181] Because chemotherapy has an established role in gastroesophageal cancer, it has been reassuring that immunotherapy may be combined with chemotherapy for these malignancies. Examples include a study of vaccination with peptides derived from vascular endothelial growth factor receptor (VEGFR)-1 and -2 combined with chemotherapy consisting of S-1 and cisplatin, which was associated with a partial response rate of 55%, higher than expected from the chemotherapy alone.[182] A peptide vaccine consisting of epitopes from the cancer-testis antigens, TTK, LY6K, and IMP-3 was used to immunize patients with advanced HLA-A2402-positive esophageal squamous cell carcinoma.[183] T cell responses against the peptide epitopes was detected in nine out of ten patients. Interestingly one patient experienced a complete response in a hepatic metastasis and one had responses in lung metastases. Three other patients had brief stability of disease. A vaccine utilizing nanoparticle complexes of cholesteryl pullulan (CHP) encapsulating NY-ESO-1 protein, designed to activate HLA class I and II responses, was tested in advanced esophageal cancer patients (histology not reported) and demonstrated dose dependent immunogenicity with all 12 patients at the high dose developing new or increased antibodies against NY-ESO-1. Despite the lack of clinical responses, survival was independently correlated with vaccine dose.[184]

There have been several studies of cytokine induced killer cells for gastric cancer. Survival improvements were reported in patients who had undergone palliative gastrectomy and received autologous cytokine-induced killer cells after chemotherapy compared with patients receiving only chemotherapy.[185–187] The need for continued treatment is suggested by the loss of the survival benefit after two years. Systemic side effects such as fever, chills, and headache were as expected, occurring in 5–20% of patients. In a randomized trial, patients with gastric cancer treated with cisplatin/5-FU in combination therapy with tumor-associated lymphocytes purified from ascites, pleural fluid, and/or lymph nodes demonstrated an increased survival compared with those treated with chemotherapy alone.[188] In a study of adoptive transfer with autologous tumor cell-stimulated peripheral blood mononuclear cells and systemic IL-2, 4 out of 11 patients with esophageal squamous cell carcinoma experienced objective responses.[189] The future of this approach will likely depend on further refinements in T cell therapeutics and demonstration of safety in ongoing studies.[190]

6.3 Most recent development: PD-1 blockade in the treatment of gastric cancer

The recent publication of a molecular classification of gastric cancer by the Cancer Genome Atlas (TCGA) Research Network[191] has highlighted the potential role of immunotherapy in at least one subtype of gastric cancer, those tumors positive for Epstein–Barr virus, which were found to have elevated PD-L1/2 expression and IL-12 mediated signaling. In some cases there were recurrent amplifications at 9p24.1 at the locus containing JAK2, CD274 (encoding PD-1L1) and PDCD1LG2 (encoding PD-L2).

In the gastric cancer cohort of the phase I KEYNOTE-012 clinical trial (presented at ESMO2014 and with additional analysis at ASCO GI 2015),[192] patients with recurrent or metastatic adenocarcinoma of the stomach or GEJ and PD-L1 expressing tumors were treated with pembrolizumab (anti-PD-1) at 10mg/Kg every two weeks. PD-L1 expression was required in the stroma or in ≥1% of tumor cells as assessed in archival tumor samples by IHC using the 22C3 antibody. Using this cut-off, 40% of assessed patients had PD-L1+ tumors. Of the 39 advanced chemotherapy refractory gastric cancer patients treated with the pembrolizumab, 22.2% had an objective response as determined by a central review and 33% as determined by the treating physicians; 14% had stable disease; and 10% were not evaluable. Overall, 41% had some decrease in tumor volume. Unfortunately, there were no complete responses but a few subjects had more than 50% shrinkage of their tumor. Many responses were ongoing but follow-up was short (the longest follow-up was 48 weeks). Benefit can be seen quickly as the median time to response was eight weeks. There was evidence of a relationship between PD-L1 expression and objective response ($p = 0.071$). Regarding toxicity in this study, 67% of subjects had a side effect with the most common fatigue (18%), decreased appetite (13%), hypothyroidism (12.8%), arthralgia (10.3%), hyperthyroidism (7.7%), nausea (7.7%), pruritus (7.7%); 4 out of 39 patients had severe adverse events of various types (pneumonitis, peripheral neuropathy, hypoxia, fatigue, decreased appetite). No patients discontinued pembrolizumab due to a treatment-related adverse events. These data support continued study of PD-1/PD-L1 blockade and a number of studies are ongoing or planned including: NCT01928394: A Phase I/II, Open-label Study of Nivolumab Monotherapy or Nivolumab Combined with Ipilimumab in Subjects with Advanced or Metastatic Solid Tumors (Gastric subgroup); NCT01772004 : Phase I, Open-label, Multiple-ascending Dose Trial to Investigate the Safety, Tolerability, Pharmacokinetics, Biological and Clinical Activity of MSB0010718C in Subjects with Metastatic or Locally Advanced Solid Tumors and Expansion to Selected Indications; NCT01375842: A Phase I, Open Label, Dose Escalation Study of the Safety and Pharmacokinetics of MPDL3280A Administered Intravenously as a Single Agent to Patients with Locally Advanced or Metastatic Solid Tumors or Hematologic Malignancies; and, NCT02340975: A Phase Ib/II Study of MEDI4736 With Tremelimumab, MEDI4736 or Tremelimumab Monotherapy in Gastric or GEJ Adenocarcinoma (see Table 1).

7 Anal Cancer

7.1 *Role of immune cell infiltrate and tumor antigens*

Comparatively, less has been reported and written about the immune cell response to anal cancer. It was reported surprisingly that among patients treated with chemoradiotherapy for anal cancer, a high number of CD3+ and CD4+ TILS in tissue microarrays was associated with a worse prognosis.[193] No prognostic influence was observed for the numbers of tumor-infiltrating CD68$^+$ macrophages and of FoxP3$^+$ regulatory T cells. The authors suggested that the reason for the unexpected effect of TILS could be that CTL-mediated killing left remaining tumor cells with a greater resistance to apoptosis. They also point out that a similar paradoxical effect of TIL is seen in another virally mediated tumor, EBV-associated nasopharyngeal cancer.[194]

Regarding potential tumor antigens, because the E6 and E7 proteins are required for the oncogenicity of HPV and because they are targets for T cell responses detected in patients with high grade anal squamous intraepithelial lesions,[195] they are the most rationale targets for immunotherapy against HPV-related neoplasms.

7.2 *Immunotherapeutic strategies for anal cancer*

Currently, there are few immunotherapy studies for anal cancer. An earlier study[196] reported the use of ZYC101, a plasmid encoding HLA-A2-restricted epitopes derived from the HPV-16 E7 protein, encapsulated in biodegradable polymer microparticles to treat patients with high-grade. Ten of the 12 immunized patients developed antigen-specific immune responses and 3 individuals experienced partial histological responses. However, the follow-up vaccine, amolimogene bepiplasmid which includes epitopes from HPV-16 and HPV-18 E6 and E7 proteins and an HLA-DRalpha intracellular trafficking peptide in women with cervical dysplasia did not show improved resolution of the dysplasia.[197] However, there have been significant strides in developing therapeutic vaccines in an attempt to treat HPV infections or early cervical and vulvar intraepithelial neoplasias which may have a role in the future for anal cancer.[198] In a study of HIV+ men with AIN1-3, HPV-16 E6E7 ISCOMATRIX vaccine was well tolerated except for injection site and systemic reactions including headache, myalgia, and fatigue. The majority of the patients were observed to have increases in antibody and T cell responses to the vaccine.[199] Ongoing studies that could enroll anal cancer patients are listed in Table 1.

8 Conclusions

The immune system responds to gastrointestinal malignancies. The presence of CD8+ cytolytic T cells, CD45RO+ memory T cells, and DCs in the tumor stroma is generally associated with improved survival. However, often there is an immuno-suppressive infiltrate or molecular expression pattern. Thus far, there have been hints of activity for vaccines in patients who obtain an immune response. Too few patients have received cellular therapies to assess their potential future benefit. Checkpoint blockade has not demonstrated the early evidence of activity as was seen with non-small cell lung cancer and melanoma. However, there are studies enrolling patients in gastroesophageal, pancreatic and colon cancer to better assess their activity and results from these signal-finding studies are expected soon. We hypothesize that combinations of more potent vaccines, targeting more relevant antigens, administered with immune modulators following or in conjunction with therapies that alter the immune environment such as chemotherapy may be required to realize a major impact of immunotherapy for gastrointestinal malignancies.

9 Addendum: PD-1 Blockade in the Treatment of MSI High Malignancies Including Colon Cancer

It has long been recognized that CRCs with MMR defects (MSI-high) have high levels of somatic mutations[200] which can encode potential antigens for immune effectors and are heavily T cell infiltrated.[201] However, this subset of colorectal cancers also displays significantly upregulated expression of the immunomodu-latory molecules PD-1, PD-L1, CTLA-4, LAG-3, and IDO[202] that may limit T cell-mediated tumor destruction. It has therefore been hypothesized that the use of checkpoint blockade might increase immune responses against these tumors. Le and colleagues[202] reported a phase II study administering the anti-PD-1 antibody pembrolizumab (10mg/kg every 14 days) to 41 patients with previously-treated, progressive metastatic disease of three subgroups: MMR-deficient CRCs (*n* = 11), MMR-proficient CRCs (*n* = 21), and MMR-deficient cancers of types other than colorectal (*n* = 9). The authors reported: "The immune-related objective response rate (irORR) and immune-related progression-free survival (irPFS) at 20 weeks for MMR-deficient CRC were 40% and 78%, respectively, and for MMR-deficient other cancers were 71% and 67%, respectively. In MMR-proficient CRC, irORR and irPFS at 20 weeks were 0% and 11%, respectively. The response rates and disease control rates (CR+PR+SD) by RECIST criteria were 40% and 90% in MMR-deficient CRC, 0% and 11% in MMR-proficient CRC, and 71% and 71% in MMR-deficient other cancers, respectively. Median PFS and OS were not reached in the MMR-deficient CRC group but was 2.2 and 5.0 months in the MMR-proficient CRC cohort." These data suggest that MMR deficient colorectal and other cancers respond to anti-PD-1 therapy.

References

1. Couzin-Frankel J. Breakthrough of the year 2013. Cancer immunotherapy. *Science* 2013;**342**(6165):1432–1433.
2. Blankenstein T, *et al.* The determinants of tumour immunogenicity. *Nat Rev Cancer* 2012 Mar 1;**12**(4):307–313.
3. Ascierto ML, *et al.* An immunologic portrait of cancer. *J Transl Med* 2011;**9**:146.
4. Pradeu T, Carosella ED. On the definition of a criterion of immunogenicity. *Proc Natl Acad Sci USA* 2006;**103**:17858–17861.
5. Overwijk WW, *et al.* Mining the mutanome: developing highly personalized Immunotherapies based on mutational analysis of tumors. *J. Immunother* 2013;**1**:11.
6. Ikushima H, *et al.* The IRF Family Transcription Factors at the Interface of Innate and Adaptive Immune Responses. *Cold Spring Harb Symp Quant Biol* 2013;**78**:105–116.
7. Bakdash G, *et al.* Crosstalk between dendritic cell subsets and implications for dendritic cell-based anticancer immunotherapy. *Expert Rev Clin Immunol* 2014;**10**:915–26.
8. Bretscher PA. A two-step, two-signal model for the primary activation of precursor helper T cells. *Proc Natl Acad Sci* 1999;**96**:185–190.
9. Maj T, *et al.* T cells and costimulation in cancer. *Cancer J.* 2013 Nov–Dec;**19**(6):473–82.
10. Bromley SK, *et al.* Orchestrating the orchestrators: chemokines in control of T cell traffic. *Nat Immunol* 2008;**9**(9):970–80.
11. Hindley JP, *et al.* T-cell trafficking facilitated by high endothelial venules is required for tumor control after regulatory T-cell depletion. *Cancer Res* 2012 Nov 1;**72**(21):5473–82.

12. Sigal LH. Basic science for the clinician 55: CTLA-4. *J Clin Rheumatol* 2012 Apr;**18**(3):155–8.
13. Pardoll DM. The blockade of immune checkpoints in cancer immunotherapy. *Nature Reviews Cancer* 2012;**12**:252–264.
14. Piccirillo CA, Thornton AM. Cornerstone of peripheral tolerance: naturally occurring CD4+CD25+regulatory Tcells. *Trends Immunol* 2004;**25**:374–80.
15. Raber PL, *et al.* Subpopulations of myeloid-derived suppressor cells impair T cell responses through independent nitric oxide-related pathways. *Int J Cancer* 2014 Jun 15;**134**(12):2853–64.
16. Bailey SR, *et al.* Th17 cells in cancer: the ultimate identity crisis. *Front Immunol* 2014 Jun 17;**5**:276.
17. Franklin RA, *et al.* The cellular and molecular origin of tumor-associated macrophages. *Science* 2014 May 23;**344**(6186):921–5.
18. Terabe M, Berzofsky JA. The immunoregulatory role of type I and type II NKT cells in cancer and other diseases. *Cancer Immunol Immunother* 2014;**63**(3):199–213.
19. Prendergast GC, *et al.* Indoleamine 2,3-dioxygenase pathways of pathogenic inflammation and immune escape in cancer. *Cancer Immunol Immunother* 2014 Jul;**63**(7):721–35.
20. Wolchok JD, *et al.* Guidelines for the evaluation of immune therapy activity in solid tumors: immune-related response criteria. *Clin Cancer Res* 2009 Dec 1;**15**(23):7412–20.
21. Shetty V, *et al.* MHC class I-presented lung cancer-associated tumor antigens identified by immunoproteomics analysis are targets for cancer-specific T cell response. *J Proteomics* 2011 May 1;**74**(5):728–43.
22. Pernot S, *et al.* Colorectal cancer and immunity: what we know and perspectives. *World J Gastroenterol* 2014 Apr 14;**20**(14):3738–50.
23. de Miranda NF, *et al.* Infiltration of Lynch colorectal cancers by activated immune cells associates with early staging of the primary tumor and absence of lymph node metastases. *Clin Cancer Res* 2012 Mar 1;**18**(5):1237–45.
24. Pagès F, *et al.* In situ cytotoxic and memory T cells predict outcome in patients with early-stage colorectal cancer. *J Clin Oncol* 2009 Dec 10;**27**(35):5944–51.
25. Nosho K, *et al.* Tumour-infiltrating T-cell subsets, molecular changes in colorectal cancer, and prognosis: cohort study and literature review. *J Pathol* 2010 Dec;**222**(4):350–66.
26. Galon J, *et al.* Towards the introduction of the 'Immunoscore' in the classification of malignant tumours. *J Pathol* 2014 Jan;**232**(2):199–209.
27. Salama P, *et al.* Low expression of Granzyme B in colorectal cancer is associated with signs of early metastastic invasion. *Histopathology* 2011 Aug;**59**(2):207–15.
28. Coca S, *et al.* The prognostic significance of intratumoral natural killer cells in patients with colorectal carcinoma. *Cancer* 1997;**79**(12):2320–2328.
29. Tachibana T, *et al.* Increased intratumor Valpha24-positive natural killer T cells: a prognostic factor for primary colorectal carcinomas. *Clin Cancer Res* 2005;**11**:7322–7327.

30. deLeeuw RJ, *et al.* The prognostic value of FoxP3+ tumor-infiltrating lymphocytes in cancer: a critical review of the literature. *Clin Cancer Res* 2012 Jun 1;**18**(11):3022–9.

31. Huang Y, *et al.* Prognostic value of tumor-infiltrating FoxP3+ T cells in gastrointestinal cancers: a meta analysis. *PLoS One* 2014 May 14;**9**(5):e94376.

32. Ladoire S, *et al.* Prognostic role of FOXP3+ regulatory T cells infiltrating human carcinomas: the paradox of colorectal cancer. *Cancer Immunol Immunother* 2011;**60**:909–18.

33. Nagorsen D, *et al.* Tumor-infiltrating macrophages and dendritic cells in human colorectal cancer: relation to local regulatory T cells, systemic T-cell response against tumor-associated antigens and survival. *J Transl Med* 2007;**5**(62):52.

34. Sandel MH, *et al.* Prognostic value of tumor-infiltrating dendritic cells in colorectal cancer: role of maturation status and intratumoral localization. *Clinical Cancer Res* 2005;**11**(7):2576–2582.

35. Kuniyasu H, *et al.* Depletion of tumor-infiltrating macrophages is associated with amphoterin expression in colon cancer. *Pathobiology* 2004;**71**(3):129–136.

36. Kimura T, *et al.* MUC1 vaccine for individuals with advanced adenoma of the colon: a cancer immunoprevention feasibility study. *Cancer Prev Res* (Phila). 2013;**6**(1): 18–26.

37. Tosolini M, *et al.* Clinical Impact of Different Classes of Infiltrating T Cytotoxic and Helper Cells (Th1, Th2, Treg, Th17) in Patients with Colorectal Cancer. *Cancer Res* 2011;**71**(4):1263–1271.

38. Galizia G, *et al.* Prognostic significance of circulating IL-10 and IL-6 serum levels in colon cancer patients undergoing surgery. *Clin Immunol* 2002;169–178.

39. Liu J, *et al.* IL-17 is associated with poor prognosis and promotes angiogenesis via stimulating VEGF production of cancer cells in colorectal carcinoma. *Biochem Biophys Res Commun* 2011 Apr 8;**407**(2):348–54.

40. Narai S, *et al.* Significance of transforming growth factor $\beta 1$ as a new tumor marker for colorectal cancer. *Int J Cancer* 2002;**97**(4):508–511.

41. Brandacher G, Perathoner A, Ladurner R, *et al.* Prognostic value of indoleamine 2, 3-dioxygenase expression in colorectal cancer: effect on tumor-infiltrating T cells. *Clin Cancer Res* 2006;**12**(4):1144–1151.

42. Cavia-Saiz M, *et al.* The role of plasma IDO activity as a diagnostic marker of patients with colorectal cancer. *Mol Biol Rep* 2014 Apr;**41**(4):2275–9.

43. Grimm MG, *et al.* Clinical significance and therapeutic potential of programmed death-1 ligand-1 and programmed death-1 ligand-2 expression in human colorectal cancer *J Clin Oncol* 2008;**26**:suppl 15005 (ASCO Meeting Abstracts).

44. Taube JM, *et al.* Association of PD-1, PD-1 Ligands, and Other Features of the Tumor Immune Microenvironment with Response to Anti-PD-1 Therapy. *Clin Cancer Res.* 2014 Apr 8. [Epub ahead of print]

45. Droeser RA, *et al.* Clinical impact of programmed cell death ligand 1 expression in colorectal cancer. *Eur J Cancer* 2013 Jun;**49**(9):2233–42.

46. Sarobe P, *et al.* Carcinoembryonic antigen as a target to induce anti-tumor immune responses. *Curr Cancer Drug Targets* 2004 Aug;**4**(5):443–54.

47. Bauer K, *et al.* T cell responses against microsatellite instability-induced frameshift peptides and influence of regulatory T cells in colorectal cancer. *Cancer Immunol Immunother* 2013;**62**(1):27–37.

48. De Weger VA, *et al.* Clinical Effects of Adjuvant Active Specific Immunotherapy Differ between Patients with Microsatellite-Stable and Microsatellite-Instable Colon Cancer. *Clinical Cancer Research* 2012;**18**(3):882–889.

49. Sandel MH, *et al.* Natural killer cells infiltrating colorectal cancer and MHC class I expression. *Mol Immunol* 2005;**42**:541–546.

50. Valdivieso M, *et al.* Chemoimmunotherapy of metastatic large bowel cancer: nonspecific stimulation with BCG and levamisole. *Cancer* 1977 Nov;**40**(5 Suppl):2731–9.

51. Windle R, *et al.* The effect of levamisole on postoperative immunosuppression. *Br J Surg* 1979 Jul;**66**(7):507–9.

52. Correale P, *et al.* Chemo-immunotherapy of metastatic colorectal carcinoma with gemcitabine plus FOLFOX 4 followed by subcutaneous granulocyte macrophage colony-stimulating factor and interleukin-2 induces strong immunologic and antitumor activity in metastatic colon cancer patients. *J Clin Oncol* 2005;**23**:8950–8958.

53. Barni S, *et al.* A randomized study of low-dose subcutaneous interleukin-2 plus melatonin versus supportive care alone in met astatic colorectal cancer patients progressing under 5-fluorouracil and folates. *Oncology* 1995;**52**:243–245.

54. Wiesenfeld M, *et al.* Controlled clinical trial of interferon-gamma as postoperative surgical adjuvant therapy for colon cancer. *J Clin Oncol* 1995;**13**(9):2324–2329.

55. Wolmark N, Smith R, Fisher B, *et al.* Adjuvant 5-fluorouracil and leucovorin with or without interferon alfa-2a in colon carcinoma: National Surgical Adjuvant Breast and Bowel Project protocol C-05. *J Nat Cancer Inst* 1998;**90**(23):1810–1816.

56. Panettiere FJ, *et al.* Adjuvant therapy in large bowel adenocarcinoma: long-term results of a Southwest Oncology Group Study. *J Clin Oncol* 1988;**6**(6):947–954.

57. Smith RE, *et al.* Randomized trial of adjuvant therapy in colon carcinoma: 10-year results of NSABP protocol C-01. *J Nat Cancer Inst* 2004;**96**(15):1128–1132.

58. Nagorsen D, Thiel E. Clinical and Immunologic Responses to Active Specific Cancer Vaccines in Human Colorectal Cancer. *Clin Cancer Res* 2006;**12**(10):3064–3069.

59. Marshall JL, *et al.* Phase I study of sequential vaccinations with fowlpox-CEA(6D)-TRICOM alone and sequentially with vaccinia-CEA(6D)-TRICOM, with and without granulocyte-macrophage colony-stimulating factor, in patients with carcinoembryonic antigen-expressing carcinomas. *J Clin Oncol* 2005;**23**(4):720–31.

60. Harris JE, *et al.* Adjuvant active specific immunotherapy for stage II and III colon cancer with an autologous tumor cell vaccine: Eastern Cooperative Oncology Group Study E5283. *J Clin Oncol* 2000;**18**:148–148.

61. Vermorken JB, *et al.* Active specific immunotherapy for stage II and stage III human colon cancer: a randomised trial. *The Lancet* 1999;**353**(9150):345–350.

62. Zheng L, *et al.* A Safety and Feasibility Study of an Allogeneic Colon Cancer Cell Vaccine Administered with a Granulocyte-Macrophage Colony Stimulating Factor-Producing Bystander Cell Line in Patients with Metastatic Colorectal Cancer. *Ann Surg Oncol* 2014 Jun 19. [Epub ahead of print].

63. Senzer N, *et al*. Phase I trial of "bi-shRNAi(furin)/GMCSF DNA/autologous tumor cell" vaccine (FANG) in advanced cancer. *Mol Ther* 2012 Mar;**20**(3):679–86.

64. Kameshima H, *et al*. Immunogenic enhancement and clinical effect by type-I interferon of anti-apoptotic protein, survivin-derived peptide vaccine, in advanced colorectal cancer patients. *Cancer Sci* 2011 Jun;**102**(6):1181–7.

65. Diaz CM, *et al*. Phase 1 studies of the safety and immunogenicity of electroporated HER2/CEA DNA vaccine followed by adenoviral boost immunization in patients with solid tumors. *J Transl Med* 2013 Mar 8;**11**:62.

66. Schulze T, *et al*. Efficiency of adjuvant active specific immunization with Newcastle disease virus modified tumor cells in colorectal cancer patients following resection of liver metastases: results of a prospective randomized trial. *Cancer Immunol Immunother* 2009 Jan;**58**(1):61–9.

67. Morse MA, *et al*. A Randomized Phase II Study of Immunization With Dendritic Cells Modified With Poxvectors Encoding CEA and MUC1 Compared With the Same Poxvectors Plus GM-CSF for Resected Metastatic Colorectal Cancer. *Annals of Surgery* 2013;**258**(6):879–886.

68. Rao B, *et al*. Clinical outcomes of active specific immunotherapy in advanced colorectal cancer and suspected minimal residual colorectal cancer: a meta-analysis and system review. *J Transl Med* 2011;9:17.

69. Marshall JL, *et al*. Phase I study in advanced cancer patients of a diversified prime and boost vaccination protocol using recombinant vaccinia virus and recombinant nonreplicating avipox virus to elicit anti-carcinoembryonic antigen immune responses. *J Clin Oncol* 2000;**18**:3964–3973.

70. Moulton HM, *et al*. Active Specific Immunotherapy with a β-Human Chorionic Gonadotropin Peptide Vaccine in Patients with Metastatic Colorectal Cancer: Antibody Response Is Associated with Improved Survival. *Clin Cancer Res* 2002;**8**(7):2044–2051.

71. Kaufman HL, *et al*. Combination Chemotherapy and ALVAC-CEA/B7.1 Vaccine in Patients with Metastatic Colorectal Cancer. *Clin Cancer Res* 2008;**14**(15):4843–4849.

72. Rocha-Lima CM, *et al*. A multicenter phase II study of G17DT immunogen plus irinotecan in pretreated metastatic colorectal cancer progressing on irinotecan. *Cancer Chemother Pharmacol* 2014 Jul 17.

73. Harrop R, *et al*. Cross-trial analysis of immunologic and clinical data resulting from phase I and II trials of MVA-5T4 (TroVax) in colorectal, renal, and prostate cancer patients. *J Immunol* 2010;**33**(9):999–1005.

74. Morse MA, *et al*. An alphavirus vector overcomes the presence of neutralizing antibodies and elevated numbers of Tregs to induce immune responses in humans with advanced cancer. *J Clin Invest* 2010;**120**(9):3234–3241.

75. Morse MA, *et al*. Novel adenoviral vector induces T-cell responses despite anti-adenoviral neutralizing antibodies in colorectal cancer patients. *Cancer Immunol Immunother*. 2013 Aug;**62**(8):1293–301.

76. Chong G, *et al*. Phase III trial of 5-fluorouracil and leucovorin plus either 3H1 anti-idiotype monoclonal antibody or placebo in patients with advanced colorectal cancer. *Annals of Oncology* 2006;**17**(3):437–442.

77. Posner M, *et al.* A Phase II Prospective Multi-institutional Trial of Adjuvant Active Specific Immunotherapy Following Curative Resection of Colorectal Cancer Hepatic Metastases: Cancer and Leukemia Group B Study 89903. *Ann Surg Oncol* 2008;**15**(1):158–164.

78. Ullenhag GJ, *et al.* A neoadjuvant/adjuvant randomized trial of colorectal cancer patients vaccinated with an anti-idiotypic antibody, 105AD7, mimicking CD55. *Clin Cancer Res* 2006;**12**(24):7389–7396.

79. Samonigg H, *et al.* A double-blind randomized-phase II trial comparing immunization with antiidiotype goat antibody vaccine SCV 106 versus unspecific goat antibodies in patients with metastatic colorectal cancer. *J Immunol* 1999;**22**:482–488.

80. Amedei A, *et al.* T cells and adoptive immunotherapy. Recent developments and future prospects in gastrointestinal oncology. *Clin Dev Immunol* 2011;**2011**:320571.

81. Karlsson M, *et al.* Pilot study of sentinel-node-based adoptive immunotherapy in advanced colorectal cancer. *Ann Surg Oncol* 2010 Jul;**17**(7):1747–57.

82. Parkhurst MR, *et al.* T cells targeting carcinoembryonic antigen can mediate regression of metastatic colorectal cancer but induce severe transient colitis. *Mol Ther* 2011 Mar;**19**(3):620–6.

83. Morgan RA, *et al.* Case report of a serious adverse event following the administration of T cells transduced with a chimeric antigen receptor recognizing ERBB2. *Mol Ther* 2010;**18**:843–851.

84. Osada T, *et al.* Metastatic colorectal cancer cells from patients previously treated with chemotherapy are sensitive to T-cell killing mediated by CEA/CD3-bispecific T-cell-engaging BiTE antibody. *Br J Cancer* 2010 Jan 5;**102**(1):124–33.

85. Punt CJ, *et al.* Edrecolomab alone or in combination with fluorouracil and folinic acid in the adjuvant treatment of stage III colon cancer: a randomised study. *Lancet* 2002 Aug 31;**360**(9334):671–7.

86. Chung KY, *et al.* Phase II study of the anti-cytotoxic T-lymphocyte-associated antigen 4 monoclonal antibody, tremelimumab, in patients with refractory metastatic colorectal cancer. *J Clin Oncol* 2010 Jul 20;**28**(21):3485–90.

87. Brahmer JR, *et al.* Phase I study of single-agent anti–programmed death-1 (MDX-1106) in refractory solid tumors: safety, clinical activity, pharmacodynamics, and immunologic correlates. *J Clin Oncol* 2010;**28**:3167–3175.

88. Topalian SL, *et al.* Safety, activity, and immune correlates of anti-PD-1 antibody in cancer. *New Engl J Med* 2012;**366**:2443–2454.

89. Brahmer JR, *et al.* Safety and Activity of Anti–PD-L1 Antibody in Patients with Advanced Cancer. *New England Journal of Medicine* 2012;**366**:2455–2465.

90. Xu Z, *et al.* Pancreatic cancer and its stroma: A conspiracy theory. *World J Gastroenterol* 2014 Aug 28;**20**(32):11216–11229.

91. Ino Y, *et al.* Immune cell infiltration as an indicator of the immune microenvironment of pancreatic cancer. *Br J Cancer* 2013 Mar 5;**108**(4):914–23.

92. Hiraoka N, *et al.* Prevalence of FOXP3+ regulatory T cells increases during the progression of pancreatic ductal adenocarcinoma and its premalignant lesions. *Clin Cancer Res* 2006;**12**:5423–34.

93. Terashima T, *et al.* P53, hTERT, WT-1, and VEGFR2 are the most suitable targets for cancer vaccine therapy in HLA-A24 positive pancreatic adenocarcinoma. *Cancer Immunol Immunother* 2014 May;**63**(5):479–89.

94. Argani P, *et al.* Mesothelin is overexpressed in the vast majority of ductal adenocarcinomas of the pancreas: identification of a new pancreatic cancer marker by serial analysis of gene expression (SAGE). *Clin Cancer Res* 2001;7:3862–8.

95. Johnston FM, *et al.* Circulating mesothelin protein and cellular antimesothelin immunity in patients with pancreatic cancer. *Clin Cancer Res* 2009;**15**(21):6511–6518.

96. Salman B, *et al.* Vaccine therapy for pancreatic cancer. *Oncoimmunology* 2013 Dec 1;**2**(12):e26662.

97. Laheru D, *et al.* Allogeneic granulocyte macrophage colony stimulating factor-secreting tumor immunotherapy alone or in sequence with cyclophosphamide for metastatic pancreatic cancer: a pilot study of safety, feasibility, and immune activation. *Clin Cancer Res* 2008;**14**:1455–63.

98. Lutz E, *et al.* A lethally irradiated allogeneic granulocyte- macrophage colony stimulating factor-secreting tumor vaccine for pancreatic adenocarcinoma. A Phase II trial of safety, efficacy, and immune activation. *Ann Surg* 2011;**253**:328–35.

99. Lutz ER, *et al.* Immunotherapy converts nonimmunogenic pancreatic tumors into immunogenic foci of immune regulation. *Cancer Immunol Res* 2014 Jul;**2**(7):616–31.

100. Le D, *et al.* A phase 2, randomized trial of GVAX pancreas and CRS-207 immunotherapy versus GVAX alone in patients with metastatic pancreatic adenocarcinoma: Updated results. *J Clin Oncol* 2014;**32**(Suppl 3; abstr 177).

101. Hardacre JM, *et al.* Addition of algenpantucel- L immunotherapy to standard adjuvant therapy for pancreatic cancer: a phase 2 study. *J Gastrointest Surg* 2013;17:94–100.

102. Geynisman DM, *et al.* A randomized pilot phase I study of modified carcinoembryonic antigen (CEA) peptide (CAP1-6D)/montanide/GM-CSF-vaccine in patients with pancreatic adenocarcinoma. *J Immunother Cancer* 2013 Jun 27;**1**:8.

103. Abou-Alfa GK, *et al.* Targeting mutated K-ras in pancreatic adenocarcinoma using an adjuvant vaccine. *Am J Clin Oncol* 2011; **34**:321–5.

104. Kameshima H, *et al.* Immunotherapeutic benefit of α-interferon (IFNα) in survivin-2Bderived peptide vaccination for advanced pancreatic cancer patients. *Cancer Sci* 2013;**104**:124–9.

105. Inderberg-Suso EM, *et al.* Widespread CD4+ T-cell reactivity to novel hTERT epitopes following vaccination of cancer patients with a single hTERT peptide GV1001. *Oncoimmunology* 2012;**1**:670–686.

106. Buanes T, *et al.* A randomized phase III study of gemcitabine (G) versus GV1001 in sequential combination with G in patients with unresectable and metastatic pancreatic cancer (PC). *J CLin Oncol* 2009;**27**:15S (May 20 Supplement): 4601.

107. Middleton G, *et al.* Gemcitabine and capecitabine with or without telomerase peptide vaccine GV1001 in patients with locally advanced or metastatic pancreatic cancer (TeloVac): an open-label, randomized, phase 3 trial. *Lancet Oncol* 2014 Jul;**15**(8):829–40.

108. Neoptolemos JP, *et al.* Predictive cytokine biomarkers for survival in patients with advanced pancreatic cancer randomized to sequential chemoimmunotherapy

comprising gemcitabine and capecitabine (GemCap) followed by the telomerase vaccine GV1001 compared to concurrent chemoimmunotherapy in the TeloVac phase III trial. *J Clin Oncol* 2014;**32**:5s, (Suppl; abstr 4121).

109. Gilliam AD, *et al*. An international multicenterrandomized controlled trial of G17DT in patients with pancreatic cancer. *Pancreas* 2012;**41**:374–9.

110. Richards D, *et al*. A Phase 2 adjuvant trial of GI-4000 plus gemcitabine vs gemcitabine alone in RAS+ patients with resected pancreas cancer: R1 subgroup analysis. *Ann Oncol* (2012) 23 (Suppl 4): iv5-iv18, O-0002.

111. Gansauge F, *et al*. Effectivity of long antigen exposition dendritic cell therapy (LANEXDC®) in the palliative treatment of pancreatic cancer. *Curr Med Chem* 2013;**20**(38):4827–35.

112. Kimura Y, *et al*. Clinical and immunologic evaluation of dendritic cell-based immunotherapy in combination with gemcitabine and/or S-1 in patients with advanced pancreatic carcinoma. *Pancreas* 2012;**41**:195–205.

113. Soulen MC, *et al*. Mesothelin-specific chimeric antigen receptor mRNA-engineered T cells induce anti-tumor activity in solid malignancies. *Cancer Immunol Res* 2014;**2**:112–20.

114. Maus MV, *et al*. T cells expressing chimeric antigen receptors can cause anaphylaxis in humans. *Cancer Immunol Res* 2013;**1**:26–31.

115. Abate-Daga D, *et al*. Pancreatic cancer: Hurdles in the engineering of CAR-based immunotherapies. *Oncoimmunology* 2014 Jun 18;**3**:e29194.

116. Beatty GL, *et al*. CD40 agonists alter tumor stroma and show efficacy against pancreatic carcinoma in mice and humans. *Science* 2011 Mar 25;**331**(6024):1612–6.

117. Beatty GL, *et al*. CD40 agonistsalter tumor stroma and show efficacy against pancreatic carcinoma in mice and humans. *Science* 2011 Mar 25;**331**(6024):1612–6.

118. Luheshi N, *et al*. Th1 cytokines are more effective than Th2 cytokines at licensing anti-tumour functions in CD40-activated human macrophages in vitro. *Eur J Immunol* 2013; 2014 Jan;**44**(1):162–72.

119. Royal RE, *et al*. Phase 2 trial of single agent Ipilimumab (anti-CTLA-4) for locally advanced or metastatic pancreatic adenocarcinoma. *J Immunother* 2010 Oct;**33**(8): 828–33.

120. Le DT, *et al*. Evaluation of ipilimumab in combination with allogeneic pancreatic tumor cells transfected with a GM-CSF gene in previously treated pancreatic cancer. *J Immunother* 2013;**36**:382–9.

121. Mossanen JC, Tacke F. Role of lymphocytes in liver cancer. *Oncoimmunology* 2013 Nov 1;**2**(11):e26468. Epub 2013 Oct 21.

122. Chew V, *et al*. Inflammatory tumour microenvironmentis associated with superior survival in hepatocellular carcinoma patients. *J Hepatol* 2010 Mar;**52**(3):370–9.

123. Shirabe K, *et al*. Tumor-infiltrating lymphocytes and hepatocellular carcinoma: pathology and clinical management. *Int J Clin Oncol* 2010 Dec;**15**(6):552–8.

124. Schneider C, *et al*. Adaptive immunity suppresses formation and progression of diethylnitrosamine-induced liver cancer. *Gut* 2012 Dec;**61**(12):1733–43.

125. Zhao F, *et al*. Cellular immune suppressor mechanisms in patients with hepatocellular carcinoma. *Dig Dis* 2012;**30**(5):477–82.

126. Kakumu S, *et al*. Decreased function of peripheral blood dendritic cells in patients with hepatocellular carcinoma with hepatitis B and C virus infection. *Journal of Gastroenterology and Hepatology* 2000;**15**(4):431–436.

127. Kelly A, *et al*. CD141$^+$ myeloid dendritic cells are enriched in healthy human liver. *J Hepatol* 2014 Jan;**60**(1):135–42.

128. Ormandy LA, *et al*. Increased populations of regulatory T cells in peripheral blood of patients with hepatocellular carcinoma. *Cancer Res* 2005 Mar;**65**:2457–2464.

129. Unitt E, *et al*. Compromised lymphocytes infiltrate hepatocellular carcinoma: the role of T-regulatory cells. *Hepatology* 2005 Apr;**41**:722–730.

130. Yang XH, *et al*. Increase of CD4+ CD25+ regulatory T-cells in the liver of patients with hepatocellular carcinoma. *J Hepatol* 2006 Aug;**45**:254–262.

131. Fu J, *et al*. Increased regulatory T cells correlate with CD8 T-cell impairment and poor survival in hepatocellular carcinoma patients. *Gastroenterology* 2007 Jun;**132**:2328–2339.

132. Gao Q, *et al*. Intratumoral balance of regulatory and cytotoxic T cells is associated with prognosis of hepatocellular carcinoma after resection. *J Clin Oncol* 2007 Jun;25:2586–2593.

133. deLeeuw RJ, *et al*. The prognostic value of FoxP3+ tumor-infiltrating lymphocytes in cancer: a critical review of the literature. *Clin Cancer Res* 2012 Jun 1;**18**(11):3022–9.

134. Cai L, *et al*. Functional impairment in circulating and intrahepatic NK cells and relative mechanism in hepatocellular carcinoma patients. *Clin Immunol* 2008 Dec;**129**(3):428–37.

135. Greten TF, *et al*. Low-dose cyclophosphamide treatment impairs regulatory T cells and unmasks AFP-specific CD4+ T-cell responses in patients with advanced HCC. *J Immunother* 2010 Jan;**33**:211–218.

136. Flecken T, *et al*. Immunodominance and functional alterations of tumor-associated antigen-specific CD8+ T-cell responses in hepatocellular carcinoma. *Hepatology* 2014 Apr;**59**(4):1415–26.

137. Hoechst B, *et al*. A new population of myeloid-derived suppressor cells in hepatocellular carcinoma patients induces CD4(+)CD25(+)Foxp3(+) T cells. *Gastroenterology* 2008 Jul;**135**:234–243.

138. Hoechst B, *et al*. Myeloid derived suppressor cells inhibit natural killer cells in patients with hepatocellular carcinoma via the NKp30 receptor. *Hepatology* 2009 Sep;**50**: 799–807.

139. Liao R, *et al*. High expression of IL-17 and IL-17RE associate with poor prognosis of hepatocellular carcinoma. *J Exp Clin Cancer Res* 2013 Jan 11;**32**:3.

140. Wu J, *et al*. Elevated pretherapy serum IL17 in primary hepatocellular carcinoma patients correlate to increased risk of early recurrence after curative hepatectomy. *PLoS One* 2012;**7**(12):e50035.

141. Kuang D-M, *et al*. Peritumoral neutrophils link inflammatory response to disease progression by fostering angiogenesis in hepatocellular carcinoma. *J Hepatol* 2011 May 1;**54**:948–955.

142. Kuang DM, *et al*. Activated monocytes in peritumoral stroma of hepatocellular carcinoma foster immune privilege and disease progression through PD-L1. *Journal of Experimental Medicine* 2009 Jun;**206**:1327–1337.

143. Gehring AJ, *et al*. Profile of tumor antigen-specific CD8 T cells in patients with hepatitis B virus-related hepatocellular carcinoma. *Gastroenterology* 2009;**137**:682–690.

144. Sprinzl MF, *et al*. Sorafenib perpetuates cellular anticancer effector functions by modulating the crosstalk between macrophages and natural killer cells. *Hepatology* 2013;**57**(6):2358–68.

145. Cabrera R, *et al*. Immune modulation of effector CD4+ and regulatory T cell function by sorafenib in patients with hepatocellular carcinoma. *Cancer Immunol Immunother* 2013;**62**(4):737–46.

146. Chen ML, *et al*. Sorafenib relieves cell-intrinsic and cell-extrinsic inhibitions of effector T cells in tumor microenvironment to augment antitumor immunity. *Int J Cancer* 2014;**134**(2):319–31.

147. Wang Q, *et al*. Sorafenib reduces hepatic infiltrated regulatory T cells in hepatocellular carcinoma patients by suppressing TGF-beta signal. *J Surg Oncol* 2013 Mar;**107**(4): 422–7.

148. Korangy F, *et al*. Spontaneous tumor-specific humoral and cellular immune responses to NY-ESO-1 in hepatocellular carcinoma. *Clin Cancer Res* 2004 Jul.10:4332–4341.

149. Zhang H-G, *et al*. Specific CD8+ T cell responses to HLA-A2 restricted MAGE-A3 p271–279 peptide in hepatocellular carcinoma patients without vaccination. *Cancer Immunol Immunother* 2007 May 24;**56**:1945–1954.

150. Behboudi S. Alpha-fetoprotein specific CD4 and CD8 T cell responses in patients with hepatocellular carcinoma. *WJH* 2010;**2**:256.

151. Nobuoka D, *et al*. Peptide vaccines for hepatocellular carcinoma. *Hum Vaccin Immunother* 2013 Jan;**9**(1):210–2.

152. Greten TF, *et al*. A phase II open label trial evaluating safety and efficacy of a telomerase peptide vaccination in patients with advanced hepatocellular carcinoma. *BMC Cancer* 2010 May 17;**10**:209.

153. Butterfield LH, *et al*. Spontaneous and vaccine induced AFP-specific T cell phenotypes in subjects with AFP-positive hepatocellular cancer. *Cancer Immunol Immunother* 2007 Dec;**56**(12):1931–43.

154. El Ansary M, *et al*. Immunotherapy by autologous dendritic cell vaccine in patients with advanced HCC. *J Cancer Res Clin Oncol* 2013 Jan;**139**(1):39–48.

155. Palmer DH, *et al*. A phase II study of adoptive immunotherapy using dendritic cells pulsed with tumor lysate in patients with hepatocellular carcinoma. *Hepatology* 2009 Jan;**49**(1):124–32.

156. Mizukoshi E, *et al*. Enhancement of tumor-specific T-cell responses by transcatheter arterial embolization with dendritic cell infusion for hepatocellular carcinoma. *Int J Cancer* 2010 May 1;**126**(9):2164–74.

157. Butterfield LH, *et al*. Alpha fetoprotein DNA prime and adenovirus boost immunization of two hepatocellular cancer patients. *J Transl Med* 2014 Apr 5;**12**:86.

158. Jäkel CE, *et al*. Clinical studies applying cytokine-induced killer cells for the treatment of gastrointestinal tumors. *J Immunol Res* 2014;**2014**:897214.

159. Shi M, *et al*. Autologous cytokine-induced killer cell therapy in clinical trial phase I is safe in patients with primary hepatocellular carcinoma. *World J Gastroenterol* 2004 Apr 15;**10**(8):1146–51.

160. Sangro B, *et al.* A clinical trial of CTLA-4 blockade with tremelimumab in patients with hepatocellular carcinoma and chronic hepatitis C. *J Hepatol* 2013; **59**:81–8.

161. Goeppert B, *et al.* Prognostic impact of tumour-infiltrating immune cells on biliary tract cancer. *Br J Cancer* 2013 Nov 12;**109**(10):2665–74.

162. Kasper HU, *et al.* Liver tumor infiltrating lymphocytes: comparison of hepatocellular and cholangiolar carcinoma. *World J Gastroenterol* 2009 Oct 28;**15**(40):5053–7.

163. Hasita H, *et al.* Significance of alternatively activated macrophages in patients with intrahepatic cholangiocarcinoma. *Cancer Sci* 2010 Aug;**101**(8):1913–9.

164. Takagi S, *et al.* Dendritic cells, T-cell infiltration, and Grp94 expression in cholangio-cellular carcinoma. *Hum Pathol* 2004 Jul;**35**(7):881–6.

165. Shimonishi T, *et al.* Up-regulation of fas ligand at early stages and down-regulation of Fas at progressed stages of intrahepatic cholangiocarcinoma reflect evasion from immune surveillance. *Hepatology* 2000 Oct;**32**(4 Pt 1):761–9.

166. Ye Y, *et al.* Interaction of B7-H1 on intrahepatic cholangiocarcinoma cells with PD-1 on tumor-infiltrating T cells as a mechanism of immune evasion. *J Surg Oncol* 2009 Nov 1;**100**(6):500–4.

167. Zhou JX, *et al.* Expression and prognostic significance of cancer-testis antigens (CTA) in intrahepatic cholagiocarcinoma. *J Exp Clin Cancer Res* 2011 Jan 6;**30**:2.

168. Mall AS, *et al.* The expression of MUC mucin in cholangiocarcinoma. *Pathol Res Pract* 2010 Dec 15;**206**(12):805–9.

169. Ross JS, *et al.* New routes to targeted therapy of intrahepatic cholangiocarcinomas revealed by next-generation sequencing. *Oncologist* 2014 Mar;**19**(3):235–42.

170. Tran E, Turcotte S, Gros A, Robbins PF, Lu YC, Dudley ME, Wunderlich JR, Somerville RP, Hogan K, Hinrichs CS, Parkhurst MR, Yang JC, Rosenberg SA. Cancer immunotherapy based on mutation-specific CD4+ T cells in a patient with epithelial cancer. *Science* 2014 May 9;**344**(6184):641–5.

171. Aruga A, *et al.* Long-term Vaccination with Multiple Peptides Derived from Cancer-Testis Antigens Can Maintain a Specific T-cell Response and Achieve Disease Stability in Advanced Biliary Tract Cancer. *Clin Cancer Res* 2013 Apr 15;**19**(8):2224–31.

172. Aruga A, *et al.* Phase I clinical trial of multiple-peptide vaccination for patients with advanced biliary tract cancer. *J Transl Med* 2014 Mar 7;**12**:61.

173. Shimizu K, *et al.* Clinical utilization of postoperative dendritic cell vaccine plus activated T-cell transfer in patients with intrahepatic cholangiocarcinoma. *J Hepatobiliary Pancreat Sci* 2012;**19**(2):171–8.

174. Kobayashi M, *et al.* DC-vaccine study group at the Japan Society of Innovative Cell Therapy (J-SICT). Dendritic cell-based immunotherapy targeting synthesized peptides for advanced biliary tract cancer. *J Gastrointest Surg* 2013;**17**(9):1609–17.

175. O'Sullivan KE, *et al.* The role of inflammation in cancer of the esophagus. *Expert Rev Gastroenterol Hepatol* 2014 Sep;**8**(7):749–60.

176. Senol K, Ozkan MB, Vural S, Tez M. The role of inflammation in gastric cancer. *Adv Exp Med Biol.* 2014;**816**:235–57.

177. Chang WJ, *et al.* Inflammation-related factors predicting prognosis of gastric cancer. *World J Gastroenterol* 2014 Apr 28;**20**(16):4586–96.

178. Kuehnle MC, *et al.* Phenotyping of peripheral blood mononuclear cells of patients with advanced heavily pre-treated adenocarcinoma of the stomach and gastro-esophageal junction. *Cancer Immunol Immunother* 2014 Aug 28. [Epub ahead of print].

179. Wang Y, *et al.* Cancer/testis antigen expression and autologous humoral immunity to NY-ESO-1 in gastric cancer. *Cancer Immun* 2004 Nov 1;**4**:11.

180. Chen YT, *et al.* Cancer-testis antigen expression in digestive tract carcinomas: frequent expression in esophageal squamous cell carcinoma and its precursor lesions. *Cancer Immunol Res* 2014 May;**2**(5):480–6.

181. Kono K, *et al.* Dendritic cells pulsed with HER-2/neu-derived peptides can induce specific T-cell responses in patients with gastric cancer. *Clin Cancer Res* 2002;**8**(11):3394–3400.

182. Masuzawa T, *et al.* Phase I/II study of S-1 plus cisplatin combined with peptide vaccines for human vascular endothelial growth factor receptor 1 and 2 in patients with advanced gastric cancer. *Int J Oncol* 2012;**41**:1297–1304.

183. Kono K, *et al.* Vaccination with multiple peptides derived from novel cancer-testis antigens can induce specific T-cell responses and clinical responses in advanced esophageal cancer. *Cancer Sci* 2009;**100**(8):1502–1509.

184. Kageyama S, *et al.* Dose-dependent effects of NY-ESO-1 protein vaccine complexed with cholesteryl pullulan (CHP-NY-ESO-1) on immune responses and survival benefits of esophageal cancer patients. *J Transl Med* 2013 Oct 5;**11**:246.

185. Jiang J, *et al.* Treatment of advanced gastric cancer by chemotherapy combined with autologous cytokine-induced killer cells. *Anticancer Research* 2006;**26**(3B):2237–2242.

186. Jiang JT, *et al.* Increasing the frequency of CIK cells adoptive immunotherapy may decrease risk of death in gastric cancer patients. *World J Gastroenterol* 2010;**16**(48):6155–6162.

187. Shi L, *et al.* Efficacy of adjuvant immunotherapy with cytokine-induced killer cells in patients with locally advanced gastric cancer. *Cancer Immunology, Immunotherapy* 2012;**61**(12):2251–2259.

188. Kono K, *et al.* Prognostic significance of adoptive immunotherapy with tumor-associated lymphocytes in patients with advanced gastric cancer: a randomized trial. *Clin Cancer Res* 2002;**8**(6):1767–1771.

189. Toh U, *et al.* Locoregional cellular immunotherapy for patients with advanced esophageal cancer. *Clin Cancer Res* 2000;**6**(12):4663–4673.

190. Cancer Genome Atlas Research Network. Comprehensive molecular characterization of gastric adenocarcinoma. *Nature* 2014 Sep 11;**513**(7517):202–9.

191. Muro K, *et al.* Relationship between PD-L1 expression and clinical outcomes in patients (Pts) with advanced gastric cancer treated with the anti-PD-1 monoclonal antibody pembrolizumab (Pembro; MK-3475) in KEYNOTE-012. *J Clin Oncol* 33, 2015 (Suppl 3; abstr 3).

192. Grabenbauer GG, *et al.* Tumor-infiltrating cytotoxic T cells but not regulatory T cells predict outcome in anal squamous cellcarcinoma. *Clin Cancer Res* 2006 Jun 1;**12**(11 Pt 1):3355–60.

193. Oudejans JJ, *et al.* High numbers of granzyme B/CD8-positive tumor-infiltrating lymphocytes in nasopharyngeal carcinoma biopsies predict rapid fatal outcome in patients treated with curative intent. *J Pathol* 2002;**198**:468–7.

194. Tong WW, *et al.*; on behalf of the Study of the Prevention of Anal Cancer (SPANC) team. Human Papillomavirus 16-Specific T-Cell Responses and Spontaneous Regression of Anal High-Grade Squamous Intraepithelial Lesions. *J Infect Dis* 2014 Aug 19.

195. Klencke B, *et al.* Encapsulated plasmid DNA treatment for human papillomavirus 16-associated anal dysplasia: a Phase I study of ZYC101. *Clin Cancer Res* 2002 May;**8**(5):1028–37.

196. Alvarez-Salas LM. Amolimogene bepiplasmid, a DNA-based therapeutic encoding the E6 and E7 epitopes from HPV, for cervical and anal dysplasia. *Curr Opin Mol Ther* 2008 Dec;**10**(6):622–8.

197. Vici P, *et al.* Immunologic treatments for precancerous lesions and uterine cervical cancer. *J Exp Clin Cancer Res* 2014 Mar 26;**33**:29.

198. Anderson JS, *et al.* A randomized, placebo-controlled, dose-escalation study to determine the safety, tolerability, and immunogenicity of an HPV-16 therapeutic vaccine in HIV-positive participants with oncogenic HPV infection of the anus. *J Acquir Immune Defic Syndr* 2009 Nov 1;**52**(3):371–81.

199. Timmermann B, *et al.* Somatic mutation profiles of MSI and MSS colorectal cancer identified by whole exome next generation sequencing and bioinformatics analysis. *PLoS One* 2010 Dec 22;**5**(12):e15661.

200. Dolcetti R, *et al.* High prevalence of activated intraepithelial cytotoxic T lymphocytes and increased neoplastic cell apoptosis in colorectal carcinomas with microsatellite instability. *Am J Pathol* 1999;**154**:1805–13.

201. Llosa NJ, *et al.* The vigorous immune microenvironment of microsatellite instable colon cancer is balanced by multiple counter-inhibitory checkpoints. *Cancer Discov* 2015 Jan;**5**(1):43–51.

202. Le DT, *et al.* PD-1 blockade in tumors with mismatch repair deficiency. *J Clin Oncol* 33, 2015 (Suppl; abstr LBA100).

Chapter 3

The Role of EMR and Ablative Therapies for Barrett's Mucosa and Early Esophageal Cancer

Kenneth Fasanella and Kevin McGrath

1 Introduction

Barrett's esophagus (BE) is a metaplastic change of the esophageal stratified squamous mucosa due to chronic gastroesophageal reflux.[1] Recognized at endoscopy as salmon-colored mucosa of any length affecting the tubular esophagus, the presence of specialized columnar epithelium with goblet cells (i.e. intestinal metaplasia) is required to make the histologic diagnosis.[2,3] BE is the main risk factor for the development of esophageal adenocarcinoma (EAC), whose rate of increase is greater than any other cancer in the Western world. This chapter will discuss the role of endoscopic therapy of BE and superficial esophageal cancer.

Given the prevalence of gastroesophageal reflux disease (GERD) in Western adults, it is estimated that BE may affect 1–2% of this population.[4,5] Fortunately, the malignant risk is exceedingly small and is estimated to be 0.12–0.6% per patient with BE per year.[6,7] However, the presence of dysplasia increases the malignant risk. In the setting of malignant progression, BE typically progresses through the metaplasia–dysplasia–carcinoma sequence, where dysplasia is graded as low grade and high grade. For non-dysplastic BE, given the small risk, endoscopic surveillance is recommended every 3 to 5 years.[8,9] Barrett's surveillance is considered not cost effective,[10] but studies have demonstrated better survival for early stage EAC discovered by surveillance endoscopy.[11–14]

For low-grade dysplasia (LGD), the annual risk for malignancy is estimated to be approximately 1.7%.[7] Given this, guidelines have recommended shorter surveillance intervals (six-month interval, and if no progression, yearly surveillance).[8,9] The histologic interpretation of LGD is quite subjective, but it has been shown that if two or more pathologists confirm the presence of LGD, the risk of progression to high-grade dysplasia (HGD) or EAC is higher (up to 14.6% per year).[15,16] A recent randomized controlled trial for treatment of LGD found a 9% malignant progression rate at three years.[17] The annual risk for malignancy for HGD is estimated to be up to 6.6%, with a five-year risk that exceeds 30%.[7,8] It is currently recommended that any grade of dysplasia be confirmed by a second pathologist, preferably one with expertise in gastrointestinal pathology.[8,9] For confirmed HGD, experts recommend intervention, with endoscopic therapy emerging as the preferred treatment. Endoscopic therapy for LGD is more controversial, with societal guidelines recommending it as a choice after consultation between the patient and the treating physician.[9] Given recent data showing a heightened risk of malignant progression for LGD, our center currently offers endoscopic therapy for all grades of confirmed dysplastic BE.

2 Ablative Therapies for Barrett's Esophagus

2.1 *Argon plasma coagulation*

Historically, esophagectomy with its associated high morbidity rate was the recommended treatment for BE with HGD. Fortunately for patients, the evolution of endoscopic technology and therapy has allowed outpatient treatment of dysplastic BE with high success rates. After a 1991 case report in abstract form,[18] Berenson *et al.* were the first to report successful restoration of squamous mucosa after ablation of BE.[19] They hypothesized that appropriate acid suppression after Barrett mucosal injury would lead to squamous mucosal regeneration. Argon plasma coagulation (APC), a focal "point-and-shoot" ablative technique where ionized argon gas coagulates tissue, was applied to a small series of patients, which led to successful reversal of Barrett's epithelium. This experience marked the age of endoscopic ablative therapy for BE.

For the next decade, many studies evaluated the use of APC to reverse both dysplastic and non-dysplastic BE. From a historical perspective, it is safe to say that this treatment has essentially been replaced by newer and more efficacious ablative therapies. The major issues with APC ablative therapy were its non-uniform treatment (due to the focal point and shoot technique) and lack of a universal recommended power setting.

2.2 *Photodynamic therapy*

Photodynamic therapy (PDT) involves systemic administration of a photosensitizing agent, followed by laser light activation. Evolved from dermatologic applications, it was investigated for potential use in the treatment of early esophageal cancer and ablation of Barrett's HGD as an alternative nonsurgical therapy. In the United States, porfimer sodium is the approved photosensitizing agent for PDT applications in the esophagus. The procedure consists of systemic injection of porfimer sodium (2 mg/ kg), which is retained preferentially by neoplastic tissue. Forty eight hours later, allowing for wash-out from normal tissue, endoscopy is performed where a low-powered tunable laser is used to generate 630-nm light, which activates the porfimer sodium. The nonthermal laser light is delivered using a cylindrical diffusing fiber, which is inserted through the endoscope into the esophageal lumen.[20,21] Laser light activation of the photosensitizer results in a photodynamic reaction, where singlet oxygen species and superoxide hydroxyl radicals are generated, resulting in cell death. The treatment is localized, as there is relatively selective retention of porfimer sodium in neoplastic tissue, and laser light is delivered selectively to the involved portion of the esophagus. A power density setting of 400 mW/cm of diffuser provides an energy density of 100 to 250 J/cm to the esophageal tissue based on the duration of laser light exposure.[20–22] This can also result in significant "peripheral" damage to normal esophageal epithelium. An optional "second-look" endoscopy can be performed 48 h after the first, whereby additional treatment can be delivered to "skip" or under-treated areas of neoplastic mucosa.

A study of 100 patients undergoing PDT (87 HGD and 13 superficial EAC) reported a dysplasia eradication rate of 78%, with complete elimination of Barrett's mucosa in 43% of patients. Ten of the 13 superficial cancers were successfully ablated. During follow-up, dysplasia developed in 23% of patients in untreated Barrett's mucosa, which required additional treatment. Esophageal strictures occurred in 34% of patients as a result of PDT.[22] During the later part of this study, the use of a windowed centering balloon was introduced, which reduced the stricture incidence. This balloon centered the diffusing fiber in the lumen, allowing for a more uniform circumferential treatment, as opposed to use of a bare fiber which can result in areas of over-treatment with resultant stricturing.

The favorable results of this single center study led to a phase III international multicenter randomized trial of PDT for ablation of HGD using the centering balloon. This study randomized 208 patients with HGD to balloon PDT or omeprazole only. The treatment dose was 130 J/cm of diffuser length, with a maximum length of 7 cm treated in one session. At the second year of follow-up, PDT resulted in complete ablation of HGD in 77% compared with 39% in the omeprazole control group, and it reduced the incidence of adenocarcinoma by 54%. Complete eradication of all Barrett's mucosa was obtained in 52% of patients, and the treatment-related stricture rate was 36%. Most patients required more than one treatment with PDT (maximum of three courses), with 69% of patients experiencing photosensitivity reactions.[23] At the fifth year of follow-up, results were durable with HGD eradication persisting at 77%, and a 48% relative risk reduction for esophageal cancer.[24]

The fact that PDT is a nonthermal easy-to-perform procedure with minimal endoscopic maneuvering is an advantage of this treatment modality. Tissue is not burned, there is no smoke generation, nor is there thermal damage to the equipment. The disadvantages include the cost of the photosensitizer and side effects of the treatment, notably the 4–6-week period of photosensitivity where the patient cannot be exposed to sunlight, significant pain as a result of the tissue necrosis, and a significant stricture rate. As technology has continued to evolve, PDT has fallen out of favor, to be replaced by better tolerated and more efficacious ablative therapies.

2.3 *Radiofrequency ablation*

Early in the first decade of the new millennium, radiofrequency ablation (RFA) for BE was developed. After animal studies to determine the appropriate dosimetry and limited human experience,[25] the AIM (ablation of intestinal metaplasia) trial was launched using first generation equipment. This multicenter study reported a 70% eradication rate of non-dysplastic BE after one year.[26] Commercially marketed in 2005, RFA now has mature data for efficacious eradication of BE (both dysplastic and non-dysplastic). Treatment catheters consist of circumferential balloon-based electrodes (3 cm in length) of varying diameters, focal electrodes of varying sizes attached to the tip of the endoscope, and even a through-the-scope focal electrode. The catheter's treatment surface consists of multiple, tightly spaced bipolar electrodes that alternate in polarity.[25] Energy in joules is delivered to the electrode by a generator, which ablates epithelium to a depth of 1 mm. As the depth of injury is very limited, the stricture rate is far less than that of PDT.

With the addition of focal RFA, small Barrett's areas or remnant Barrett's mucosa after circumferential RFA are easily treated. The original AIM trial extended follow-up to five years, allowing for stepwise focal ablation. The results demonstrated treatment durability, with a 92% complete eradication rate, and all initial treatment "failures" were converted to complete eradication with one focal ablation treatment.[27]

Given the low risk of incident EAC, current societal guidelines do not recommend or support endoscopic ablation of non-dysplastic BE.[9] With the hope of successful ablation of dysplastic BE and resultant cancer reduction, RFA was evaluated in this regard. Prior to the introduction of focal ablation, a U.S.

multicenter registry study reported a 90% eradication rate for HGD at the 12th month of follow-up.[28] Although impressive results were shown, this study was fraught with the typical limitations of a registry experience, notably lack of standardization of treatment and follow-up, lack of a centralized pathologist, and a nonrandomized design without a control arm. These limitations were soon addressed by the AIM dysplasia trial, which was a multicenter, randomized, sham-controlled trial of RFA for BE with dysplasia. Patients were randomized to balloon-based RFA with stepwise focal treatment (if necessary) versus sham endoscopy/catheter insertion and proton pump inhibition. The LGD and HGD study arms reported dysplasia eradication rates of 90% and 81%, respectively, at one-year follow up. The esophageal stricture rate was 6%. In the HGD arm, RFA reduced the risk of cancer development as compared to the sham cohort (2% *vs.* 19%). All patients enrolled had long-segment BE, with the vast majority harboring multifocal dysplasia. Within the LGD sham cohort, 14% progressed to HGD during the 12-month follow-up.[29] At the conclusion of the study, all patients in the sham cohorts were offered RFA treatment. The continuation phase of the study, planned for five years, has reported three-year durability results thus far. The complete eradication of dysplasia was 98%, with a complete eradication of intestinal metaplasia (all Barrett's epithelium) of 91%, allowing for interim focal ablation.[30] This experience has proven the efficacy of RFA for HGD with resultant cancer reduction, and it is now considered primary therapy at many expert centers, replacing esophagectomy.

Treatment of LGD has been more controversial, for reasons stated earlier. Our center offers RFA for patients with LGD confirmed by an expert pathologist, given the increased cancer risk. The recently reported SURF (Surveillance *vs.* Radiofrequency ablation) study, in the authors' opinion, puts an end to the controversy. This was a study randomizing patients with confirmed LGD to RFA versus endoscopic surveillance. The complete eradication of dysplasia was 93%, with an 88% complete eradication of IM. The risk of progression to HGD or EAC in the surveillance arm was 26.5%, compared to 1.5% in the RFA arm. The absolute risk reduction (ARR) was 25%, with a number needed to treat (NNT) of four patients with LGD to prevent one case of neoplastic progression. The progression rate to EAC was 8.8% in the surveillance arm compared to 1.5% in the treatment arm (ARR 7.4%; NNT 13.6). Given the significant findings, the data safety and monitoring board recommended early termination of this trial prior to the planned three-year follow-up. This was due to the superiority of ablation for the primary outcome of neoplastic progression, and for potential patient safety concerns (in the surveillance arm) if the trial continued.[17] This experience solidifies the data that LGD, confirmed by an expert pathologist, harbors significant risk for neoplastic progression. We anticipate that the next versions of societal guidelines for management of BE will recommend ablation for confirmed LGD.

RFA is more efficacious and better tolerated than PDT. The dysplasia and IM eradication rates of RFA exceed that of PDT, with similar cancer risk reductions. The majority of patients treated with RFA will experience self-limited chest pain and odynophagia. In our experience, this usually lasts for approximately one week, and is subjectively related to the length of Barrett's treated. Patients are counseled to adhere to a soft diet for three days, and then advance their diet as tolerated. Sucralfate suspension is used prior to meals, and acetaminophen (with or without codeine) is recommended for pain. In contrast, patients treated with PDT were all given morphine elixir and told to start it immediately given the very significant resultant chest pain. The esophageal stricture rate is 5–6% for RFA,[29,31] compared to 34–36% for PDT.[22,23] Hence the old saying, "out with the old and in with the new."

2.4 *Cryotherapy*

Cryotherapy has also been evaluated in the treatment of dysplastic BE and early EAC. Endoscopic spray cryotherapy utilizes low-pressure medical-grade liquid nitrogen ($-196°C$) sprayed through a 7Fr disposable catheter to freeze the target epithelium. Treatment dosimetry is related to the duration of tissue freeze time (seconds) and the number of freeze/thaw cycles. After a visible "cryofrost" forms on the target area, treatment continues for a set amount of time. The treatment area is limited to several centimeters (1/3 or hemi-circumferential) to maintain an adequate tissue freeze for the treatment duration. For dysplastic BE, accepted treatment is generally two cycles of 20 s or four cycles of 10 s.[32] Thaw time is usually 60 s, and the mucosa returns to its normal color. An oro-gastric (OG) decompression tube is placed during treatment to evacuate gas pumped into the stomach. An assistant will monitor the patient's abdomen for distension, and if significant distension occurs, treatment may need to be temporary discontinued. This is less of a problem with the introduction of a new-generation lower-pressure cryotherapy system.

Compared to RFA, the experience with cryotherapy is limited with a less uniform dosimetry. Although better tolerated than RFA due to less chest pain, the treatment can be more cumbersome and difficult due to the presence of the OG tube, the catheter freezing to the mucosa, and poor visualization due to moisture freezing on the lens and "fog" generated by the cryogen.

The initial clinical work by Johnston *et al.* was a small single-center study which treated 11 patients with variable grades of BE. There was complete endoscopic and histologic reversal of BE in 78%.[33] Based on this early yet positive experience, several small single-center studies were reported as the technology evolved.

The largest experience to date is a multicenter, retrospective cohort study, where 98 patients with HGD were treated with endoscopic spray cryotherapy. Only 60 patients completed all planned treatments (mean four per patient) at the time of analysis. The complete eradication rate of HGD was 97%, of all dysplasia 87%, and of IM 57%, respectively, after 10.5 months of follow-up. The stricture rate was 3%.[32]

A single-center study with a two-year follow-up reported a complete eradication rate for HGD of 100%, and an 84% eradication rate for IM. This was a 32-patient experience, with an 18% HGD recurrence rate. Repeat therapy led to eradication in all but one recurrence.[34] Thus, it appears that cryotherapy has potential durability.

2.5 *Acid reduction*

Aggressive treatment of reflux disease is paramount to the success of endoscopic ablation, regardless of the ablative technique. The equivalent of omeprazole 40 mg twice daily is generally sufficient to control acid exposure, heal treatment-induced injury, and allow squamous mucosal regeneration. Occasionally, further escalation of pharmacotherapy (PPI TID, additional of bedtime H_2 blocker) is necessary, and at times, anti-reflux surgery must be performed to allow mucosal healing.

2.6 *Post-ablation surveillance*

When treating dysplastic BE, the goal is complete eradication of all IM. Leaving residual IM allows premalignant mucosa to persist, which could give rise to metachronous neoplasia in the future. Additionally, continued endoscopic surveillance is still necessary after complete eradication, as recurrences do occur. Fortunately, recurrences of dysplasia or IM can be easily treated with repeat focal RFA. The surveillance intervals for the original dysplastic grade are generally followed, and increased with time. As ablation is still in its infancy, post-treatment surveillance is not standardized, and continues to evolve as longer durability studies are completed.

3 Endoscopic Treatment of Early Esophageal Cancer

As previously mentioned, EAC is the fastest-rising cancer in the United States, having risen six-fold in incidence over the last three decades.[35] Its prognosis is typically poor, with a 19% five-year survival due to typical presentation in the setting of advanced disease.[36] Early detection is critical to improving disease survival, with resectable stage II and III disease demonstrating improved outcomes with neoadjuvant chemo-radiation.[37] Until the last decade, esophagectomy was the dominant treatment for not only early EAC, but also BE with HGD. This recommendation for resection in BE with HGD was primarily due to concern of prevalent carcinoma based upon "prospective" surgical cohorts with retrospective review of preoperative data. One study, published by Hietmiller *et al.*, reported a 43% rate of "occult" adenocarcinoma found on esophagectomy specimens of patients undergoing esophagectomy for HGD.[38] These studies were unfortunately limited by the retrospective nature of their preoperative data, without rigorous endoscopic biopsy protocols or centralized pathology review, highlighted by the fact that 5 of the 13 "occult" cancers in Heitmiller's study were at stage II or III. Additionally, they took place at a time when endoscopic imaging was fiber-optic, limiting high-quality inspection of the esophageal mucosa. Subsequent introduction of improved, high-definition video endoscopes and more widespread adoption of rigorous surveillance biopsy protocols have made this a very dated recommendation. As reviewed in the previous section, thanks to the excellent results of the AIM dysplasia trial, endoscopic ablation has replaced esophagectomy in the treatment of HGD. Fortunately, in addition to expanding data on endoscopic treatment of dysplastic BE, the last decade has brought with it a plethora of data demonstrating efficacy of endoscopic treatment for early or superficial EAC.

The main concern regarding endoscopic therapy for superficial cancer is the risk of subsequent development of lymph node metastases (LNM). However, there is significant literature for such risk based on the depth of invasion. T1a lesions are limited to the mucosa, whereas T1b lesions invade into the submucosa where there is a rich lymphatic and vascular network. Based on eight of the largest surgical series of T1 EAC, only 8 of 317 patients (2.5%) with T1a cancer had LNM on surgical pathology compared to a 12–37% LNM rate for T1b lesions.[39–47] Among those eight patients with T1a LNM, only one had available pathology information, which demonstrated the lesion to have poor differentiation and angiolymphatic invasion, both features associated with higher risk of LNM. In the setting of significant morbidity (30–40%)[39–41] and mortality (0–4%) for esophagectomy among even high-volume surgery centers, the (likely inflated) risk of LNM in low-risk T1a cancers appears quite acceptable to recommend endotherapy with the goal of cure and esophageal preservation. Low-risk features are defined as well to moderate tumor differentiation, limited to the mucosa, with no evidence of angiolymphatic invasion.

3.1 *Endoscopic mucosal resection techniques*

Techniques for endoscopic mucosal resection (EMR) have evolved over the last two decades (Figure 1). Initial techniques utilized submucosal saline injections to lift the lesion to make it easier to snare, akin to polypectomy. The "inject and cut"

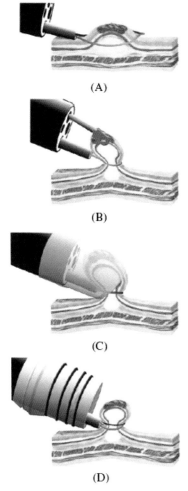

Figure 1 (A) Inject and cut EMR; (B) inject, lift, and cut EMR; (C) cap-assisted EMR; and (D) band-assisted EMR.

Reprinted from *Gastrointestinal Endoscopy*, **57**(4), Soetikno RM, Gotada T, Yukihiro N, Soehendra N. Endoscopic mucosal resection. pp. 567–579, 2003, with permission from Elsevier.

method utilizes standard endoscopic snares with saline injection, and the "inject, lift, and cut" technique (strip biopsy) employs a double-channel endoscope, where forceps are passed through one channel to grasp and lift the lesion while it is ensnared using the other channel. Disadvantages of these techniques include relatively small resection specimens, and difficulty ensnaring flat lesions despite submucosal injection. In the early 1990s, the first suction-assisted, or "suck and cut" mucosal resection technique was introduced using a clear plastic cap fixed to the tip of the endoscope.[48] The cap has a ridge at its base, and after submucosal injection to lift the lesion, a small polypectomy snare is fully opened along the circumference of the ridged cap. The lesion to be resected is then suctioned into the cap through the snare. The snare is tightened around the lesion's base, forming a pseudopolyp, which is subsequently removed via electocautery. There are commercially available kits with different cap sizes and firmness (Olympus EMR Kit, Olympus America Inc, Center Valley, PA). The cap-assisted technique allows for specimens up to 2 cm in diameter to be removed *en bloc*. While this technique can be very effective, we find it technically demanding and laborious. It also requires significant experience to minimize complication rates.[49]

Subsequently, a technique was introduced using band ligation to create a pseudopolyp, followed by snare resection. We find this band-assisted technique easier, as most gastroenterologists are familiar with band ligation to control variceal hemorrhage. With this technique, the target lesion is suctioned into the banding cap affixed to the tip of the endoscope. The band is then "fired" by turning a small hand wheel that releases the band and creates the pseudopolyp. The pseudopolyp is resected below the band without the need for submucosal injection, as the band is not strong enough to entrap the muscularis propria. A commercially available device (Duette Multiband Mucosectomy Device, Cook Ireland, Limerick, Ireland) allows for six mucosal resections, as the cap is outfitted with six bands. Subjectively, it was felt that band-assisted EMR was as effective as the cap-assisted method, but was technically easier and associated with lower complication rates. Given this anecdotal experience, cap-assisted EMR was compared in a randomized, prospective manner to "multiband mucosectomy" (MBM). The cap-assist technique was able to remove lesions or target mucosa with less resections (three *vs.* five) but required more time and had a higher perforation rate (7% *vs.* 2%).[50] A Dutch study compared 80 MBMs to 86 cap-assist resections and found that the former took 13 min less per procedure, resulted in less bleeding (6% *vs.* 20%), and the only perforation occurred in the cap-assist resection group.[51] A subsequent larger trial evaluated the safety of MBM in 243 patients who underwent 1,060 mucosal resections, reporting a 3% clinically significant bleeding rate and no perforations.[52] Given this experience, most therapeutic endoscopists currently employ the band-assisted technique for EMR of EAC or nodular HGD.

3.2 Endoscopic mucosal resection for cure

Utilizing the aforementioned techniques, there has been a growing body of literature over the past decade, mainly out of European centers, demonstrating this to be not only a safe method of mucosal resection, but also effective for primary endo-therapy of carefully selected cases of superficial EAC. The first large series (100 patients) using EMR with curative intent for low-risk T1a EAC was published by the Weisbaden group in 2007.[53] Inclusion was limited to tumors confined to the mucosa with well to moderate differentiation, <2 cm in size, and without lympho-vascular invasion. Complete remission (CR) was achieved within a year in 99%, and during a median follow up period of 33 months, there were no deaths due to esophageal cancer. In fact, the calculated five-year survival of 98% was better than an age-matched German population. The metachronous cancer or recurrence rate was 11%, and all lesions were successfully treated endoscopically.

A subsequently-published American study compared two cohorts treated endo-scopically or surgically for mucosal-based EAC.[54] The endotherapy cohort com-prised 132 patients treated for T1a EAC with EMR or EMR and PDT, followed for a median of 43 months. CR was achieved in 94%, but 12% developed metachro-nous cancer. However, complete eradication of Barrett's mucosa was not a goal of this study, and 92% had residual BE or dysplasia. Overall five-year survival was better in the surgery group but was not significant when adjusted for age and comorbidities. The study was limited by heterogeneous inclusion, with some T1b EACs and some squamous carcinomas, as well as its retrospective nature and evolving treatment protocol.

To address the concern of residual tissue at risk after endoscopic removal of Barrett's neoplasia, Peters *et al.* published a study on a series of nine patients who underwent stepwise radical endoscopic resection (SRER) of not only the neoplasia, but all remaining IM.[55] After successful eradication, neosquamous tissue was ana-lyzed for pre-existing genetic risk factors (p16, p53, and aneuploidy for chromo-somes 1 and 9) and found none remained. The same group subsequently reported using the SRER technique to treat early Barrett's neoplasia in 169 patients.[56] With an intention-to-treat analysis, CR for neoplasia was achieved in 97.6% and CR-IM in 85.2%, which was sustained after 27 months median follow-up. Unfortunately, this treatment was associated with a 49.7% rate of esophageal stricturing. One third of these were difficult-to-treat strictures (more than five dilations, stent placement, incisional therapy) complicated by two perforations. Given the excellent BE eradi-cation results and safety record of RFA, it is currently the recommended ablation modality for the eradication of residual BE after EMR of early neoplasia, as opposed to SRER.[57]

Our group has also reported experience with endotherapy for treatment of superficial EAC.[47] Fifty-four patients underwent EMR of T1a lesions, followed by ablation of remaining BE (PDT 2%, cryotherapy 9%, RFA 95%). At a mean 23 months follow-up, CR for cancer was 96%, CR for dysplasia was 87%, and CR for IM was 59%. One patient developed a metachronous T1b cancer and underwent esophagectomy. The same year, the Amsterdam group reported a five-year follow-up study of 54 patients who underwent RFA +/- EMR for Barrett's with early neoplasia, revealing CR rates for neoplasia and IM of 90%.[58] There was a 6% incidence of metachronous cancer in this cohort, highlighting the need for strict endoscopic surveillance, as the majority of these can be managed with repeat endotherapy.

The Weisbaden group has been the world authority on endotherapy for superficial EAC. As their experience grows, they have periodically updated their work, the most recent of which reported on 1,000 patients with a mean follow-up of 57 months.[59] CR was achieved in 96.3%, and overall five-year survival was 92%. Metachronous lesions or recurrence developed in 14.5%, with most successfully managed via endoscopic retreatment. Twelve patients (3.7%) required surgery due to endoscopic failure. The major complication rate was 1.5% (14 bleeds and one perforation), and two patients died of metastatic EAC (0.2%), one of whom was non-compliant with follow-up. Risk factors for endoscopic failure included poorly differentiated tumor grade and long segment BE.[59]

The development of metachronous neoplasia or recurrence has plagued endotherapy and highlights the need for onging surveillance. With experience, the Weisbaden group's practice pattern shifted to ablation of all remaining BE after EMR. Over 10 years ago, they recognized that ablation of remnant "at-risk" BE would reduce metachronous cancer development. They even proved this in a randomized study of ablation or observation after EMR; there was a 37% metachronous lesion rate in the observation arm compared to only a 3% rate in the ablation arm.[60] Current experience supports a two-stage treatment consisting of EMR of all neoplastic lesions followed by ablation of all residual BE, with RFA being the preferred ablation technique.[47,57–59]

As EMR is recommended for definitive diagnosis and/or staging of visible lesions within BE, occasionally one receives a pathology report noting submucosal invasion (T1b EAC). Generally, this calls for surgical referral for esophagectomy given the increased LNM risk with deeper invasion. However, there is a small but growing experience managing low-risk T1b lesions with EMR.[61,62] Low-risk is defined by invasion limited to the top third of the submucosal layer (SM1), well to moderate tumor differentiation, and lack of angiolymphatic invasion. In a series of 61 patients, there was an 84% long-term remission at mean 47 months follow-up (90% for those with lesions <2 cm). One patient (1.9%) developed a LNM. There were no tumor-associated deaths, and the estimated five-year survival was 84%.[63] Therefore, in highly select patients with low-risk T1b EAC, endotherapy may be an acceptable alternative to esophagectomy.

4 Conclusion

Given the existing evidence, we believe endotherapy is the treatment of choice for dysplastic BE and low risk T1a EAC. RFA is the preferred ablation modality for treatment of dysplastic BE and for eradicating residual BE after EMR of superficial low risk cancer; however it is only efficacious for flat Barrett's mucosa given the limited injury depth. Therefore, if present, nodular HGD should be removed via EMR prior to treatment with RFA. EMR provides accurate histologic staging which is better than endoscopic ultrasound (EUS) for superficial cancer, and allows for appropriate patient selection for continued endotherapy. Treating patients in this manner requires endoscopists experienced in therapeutic endoscopy, expert pathologists, careful processing of pathology specimens, and close endoscopic surveillance. For low-risk T1a cancers undergoing EMR for cure, our surveillance program entails EUS every three months for the first year after resection, every six months for the second year, and annually thereafter for a total of five years. We also perform annual PET/CT scans, but evidence for the utility of this is lacking. We believe gastrointestinal societal guidelines will soon follow suit regarding primary endotherapy for cure in these select cases, but appropriate surveillance still requires further study. Esophagectomy should be reserved for cases of endotherapy failure, as the surgical mortality rate is greater than the LNM rate (0.2%) in the largest experience to date.[59]

References

1. Sharma P. Clinical practice. Barrett's esophagus. *N Engl J Med* 2009;**361**:2548–2556.
2. Odze RD. Update on the diagnosis and treatment of Barrett's esophagus and related neoplastic precursor lesions. *Arch Pathol Lab Med* 2008;**32**:1577–1585.
3. Riddell RH, Odze RD. Definition of Barrett's esophagus: Time for a rethink — is intestinal metaplasia dead? *Am J Gastroenterol* 2009;**104**:2588–2594.
4. Ronkainen J, *et al*. Prevalence of Barrett's esophagus in the general population: an endoscopic study. *Gastroenterology* 2005;**129**:1825–1831.
5. Sampliner RE. A population prevalence of Barrett's esophagus — finally. *Gastroenterology* 2005;**129**:2101–2113.
6. Hvid-Jensen F, *et al*. Incidence of adenocarcinoma among patients with Barrett's esophagus. *N Engl J Med* 2001;**365**:1375–1383.
7. Wani S, *et al*. Esophageal adenocarcinoma in Barrett's esophagus after endoscopic ablative therapy: A meta-analysis and systemic review. *Am J Gastroenterol* 2009;**104**:502–513.
8. Wang KK, Sampliner RE. Updated guidelines for the diagnosis, surveillance and therapy of Barrett's esophagus. *Am J Gastroenterol* 2008;**103**:788–797.
9. Spechler SJ, *et al*. American Gastroenterological Association medical position statement on the management of Barrett's esophagus. *Gastroenterology* 2011;**140**:1084–1091.

10. Fleischer DE, *et al*. The case for endoscopic treatment of non-dysplastic and low-grade dysplastic Barrett's esophagus. *Dig Dis Sci* 2010;**55**:1918–1931.

11. Corley DA, *et al*. Surveillance and survival in Barrett's adenocarcinomas: A population-based study. *Gastroenterology* 2012;**122**:633–640.

12. Streitz Jr, JM, *et al*. Endoscopic surveillance of Barrett's esophagus. Does it help? *J Thorac Cardiovasc Surg* 1993;**105**:383–387.

13. Peters JH, *et al*, DeMeester TR. Outcome of adenocarcinoma arising in Barrett's esophagus in endoscopically surveyed and nonsurveyed patients. *J Thorac Cardiovasc Surg* 1994;**108**:813–821.

14. Fountoulakis A, *et al*. Effect of surveillance of Barrett's oesophagus on the clinical outcome of oesophageal cancer. *Br J Surg* 2004;**91**:997–1003.

15. Skacel M, *et al*. The diagnosis of low-grade dysplasia in Barrett's esophagus and its implications for disease progression. *Am J Gastroenterol* 2000;**95**:3383–3387.

16. Curvers WL, *et al*. Low-grade dysplasia in Barrett's esophagus: overdiagnosed and underestimated. *Am J Gastroenterol* 2010;**105**:1523–1530.

17. Phoa KN, *et al*. Radiofrequency ablation *vs*. endoscopic surveillance for patients with Barrett's esophagus and low-grade dysplasia: A randomized clinical trial. *JAMA* 2014;**311**:1209–1217.

18. Johnson TD, *et al*. Restoration of normal esophageal mucosa after argon laser photoablation and omeprazole treatment of esophageal columnar epithelium. *Clin Res* 1991;**39**:93A.

19. Berenson MM, *et al*. Restoration of squamous mucosa after ablation of Barrett's esophageal epithelium. *Gastroenterology* 1993;**104**:1686–1691.

20. Overholt BF, Panjehpour M. Photodynamic therapy for Barrett's esophagus: clinical update. *Am J Gastroenterol* 1996;**91**:1719–1723.

21. Overholt BF, Panjehpour M. Photodynamic therapy for Barrett's esophagus. *Gastroenterol Clin North Am* 1997;**7**:207–220.

22. Overholt BF, *et al*. Photodynamic therapy for Barrett's esophagus: follow-up in 100 patients. *Gastrointest Endosc* 1999;**49**:1–7.

23. Overholt BF, *et al*. Photodynamic therapy with porfimer sodium for ablation of high-grade dysplasia in Barrett's esophagus: International, partially blinded, randomized phase III trial. *Gastrointest Endosc* 2005;**62**:488–498.

24. Overholt BF, *et al*. Five-year efficacy and safety of photodynamic therapy with Photofrin in Barrett's high-grade dysplasia. *Gastrointest Endosc* 2007;**66**:460–468.

25. Ganz RA, *et al*. Complete ablation of esophageal epithelium with a balloon-based bipolar electrode: A phased evaluation in the porcine and in the human esophagus. *Gastrointest Endosc* 2004;**60**:1002–1010.

26. Sharma VK, *et al*. Balloon-based, circumferential, endoscopic radiofrequency ablation of Barrett's esophagus: 1-year follow-up of 100 patients (with video). *Gastrointest Endosc* 2007;**65**:185–195.

27. Fleischer DE, *et al*. Endoscopic radiofrequency ablation for Barrett's esophagus: 5-year outcomes from a prospective multicenter trial. *Endoscopy* 2005;**42**:781–789.

28. Ganz RA, *et al*. Circumferential ablation of Barrett's esophagus that contains high-grade dysplasia; a U.S. multicenter registry. *Gastrointest Endosc* 2008;**68**:35–40.

29. Shaheen NJ, *et al*. Radiofrequency ablation in Barrett's esophagus with dysplasia. *N Engl J Med* 2009;**360**:2277–2288.

30. Shaheen NJ, *et al*. Durability of radiofrequency ablation in Barrett's esophagus with dysplasia. *Gastroenterology* 2011;**141**:460–468.

31. Orman ES, *et al*. Efficacy and durability of radiofrequency ablation for Barrett's esophagus: Systematic review and meta-analysis. *Clin Gastroenterol Hepatol* 2013; **11**:1245–1255.

32. Shaheen NJ, *et al*. Safety and efficacy of endoscopic spray cryotherapy for Barrett's esophagus with high-grade dysplasia. *Gastrointest Endosc* 2010;**71**:680–685.

33. Johnston MH, *et al*. Cryoablation of Barrett's esophagus: A pilot study. *Gastrointest Endosc* 2005;**62**:842–848.

34. Gosain S, *et al*. Liquid nitrogen spray cryotherapy in Barrett's esophagus with high-grade dysplasia: Long-term results. *Gastrointest Endosc* 2013;**78**:260–265.

35. Pohl H, *et al*. Esophageal adenocarcinoma incidence: Are we reaching the peak? *Cancer Epidemiol Biomarkers Prev* 2010;**19**:1468–1470.

36. Siegel R, *et al*. Cancer statistics, 2012. *CA Cancer J Clin* 2012;**62**:10–29.

37. Van Hagen P, *et al*. Preoperative chemoradiotherapy for esophageal or junctional cancer. *N Engl J Med* 2012;**366**:2074–2084.

38. Heitmiller RF, *et al*. Barrett's esophagus with high grade dysplasia: an indication for prophylactic esophagectomy. *Ann Surg* 1996;**224**:66–71.

39. Altorki NK, *et al*. Multifocal neoplasia and nodal metastases in T1 esophageal carcinoma: implications for endoscopic treatment. *Ann Surg* 2008;**247**:434–439.

40. Griffin SM, *et al*. Lymph node metastases in early esophageal adenocarcinoma. *Ann Surg* 2011;**254**:731–737.

41. Pennathur A, *et al*. Esophagectomy for T1 esophageal cancer: outcomes in 100 patients and implications for endoscopic therapy. *Ann Thorac Surg* 2009;**87**:1048–1055.

42. Rice TW, *et al*. Esophageal carcinoma: depth of tumor invasion is predictive of regional lymph node status. *Ann Thorac Surg* 1998;**65**:787–792.

43. Stein HJ, *et al*. Limited resection for early adenocarcinoma in Barrett's esophagus. *Ann Surg* 2000;**232**:733–742.

44. Liu L, *et al*. Significance of the depth of tumor invasion and lymph node metastasis in superficially invasive (T1) esophageal adenocarcinoma. *Am J Surg Pathol* 2005;**29**: 1079–1085.

45. Sepesi B, *et al*. Are endoscopic therapies appropriate for superficial submucosal esophageal adenocarcinoma? An analysis of esophagectomy specimens. *J Am Coll Surg* 2010; **210**:418–427.

46. Leers JM, *et al*. The prevalence of lymph node metastases in patients with T1 esophageal adenocarcinoma: A retrospective review of esophagectomy specimens. *Ann Surg* 2011;**253**:271–278.

47. Saligram S, *et al*. Endotherapy for superficial adenocarcinoma of the esophagus: an American experience. *Gastrointest Endosc* 2013;**77**:872–876.

48. Inoue H, Endo M. A new simplified technique of endoscopic esophageal mucosal resection using a cap-fitted panendoscope. *Surg Endosc* 1993;**6**:264–265.

49. van Vilsteren FG, *et al.* Learning to perform endoscopic resection of esophageal neoplasia is associated with significant complications even within a structured training program. *Endoscopy* 2012;**44**:4–14.

50. Pouw RE, *et al.* Randomized trial on endoscopic resection-cap versus multiband mucosectomy for piecemeal endoscopic resection of early Barrett's neoplasia. *Gastrointest Endosc* 2011;**74**:35–43.

51. Peters FP, *et al.* Multiband mucosectomy for endoscopic resection of Barrett's esophagus: feasibility study with matched historical controls. *Eur J Gastroenterol Hepatol* 2007;**19**:311–315.

52. Alvarez Herrero L, *et al.* Safety and efficacy of multiband mucosectomy in 1060 resections in Barrett's esophagus. *Endoscopy* 2011;**43**:177–183.

53. Ell C, *et al.* Curative endoscopic resection of early esophageal adenocarcinomas (Barrett's cancer). *Gastrointest Endosc* 2007;**65**:3–10.

54. Prasad GA, *et al.* Endoscopic and surgical treatment of mucosal (T1a) esophageal adenocarcinoma in Barrett's esophagus. *Gastroenterology* 2009;**137**:815–823.

55. Peters FP, *et al.* Stepwise radical endoscopic resection of the complete Barrett's esophagus with early neoplasia successfully eradicates pre-existing genetic abnormalities. *Am J Gastroenterol* 2007;**102**:1853–1861.

56. Pouw RE, *et al.* Stepwise radical endoscopic resection for eradication of Barrett's oesophagus with early neoplasia in a cohort of 169 patients. *Gut* 2010;**59**:1169–1177.

57. Van Vilsteren FG, *et al.* Stepwise radical endoscopic resection versus radiofrequency ablation for Barrett's oesophagus with high-grade dysplasia or early cancer: a multicenter randomized trial. *Gut* 2011;**60**:765–773.

58. Phoa, KN, *et al.* Remission of Barrett's esophagus with early neoplasia 5 years after radiofrequency ablation with endoscopic resection: A Netherlands cohort study. *Gastroenterology* 2013;**145**:96–104.

59. Pech O, *et al.* Long-term efficacy and safety of endoscopic resection for patients with mucosal adenocarcinoma of the esophagus. *Gastroenterology* 2014;**146**:652–660.

60. Manner H, *et al.* Ablation of residual Barrett's epithelium after endoscopic resection: A randomized long-term follow-up study of argon plasma coagulation *vs.* surveillance (APE study). *Endoscopy* 2014;**46**:6–12.

61. Manner H, *et al.* Early Barrett's carcinoma with "low-risk" submucosal invasion: long-term results of endoscopic resection with a curative intent. *Am J Gastroenterol* 2008; **103**:2589–2597.

62. Alvarez Herrero L, *et al.* Risk of lymph node metastasis associated with deeper invasion by early adenocarcinoma of the esophagus and cardia: study based on endoscopic resection specimens. *Endoscopy* 2010;**42**:1030–1036.

63. Manner H, *et al.* Efficacy, safety, and long-term results of endoscopic treatment for early stage adenocarcinoma of the esophagus with low-risk sm1 invasion. *Clin Gastroenterol Hepatol* 2013;**11**:630–635.

Chapter 4

The Role of Peri-Operative Therapy in Esophageal and Gastric Cancers

Jennifer Eads and Michael K. Gibson

1 Esophageal Cancer

1.1 *Introduction*

Locally advanced esophageal cancer remains one of a limited number of solid malignancies for which multimodality care is reality. This provides a variety of options for therapy while simultaneously adding to the complexity of both planning and executing treatment. The aim of the first part of this chapter is to provide a concise review of the state of the art multimodality approaches to locally advanced squamous cell carcinoma (SCC) and adenocarcinoma (AC) of the esophagus. To that end, this summary will touch on: epidemiology, presentation and staging, approaches to operable and inoperable cancers as well as future directions for treatment.

1.2 *Epidemiology*

The incidence of the combination of AC and SCC of the esophagus is estimated to exceed 18,000 cases in 2014, with the majority of patients being men. Overall survival (OS) is approximately 15–20% with best available care, an improvement from 5% in 1975.[1] Regarding subtype, in the United States and the Western world, most cases (80%) are AC and are thought to be related to obesity and reflux. However, in developing countries and Asia, SCC predominates and is likely related to dietary factors.[2]

1.3 *Presentation and staging*

The most common presenting symptoms are weight loss, dysphagia and, to a lesser extent, abdominal pain. Given that such symptoms are non-specific and often insidious, patients frequently present with advanced stage disease. In fact, approximately 50% of patients present with inoperable disease. There are screening tests with efficacy, but they lack effectiveness.[3] Furthermore, physical examination and lab testing is generally unhelpful.

Upon the onset of clinical suspicion, the most efficient test is upper endoscopy. In most cases, a lesion can be both visualized and biopsied. Trans-axial imaging (computed tomography) is also useful; however, an intervention is not possible concurrent with this test. Following biopsy proof of either AC or SCC, staging is approached by the use of endoscopic ultrasound (EUS), PET imaging, and on occasion, laparoscopy.[4] The first decision point for treatment and prognosis is made with these tests — the presence or absence of resectability.

EUS is the best modality for local staging, including depth of penetration through the esophageal wall and presence of malignant loco-regional lymph nodes. It has an overall accuracy for tumor (T) and nodal (N) staging of 80–90%.[5] Staging accuracy may be less reliable in patients with early superficial esophageal cancer than in those with more advanced esophageal cancer.

To complement local staging, PET (positron emission tomography) imaging is the best approach to evaluating for distant metastatic disease. PET scans are more sensitive than CT (computed tomography) and are now preferred for preoperative staging in patients who lack evidence of distant disease on CT. Preoperative PET imaging results in a change in management (usually avoidance of unnecessary surgery) in up to 20% of patients with esophageal cancer.[6] Laparoscopic evaluation of the peritoneum is done in select circumstances in which peritoneal seeding is suspected, such as for bulky gastroesophageal junction (GEJ) or cardia disease or significant regional nodal involvement.

1.4 *Approaches to therapy*

The three modalities — surgery, radiotherapy, and chemotherapy — from which one can choose, may be sequenced and combined in a number of ways. However, before determining this, resectability of locally advanced disease must be determined. The definition of an operable tumor is different from operability, meaning that a tumor may be resectable but surgery is not an option. For example this may be due to comorbid conditions or patient preference. Short of medical and patient variables, technical issues also arise. In general, all stages short of metastatic disease qualify for resection. However, T4 lesions represent a special situation.

Locally invasive disease is non-operable with the surgeon's assessment of subsets of disease that involves the pleura, pericardium and diaphragm.[3]

1.4.1 *Unresectable*

Locally advanced disease that cannot be resected is treated with either concurrent chemoradiotherapy (CRT) or palliative chemotherapy. The paradigm evaluation for this approach for SCC was published by Herskovic and colleagues (RTOG 85-01).[7] This trial demonstrated that the addition of concurrent cisplatin-based chemotherapy to conventional fractionation radiotherapy (RT) provided a significant OS benefit compared to treatment with RT alone. Patients with T4 disease were not included and unresectability was not required. The percentage of patients having squamous histology was roughly 90%, and patients with cervical esophageal cancer were not included. CRT was associated with a significantly better median OS (14 vs. 9 months) and five-year OS (27% *vs.* 0%). These data resulted in the widespread adoption of CRT rather than RT alone for definitive non-operative treatment of locoregional esophageal cancer of both SCC and AC subtypes.

1.4.2 *Cervical esophagus*

SCC of the cervical esophagus is a rare but challenging situation. Given the location (essentially an extension of the hypopharynx), extensive surgery in the form of a laryngopharyngectomy is required to achieve an R0 resection. As such, definitive CRT is preferred, with special attention applied to treatment related dysphagia and aspiration. Often, a head and neck cancer multidisciplinary team is involved.

1.4.3 *Resectable*

For years, the only option for definitive therapy was primary surgery. Several approaches were used, including trans-hiatal and Ivor Lewis as well as more recently minimally invasive Ivor Lewis esophagectomy.[8,9] It is clear that complete resection is necessary for cure, but long-term outcomes are not satisfactory with resection alone, even if it is microscopically complete (R0). As such, with the exception of stage I disease, chemotherapy and radiotherapy are added to achieve cure rates beyond that obtained with surgery alone.

1.5 *Pre-operative chemotherapy*

Several randomized trials have evaluated preoperative chemotherapy versus surgery alone in patients with locally advanced esophageal cancer.[10–15] In the U.S.

Intergroup trial, 467 patients with potentially resectable esophageal or GEJ cancer were assigned to surgery or preoperative chemotherapy with cisplatin and 5-FU followed by surgery.[10] The majority of patients had adenocarcinoma (55%), and outcomes were similar for both histologies. Preliminary results showed no difference in survival. In an update (median follow-up of 8.8 years), preoperative chemotherapy decreased the incidence of R1 resection (4% *vs*.15% in the surgery alone group); however, no improvement was seen in overall survival between the groups.

In contrast, several studies demonstrated a survival benefit. The Medical Research Council (MRC) OEO2 trial randomly assigned 802 patients with AC (69%) or SCC (31%) to surgery alone or preoperative chemotherapy with cisplatin and 5-FU.[15] At a median follow-up of six years, disease-free and OS were significantly longer for the preoperative chemotherapy group. The 16% reduction in risk of death favoring chemotherapy translated into an improvement in five-year OS as well (23 *vs.* 17%).

The French Study group (FNLCC ACCORD07-FFCD 9703) compared preoperative chemotherapy (5-FU and cisplatin) followed by surgery with surgery alone.[16] A total of 224 patients with stage II or greater AC of the GEJ (n = 144), distal esophagus (n = 25), or stomach (n = 55) were randomly assigned. At a median follow-up of 5.7 years, three- and five-year OS rates were 48% and 38%, respectively, for patients receiving preoperative chemotherapy compared with 35% and 21%, respectively, for those receiving surgery alone.

A meta-analysis of eight randomized trials (1,724 patients, any histology, excluding cervical esophageal cancers) suggested a small survival benefit for preoperative chemotherapy.[17] The hazard ratio for all cause survival at two years favored chemotherapy followed by surgery (hazard ratio for all-cause mortality 0.90, 95% CI 0.81–1.0). There was no significant benefit for patients with SCC.

1.6 *Peri-operative chemotherapy*

The UK MAGIC trial evaluated the effect of perioperative chemotherapy with ECF (epirubicin, cisplatin, and 5-FU) given before and after surgery in resectable gastric (74%), GEJ (15%), or distal esophageal adenocarcinomas (11%).[14] A total of 503 patients were randomly assigned to surgery with or without perioperative chemotherapy. At a median follow-up of four years, five-year OS was significantly better in the perioperative chemotherapy group compared with surgery alone (36 *vs.* 23%).

1.7 *Pre-operative concurrent chemoradiotherapy*

As mentioned above, concurrent CRT in the RTOG 85-01[7] and Intergroup 0123 trials[18] demonstrated the superiority of CRT versus surgery alone as definitive therapy for locally advanced disease. The benefit of radiosensitization was studied pre-operatively with the goal of downstaging disease, facilitating surgery and increasing survival. Two randomized trials provide support for this approach.

A Dutch group tested the effect of surgery alone versus preoperative concurrent CRT prior to surgery.[19] In the CROSS trial, 366 patients from the Netherlands were randomized to two groups, surgery alone ($n = 188$) or CRT with weekly paclitaxel (50 mg/m^2) plus carboplatin (AUC = 2) plus concurrent RT (41.4 Gy in five weeks) followed by surgery ($n = 178$). Overall survival was significantly higher in patients receiving neoadjuvant chemoradiation (49.4 months) *vs.* patients receiving surgery alone (24 months). A higher R0 resection rate was also observed in the chemoradiation group (92% *vs.* 69%). In the chemoradiation group, a pathologic complete response rate of 29% was observed.

CALGB 9781 was closed early due to poor enrollment (only 12% of planned).[20] Patients were randomly assigned to surgery with or without preoperative chemoradiotherapy (50.4 Gy external beam RT in 1.8 daily fractions, five days per week, and concurrent cisplatin [100 mg/m^2 on days 1 and 29] and infusion 5-fluorouracil [1,000 mg/m^2 per day by continuous infusion for 96 h, days 1 through 4 and 29 through 32, after cisplatin]). Only 56 patients were enrolled (76% AC), all from North America. However, after six years of median follow-up, the primary objective was met. The median OS was 4.48 years in tri-modality *vs.* 1.79 years in the surgery alone group. Survival at five years was also superior — 39% *vs.* 16% in favor of the tri-modality group.

These two definitive trials support pre-operative CRT as the standard approach for resectable disease.

1.8 *Adjuvant therapy*

For patients with completely resected node-positive or T4 esophageal cancer who did not receive neoadjuvant or perioperative therapy, adjuvant treatment is suggested in an attempt to improve outcomes. It is difficult to come to any conclusions as to whether there are specific advantages for adjuvant chemoradiotherapy over chemotherapy alone, and either approach is reasonable.

1.8.1 *Chemoradiotherapy*

The Intergroup SWOG 9008/INT-0116 trial investigated the benefit of surgery followed by postoperative CRT on the OS of patients with AC of the stomach (80%) or GEJ (20%).[21] It is important to point out that this study did not assess patients with cancer of the distal esophagus. A total of 556 patients were randomly assigned to surgery plus leucovorin/5-FU based postoperative CRT or surgery alone. Median

OS with surgery alone was 27 months compared with 36 months in the postoperative CRT group despite the fact that only 64% of patients completed all of the planned adjuvant treatment. Extent of resection varied, with 54% of patients having a D0 resection, 36% with a D1 resection, and 10% with a D2 resection. Nevertheless, this study established postoperative CRT therapy as a reasonable option of patients with gastric and GEJ AC.

With the associated success of the MAGIC trial to improve OS with perioperative ECF chemotherapy, the CALGB 80101 study was launched to investigate the benefit of using ECF with adjuvant CRT versus the INT-0116 approach. Patients with resected gastric or GEJ AC were randomly assigned to either (a) one cycle of 5-FU/LV for five days per month, followed by 45 Gy (1.8 Gy/day) of RT and concurrent with 5FU throughout RT, followed by an additional two cycles of 5-FU/LV or (b) one cycle of epirubicin/cisplatin/5-FU (ECF) throughout RT, followed by two cycles of reduced dose ECF. Preliminary data presented at ASCO 2011 showed that the ECF-containing arm had lower rates of diarrhea, mucositis, and grade 4 or worse neutropenia. However, OS was not significantly better with ECF (at three years, 52% vs. 50% for 5-FU/LV).

1.8.2 Chemotherapy

Adjuvant chemotherapy was studied for both AC and SCC of the esophagus, with the major studies carried out in Japan, Korea, and the United States.

The benefit for adjuvant chemotherapy alone was suggested in a single-arm trial conducted by the Eastern Cooperative Oncology Group that included patients with AC of the distal esophagus ($n = 9$), GEJ ($n = 34$), and cardia ($n = 12$), of which 89% were node positive.[22] After treatment with four three-weekly cycles of paclitaxel (175 mg/m^2) and cisplatin (75 mg/m^2) and at a median follow-up of four years, the two- and three-year survival rates were 60% and 44%. The lack of a surgery alone control group precludes interpretation of these data.

SCCs were evaluated in the Japanese Clinical Oncology Group (JCOG) phase III trial which compared surgery alone versus surgery followed by adjuvant chemotherapy (two courses of cisplatin 80 mg/m^2 on day 1 and 5-FU 800 mg/m^2 daily for five days).[23] Treatment of 242 patients with esophageal SCC resulted in a five-year disease-free survival (primary endpoint) that was significantly better in the chemotherapy arm (55% *vs.* 45%). However, OS did not differ (61% *vs.* 52%).

1.9 Summary

Locally advanced esophageal cancer, both squamous and adenocarcinoma histologies, are best managed with multimodality care. For resectable adenocarcinoma of the esophagus and GEJ, level 1 evidence supports (1) pre-operative chemotherapy, (2) peri-operative chemotherapy, (3) pre-operative concurrent chemoradiotherapy (CRT), and (4) adjuvant concurrent CRT. There are phase II studies that support adjuvant chemotherapy as well. Major unanswered questions for adenocarcinoma include the lack of level 1 evidence for adjuvant chemotherapy, the role of adjuvant chemotherapy following pre-operative CRT, the cure rate for definitive CRT and the use of molecular/targeted therapies in the curative setting. SCC may be managed with definitive CRT with or without surgery followed by adjuvant chemotherapy.

2 Gastric Cancer

2.1 *Introduction*

As is the case for localized esophageal cancer, localized gastric cancer is also a solid tumor malignancy for which a multimodality approach is commonly used. Historically the use of radiation therapy has been included in the management of this disease, and often still is. However, more recent studies assessing exclusive chemotherapeutic management strategies have demonstrated that an approach inclusive of chemotherapy only is equally acceptable in particular settings. It is often nuances of a particular patient's case that guide the management strategy and it is not uncommon for single practitioners to utilize a broad range of management strategies as part of their practice. In the second part of this chapter, an overview of the various approaches to the management of localized gastric cancer will be provided including the roles of chemotherapy, radiation and surgery in both the peri-operative and adjuvant settings.

2.2 *Epidemiology*

Gastric cancer is one of the most common cancer diagnoses worldwide and is thought to be the 5th most commonly diagnosed cancer.[24] Most cases occur in Asia and it is far less common in the United States where an estimated 22,220 new gastric cancer cases and 10,990 gastric cancer related deaths were predicted in 2014.[1] It is more common in males who account for approximately 60% of all patients afflicted with this disease. Unfortunately, it is often diagnosed at a late stage where palliative chemotherapy is the only treatment option. Greater than a third of patients (35%) are diagnosed with metastatic disease with an additional 29% having regional disease at diagnosis (involvement of regional lymph nodes) and 26% having localized disease (confined to the primary tumor site). Unfortunately, the five-year survival for each of these groups are 4.2%, 28.8%, and 64.1% respectively, rendering this disease highly fatal.[25]

2.3 *Presentation and staging*

2.3.1 *Presenting symptoms*

The most common presenting symptoms of patients with gastric cancer are weight loss and abdominal pain, most often in the epigastric area. Patients may have nausea, early satiety, anorexia or dysphagia depending on the location of the primary tumor. Many patients (25%) have a history of a prior gastric ulcer. Iron deficiency anemia may also be observed and particularly for earlier stage cancers, is more likely than overt blood loss.[26]

2.3.2 *Endoscopy*

If a diagnosis of gastric cancer is suspected, pathologic confirmation for the presence of cancer is required and is obtained via a tissue biopsy. This is most often obtained by performing an upper endoscopy which allows for collection of diagnostic material and also for identification of the location of the primary tumor. For this, the Siewert classification is used and is important (particularly for localized disease) as it determines if a lesion will be treated as an esophageal/gastroesophageal junctional cancer versus a gastric cancer.[27,28] The Siewert classification system is outlined in Table 1.

Tumors identified as Siewert types I and II are treated as esophageal cancers (see section on esophageal cancer) while Siewert type III tumors are treated as gastric cancers.[29]

Provided there is no evidence of metastatic disease, an EUS is warranted. Conduct of this procedure allows for determination of the depth of invasion of the primary tumor through the gastric wall and is useful in identifying any regional lymph nodes that appear pathologically enlarged and therefore concerning for disease involvement.[30,31] Both of these findings will guide the therapeutic approach, i.e. if surgery alone is indicated versus surgery in combination with chemotherapy with or without radiation therapy versus systemic chemotherapy only.

Table 1   Siewert classification.

Siewert Type I	Adenocarcinoma of the lower esophagus (often associated with Barrett's esophagus) with the center located within 1 cm to 5 cm above the anatomic EGJ
Siewert Type II	True carcinoma of the cardia at the EGJ, with the tumor center within 1 cm above and 2 cm below the EGJ
Siewert Type III	Subcardial carcinoma with the tumor center between 2 and 5 cm below the EGJ, which infiltrates the EGJ and lower esophagus from below

2.3.3 *Pathology*

Pathologic confirmation of the presence of invasive adenocarcinoma is required. There are currently no recommended standard molecular assessments that are performed in the setting of localized disease. It is standard to perform a Her2 assessment in patients with metastatic disease, however in patients with localized disease, it is not standard to perform Her2 testing outside the context of a clinical trial.

2.3.4 *Staging*

In addition to endoscopic evaluation and pathological assessment, staging procedures involved for patients with gastric cancer include a basic laboratory assessment, imaging and in some cases a staging laparoscopy. CT imaging of the chest, abdomen, and pelvis with intravenous and oral contrast is considered the standard imaging modality for gastric cancer. If no evidence of metastatic disease is identified but the primary tumor appears to be a T1b lesion (invades the submucosa) or higher, or there is concern for possible nodal involvement based on either imaging or EUS, a diagnostic laparoscopy for assessment of occult metastases should be performed. This includes direct visualization of the peritoneal cavity for small peritoneal deposits as well as peritoneal washings with a cytological assessment.

2.4 *Approaches to management*

2.4.1 *Surgical resection*

The role for surgery is variable depending on the extent of disease and is most often reserved for management of localized disease. For patients with very early cancers (Tis or T1b), tumor removal using endoscopic mucosal resection (EMR) is a consideration. This procedure should be performed only by an advanced endoscopist at an experienced center.[32,33] More advanced tumors (T1b–T3) require more extensive surgery with the approach depending on the site of the primary lesion. Distal tumors are removed primarily with a subtotal gastrectomy while more proximal tumors require either a proximal gastrectomy or a total gastrectomy. With any of these surgical approaches, a margin of 4 cm that is clear or microscopic tumor is recommended.[34] In the case of T4 tumors (tumors that invade the visceral peritoneum or adjacent structures), an en bloc removal of involved structures is indicated. In the case of metastatic disease, any surgery performed will be with palliative intent only. The primary indications for surgery in this setting are for management of bleeding or obstruction.

2.4.1.1 Importance of nodal dissection

Aside from endoscopic mucosal resection, any gastric surgical resection should also include an appropriate lymph node dissection. A D1 lymph node dissection is defined as one involving the removal of the greater and lesser omental lymph nodes (right and left cardiac lymph nodes along the lesser and greater curvatur; suprapyloric lymph nodes along the right gastric artery and infrapyloric area) along with the chosen gastrectomy method. A D2 lymph node dissection is defined as a D1 plus the additional removal of all lymph nodes along the left gastric artery, common hepatic artery, celiac artery, splenic hilum, and splenic artery. A D2 lymph node dissection is therefore more extensive and also associated with a greater complication rate. It should be performed only by surgeons with extensive training in this procedure.

Weather a D1 or a D2 lymph node dissection needs to be performed is somewhat controversial. In Asia, a D2 lymph node dissection is considered the standard of care and there have been additional non-Asian studies that demonstrate an improved survival benefit with a D2 resection.[35,36] Several larger studies have shown no overall survival benefit with performance of a D2 lymph node dissection over a D1 dissection. In a randomized study of 400 patients undergoing curative resection for gastric cancer, no survival benefit was observed between patients undergoing a D1 *vs.* a D2 lymph node dissection (five-year survival rate 35% *vs.* 33% in favor of D1; HR 1.10; 95% CI 0.87–1.39).[37] A randomized phase II study of 267 patients assigned to either D1 ($n = 133$) or D2 ($n = 134$) lymph node dissection reported no significant difference in five-year survival (66.5% with a D1 dissection *vs.* 64.2% with a D2 dissection; $p = 0.695$); however, patients with a T2-4 lesion and nodal involvement did appear to derive an additional five-year survival benefit (59% with a D2 dissection *vs.* 38% with a D1 dissection).[38] The largest randomized trial of 711 patients undergoing gastrectomy with curative intent (380 assigned to have a D1 lymph node dissection; 331 assigned to have a D2 lymph node dissection) showed no overall survival benefit after 11 years of follow-up (30% for D1 *vs.* 35% for D2; $p = 0.53$). There was however a greater morbidity (25% *vs.* 43%; $p < 0.001$) and mortality (4% *vs.* 10%; $p = 0.004$) rate in patients undergoing a D2 lymph node dissection.[39] After 15 years of follow-up however, results of this trial reported that a D1 lymph node dissection is associated with a greater gastric cancer related death rate than a D2 lymph node dissection (hazard ratio [HR] 0.74 for D2 lymph node dissection *vs.* D1; 95% CI 0.59–0.93).

Based on these mixed results, it remains controversial as to whether or not there is a survival benefit associated with more extensive lymph node dissection at the time of gastrectomy. In a pathologic analysis of lymph node status in 1,038 patients who had undergone gastrectomy for gastric cancer, it was found that the number of positive lymph nodes has a greater influence on prognosis and survival than the location of those lymph nodes when at least 15 lymph nodes are evaluated.[40] In a SEER database analysis of 1,377 patients with gastric cancer who had undergone surgical resection it was found that analysis of greater than 15 negative N2 lymph nodes or greater than 20 negative N3 lymph nodes was associated with improved survival.[41] Based on these results, it is recommended by the National Comprehensive Cancer Network (NCCN) that at least 15 lymph nodes be assessed at the time of gastrectomy regardless of whether a D1 or D2 lymph node dissection is performed. While a D2 lymph node dissection is the standard of care in Asia, in Western countries an extended lymph node dissection is considered acceptable as long as adequate lymph node sampling is performed.[29]

For patients with more than stage IA disease and for which surgical resection alone is considered inadequate therapy, there are several approaches that may be taken including peri-operative chemotherapy (chemotherapy before and after surgical resection), adjuvant chemoradiation therapy or adjuvant chemotherapy. The decision as to which approach to take is often based on physician preference; however, there are some circumstances in which it may be preferable to pursue one approach over another. In cases of bleeding or obstruction, an upfront surgical approach is typically taken. It is important to consider that patient tolerance of chemotherapy is often better prior to surgery as patients are less physically debilitated and generally have a better nutritional status. A summary of the various options is discussed below.

2.4.2 *Peri-operative chemotherapy*

The main trial establishing peri-operative chemotherapy as a standard approach to the management of gastric cancer was the MAGIC trial.[14] This trial was conducted in patients with localized gastric cancer after a study in the metastatic setting demonstrated a survival benefit with the use of combination chemotherapy with epirubicin, cisplatin and 5-fluorouracil (ECF). In this trial, 503 patients with resectable gastric cancer (74%), GEJ cancer (11.5%), or distal esophageal cancer (14.5%) were randomized to receive three cycles of ECF chemotherapy both before and after surgery ($n = 250$) *vs.* surgery alone ($n = 253$). The primary endpoint for the study was OS and investigators found that there was a statistically significant improvement in overall survival with a five-year survival rate of 36% in the chemotherapy-containing arm *vs.* 23% in the surgery only arm (HR 0.75; 95% CI 0.60–0.93; $p = 0.009$). A significant improvement in progression-free survival was also observed in the chemotherapy-containing arm (HR 0.66; 95% CI 0.53–0.81; $p < 0.001$). With the publication of these results, the approach of peri-operative ECF in the management of localized gastric cancer was adopted and is considered a category 1 recommendation in the NCCN guidelines.[29]

The benefit of peri-operative chemotherapy was also observed in a French study of patients with lower esophageal cancer (11%), GEJ cancer (64%), or gastric cancer (25%).[42] In this randomized phase III study, 224 patients were assigned to receive either two-three cycles of pre-operative cisplatin and infusional 5-fluorouracil chemotherapy along with another three-four cycles of the same chemotherapy following surgical resection ($n = 113$) *vs.* surgery alone ($n = 111$). Patients receiving cisplatin and 5-fluorouracil in addition to surgical resection were found to have a significantly improved overall survival as compared to patients undergoing surgery alone (five-year survival rate 38% *vs.* 24%, respectively; HR 0.69; 95% CI 0.50–0.95; $p = 0.02$). They were also observed to have an improved disease free survival (five-year disease free survival rate 34% *vs.* 19%, respectively; HR 0.65, 95% CI 0.48–0.89; $p = 0.003$) and an improved curative resection rate (84% *vs.* 73%; $p = 0.04$). In a multivariable analysis, location of the primary tumor in the stomach was associated with a favorable prognosis.

With the publication of these two trials, peri-operative chemotherapy has been accepted as a reasonable alternative to administration of adjuvant chemoradiation. While the regimens used have not been directly compared, reported survival outcomes and toxicity profiles are similar between the two regimens.

2.4.3 *Surgery followed by adjuvant therapy*

The most widely accepted adjuvant therapy approach within the United States is based on results reported from the INT-0116 trial.[21] This trial established adjuvant chemoradiation as a standard of care for patients with stage Ib or greater gastric or gastroesophageal junctional adenocarcinoma who had undergone a curative surgical resection with clear surgical margins. A total of 556 patients meeting these pathologic and surgical criteria were randomly assigned to either fluoropyrimidine chemotherapy with 5-fluorouracil and leucovorin, followed by combined fluoropyrimidine/leucovorin and radiation therapy to a total of 45 Gy followed by an additional two months of fluoropyrmidine/leucovorin therapy ($n = 281$) *vs.* surgery alone ($n = 275$). The study was powered to detect statistically significant differences in median overall survival and relapse-free survival between the two treatment arms and both were found to be significant. Median overall survival was 27 months in the surgery alone arm *vs.* 36 months in the chemoradiation arm (HR for death 1.35; 95% CI 1.09–1.66; $p = 0.005$). Relapse-free survival was 19 months in the surgery only group *vs.* 30 months in the chemoradiation group (HR for relapse 1.52; 95% CI 1.23–1.86; $p < 0.001$). Amongst patients in the chemoradiation group, only 64% of them were able to receive the full planned adjuvant regimen, primarily due to side effects. Of the 273 patients who received chemoradiation, 54% experienced at least grade 3 hematologic side effects and 33% experienced at least grade

3 gastrointestinal side effects, suggesting some toxicity associated with use of this regimen. Also of note, only 10% of patients underwent a D2 resection with 36% undergoing a D1 resection and the majority (54%) undergoing a D0 resection, thus all assessments were performed in an era of suboptimal surgical resection for patients with gastric cancer.

An acceptable alternative of chemotherapy without radiation therapy has been more recently established, provided that patients have undergone a D2 lymph node dissection. The CLASSIC trial was a randomized, open-label, multicenter phase III clinical trial that evaluated 1,035 patients with stage II–IIIB gastric cancer who had undergone a surgical resection inclusive of a D2 lymphadenectomy. Patients were randomized to receive either six months of capecitabine and oxaliplatin ($n = 520$) *vs.* observation alone ($n = 515$). Results demonstrated a significant improvement in three-year disease-free survival of 74% *vs.* 59% in favor of the chemotherapy arm (HR 0.56; 95% CI 0.44–0.72; $p < 0.0001$). Of patients assigned to receive chemotherapy, approximately two thirds of them were able to complete the full course of adjuvant treatment.[43]

In the Eastern part of the world, primarily Asia, adjuvant chemotherapy is considered an appropriate standard treatment option and is used more commonly than adjuvant regimens, including radiation. It is standard in Asian countries for a D2 lymphadenectomy to be performed at the time of surgical resection. The ACTS-GC study (Adjuvant Chemotherapy Trial of S-1 for Gastric Cancer) was a randomized phase III trial assessing adjuvant S-1 chemotherapy vs. surgery alone in patients diagnosed with a stage II or III gastric adenocarcinoma who had undergone a D2 lymphadenectomy at the time of surgical resection.[44,45] A total of 1,059 patients were randomly assigned to receive either the oral fluoropyrimidine S-1 twice daily for four weeks followed by a two-week break for a total treatment duration of one year ($n = 529$) *vs.* surgery alone ($n = 530$). The primary endpoint for the study was OS. This trial demonstrated a significant overall survival benefit for patients receiving S-1 with a five-year survival rate of 71.7% for patients receiving S-1 (95% CI 67.8%–75.7%) *vs.* 61.1% for patients receiving surgery alone (95% CI 56.8%–65.3%) with a HR for death favoring the S-1 group (HR 0.669; 95% CI 0.540–0.828).

It is important to note for both of these large adjuvant trials that even when an extensive lymphadenectomy is conducted, there does appear to be additional benefit derived from receipt of adjuvant chemotherapy.

There have been several additional adjuvant studies that have reported conflicting results regarding a benefit from adjuvant therapy and because of this, the GASTRIC meta-analysis was performed.[46] This study evaluated 17 of 31 previously conducted randomized controlled trials of patients with gastric cancer receiving adjuvant therapy *vs.* undergoing surgery alone. This was an individual patient level analysis of 3,838 patients and reported an OS benefit with administration of adjuvant chemotherapy. The median overall survival of patients receiving chemotherapy was 7.8 years *vs.* 4.9 years for patients undergoing surgery alone and this benefit was independent of the adjuvant regimen received.

The question of whether adjuvant chemotherapy *vs.* adjuvant chemoradiation is superior is unclear. The ARTIST (Adjuvant Chemoradiation Therapy in Stomach Cancer) trial sought to assess six cycles of adjuvant cisplatin and capecitabine ($n = 228$) versus two cycles of cisplatin and capecitabine before and after a five-week course of chemoradiation with capecitabine ($n = 230$) in patients with localized gastric cancer who had undergone surgical resection with a D2 lymph node dissection.[47] The primary endpoint of the study was disease-free survival, which was not significantly improved by the addition of radiation (three-year disease-free survival of 78.2% and 74.2% in the chemoradiation and chemotherapy arms, respectively; $p = 0.0862$). In a subgroup analysis, however, of 396 patients identified as lymph-node-positive at the time of surgery, three-year disease free survival was significantly improved in the chemoradiation therapy group (77.5%) *vs.* the chemotherapy only group (72.3%); $p = 0.0365$. Therefore, patients with positive lymph nodes following surgery may benefit more from the addition of radiation therapy although there is not yet definitive data to support this.

2.5 Conclusions

Gastric cancer, even in the localized setting, is associated with high mortality and is often quite advanced at the time of initial diagnosis. Curative surgical resection should be included as part of the treatment strategy; however the roles of chemotherapy *vs.* chemoradiation are less clear. Peri-operative chemotherapy with epirubicin, a platinum agent and a fluoropyrimidine (per the MAGIC trial) and adjuvant chemoradiation (per the MacDonald regimen) are the most broadly used treatment approaches. More recent data suggest that adjuvant chemotherapy is also an appropriate management strategy for patients who have undergone an extensive D2 lymph node dissection. Results of ongoing trials should shed additional light on the optimal management approach for these patients.

3 Unanswered Questions and Ongoing Studies

The ongoing NEOPECX study, titled 'An Open Labeled Randomized Controlled Phase II Trial of Panitumumab in Combination with Epirubicin, Cisplatin and Capecitabine (ECX) versus ECX Along in Subjects with Locally Advanced Gastric Cancer or Cancer of the Gastroesophageal Junction (NCT01234324)' is investigating the addition of panitumumab to the MAGIC regimen. Given the worse outcome seen in the REAL-3 trial with the addition of panitumumab to chemotherapy, the results of NEOPECX are expectantly awaited.[48]

Several studies are investigating the role of predictive markers (both imaging and molecular) in directing therapy for resectable adenocarcinomas. CALGB 80803 (NCT01333033) uses PET guided selection of therapy. Patients are randomly assigned to either mFOLFOX6 or carboplatin and paclitaxel. A repeat PET scan following several cycles of chemotherapy is used to measure response. Patients considered as "responders" continue on the same chemotherapy with radiation therapy, while "non-responders" switch to the alternative chemotherapeutic regimen during their chemoradiation period.

Overexpression of Her2 predicts for response to trastuzumab-based chemotherapy in patients with metastatic disease (ToGA trial).[49] Clinical trial RTOG 1010 is underway (NCT01196390) with the goal of testing the benefit of adding trastuzumab to pre-operative carboplatin/paclitaxel/radiation therapy as per the CROSS trial regimen.[19] The follow-up to the UK MAGIC trial adds bevacizumab to peri-operative chemotherapy, and results are pending. Investigators and clinicians alike are awaiting validation of other predictive biomarkers in anticipation of designing future trials.

Given the option of peri-operative chemotherapy *vs.* surgery followed by adjuvant radiation therapy, the question of whether a combination of the two would improve overall survival as compared to either approach alone arises. In the ongoing CRITICS (Chemoradiotherapy after Induction Chemotherapy in Cancer of the Stomach) trial (NCT00407186), patients who have undergone surgical resection following neoadjuvant chemotherapy with ECX (epirubicin, cisplatin, and capecitabine) will be randomly assigned to three additional cycles of ECX *vs.* chemoradiation with cisplatin and capecitabine in combination with 45 Gy of radiation therapy. This trial will determine if there is an added benefit to receipt of radiation therapy over peri-operative chemotherapy alone.

Looking at the question of the role of radiation therapy from more of an esophageal approach, the TOPGEAR trial (NCT01924819) is assessing the role for neoadjuvant chemoradiotherapy for patients with resectable gastric cancer. In this trial, patients are assigned to receive either three cycles of ECF or ECX followed by surgery then an additional three cycles of ECF/ECX *vs.* two cycles of ECF/ECX followed by chemoradiation with a fluoropyrimidine, then surgery with three cycles of ECF/ECX post-operatively. The primary objective of this study is to determine if there is an improvement in the achievement of a pathologic complete response along with secondary survival endpoints.

The question of chemotherapy *vs.* chemoradiation therapy use in the adjuvant setting following surgical resection with a D2 lymph node dissection remains unclear. The ARTIST trial reported that a subgroup of patients with lymph-node-positive disease did appear to significantly benefit from the addition of radiation therapy to their chemotherapeutic regimen. To further investigate this, the ARTIST-II trial (NCT01761461) is underway where patients known to have lymph-node-positive disease are randomly assigned to oxaliplatin plus S-1 *vs.* S-1 *vs.* oxaliplatin and S-1 sandwiched around S-1 with radiation therapy. The results of this trial should provide guidance as to what is the optimal treatment approach in this especially high risk population.

References

1. Siegel R, *et al.* Cancer statistics, 2014. *CA Cancer J Clin* 2014;**64**:9–29.
2. Merkow RP, *et al.* Effect of histologic subtype on treatment and outcomes for esophageal cancer in the United States. *Cancer* 2012;**118**:3268–3276.
3. Singal AG, *et al.* A primer on effectiveness and efficacy trials. *Clin Transl Gastroenterol* 2014;**5**:e45.
4. Edge SB BD, Compton CC. A*merican Joint Committee on Cancer Staging Manual*, 7th Ed., New York: Springer, 2010, p. 103.
5. Rosch T. Endosonographic staging of esophageal cancer: A review of literature results. *Gastrointest Endosc Clin N Am* 1995;**5**:537–547.
6. Meyers BF, *et al.* The utility of positron emission tomography in staging of potentially operable carcinoma of the thoracic esophagus: results of the American College of Surgeons Oncology Group Z0060 trial. *J Thorac Cardiovasc Surg* 2007;**133**:738–745.
7. Herskovic A, *et al.* Combined chemotherapy and radiotherapy compared with radiotherapy alone in patients with cancer of the esophagus. *N Engl J Med* 1992;**326**:1593–1598.
8. Orringer MB, *et al.* Transhiatal esophagectomy: Clinical experience and refinements. *Ann Surg* 1999;**230**:392–400; discussion 400-403.
9. Luketich JD, *et al.* Outcomes after minimally invasive esophagectomy: review of over 1000 patients. *Ann Surg* 2012;**256**:95–103.
10. Kelsen DP, *et al.* Chemotherapy followed by surgery compared with surgery alone for localized esophageal cancer. *N Engl J Med* 1998;**339**:1979–1984.
11. Ancona E, *et al.* Only pathologic complete response to neoadjuvant chemotherapy improves significantly the long term survival of patients with resectable esophageal squamous cell carcinoma: Final report of a randomized, controlled trial of preoperative chemotherapy versus surgery alone. *Cancer* 2001;**91**:2165–2174.
12. Medical Research Council Oesophageal Cancer Working Group. Surgical resection with or without preoperative chemotherapy in oesophageal cancer: A randomised controlled trial. *Lancet* 2002;**359**:1727–1733.
13. Roth JA, *et al.* Randomized clinical trial of preoperative and postoperative adjuvant chemotherapy with cisplatin, vindesine, and bleomycin for carcinoma of the esophagus. *J Thorac Cardiovasc Surg* 1988;**96**:242–248.

14. Cunningham D, *et al*. Perioperative chemotherapy versus surgery alone for resectable gastroesophageal cancer. *N Engl J Me*d 2006;**355**:11–20.

15. Allum WH, *et al*. Long-term results of a randomized trial of surgery with or without preoperative chemotherapy in esophageal cancer. *J Clin Oncol* 2009;**27**:5062–5067.

16. Boige V PJ, Saint-Aubert B. Final results of a randomized trial compareing preoperative 5-fluorouracil (F)/cisplatin (P) to surgery alone in adenocarcinoma of stomach and lower esophagus (ASLE): FNLCC ACCORD07-FFCD9703 trial. *J Clin Oncol* 2007;**25** [abstract].

17. Gebski V, *et al*. Survival benefits from neoadjuvant chemoradiotherapy or chemotherapy in oesophageal carcinoma: A meta-analysis. *Lancet Oncol* 2007;**8**:226–234.

18. Minsky BD, *et al*. INT 0123 (Radiation Therapy Oncology Group 94-05) phase III trial of combined-modality therapy for esophageal cancer: high-dose versus standard-dose radiation therapy. *J Clin Oncol* 2002;**20**:1167–1174.

19. Van Hagen P, *et al*. Preoperative chemoradiotherapy for esophageal or junctional cancer. *N Engl J Me*d 2012;**366**:2074–2084.

20. Tepper J, *et al*. Phase III trial of trimodality therapy with cisplatin, fluorouracil, radiotherapy, and surgery compared with surgery alone for esophageal cancer: CALGB 9781. *J Clin Oncol* 2008;**26**:1086–1092.

21. Macdonald JS, *et al*. Chemoradiotherapy after surgery compared with surgery alone for adenocarcinoma of the stomach or gastroesophageal junction. *N Engl J Med* 2001; **345**:725–730.

22. Armanios M, *et al*. Adjuvant chemotherapy for resected adenocarcinoma of the esophagus, gastro-esophageal junction, and cardia: Phase II trial (E8296) of the Eastern Cooperative Oncology Group. *J Clin Oncol* 2004;**22**:4495–4499.

23. Ando N, *et al*. Surgery plus chemotherapy compared with surgery alone for localized squamous cell carcinoma of the thoracic esophagus: A Japan Clinical Oncology Group Study--JCOG9204. *J Clin Oncol* 2003;**21**:4592–4596.

24. GLOBOCAN 2012: Estimated cancer incidence, mortality and prevalence worldwide in 2012. Available at: http://globocan.iarc.fr/Pages/fact shees cancer.aspx. Accessed Jan 31, 2015.

25. Surveillance, Epidemiology, and End Results Program (SEER) Stat Fact Sheets: Stomach Cancer. Available at http://seer.cancer.gov/statfacts/html/stomach.html. Accessed Jan 31, 2015.

26. Wanebo HJ, *et al*. Cancer of the stomach. A patient care study by the American College of Surgeons. *Ann Surg* 1993;**218**:583.

27. Siewert JR, Stein HJ. Adenocarcinoma of the gastroesophageal junction: classification, pathology and extent of resection. *Dis Esophagus* 1996;**9**:173–182.

28. Siewert JR, *et al*. Adenocarcinoma of the esophagogastric junction. Results of surgical therapy based on anatomical/topographic classification in 1,002 consecutive patients. *Ann Surg* 2000;**232**:353–361.

29. National Comprehensive Cancer Network (NCCN) Clinical Practice Guidelines in Oncology (NCCN Guidelines): Gastric Cancer, version 1.2015.

30. Botet JF, *et al*. Endoscopic ultrasound in the pre-operative staging of gastric cancer. A comparative study with dynamic CT. *Radiology* 1991;**181**:426–432.

31. Bentrem D, *et al*. Clinical correlation of endoscopic ultrasonography with pathologic stage and outcome in patients undergoing curative resection for gastric cancer. *Ann Surg Oncol* 2007;**14**:1853–1859.

32. Soetikno R, *et al*. Endoscopic mucosal resection for early cancers of the upper gastrointestinal tract. *J Clin Oncol* 2005;**23**:4490–4498.

33. Ono H, *et al*. Endoscopic mucosal resection for treatment of early gastric cancer. Gut 2001;**48**:225–229.

34. Rusch VW. Are cancers of the esophagus, gastroesophageal junction, and cardia one disease, two, or several. *Semin Oncol* 2004;**31**:444–449.

35. Jatzko GR, *et al*. A 10-year experience with Japanese-type radical lymph node dissection for gastric cancer outside of Japan. *Cancer* 1995;**76**:1302–1312.

36. Sierra A, *et al*. Role of the extended lymphadenectomy in gastric cancer surgery: experience in a single institution. *Ann Surg Oncol* 2003;**10**:219–226.

37. Cuschieri A, *et al*. Patient survival after D1 and D2 resections for gastric cancer: long-term results of the MRC randomized surgical trial. Surgical Co-operative Group. *Br J Cancer* 1999;**79**:1522–1530.

38. Degiuli M, *et al*. Randomized clinical trial comparing survival after D1 of D2 gastrectomy for gastric cancer. *Br J Surg* 2014;**101**:23–31.

39. Hartgrink HH, *et al*. Extended lymph node dissection for gastric cancer: Who may benefit? Final results of the randomized Dutch gastric cancer group trial. *J Clin Oncol* 2004;**22**:2069–2077.

40. Karpeh MS, *et al*. Lymph node staging in gastric cancer: is location more important than number? An analysis of 1,038 patients. *Ann Surg* 2000;**232**:362–371.

41. Schwarz RE, Smith DD. Clinical impact of lymphadenectomy extent in resectable gastric cancer of advanced stage. *Ann Surg Oncol* 2007;**14**:317–328.

42. Ychou M, *et al*. Perioperative chemotherapy comparted with surgery alone for resectable gastroesophageal adenocarcinoma: An FNCLCC and FFCD multicenter phase III trial. *J Clin Oncol* 2011;**29**:1715–1721.

43. Bang YJ, *et al*. Adjuvant capecitabine and oxaliplatin for gastric cancer after D2 gastrectomy (CLASSIC): A phase 3 open-label, randomised controlled trial. *Lancet* 2012;**379**:315–321.

44. Sakuramoto S, *et al*. Adjuvant chemotherapy for gastric cancer with S-1, an oral fluoropyrimidine. *N Engl J Med* 2007;**357**:1810–1820.

45. Sasako M, *et al*. Five-year outcomes of a randomized phase III trial comparing adjuvant chemotherapy with S-1 versus surgery alone in stage II or III gastric cancer. *J Clin Oncol* 2011;**29**:4387–4393.

46. Paoletti X, *et al*. Role of chemotherapy for advanced/recurrent gastric cancer: An individual-patient-data meta-analysis. *Eur J Cancer* 2013;**49**:1565–1577.

47. Lee J, *et al*. Phase III trial comparing capecitabine plus cisplatin versus capecitabine plus cisplatin with concurrent capecitabine radiotherapy in completely resected gastric

cancer with D2 lymph node dissection: The ARTIST trial. *J Clin Oncol* 2012;**30**: 268–273.

48. Waddell T, *et al.* Epirubicin, oxaliplatin, and capecitabine with or without panitumumab for patients with previously untreated advanced oesophagogastric cancer (REAL3): A randomized, open label phase 3 trial. *Lancet Oncol* 2013;**14**:481–489.

49. Bang YJ, *et al.* Trastuzumab in combination with chemotherapy versus chemotherapy alone for treatment of HER2-positive advanced gastric or gastro-esophageal junction cancer (ToGA): A phase 3, open-label, randomized controlled trial. *Lancet* 2010; **376**:687–697.

Chapter 5

Surgical Treatment
of Esophagogastric Junction Tumors

Manuel Villa Sanchez, Arjun Pennathur and James D. Luketich

1 Introduction

Multiple and distinct carcinogenic pathways likely occur at the esophagogastric junction (EGJ) resulting in cancers with unique features and a spectrum of characteristics — some typical of distal esophageal adenocarcinoma and some typical of proximal gastric cancer. The most recent American Joint Committee on Cancer (AJCC) staging system (7th edition, 2010) classifies tumors in the EGJ and tumors in the proximal 5 cm of the stomach with involvement of the EGJ as esophageal cancer.[1] Because EGJ tumors are in the transition zone between two organs located in different body cavities with different lymphatic drainage, surgical treatment is complex and technically challenging with significant physiologic burden to the patient.

2 Staging

Before surgery for an EGJ tumor can be considered, thorough staging must be performed to determine tumor location, depth of tumor invasion, and whether lymph node metastases or other metastases are present. An appropriate treatment plan cannot be devised without this information. Primary staging modalities include upper-gastrointestinal endoscopy (esophagogastroduodenoscopy; EGD), endoscopic ultrasonography (EUS), computed tomography (CT), and positron emission tomography (PET). Minimally invasive staging by laparoscopy is performed selectively by surgeons at some institutions. We have found that minimally invasive staging is particularly useful in the detection of small distant metastases.[2,3]

3 Tumor Classification

Traditionally, adenocarcinoma of the EGJ has been defined using the Siewert classification. Three Siewert types were defined according to their anatomic relationship with the EGJ: type I distal esophageal adenocarcinoma, type II arising from the cardia, and type III arising from subcardial region and infiltrating to the EGJ and distal esophagus.[4,5]

Previously, it was proposed that this classification guide treatment and the extent of surgical resection.[5–9] However, the necessity of this classification system in determining treatment has been questioned. Leers and colleagues[8] demonstrated that Siewert classification was not associated with the prevalence and distribution of nodal metastases, prevalence and type of recurrence, or overall and disease-specific survival. Additionally, Leers noted the difficulty in identifying the EGJ and clearly classifying by Siewert type in some patients, encountering this problem in 96 of 613 patients assessed retrospectively in their study. Others have also noted similarities in key parameters that determine clinical outcome and argue that subdividing tumors of the distal esophagus, EGJ, and gastric cardia by Siewert type is not relevant to treatment.[10,11] In the latest AJCC classification (7th edition, 2010), cancers of the distal esophagus and the EGJ are classified as esophageal cancer and this is discussed in more detail below. The findings on endoscopy are important and allow the surgeon to evaluate the extent of the tumor and the margins needed for complete resection, and tailor the gastric conduit after esophagectomy and the location of the anastomosis. In general, for distal and EGJ tumors, our approach is an Ivor Lewis minimally invasive esophagectomy with an anastomosis in the chest. This is detailed below.

3.1 *TNM classification*

The TNM (tumor, node, metastasis) staging system takes into account the depth of tumor invasion, the nodal status, and the presence or absence of metastatic disease. The 7th edition of the AJCC and the International Union Against Cancer (AJCC/ UICC) cancer staging system defined EGJ cancers as cancers with an epicenter in the lower thoracic esophagus or EGJ or located within the proximal 5 cm of the stomach (cardia) that extend into the EGJ or esophagus.[1] These tumors were stage-grouped similar to adenocarcinoma of the esophagus. A data-driven analysis was

Table 1   Staging of esophageal adenocarcinoma as defined by the AJCC 7th Edition Staging Manual.

Stage	T	N	M	G
0	Tis (HGD)	0	0	1
IA	1	0	0	1–2
IB	1	0	0	3
	2	0	0	1–2
IIA	2	0	0	3
IIB	3	0	0	Any
	1–2	1	0	Any
IIIA	1–2	2	0	Any
	3	1	0	Any
	4a	0	0	Any
IIIB	3	2	0	Any
IIIC	4a	1–2	0	Any
	4b	Any	0	Any
	Any	3	0	Any
IV	Any	Any	1	Any

T indicates tumor classification; N, lymph node status; M. metastasis; G, histologic grade; Tis, Tumor in situ; HGD, high-grade dysplasia. Further detail can be found in Ref. 1.

Reprinted from Ref. 12, Copyright 2010, used with Permission from Wiley and Sons.

used to identify TNM criteria that influenced survival and create stage groupings, from stage 0 to stage IV with further subdivision of stages II and III.[12] A regional lymph node was redefined to include any paraesophageal node extending from the cervical nodes to the celiac nodes (Table 1).

4 Principles of Surgical Resection

Surgical resection, either as initial therapy or after neoadjuvant treatment, is an essential part of any curative attempt for localized adenocarcinoma of the EGJ. Although there are controversies and personal preferences regarding which surgical approach to apply, it is accepted that complete resection is essential for any potentially curative surgery.[13–16] Obtaining tumor-free resection margins (an R0 resection) is a key determinant that limits recurrence and is associated with improved oncologic outcomes. Adequate lymphadenectomy is also an important component of resection. The definition of an adequate lymph node dissection is an area of active investigation and debate. Appropriate patient selection, accurate staging, risk assessment, and selection of an appropriate surgical approach are necessary to optimize surgical treatment. The risks of esophagectomy can be significantly reduced by a variety of factors that include having the surgery performed in a high-volume hospital, by a high-volume surgeon, by a surgeon with specialty training, in a hospital with the daily involvement of critical care specialists, and in some centers, using a minimally invasive approach.[17–19]

4.1 *Types of resection*

Different surgical approaches for resection of EGJ tumors have been described. When the stomach or a gastric tube is used as a replacement esophageal conduit, approaches include abdominal only, Ivor Lewis (combined abdominal and right thoracotomy), McKeown (three-incision), transhiatal resection, left thoracoabdominal, and left thoracotomy. The single anastomosis needed to reconstruct the conduit can be placed in either the neck or the chest. The jejunum and colon can also be used as conduits using approaches such as Merendino jejunal interposition, long-segment reconstruction with a jejunal pedicle, and short- or long-segment colon interposition with either the transverse colon or the right colon. Because the stomach is used most often as a replacement conduit and is our preferred approach, we will limit discussion in this chapter to these approaches. Approaches using the jejunum or colon are described in detail elsewhere (see Chapters 26–28 in Ref. 20).

Some studies have demonstrated that transhiatal esophagectomy is associated with lower 30-day morbidity and mortality when compared with transthoracic esophagectomy, although there is some evidence showing a trend toward better oncologic outcome with *en bloc* transthoracic esophagectomy.[21–24] Since the introduction of minimally invasive esophagectomy (MIE), it has become evident that MIE combines the reduced short-term morbidity and mortality of the transhiatal approach with the potential oncologic advantages of *en bloc* transthoracic resection.[25–27] Additionally improved surgical outcomes are associated with surgery performed at a high-volume center with dedicated surgical and support teams.[28–30] The Department of Thoracic Surgery at the University of Pittsburgh Medical Center (UPMC) has embraced the minimally invasive Ivor Lewis esophagectomy as their surgical approach of choice for cancers of the EGJ.

4.2 Resection margins

Given the rich, submucosal, longitudinal lymphatic network in the esophagus, the resection margin has always been a specific point of concern due to worse prognosis associated with R1 resections. The incidence of R1 resections reported varies widely from 2.5 to 51%.[31–33] The prognostic significance of positive margins has been investigated.[13,34–42] At UPMC, we examine the specimen at the back table and obtain frozen sections of both the proximal and the distal margins.

4.2.1 Proximal (esophageal) resection margin

Several retrospective studies have assessed the importance of the proximal (esophageal) resection margin to cancer recurrence and survival in patients with EGJ tumors. A proximal esophageal margin of at least 5 cm is widely accepted as adequate. Barbour and colleagues[34] reported on 505 patients with EGJ tumors with R0 or R1 resection and no neoadjuvant therapy. Kaplan–Meier survival analysis demonstrated that patients with grossly normal proximal margin lengths greater than 3.8 cm experienced significantly improved survival (median overall survival 54 months *vs.* 29 months if the proximal margin was <3.8 cm; five-year overall survival 47% *vs.* 29%). Since the 3.8 cm length was determined in specimens that had been stretched, pinned to a cork board and fixed with formalin, the authors extrapolated that the margin length *in situ* would need to be at least 5 cm to improve survival. Multivariate analysis showed that a proximal margin >3.8 cm, along with the number of positive lymph nodes, T stage, and poor differentiation, was independently associated with survival. Subgroup analysis revealed that in patients with an R0 resection, the length of the proximal margin was a significant predictor of survival in patients with tumors more advanced than or at stage T2 or with six or fewer positive lymph nodes, but not in patients with T1 tumors or with more than six positive lymph nodes. Mariette *et al.*[13] reported outcomes in 94 patients who underwent resection for EGJ tumors. Of the 94 patients, eight patients were found with positive histologic involvement of the proximal margin. Median survival was 11.1 months in patients with a positive proximal resection margin compared with 36.3 months in patients with a negative proximal resection margin. Recurrence occurred in 9.5% of the patients with a positive margin and none (0%) of the patients with a negative margin. No R1 resections were seen in specimens with a proximal margin >7 cm from the tumor.

4.2.2 Distal (gastric) resection margin

Obtaining an R0 resection at the distal (gastric) resection margin is also associated with improved survival. Casson,[35] using a left thoracoabdominal approach, found a positive distal margin in 12% of patients with esophageal adenocarcinoma and in 28% of patients with adenocarcinoma of the gastric cardia. An R0 resection was significantly more likely if the distal margin was 4 cm as compared with 2 cm in patients with esophageal cancer and 3 cm as compared with 1 cm in patients with adenocarcinona of the gastric cardia. In patients with adenocarcinoma of the cardia and a negative distal resection margin, there was a significantly improved survival (15.4 months for R0 compared with 5.7 months for R1 resection). DiMusto and Orringer[36] reported a 2.5% incidence (26 patients) of histologically positive distal resection margins in 1,044 patients who underwent transhiatal esophagectomy for distal esophageal or EGJ cancer. The stomach was routinely divided 4–6 cm from the tumor. Of the 26 patients, nine underwent adjuvant therapy and 11 were followed with observation only. There were no differences in survival or local recurrence between the two groups.

4.3 *Lymph node involvement*

The involvement of the lymph nodes in patients with EGJ tumors influences both treatment and prognosis. Lymph nodes are affected in two different body cavities reflecting the nature of EGJ tumors. Thus, significant attention has been directed toward understanding patterns of lymph node involvement in patients with EGJ tumors and examining whether or not Siewert type I, II, and III tumors have different distributions of lymph node involvement at the mediastinal and abdominal lymph node stations.[6,8,43,44] There is evidence of increased mediastinal lymph node involvement in patients with Siewert type I tumors than in patients with type II or type III tumors.[6,43,44] However, the clinical significance of this difference is unclear. Leers and colleagues[8] found that the mediastinal lymph nodes (primarily the paraesophageal nodes) were involved in 25% of patients with distal esophageal tumors and 24% of patients with EGJ tumors, an incidence that justifies lower mediastinal node dissection for all EGJ tumors regardless of their Siewert classification. The abdominal lymph nodes seem to be affected independently from the localization of the primary tumor with involved abdominal lymph nodes, particularly those along the lesser curvature of the stomach, in >50% of patients with distal esophageal or EGJ carcinoma (Figure 1).[6,8,43,44]

Schurr[45] assessed the significance of microscopic involvement of the lymph nodes (detected using immunostaining) in 85 patients with resectable EGJ carcinoma who underwent curative surgery. There was a significant impact of nodal microinvolvement on disease-specific survival. The estimated two- and five-year overall survival rates were 77% and 39% for patients without nodal microinvolvement and 62% and 21% for patients with nodal microinvolvement.

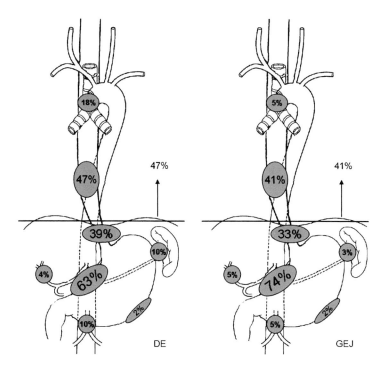

Figure 1 Lymph node involvement after *en bloc* esopahgectomy in 144 patients with distal esophageal (DE) or gastroesophageal (GEJ/ EGJ) tumors (reprinted from Ref. 8 , copyright 2009 with permission from Elsevier).

4.4 *Optimal lymphadenectomy*

The optimal number of lymph nodes to remove during potentially curative resection of esophageal cancer has been an area of active investigation. Although most studies have been done on patients without neoadjuvant therapy, there is evidence that adequate lymphadenectomy is also important in patients who receive neoadjuvant therapy with editorials and warnings from experts that neoadjuvant therapy is not a replacement for lymphadenectomy.[46,47]

Two studies have suggested that at least 18 lymph nodes should be removed and examined when curative resection is attempted. Rizk and colleagues[48] retrospectively reviewed 336 patients who underwent esophagectomy for cancer without neoadjuvant therapy during an eight-year period; 87% of the patients had EGJ tumors. Using recursive partitioning analyses, they identified 18 lymph nodes as the minimal number required for accurate staging. They further found that in patients with T2 or T3 tumors and fewer than four involved lymph nodes, survival was improved if >18 lymph nodes were examined at the time of resection. Greenstein[49] searched the SEER (Surveillance, Epidemiology, and End Results) database to identify 972 patients who had undergone esophagectomy for cancer, were node negative, and received no neoadjuvant therapy. The patients were then classified by the number of negative lymph nodes recorded: ≤10 negative lymph nodes (70% of patients), 11–17 negative lymph nodes (19% of patients), or ≥18 negative lymph nodes (11% of patients). Esophageal cancer-specific survival was significantly higher with an increasing number of negative lymph nodes. The five-year cancer-specific survival rate was 55% for patients with ≤10 negative nodes, 66% for 11–17 negative nodes, and 75% for ≥18 negative lymph nodes. The minimal number of negative lymph nodes associated with improved survival depended on the T classification of the esophageal cancer. For T1 tumors, ≥18 negative lymph nodes was associated with improved survival and for T2 or T3 ≥10 negative lymph nodes. Both studies provide evidence that at least 18 nodes should be examined to accurately stage EGJ cancer.

In another study, Rizk[50] examined data from the Worldwide Esophageal Cancer Collaboration on 4,627 patients who underwent esophagectomy for cancer using risk-adjusted five-year survival to determine the optimum number of nodes that should be resected to maximize five-year survival; 69% (2,995 patients) had distal esophageal or EGJ tumors. The study found that T status affected the number of lymph nodes required for optimal lymphadenectomy. For pN0M0 cancers, optimum lymphadenectomy was 10–12 nodes for pT1, 15–22 for pT2, and 31–42 for pT3/T4. For pN+M0 cancers with 1–6 positive nodes, optimum lymphadenectomy was 10 for pT1, 15 for pT2, and 29–50 for pT3/T4. Mariette and colleagues[51] reviewed 536 patients who underwent *en bloc* esophagectomy with an R0 resection; ~50% of the patients received neoadjuvant therapy. Patients with more than four positive lymph nodes or a lymph node ratio >0.2 experienced more recurrence and worse survival. When fewer than 15 lymph nodes were examined, the lymph node ratio predicted survival more accurately than the number of positive lymph nodes. In contrast, when 15 or more nodes were examined, such that the patient was considered adequately staged, the number of positive lymph nodes predicted survival more accurately than the lymph node ratio. Peyre and colleagues[52] studied 2,303 patients at multiple centers who underwent R0 esophagectomy, were node negative and received no neoadjuvant therapy. The number of lymph nodes removed was an independent predictor of survival, as were the presence of nodal metastasis, the number of involved nodes, tumor depth, and the histologic cancer type. Sampling at least 23 lymph nodes was associated with increased survival.

Using the National Comprehensive Cancer Network (NCCN) guideline that at least 15 lymph nodes should be dissected and assessed during an adequate lymphadenectomy, the adequacy of lymphadenectomy as performed by surgeons in the United States was assessed by Merkow and colleagues.[53] They examined data from the National Cancer Database. From 1998 to 2007, 13,995 patients from 639 hospitals underwent esophagectomy for cancer; only 28.7% (4,014 patients) had at least 15 lymph nodes examined. When examined by center, 45 centers (7%) examined a median of at least 15 lymph nodes, comprising 8.7% of academic hospitals and 6.2% of community hospitals. These numbers improved when only the most recent data (2005–2007) was examined with 38.9% of academic centers and 28.0% of community hospitals examining a median of at least 15 nodes. Patients treated at high-volume centers (defined as more than 12 cases per year) had 15 or more nodes examined significantly more often than patients treated at low-volume centers.

4.5 *Extent of lymphadenectomy*

While the number of lymph nodes that constitute an adequate dissection is slowly being defined, there remains controversy regarding the extent of lymphadenectomy when considering a two-field (abdominal and thoracic) *vs.* a three-field (abdominal, thoracic and cervical) dissection. Most of the experience with three-field lymph node dissection comes from Japan where the spectrum of disease is mainly squamous cell carcinoma, which is typically located more proximally in the esophagus. In the Western hemisphere, distal esophageal and EGJ adenocarcinoma is the predominant presentation of esophageal cancer, two-field dissection is most commonly performed, and fewer surgeons advocate a three-field dissection.[54–56]

The only randomized study comparing three-field and two-field lymph node dissection failed to show any survival advantage and found significant morbidity associated with the three-field dissection. Nishihara and colleagues[56] randomized 32 patients to receive three-field (extended) lymphadenectomy and 30 patients to receive two-field lymphadenectomy; all the patients had squamous cell esophageal carcinoma. Of the patients who underwent three-field lymphadenectomy, 18 patients (56%) experienced recurrent laryngeal nerve palsy and 17 (53%) required tracheostomy. In contrast, only 9 of the 30 patients who underwent two-field lymphadenectomy experienced recurrent laryngeal nerve palsy (30%) and only three (10%) required tracheostomy. The three-field lymphadenectomy group showed improved, but not significantly different, five-year survival (66.2% *vs.* 48%). Another argument in favor of two-field lymph node dissection comes from the low observed esophageal cancer recurrence rate (6–9%) to the cervical nodes.[57–59]

5 Surgical Approaches

A gastric tube constructed from the proximal portion of the stomach is the most frequently used replacement conduit during esophagectomy and is a logical replacement after resection of most EGJ tumors. A left thoractomy approach was first introduced more than 60 years ago and was the standard approach for more than 30 years. Other approaches for open esophagectomy include the Ivor Lewis approach, the McKeown (three-incision) approach, and the left thoracoabdominal approach. To minimize the morbidity associated with thoracotomy, transhiatal esophagectomy is favored by some surgeons. We utilize a minimally invasive laparoscopic and thoracoscopic approach to reduce the morbidity associated with open esophectomy. These approaches are summarized below.

5.1 *Ivor Lewis esophagectomy*

Considered a transthoracic approach, the Ivor Lewis esophagectomy encompasses abdominal and right thoracotomy incisions. After tumor excision, the esophageal continuity is reestablished using a gastric tube constructed from the proximal portion of the stomach. A single anastomosis is performed in the chest. The Ivor Lewis esophagectomy was initially described as a two-stage procedure and has evolved to a single stage.[60–62] The Ivor Lewis esophagectomy permits *en bloc* resection of midesophageal, distal esophageal, and EGJ tumors and facilitates completion of a two-field lymphadenectomy. It is very well suited for resection of EGJ tumors. Complications which may be associated with Ivor Lewis esophagectomy include anastomotic leak, delayed gastric emptying, gastroesophageal reflux, respiratory failure, and pneumonia.[63,64]

5.2 *McKeown (three-incision) esophagectomy*

This transthoracic approach encompasses cervical, abdominal, and right thoracotomy incisions. After tumor excision, the esophageal continuity is reestablished using a gastric tube constructed from the proximal portion of the stomach, similar to the Ivor Lewis technique. A single anastomosis is performed at the neck.[65,66] *En bloc* resection of midesophageal, distal esophageal, and EGJ tumors and three-field lymphadenectomy are possible using the McKeown approach. Benefits of the McKeown approach include the ability to resect the proximal margin higher on the esophagus and easier management of anastomotic leaks if they occur. Recurrent laryngeal nerve injury as a result of the cervical anastomosis can be a significant complication.[66,67] Other complications include anastomotic leak, delayed gastric emptying, respiratory failure, and pneumonia.

5.3 *Left thoracoabdominal esophagectomy*

Although the left thoracoabdominal esophagectomy (sometimes called the Sweet procedure) is not used as commonly as the Ivor Lewis or McKoewn approaches, it is a useful option especially for tumors of the EGJ.[68–70] The left thoracoabdominal approach can be used for esophagectomy, total gastrectomy, or roux-en-Y reconstruction. It provides excellent exposure using a single incision with the ability to access the superior mediastinum from inferior pulmonary ligament to the aortic arch. The thoracoabdominal approach can be used with or without a neck incision to resect EGJ tumors allowing placement of the anastomosis in either the chest or the neck. Typical complications include anastomotic leak and chylothorax.[68,71,72]

5.4 *Transhiatal esophagectomy*

Transhiatal esophagectomy was first introduced in 1933 by Turner but was not commonly used until 1978 when Orringer and Sloan showed it was feasible and could be associated with lower morbidity and mortality than transthoracic approaches.[73,74] This reduction in morbidity was mainly because the use of a cervical anastomosis prevented mediastinitis caused by leaks of intrathoracic anastomoses. The transhiatal esophagectomy is performed through a laparotomy and a cervical incision. The anastomosis is performed at the neck. *En bloc* esophagectomy can be accomplished for distal esophageal and EGJ tumors. Avoidance of a thoracotomy is thought to be the primary benefit of the transhiatal approach. Other benefits include the ability to maximize the proximal resection margin, fewer pulmonary complications, and the ability to better manage an anastomotic leak should one occur. Additionally, gastroesphageal reflux is not a common side effect of the surgery. However, the ability to perform adequate two-field lymphadectomy is limited using the transhiatal approach. Complications typically associated with transhiatal esophagectomy include recurrent laryngeal nerve injury, bleeding, airway injuries, chylothorax, and anastomotic leak.[75]

5.5 *Transhiatal extended total gastrectomy*

Transhiatal extended total gastrectomy is considered useful for proximal gastric cancers involving the EGJ and for transhiatal resection of distal esophagus.[14,76]

5.6 *Minimally invasive esophagectomy*

MIE was initially described by Cuschieri, DePaula, and their colleagues and represents one of the most recent developments in the natural evolution of esophageal surgery. Although it requires advanced and complex laparoscopic and thoracoscopic skills, MIE has been adopted by the thoracic surgical community due to the many potential benefits derived from the minimally invasive approaches.[77–81] Based on our experience, our current, preferred approach is to perform a minimally invasive Ivor Lewis esophagectomy with two-field lymph node dissection in patients with resectable esophageal cancer. The advantages of this approach include better exposure and access in the chest, the potential for an improved rate of complete resection, the potential for better gastric margins, improved lymph node dissection in the mediastinum, and lower rates of anastomotic and recurrent laryngeal nerve complications. Minimally invasive esophagectomy using a transhiatal approach or modified McKoewn techniques have also been utilized.[27,79,80] Additionally, gastrectomy and roux-en-Y reconstruction can be performed as minimally invasive surgeries.[82,83]

5.6.1 *Surgical procedure for Ivor Lewis MIE*

- Laparoscopic phase
  - Port placement (Figure 2(A))
  - Exploration
    - On-table endoscopy to confirm preoperative findings and ensure that the stomach is suitable as a gastric conduit
  - Division of gastrohepatic ligament
  - *En bloc* lymph node dissection
  - Isolation and division of left gastric artery/vein pedicle
  - Esophageal dissection from hiatus
  - Posterior mobilization of the stomach
  - Dissection along greater curvature
    - Preserving gastroepiploic arcade
    - Dividing short gastric vessels
  - Creation of the gastric tube (Figure 2(B))
  - Pyloroplasty
  - Placement of feeding jejunostomy tube
- Thoracoscopic phase
  - Mobilization of thoracic esophagus
  - Division of the azygos vein

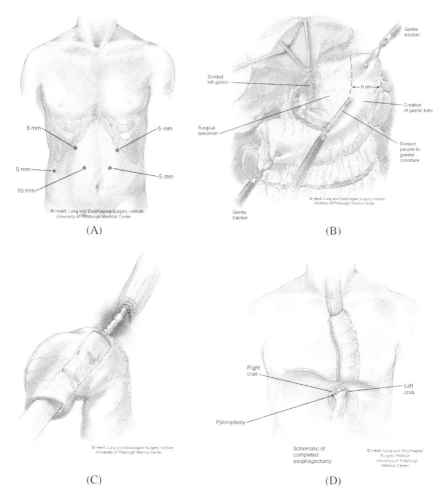

Figure 2 Ivor Lewis minimally invasive esophagectomy (MIE). (A) Port placement for laparoscopy; (B) gastric mobilization and creation of the gastric tube; (C) stapled esophagogastric anastomosis; and (D) the completed Ivor Lewis MIE.

- ○ *En bloc* dissection
  - ▪ Includes the paraesophageal and subcarinal lymph nodes
- ○ Division of the esophagus above the level of the azygos vein
- ○ Creation of gastroesophageal anastomosis (Figures 2(C,D))
- ○ Drain placement

After the introduction of MIE, studies were performed to show it was safe and that perioperative outcomes were not inferior to the standard open esophagectomy.[79,84] As a result, MIE is now widely accepted as a safe procedure with similar oncological outcomes in the intermediate-term as open esophagectomy and with some benefits from its minimally invasive nature. Our successful outcomes with MIE in more than 1,000 patients treated at our institution and in patients treated in a prospective, phase II, multicenter trial are discussed in detail below (in the subsection on survival as an oncologic outcomes after surgical treatment).[27,84]

6 Oncologic Outcomes After Surgical Treatment

6.1 *Survival*

Several large case series have demonstrated that surgical resection of EGJ tumors is feasible and can be done with good outcomes and low morbidity and mortality. Although most studies have not focused on survival specifically in patients with EGJ tumors, the studies define the approaches available for surgical treatment of all types of esophageal carcinoma. Siewert[6] presented his 23-year experience (1982–2005) and assessed outcomes in 1,602 patients with adenocarcinoma of the EGJ who underwent surgical resection as according to the Siewert tumor classification: type I, radical transmediastinal or transthoracic *en bloc* esophagectomy with resection of the proximal stomach; type II, extended gastrectomy with transhiatal resection of the distal esophagus (most frequently) or esophagectomy (occasionally); and type III, extended total gastrectomy with transhiatal resection of the distal esophagus. Patients with R0 resections had significant better survival (five-year survival 43.2%; 10-year survival 32.7%) than patients with R1 resection (five-year survival 13%; 10-year survival 11%). The 30-day mortality was higher with transthoracic esophagectomy (6.9%) than with transmediastinal esophagectomy (4.8%). Overall 30-day mortality was 3.8%, with mortality of 1.9% in the last part of the study period. Orringer[75] presented a 30-year experience (1976–2006) in over 2,000 patients who underwent transhiatal esophagectomy; 1,525 patients had malignant disease including 1,204 with distal esophageal or EGJ cancers. Orringer divided patients treated during the 30-year study period into 2 groups (group 1, 1976–1998, 1,063 patients; group 2, 1998–2006, 944 patients). The hospital mortality was 4% for group 1 and decreased to 1% for group 2. Overall five-year survival was 31%.

We have reported the long-term results (median follow-up 62.8 months) of a prospective phase II trial of neoadjuvant chemotherapy, followed by esophagectomy and adjuvant chemotherapy for locally advanced (99% with T3 and/or node positive disease) esophageal carcinoma at the University of Pittsburgh Cancer Institute.[85] The majority of patients underwent a transthoracic esophagectomy and 94% of patients had adenocarcinoma. The median overall survival of the entire group was 27.4 months. Nodal status was an important predictor of overall survival.

In a recent publication,[27] we reported our experience performing MIEs from 1996 to 2011. A total of 1,011 patients underwent MIE including 960 patients with malignant disease. We initially adopted a modified McKeown, three-incision MIE and gradually evolved to a modified minimally invasive Ivor Lewis esophagectomy. Therefore, 481 patients underwent McKeown MIE and 530 underwent Ivor Lewis MIE. The tumor was located in the distal esophagus or at the EGJ in 849 patients, and distal/EGJ tumors comprised 90% of those removed using the McKeown MIE and 97% of the tumors removed using the Ivor Lewis MIE. The total 30-day operative mortality was 1.7%, and in the later part of the study period, when Ivor Lewis MIE was performed almost exclusively, 30-day mortality dropped to 0.9%. An R0 resection was achieved in 98% of the patients. The median number of resected lymph nodes was 21. The median ICU stay was two days, and the median hospital stay was eight days. The incidence of recurrent laryngeal nerve injury was significantly lower in the Ivor Lewis group. At a median follow-up of 20 months, survival varied by tumor stage and was comparable to open series. Further proof that MIE can be performed with low morbidity and mortality and good oncologic results was provided in a recently published multicenter clinical trial coordinated by the Eastern Cooperative Oncology Group (ECOG).[84] Patients were enrolled at 17 centers with surgeons who were credentialed as having experience with both esophagetomy and minimally invasive surgery. Using MIE with either an Ivor Lewis or modified McKeown approach, an R0 resection was accomplished in 96% of patients (99/104) and a median of 19 lymph nodes were retrieved per patient. Median hospital stay was nine days, and 30-day mortality in eligible patients who underwent MIE was 2.1%. At a median follow-up of 35.8 months, estimated three-year overall survival was 58.4%. Survival by pathologic stage was similar to that seen after open esophagectomy.

6.2 *Recurrence*

Because a large number of patients experience recurrence after radical resection of esophageal cancer, it is important to understand the recurrence patterns of EGJ tumors. Wayman and colleagues[86] assessed recurrence of EGJ carcinoma classified by Siewert type. They found that type I and type II adenocarcinoma of the EGJ both have a predominantly early, hematogenous pattern of recurrence. Of 169 patients with EGJ tumors, 103 patients developed proven recurrent disease with no significant difference in recurrence between the Siewert types. The median time to recurrence was 23.3 months (range 14.2–32.4 months) for patients with type I tumors and 20.5 months (range 11.6–29.4 months) for patients with type II tumors. The most frequent type of recurrence was hematogenous, and most (56%) were detected within a year of surgery. The most frequent sites of hematogenous recurrence were the liver (27%), bone (18%), brain (11%), and lung (11%). Local recurrence occurred in 33% of patients with type I tumors and 29% of patients with type II tumors. Nodal recurrence occurred in 18% of patients with type I tumors and 25% of patients with type II tumors. Peritoneal dissemination led to recurrence in 11 patients (11%) — four with type I tumors and seven with type II. De Manzoni[87] reviewed patterns of recurrence in 92 patients with EGJ tumors who underwent R0 resection. There were 55 patients with recurrence; most (80%) within two years of resection. Recurrence was systemic in 49%, locoregional in 42%, and peritoneal in 18%. Lymph node involvement was the only predictor of recurrence. Dresner[58] examined recurrence in 176 patients who underwent an R0 resection; 64% had adenocarcinoma. Overall recurrence rate was 48%, of which 27% were locoregional (21% mediastinal and 6% cervical), 18% were distant, and 3% were synchronous. Predictors of recurrence were T and N stage. Similarly, Mariette[88] examined recurrence in 439 patients after R0 transthoracic resection and two-field lymphadenectomy. Overall, there was 52% recurrence rate: 12% local, 20% regional (cervical 3.6%, mediastinal 14%, and abdominal 2%), and 19.8% distant. The median time to recurrence was 12 months. In the multicenter ECOG 2202 trial investigating MIE, the estimated 3-year recurrence rate was 33.8%. Locoregional recurrence occurred in 6.9%, distant recurrence in 18.6%, and both locoregional and distant recurrence in 2.0% of patients.[84]

The completeness of the resection and status of the resection margins are a critical determinants of recurrence. Smit[89] reported on 220 patients with esophageal and EGJ tumors (85% with adenocarcinoma) who underwent resection with curative intent. Radical transthoracic resection with two-field lymph node dissection was performed for proximal tumors and left thoracolaparotomy approach was used for distal and EGJ tumors. An R0 resection was possible in 87%; the average number of resected lymph nodes was 11. The overall recurrence rate was 28% after a year, 44% after two years, and 64% after five years. Locoregional recurrences were found in 17% after a year, 27% after two years, and 43% after five years. Recurrence significantly impacted survival with five-year survival in 73% of patients with no recurrence versus 8% for patients with recurrence. Prognostic factors for recurrence were pT, pN (>4 nodes), positive lymph node ratio>0.2, and an R1 resection. Hulscher[59] examined recurrence after transhiatal esophagectomy in 137 patients with distal or midesophageal tumors of which 69% were adenocarcinoma. The overall recurrence rate in these patients was 52%, distributed as follows: 23% locoregional, 15% systemic, 13.9% both locoregional and systemic, and 8% cervical lymph node recurrence. Bone, liver, and lung were the most frequent sites of recurrence. The median time to recurrence was 11 months (range 1.4–62.5 months). Of the 137 patients, 28 patients had an R1 resection and were more likely to have recurrence (78.6% recurrence as compared with 45% recurrence when an R0 resection was accomplished). In multivariate analysis, an R1 resection was a significant prognostic indicator for recurrence.

7 Comparative Studies of Surgical Approaches

A single optimal surgical approach for esophagectomy has not been identified, and no single approach can be expected to fit all the possible clinical presentations of EGJ tumors. Nonetheless, some comparative studies have been performed, which inform the esophageal surgeon on the strengths and weaknesses of each approach.

7.1 *Transhiatal versus transthoracic esophagectomy*

Most studies comparing transthoracic and transhiatal esophagectomy are retrospective, and many assess a small number of patients treated over a long period of time. There are very few randomized studies, and leak definitions vary from study to study. The studies show a trend toward lower early postoperative morbidity with transhiatal esophagectomy, but no difference in long-term survival between the two techniques.[21–24,90–93] Systematic reviews, meta-analyses, and analyses of large databases have also been performed to compare transhiatal and transthoracic esophagectomy. Rindani[94] published a review of the literature from 1986 to 1996 compiling 2,675 patients who underwent transhiatal esophagectomy and 2,808 patients underwent Ivor Lewis esophagectomy. No differences in pulmonary or cardiovascular complications, wound infection, or the incidence of chylothorax were seen, but there seemed to be an increased risk of anastomotic complications and recurrent laryngeal nerve injury with the transhiatal approach. The two approaches had similar short-term and long-term mortality. Hulscher and colleagues[21] performed a meta-analysis of 50 studies published between 1990 and 1999, totaling 7,527 patients. Twenty-four studies compared the two techniques directly but only three were randomized; 15 studies assessed transthoracic esophagectomy only, and 11 reported on only transhiatal esophagectomy. In the meta-analysis, there were no significant differences identified in three- and five-year survival rates between the two approaches. Short-term mortality was significantly higher in patients who received transthoracic resection (9.2% *vs.* 5.7%), and transthoracic resections had a higher risk of pulmonary complications, chylous leak, and wound infection. Anastomotic leak and vocal cord paralysis were more frequent after transhiatal resection. Chang[90] reviewed the SEER-Medicare database from 1992 to 2002 to identify 868 patients, 225 who underwent transhiatal esophagectomy and 643 who underwent transthoracic esophagectomy. Short-term mortality was significantly lower after transhiatal resection (6.7% *vs.* 13.1%), but there was no difference in long-term survival.

In a landmark study published in the *New England Journal of Medicine*, Hulscher and colleagues[22] randomized 220 patients with distal esophageal or EGJ adenocarcinoma to undergo either transhiatal esophagectomy (106 patients) or transthoracic esophagectomy (114 patients). The transthoracic approach was associated with higher perioperative morbidity, but there were no differences short-term mortality between the two approaches. Additionally, there was a trend toward improved long-term survival at five years with the extended transthoracic approach. A second analysis was performed when five-year follow-up was complete on all patients and assessed survival differences between the two approaches as a function of tumor location and lymph node status.[23] There were no differences in survival based on surgical approach in patients with either negative lymph nodes or with more than eight involved lymph nodes at the time of the resection. However, in patients with 1–8 positive lymph nodes, increased disease-free survival was seen in patients who underwent transthoracic resection.

As demonstrated by Hulscher's study,[23] adequate lymph node removal is an important consideration when comparing transthoracic and transhiatal esophagectomy. Wolff[95] retrospectively reviewed outcomes of esophagectomy in 517 patients who underwent esophagectomy over a 10-year period (1994–2004). The surgical approach was transhiatal in 68 patients and transthoracic via either an Ivor Lewis esophagectomy or extended Ivor Lewis esophagectomy in 449 patients. Significantly more lymph nodes were retrieved with the Ivor Lewis approaches (mean 18.5 lymph nodes) than with the transhiatal approach (mean nine lymph nodes). This is an important consideration given the emerging importance of adequate lymph node dissection. Leers[8] found mediastinal lymph node involvement in 41% of patients with EGJ tumors and 47% of patients with distal esophageal adenocarcinoma. Based on this observation, they recommended transthoracic esophagectomy for distal esophageal and EGJ tumors in order to achieve adequate mediastinal lymph node removal.

7.2 *Minimally invasive versus open esophagectomies*

Several systematic reviews and meta-analyses have been conducted to assess the differences between open esophagectomy and MIE. In 2009, Biere[96] reviewed 10 studies (one controlled but not randomized clinical trial and nine case-control studies) for a total of 1,061 patients. There was no difference in morbidity, anastomotic leak, or lymph node retrieval between the two approaches. A trend toward fewer pulmonary complications with MIE was noted. Nagpal[97] reviewed 12 studies compiling 672 patients who underwent MIE and 612 patients who underwent open esophagectomy. There was no significant difference in 30-day mortality between the open esopahectomy and MIE groups. The MIE group had less blood loss, shorter hospital stays, reduced morbidity, and fewer respiratory complications. The complications of anastomotic leak, gastric conduit ischemia, chyle leak, and recurrent laryngeal nerve injury occurred at similar frequencies in each group. No difference in lymph node retrieval was detected. Sgourakis[98] reviewed eight trials for a total of 1,008 patients in a meta-analysis. The patients who underwent MIE had less morbidity overall but higher incidence of anastomotic stricture. Dantoc,[99] in another meta-analysis, reviewed literature published from 1950 to 2012 comparing open esophagectomy and MIE. Dantoc identified 16 case-control studies for a total of 1,212 patients. No statistically significant differences were found in short-term or long-term survival. Significantly more lymph nodes were retrieved with MIE (median of 16 nodes with MIE as compared with 10 nodes with open surgery). The authors concluded that open esophagectomy and MIE had equivalent oncologic outcomes.

Biere[100] recently published the first randomized, controlled trial directly comparing open esophagectomy and MIE that took place at five centers in three countries. Fifty-six patients underwent open esophagectomy, and 59 underwent MIE. For the MIE group, there was significant less postoperative pain, less pneumonia (34% *vs.* 12%), shorter median hospital stay, and better short-term quality of life as compared with the open esophagectomy group. These findings are concordant with the findings of the previous case-control series and meta-analyses.

8 Conclusions

Accurate preoperative staging is important for selection of appropriate treatment options. Surgical resection is an essential element of any potentially curative strategy to treat EGJ cancers. An R0 resection is essential to maximize survival and minimize recurrence. It is becoming increasingly clear that adequate lymph node dissection is an important component of resection, and is needed for accurate staging. Each surgeon will have preferences regarding approach based on his or her training, experience, and typical case referral pattern. We favor the MIE using an Ivor Lewis approach with a two-field lymphadenectomy, as we have found that this approach gives excellent exposure and access in chest, which increases the likelihood of a complete resection and facilitates lymph node dissection in the mediastinum. We have encountered fewer anastomotic complications and practically eliminated complications associated with recurrent laryngeal nerve injury using this approach. MIE is a viable approach to reduce the morbidity of esophagectomy while maintaining sound oncologic principles of resection and lymph node dissection to optimize outcomes.

References

1. Esophagus and esophagogastric junction. In: Edge SB, American Joint Committee on Cancer, eds. *AJCC Cancer Staging Manual*, 7th edn. New York: Springer; 2010, pp. 103–115.

2. Luketich JD, *et al*. Evaluation of distant metastases in esophageal cancer: 100 consecutive positron emission tomography scans. *Ann Thorac Surg* 1999;**68**:1133–1136; discussion 1136–1137.

3. Varghese Jr, *et al*. The society of thoracic surgeons guidelines on the diagnosis and staging of patients with esophageal cancer. *Ann Thorac Surg* 2013;**96**:346–356.

4. Siewert JR, Stein HJ. Classification of adenocarcinoma of the oesophagogastric junction. *Br J Surg* 1998;**85**:1457–1459.

5. Siewert JR, *et al*. Biologic and clinical variations of adenocarcinoma at the esophago-gastric junction: Relevance of a topographic-anatomic subclassification. *J Surg Oncol* 2005;**90**:139–146; discussion 146.

6. Feith M, *et al*. Adenocarcinoma of the esophagogastric junction: Surgical therapy based on 1602 consecutive resected patients. *Surg Oncol Clin North Am* 2006;**15**: 751–764.

7. Harrison LE, *et al*. Total gastrectomy is not necessary for proximal gastric cancer. *Surgery* 1998;**123**:127–130.

8. Leers JM, *et al*. Clinical characteristics, biologic behavior, and survival after esophagectomy are similar for adenocarcinoma of the gastroesophageal junction and the distal esophagus. *J Thorac Cardiovasc Surg* 2009;**138**:594–602; discussion 601–592.

9. Curtis NJ, *et al*. The relevance of the siewert classification in the era of multimodal therapy for adenocarcinoma of the gastro-oesophageal junction. *J Surg Oncol* 2014; **109**:202–207.

10. Van de Ven C, *et al*. Three-field lymphadenectomy and pattern of lymph node spread in t3 adenocarcinoma of the distal esophagus and the gastro-esophageal junction. *Eur J Cardiothorac Surg* 1999;**15**:769–773.

11. Wijnhoven BP, *et al*. Adenocarcinomas of the distal oesophagus and gastric cardia are one clinical entity. Rotterdam oesophageal tumour study group. *Br J Surg* 1999;**86**: 529–535.

12. Rice TW, *et al*. Worldwide Esophageal Cancer C. Cancer of the esophagus and esophagogastric junction: Data-driven staging for the 7th edition of the American Joint Committee on Cancer/International Union Against Cancer Staging Manuals. *Cancer* 2010;**116**:3763–3773.

13. Mariette C, *et al*. Extent of oesophageal resection for adenocarcinoma of the oesophagogastric junction. *Eur J Surg Oncol* 2003;**29**:588–593.

14. Papachristou DN, Fortner JG. Adenocarcinoma of the gastric cardia. The choice of gastrectomy. *Ann Surg* 1980;**192**:58–64.

15. Stipa S, *et al*. Surgical treatment of adenocarcinoma of the cardia. *Surgery* 1992;**111**:386–393.

16. von Rahden BH, *et al*. Surgical management of esophagogastric junction tumors. *World J Gastroenterol* 2006;**12**:6608–6613.

17. Pennathur A, *et al*. Surgical aspects of the patient with high-grade dysplasia. *Semin Thorac Cardiovasc Surg* 2005;**17**:326–332.

18. Pennathur A, Luketich JD. Resection for esophageal cancer: Strategies for optimal management. *Ann Thorac Surg* 2008;**85**:S751–S756.
19. Pennathur A, *et al*. The "best operation" for esophageal cancer? *Ann Thorac Surg* 2010;**89**:S2163–S2167.
20. Luketich JD, *et al*. Master Techniques in Surgery: Esophageal Surgery. 1st edition. Philadelphia, PA: Wolters Kluwer Health; 2014.
21. Hulscher JB, *et al*. Transthoracic versus transhiatal resection for carcinoma of the esophagus: A meta-analysis. *Ann Thorac Surg* 2001;**72**:306–313.
22. Hulscher JB, *et al*. Extended transthoracic resection compared with limited transhiatal resection for adenocarcinoma of the esophagus. *N Engl J Med* 2002;**347**:1662–1669.
23. Omloo JM, *et al*. Extended transthoracic resection compared with limited transhiatal resection for adenocarcinoma of the mid/distal esophagus: Five-year survival of a randomized clinical trial. *Ann Surg* 2007;**246**:992–1000; discussion 1000–1001.
24. Omloo JM, *et al*. Short and long-term advantages of transhiatal and transthoracic oesophageal cancer resection. *Eur J Surg Oncol* 2009;**35**:793–797.
25. Berger AC, *et al*. Oncologic efficacy is not compromised, and may be improved with minimally invasive esophagectomy. *J Am Coll Surg* 2011;**212**:560–566; discussion 566–568.
26. Carr SR, Luketich JD. Minimally invasive esophagectomy. An update on the options available. *Minerva Chir* 2008;**63**:481–495.
27. Luketich JD, *et al*. Outcomes after minimally invasive esophagectomy: Review of over 1000 patients. *Ann Surg* 2012;**256**:95–103.
28. Birkmeyer JD, *et al*. Hospital volume and surgical mortality in the united states. *N Engl J Med* 2002;**346**:1128–1137.
29. Birkmeyer JD, *et al*. Surgeon volume and operative mortality in the United States. *N Engl J Med* 2003;**349**:2117–2127.
30. Swisher SG, *et al*. Effect of operative volume on morbidity, mortality, and hospital use after esophagectomy for cancer. *J Thorac Cardiovasc Surg* 2000;**119**:1126–1132.
31. Law S, *et al*. The significance of histologically infiltrated resection margin after esophagectomy for esophageal cancer. *Am J Surg* 1998;**176**:286–290.
32. Mattioli S, *et al*. Surgical therapy for adenocarcinoma of the cardia: Modalities of recurrence and extension of resection. *Dis Esophagus* 2001;**14**:104–109.
33. Papachristou DN, *et al*. Histologically positive esophageal margin in the surgical treatment of gastric cancer. *Am J Surg* 1980;**139**:711–713.
34. Barbour AP, *et al*. Adenocarcinoma of the gastroesophageal junction: Influence of esophageal resection margin and operative approach on outcome. *Ann Surg* 2007;**246**:1–8.
35. Casson AG, *et al*. What is the optimal distal resection margin for esophageal carcinoma? *Ann Thorac Surg* 2000;**69**:205–209.
36. DiMusto PD, Orringer MB. Transhiatal esophagectomy for distal and cardia cancers: Implications of a positive gastric margin. *Ann Thorac Surg* 2007;**83**:1993–1998; discussion 1998–1999.

37. Dexter SP, *et al.* Circumferential resection margin involvement: An independent predictor of survival following surgery for oesophageal cancer. *Gut* 2001;**48**:667–670.

38. Griffiths EA, *et al.* The prognostic value of circumferential resection margin involvement in oesophageal malignancy. *Eur J Surg Oncol* 2006;**32**:413–419.

39. Chan DS, *et al.* Systematic review and meta-analysis of the influence of circumferential resection margin involvement on survival in patients with operable oesophageal cancer. *Br J Surg* 2013;**100**:456–464.

40. Khan OA, *et al.* Prognostic significance of circumferential resection margin involvement following oesophagectomy for cancer. *Br J Cancer* 2003;**88**:1549–1552.

41. Scheepers JJ, *et al.* Influence of circumferential resection margin on prognosis in distal esophageal and gastroesophageal cancer approached through the transhiatal route. *Dis Esophagus* 2009;**22**:42–48.

42. Gilbert S, *et al.* Prognostic significance of a positive radial margin after esophageal cancer resection. *J Thorac Cardiovasc Surg* 2015;**149**:548–555.

43. Dresner SM, *et al.* The pattern of metastatic lymph node dissemination from adenocarcinoma of the esophagogastric junction. *Surgery* 2001;**129**:103–109.

44. Monig SP, *et al.* Topographical distribution of lymph node metastasis in adenocarcinoma of the gastroesophageal junction. *Hepato-gastroenterology* 2002;**49**: 419–422.

45. Schurr PG, *et al.* Lymphatic spread and microinvolvement in adenocarcinoma of the esophago-gastric junction. *J Surg Oncol* 2006;**94**:307–315.

46. Stiles BM, *et al.* Worldwide oesophageal cancer collaboration guidelines for lymphadenectomy predict survival following neoadjuvant therapy. *Eur J Cardiothorac Surg* 2012;**42**:659–664.

47. Lerut T. Cancer of the oesophagus and gastrooesophageal junction: Neoadjuvant therapy should not be a surrogate for suboptimal lymphadenectomy. *Eur J Cardiothorac Surg* 2012;**42**:664–666.

48. Rizk N, *et al.* The prognostic importance of the number of involved lymph nodes in esophageal cancer: Implications for revisions of the american joint committee on cancer staging system. *J Thorac Cardiovasc Surg* 2006;**132**:1374–1381.

49. Greenstein AJ, *et al.* Effect of the number of lymph nodes sampled on postoperative survival of lymph node-negative esophageal cancer. *Cancer* 2008;**112**:1239–1246.

50. Rizk NP, *et al.* Optimum lymphadenectomy for esophageal cancer. *Ann Surg* 2010;**251**:46–50.

51. Mariette C, *et al.* The number of metastatic lymph nodes and the ratio between metastatic and examined lymph nodes are independent prognostic factors in esophageal cancer regardless of neoadjuvant chemoradiation or lymphadenectomy extent. *Ann Surg* 2008;**247**:365–371.

52. Peyre CG, *et al.* The number of lymph nodes removed predicts survival in esophageal cancer: An international study on the impact of extent of surgical resection. *Ann Surg* 2008;**248**:549–556.

53. Merkow RP, *et al.* Variation in lymph node examination after esophagectomy for cancer in the united states. *Arch Surg* 2012;**147**:505–511.

54. Altorki N, *et al.* Three-field lymph node dissection for squamous cell and adenocarcinoma of the esophagus. *Ann Surg* 2002;**236**:177–183.

55. Lerut T, *et al.* Three-field lymphadenectomy for carcinoma of the esophagus and gastroesophageal junction in 174 r0 resections: Impact on staging, disease-free survival, and outcome: A plea for adaptation of tnm classification in upper-half esophageal carcinoma. *Ann Surg* 2004;**240**:962–972; discussion 972–964.

56. Nishihira T, *et al.* A prospective randomized trial of extended cervical and superior mediastinal lymphadenectomy for carcinoma of the thoracic esophagus. *Am J Surg* 1998;**175**:47–51.

57. Clark GW, *et al.* Nodal metastasis and sites of recurrence after *en bloc* esophagectomy for adenocarcinoma. *Ann Thorac Surg* 1994;**58**:646–653; discussion 653–644.

58. Dresner SM, Griffin SM. Pattern of recurrence following radical oesophagectomy with two-field lymphadenectomy. *Br J Surg* 2000;**87**:1426–1433.

59. Hulscher JB, *et al.* The recurrence pattern of esophageal carcinoma after transhiatal resection. *J Am Coll Surg* 2000;**191**:143–148.

60. Lewis I. Carcinoma of the oesophagus. Radical resection with oesophagogastrotomy for a midthoracic growth by a right transpleural approach. *J R Soc Med* 1945;**38**:482–483.

61. Lewis I. The surgical treatment of carcinoma of the esophagus with special reference to a new operation for growths of the middle third. *Br J Surg* 1946;**34**:18–31.

62. Visbal AL, *et al.* Ivor lewis esophagogastrectomy for esophageal cancer. *Ann Thorac Surg* 2001;**71**:1803–1808.

63. Mathisen DJ, *et al.* Transthoracic esophagectomy: A safe approach to carcinoma of the esophagus. *Ann Thorac Surg* 1988;**45**:137–143.

64. Reed CE. Technique of open Ivor Lewis esophagectomy. *Oper Tech Thorac Cardiovasc Surg* 2009;**14**:160–175.

65. McKeown KC. Total three-stage oesophagectomy for cancer of the oesophagus. *Br J Surg* 1976;**63**:259–262.

66. Swanson SJ, Sugarbaker DJ. The three-hole esophagectomy. The Brigham and Women's Hospital approach (modified Mckeown technique). *Chest Surg Clin North Am* 2000;**10**:531–552.

67. Bakhos CT, *et al.* Impact of the surgical technique on pulmonary morbidity after esophagectomy. *Ann Thorac Surg* 2012;**93**:221–226; discussion 226–227.

68. Forshaw MJ, *et al.* Left thoracoabdominal esophagogastrectomy: Still a valid operation for carcinoma of the distal esophagus and esophagogastric junction. *Dis Esophagus* 2006;**19**:340–345.

69. Garlock JH, Klein SH. The surgical treatment of carcinoma of the esophagus and cardia; an analysis of 457 cases. *Ann Surg* 1954;**139**:19–34.

70. Sweet RH. The treatment of carcinoma of the esophagus and cardiac end of the stomach by surgical extirpation: 203 cases of resection. *Surgery* 1948;**23**:952–975.

71. Kirby TJ. Pitfalls and complications of left thoracoabdominal esophagectomy. *Chest Surg Clin North Am* 1997;**7**:613–622.

72. Heitmiller RF. Results of standard left thoracoabdominal esophagogastrectomy. *Semin Thorac Cardiovasc Surg* 1992;**4**:314–319.

73. Orringer MB, Sloan H. Esophagectomy without thoracotomy. *J Thorac Cardiovasc Surg* 1978;**76**:643–654.
74. Turner G. Excision of the thoracic œsophagus for carcinoma: With construction of an extra-thoracic gullet. *Lancet* 1933;**222**:1315–1316.
75. Orringer MB, *et al.* Two thousand transhiatal esophagectomies: Changing trends, lessons learned. *Ann Surg* 2007;**246**:363–372; discussion 372–364.
76. Rudiger Siewert J, *et al.* Adenocarcinoma of the esophagogastric junction: Results of surgical therapy based on anatomical/topographic classification in 1,002 consecutive patients. *Ann Surg* 2000;**232**:353–361.
77. Cuschieri A, *et al.* Endoscopic oesophagectomy through a right thoracoscopic approach. *J R Coll Surg Edinb* 1992;**37**:7–11.
78. DePaula AL, *et al.* Laparoscopic transhiatal esophagectomy with esophagogastroplasty. *Surg Laparosc Endosc* 1995;**5**:1–5.
79. Luketich JD, *et al.* Minimally invasive esophagectomy: Outcomes in 222 patients. *Ann Surg* 2003;**238**:486–494; discussion 494–485.
80. Luketich JD, *et al.* Minimally invasive esophagectomy. *Ann Thorac Surg* 2000;**70**: 906–911; discussion 911–902.
81. Pennathur A, *et al.* Technique of minimally invasive Ivor Lewis esophagectomy. *Ann Thorac Surg* 2010;**89**:S2159–S2162.
82. Awais O, *et al.* Roux-en-y near esophagojejunostomy for intractable gastroesophageal reflux after antireflux surgery. *Ann Thorac Surg* 2008;**85**:1954–1959; discussion 1959–1961.
83. Choi YY, *et al.* Laparoscopic gastrectomy for advanced gastric cancer: Are the long-term results comparable with conventional open gastrectomy? A systematic review and meta-analysis. *J Surg Oncol* 2013;**108**:550–556.
84. Luketich JD, Pennathur A, Franchetti Y, Catalano PJ, Swanson S, Sugarbaker DJ, De Hoyos A, Maddaus MA, Nguyen NT, Benson AB, Fernando HC. Minimally Invasive esophagectomy: Results of a prospective phase II multicenter trial — the Eastern Cooperative Oncology Group (E2202) study. *Ann Surg.* 2015;**261**(4):702–707.
85. Pennathur A, Luketich JD, Landreneau RJ, Ward J, Christie NA, Gibson MK, Schuchert M, Cooper K, Land SR, Belani CP. Long-term results of a phase II trial of neoadjuvant chemotherapy followed by esophagectomy for locally advanced esophageal neoplasm. *Ann Thorac Surg.* 2008;**85**(6):1930–1936.
86. Wayman J, *et al.* The pattern of recurrence of adenocarcinoma of the oesophagogastric junction. *Br J Cancer* 2002;**86**:1223–1229.
87. de Manzoni G, *et al.* Pattern of recurrence after surgery in adenocarcinoma of the gastro-oesophageal junction. *Eur J Surg Oncol* 2003;**29**:506–510.
88. Mariette C, *et al.* Pattern of recurrence following complete resection of esophageal carcinoma and factors predictive of recurrent disease. *Cancer* 2003;**97**:1616–1623.
89. Smit JK, *et al.* Prognostic factors and patterns of recurrence in esophageal cancer assert arguments for extended two-field transthoracic esophagectomy. *Am J Surg* 2010;**200**:446–453.

90. Chang AC, *et al*. Outcomes after transhiatal and transthoracic esophagectomy for cancer. *Ann Thorac Surg* 2008;**85**:424–429.

91. Chu KM, *et al*. A prospective randomized comparison of transhiatal and transthoracic resection for lower-third esophageal carcinoma. *Am J Surg* 1997;**174**:320–324.

92. Goldminc M, *et al*. Oesophagectomy by a transhiatal approach or thoracotomy: A prospective randomized trial. *The Br J Surg* 1993;**80**:367–370.

93. Jacobi CA, *et al*. Surgical therapy of esophageal carcinoma: The influence of surgical approach and esophageal resection on cardiopulmonary function. *Eur J Cardiothorac Surg* 1997;**11**:32–37.

94. Rindani R, *et al*. Transhiatal versus ivor-lewis oesophagectomy: Is there a difference? *Aust N Z J Surg* 1999;**69**:187–194.

95. Wolff CS, *et al*. Ivor lewis approach is superior to transhiatal approach in retrieval of lymph nodes at esophagectomy. *Dis Esophagus* 2008;**21**:328–333.

96. Biere SS, *et al*. Minimally invasive versus open esophagectomy for cancer: A systematic review and meta-analysis. *Minerva Chir* 2009;**64**:121–133.

97. Nagpal K, *et al*. Is minimally invasive surgery beneficial in the management of esophageal cancer? A meta-analysis. *Surg Endosc* 2010;**24**:1621–1629.

98. Sgourakis G, *et al*. Minimally invasive versus open esophagectomy: Meta-analysis of outcomes. *Dig Dis Sci* 2010;**55**:3031–3040.

99. Dantoc M, *et al*. Evidence to support the use of minimally invasive esophagectomy for esophageal cancer: A meta-analysis. *Arch Surg* 2012;**147**:768–776.

100. Biere SS, *et al*. Minimally invasive versus open oesophagectomy for patients with oesophageal cancer: A multicentre, open-label, randomised controlled trial. *Lancet* 2012;**379**:1887–1892.

Chapter 6

Gastric Cancer Management: East *vs*. West?

Sook Ryun Park and Yoon-Koo Kang

1 Introduction

Almost 1 million people are newly diagnosed with gastric cancer annually, and about 75% of these die of the disease, making gastric cancer the second leading cause of cancer death worldwide.[1] Surgical resection remains the only curative treatment for gastric cancer, and locoregional and distant recurrence are still common after curative intent surgical resection, which underscores the importance of a multimodal approach. Notable improvements in multidisciplinary treatments in gastric cancer that include surgery, chemotherapy, and radiotherapy have achieved in the recent decades, which influences clinical decision and treatment algorithms. However, the multimodality, multidisciplinary approaches for gastric cancer have developed in various ways according to geographical regions in the context of variations in disease incidences, etiology/epidemiology, histology, clinical features, and treatment outcomes.

2 Differences in Epidemiology Between the East and the West

The incidence of gastric cancer markedly differs according to geographical regions. The East Asia including South Korea and Japan, shows the highest incidence (~70 cases per 100,000 people annually), almost comprising half the world total, with Europe and South America showing intermediate incidence rates and North

America, Africa, South Asia, and Eastern Mediterranean regions having the lowest incidence (3–10 cases per 100,000) (http://globocan.iarc.fr).

In addition, there are significant differences in clinicopathological characteristics between Eastern and Western countries. In South Korea and Japan, where nationwide mass cancer-screening programs for early detection have been adopted, over half of gastric cancer patients are diagnosed at an early stage.[2,3] In contrast, gastric cancer often presents at an advanced stage in the West, where approximately two-thirds of patients have regional or distant metastasis at diagnosis (http://seer. cancer.gov/statfacts/html/stomach.html). Another major difference between Eastern and Western gastric cancer is the location of the primary tumor. Comparing with the East, there are much higher incidences of proximal stomach or the gastroesophageal junction (GEJ) cancers in the Western countries.[4,5] Furthermore, the incidences of proximal gastric cancer and GEJ cancer have been steadily increasing in Western populations, even with the declining of the overall gastric cancer cases.[6,7] Generally, proximal tumors are associated with more advanced stages and less likely to be resected completely therefore, worse overall outcomes.[8–10] Interestingly, different anatomic locations of gastric cancer are associated with distinct etiology. Whereas the major risk factors for distal gastric cancer include *Helicobacter pylori* infection and dietary factors, gastroesophageal reflux disease and obesity play important roles in the development of proximal gastric cancer.

These geographical variations in the epidemiology of gastric cancer are accompanied by differences in long-term survival. The overall five-year survival rate for gastric cancer population is 60% or higher in South Korea and Japan, whereas the overall five-year survival rate is approximately 20% in the West, and most areas in the rest of the world.[11,12]

3 Localized Gastric Cancer

3.1 *Differences in surgical approach*

Surgical resection remains the primary therapy for gastric cancers when the goal of treatment is curative, and it seems the difference of surgical techniques between the East and West in the management of gastric cancer may have an impact in the patient survival. The earlier stage at diagnosis has been suggested as a major reason for the better patient survival in the Eastern countries; however, several series have demonstrated that the survival advantages of the East still exist after stage stratification.[4,13] Whether the better surgical outcome in the East is due to the more extensive D2 resection or differences in tumor biology or simply because of stage migration associated with more lymph node sampling and retrieval has been controversial.

Gastric cancer shows a high tendency for lymph node metastasis. Therefore, regional lymph node dissection is an imperative part of radical gastrectomy. Over the past 30 years, the extent of lymph node dissection has been the major contro-versial area in the surgical management of gastric cancer worldwide. The Japanese Classification of Gastric Cancer defines 16 different lymph node stations that drain the stomach: stations 1–6 are perigastric, whereas the remaining 10 are located to the side of the major vessels, posterior to the pancreas, and along the aorta.[14] D1 lymphadenectomy involves limited dissection of only the perigastric lymph nodes, while D2 lymphadenectomy involves extended dissection that encompasses the removal of nodes located along the common hepatic, left gastric, celiac and splenic arteries, and splenic hilum as well as the perigastric nodes (stations 1–11). D3 lymphadenectomy involves super-extended lymph node dissection that includes the paraaortic lymph nodes as well as those mentioned above.

In East Asian countries, D2 lymphadenectomy is considered the standard of care associated with curative gastric resection. However, in Western countries, less extensive lymph node dissection has been performed traditionally. A multitude of studies has attempted to delineate the optimal extent of lymphadenectomy in terms of potential value versus perioperative morbidity and mortality. Two large randomized clinical trials (MRC STO1 and Dutch D1D2) compared D1 with D2 lymphadenectomy in advanced gastric cancer in Western countries but no survival benefit was found for D2 over D1 dissection.[15–18] This result might be explained by the increased postoperative mortality in the D2 groups (4–6.5% in D1 *vs.* 10–13% in D2), which might be the result of concomitant pancreaticosplenectomy as part of a D2 resection and less experience with D2 dissections, along with a low case volume of the hospitals and surgeons involved. These mortality and morbidity rates (25–28% in D1 *vs.* 43–46% in D2) from these studies were much higher than the rates reported from South Korea and Japan, which showed less than 1% mortality and about 20% morbidity with D2 dissection.[19,20] In the MRC STO1 study, a better long-term survival was observed in patients who underwent D2 resection without pancreatectomy or splenectomy.[16] In addition, at a median follow-up of 15 years, the Dutch D1D2 trial recently reported a significant benefit of D2 lymphadenec-tomy over D1 surgery in terms of locoregional recurrence (12% *vs.* 22%) and gas-tric cancer-related death rate (37% *vs.* 41%; $p = 0.01$).[21] Patients who underwent D2 resection without pancreaticosplenectomy had a significantly higher 15-year over-all survival (OS) than patients who underwent D1 resection (35% *vs.* 22%; $p = 0.006$). A multicenter randomized controlled trial by the Italian Gastric Cancer Study Group compared the short-term results of D1 and D2 gastrectomy where pancreaticosplenectomy was performed only when indicated rather than as a rou-tine part of the D2 gastrectomy.[22] The study was performed in those Western centers where the participating surgeons received specialized training for D2 lymphadenec-tomy. The study found no significant differences between D1 and D2 dissection in terms of operative mortality (3.0% *vs.* 2.2%; $p = 0.722$) or morbidity (12.0% *vs.* 17.9%; $p = 0.178$). These much lower rates of surgical mortality and morbidity compared with the values observed in the previous MRC STO1 and Dutch D1D2 trials suggest that D2 dissection, if performed in experienced and specialized centers, is a safe option for the radical management of gastric cancer in Western patients. Indeed, there is evidence of lower short- and long-term mortality for patients with gastric cancer resected in high-volume hospitals.[23,24]

With the belief of more extensive lymphadenectomy improving survival in the East, there have been very few studies comparing D1 and D2 dissection except one from Taiwan. This study compared D1 with D3 dissection (equivalent to D2 in the current Japanese criteria) by highly experienced surgeons.[25] The study results demonstrated a survival advantage for more extensive lymphadenectomy over D1 lymphadenectomy, with five-year OS rates of 59.5% *vs.* 53.6%, respectively ($p = 0.041$), which suggests that D2 surgery is superior to D1 when performed by well-trained surgeons.

As to whether even more extended lymph node dissection than D2 provides a survival benefit for Eastern patients, a randomized trial comparing D2 alone with D2 plus paraaortic lymph node dissection (D3) was conducted by the Japanese Clinical Oncology Group (JCOG 9501). The five-year OS (69.2% *vs.* 70.3%) and five-year disease-free survival (DFS) (62.6% *vs.* 61.7%) did not differ between D2 and D3 dissection, whereas postoperative morbidity, duration of surgery, and intraoperative blood loss were higher for D3 dissection.[19,26]

In summary, after a long period of debate, both East and West appear to be finally harmonizing on the extent of lymphadenectomy in curative gastrectomy. Western surgeons have increasingly accepted the importance of performing more than a D1 dissection for the oncologic benefit and Eastern surgeons are accepting that more than a D2 dissection does not provide a further survival benefit. Considering the impact of D2 lymphadenectomy on disease-specific survival and adequate staging, D2 dissection should be the standard procedure not only in the East, but also in the West, when applied in experienced centers.

3.2 *Differences in surgical outcomes and recurrence patterns*

In Western countries, the five-year OS rates for advanced gastric cancer with potentially curative surgery alone range from 25% to 30%.[27–30] In contrast, in Eastern countries, the five-year OS rates for advanced gastric cancer after curative surgery alone range from 60% to 70%.[31,32] When gastric cancer-specific survival was compared on a stage-by-stage basis after curative resection, it was significantly better in Eastern than in Western countries. This improved survival persisted after adjusting for other potential biases, such as age, sex, body mass index, differentiation, tumor location, type of gastrectomy, and chemotherapy.[4,13] Furthermore, recurrence patterns following potentially curative surgery alone have been different between the East and West. Notably, locoregional recurrences at the first relapse, both as the only site and as part of a systemic spread of disease, were more common in Western countries (20–30% of the cases)[27,29,30] than in Eastern countries (less than 10%).[31–33]

Another important difference between the East and West is the curative resection rate in patients who were considered to have potentially resectable gastric cancer in preoperative staging. Whereas it has been reported as about 90% in Eastern series,[34,35] only 66–74% of patients achieved curative resection in Western countries.[21,29,30]

3.3 *Differences in perioperative therapies*

Differences in surgical techniques, curative resection rate, survival outcomes after curative resection, and relapse patterns between the East and West lead to different perioperative multidisciplinary strategies. Low rates of curative resection and high rates of locoregional recurrences from suboptimal surgery in Western countires, in addition to systemic spread after surgery, provide the rationale for perioperative chemotherapy (pre- and postoperative chemotherapy) and postoperative chemoradiation. In contrast, Eastern countries have focused on reducing systemic failures through postoperative chemotherapy after curative resection.

3.3.1 *Postoperative adjuvant chemoradiation*

Adjuvant chemoradiation for gastric cancer was established as the standard of care in North America through the results of the SWOG 9008/Intergroup 0116 study that randomized 556 patients with completely resected stage IB–IV(M0) gastric or GEJ cancer into observation versus adjuvant chemoradiation.[27,28] Adjuvant chemoradiation consisted of five-monthly cycles of chemotherapy (bolus 5-fluorouracil [5-FU] plus leucovorin [LV]) with concurrent radiotherapy (45 Gy) during cycles 2 and 3. With a median follow-up of five years, the median OS was 27 months in the surgery alone group and 36 months in the adjuvant chemoradiation group (hazard ratio [HR] 1.35; 95% confidence interval [CI] 1.09–1.66; $p = 0.005$), and the median relapse-free survival (RFS) was 19 months and 30 months (HR 1.52; 95% CI 1.23–1.86; $p < 0.001$), respectively.[27] Local failure was reduced from 29% to 19% with adjuvant chemoradiation. Recently updated results with a 10-year follow-up continue to demonstrate suspend survival improvement with adjuvant chemoradiation.[28]

This trial has, however, been criticized for an inadequate quality control of surgery, since only 10% of patients had the recommended D2 dissection and more than 50% underwent D0 dissection. It was suggested that the survival improvement with chemoradiation resulted from improved local control in the setting of inadequate surgery. In East Asia, such as South Korea and Japan, where D2 lymphadenectomy provides good local tumor control, adjuvant chemoradiation is usually not recommended. Furthermore, a recent randomized phase III trial in Korea (ARTIST) comparing adjuvant chemoradiation with adjuvant chemotherapy after curative D2 dissection of gastric cancer did not show benefit with adding radiation to adjuvant chemotherapy (with three-year DFS rate 78.2% in the chemoradiation group *vs.* 74.2% in the chemotherapy group; $p = 0.0862$).[36]

3.3.2 *Perioperative therapy including neoadjuvant chemotherapy*

The main aim of neoadjuvant therapy is to downsize or downstage the tumor to facilitate its complete resection and to eliminate occult systemic micrometastases. A perioperative chemotherapy approach comprising neoadjuvant and adjuvant therapy has been mainly pursued in Western Europe where locally advanced gastric and GEJ cancer are common and curative resection rates are relatively low. Two large randomized phase III trials (MAGIC and FNCLCC/FFCD) comparing perioperative chemotherapy before and after surgery with surgery alone in resectable gastric, GEJ, or esophageal adenocarcinoma established the evidence for the use of perioperative chemotherapy over surgery alone in the West.[29,30] The U.K. MAGIC trial randomized 503 patients with T2 or higher disease (74% gastric, 11% distal esophagus, and 15% GEJ adenocarcinoma) to surgery alone versus surgery plus perioperative epirubicin, cisplatin, and 5-FU (ECF).[29] The results showed a significant improvement in the perioperative chemotherapy group in progression-free survival (PFS) (HR 0.66; 95% CI 0.53–0.81; $p < 0.001$) and OS (HR 0.75; 95% CI 0.60–0.93; five-year OS 36.3% *vs.* 23.0%; $p = 0.009$). The resected tumors were significantly smaller and had a lower pathologic stage in the perioperative chemotherapy group. The French FNCLCC/FFCD study in which 224 patients (25% gastric, 11% distal esophagus, and 64% GEJ adenocarcinoma) were randomized to surgery alone versus perioperative cisplatin/5-FU before and after surgery also showed a significant improvement in DFS (five-year DFS 34% *vs.* 19%; HR 0.65; 95% CI 0.48–0.89; $p = 0.003$), OS (five-year OS 38% *vs.* 24%; HR 0.69; 95% CI 0.50–0.95; $p = 0.02$), and the curative resection rate (87% *vs.* 74%; $p = 0.04$) in the perioperative chemotherapy group.

3.3.3 *Postoperative adjuvant chemotherapy*

Adjuvant chemotherapy is the main strategy adopted for curatively resected gastric cancer in the East, where relatively high curative resection rates are achieved and local tumor control is adequate with standard D2 lymphadenectomy. In recent decades, many phase III trials have investigated the role of adjuvant chemotherapy versus surgery alone, but conflicting results have been obtained because of the large heterogeneity of study populations, the small sample sizes, the different surgical quality, and the different chemotherapy regimens used. A recent individual patient-level meta-analysis performed by the GASTRIC group, which included 3,838 patients from 17 randomized trials of adjuvant chemotherapy, demonstrated a significant benefit from chemotherapy compared with surgery alone for OS (HR 0.82 [95% CI 0.76–0.90]; $p < 0.001$) and DFS (HR 0.82 [95% CI 0.75–0.90]; $p < 0.001$). Absolute benefits of OS were 5.8% at five years (from 49.6% to 55.3%) and 7.4% at 10 years (from 37.5% to 44.9%).[37]

Two large randomized phase III trials (ACTS-GC and CLASSIC) performed in East Asia have demonstrated survival benefits from adjuvant chemotherapy after D2 surgery.[31,38] The ACTS-GC trial conducted in Japan randomized 1,059 patients with curatively resected stage II/III by the Japanese staging system to observation versus adjuvant S-1 for one year.[31,38] A significant advantage in terms of OS (five-year OS 71.7% *vs.* 61.1%; HR 0.669; 95% CI 0.540–0.828) and RFS (five-year RFS 65.4% *vs.* 53.1%; HR 0.653; 95% CI 0.537–0.793) was observed in the chemotherapy group over the surgery alone group.[31] The CLASSIC trial performed in South Korea, China, and Taiwan in which 1,035 patients who had curatively resected stage II/III gastric cancer by the American Joint Committee on Cancer (AJCC; 6th edition, 2002) were randomized to observation alone versus adjuvant capecitabine/oxaliplatin for six months also demonstrated a survival benefit of adjuvant chemotherapy.[39] During an interim analysis, the three-year DFS rate was 74% (95% CI 69%–79%) in the chemotherapy group and 59% (95% CI 53%–64%) in the surgery alone group (HR 0.56; 95% CI 0.44–0.72; $p < 0.0001$).[39] Data from the five-year follow-up continued to demonstrate survival improvement with adjuvant chemotherapy: a five-year DFS of 68% *vs.* 53% (HR 0.58; 95% CI 0.47–0.72; $p < 0.0001$) and a five-year OS of 78% *vs.* 69% (HR 0.66; 95% CI 0.51–0.85; $p = 0.0015$).[32]

3.3.4 *Different strategies to improve perioperative therapy*

In an attempt to further improve survival in localized gastric cancer, various strategies have been tested on the basis of the different perioperative therapy backbones among regions. In North America, the combination of more intensified systemic chemotherapy with radiation after surgery was evaluated in the CALGB 80101 trial, in which adjuvant chemotherapy with ECF before and after chemoradiation (concurrent infusional 5-FU) was compared with adjuvant chemotherapy bolus 5-FU/LV before and after chemoradiation (concurrent infusional 5-FU) (Intergroup regimen).[40] Intensified adjuvant chemoradiation with ECF did not, however, improve DFS (HR 1.00; 95% CI 0.79–1.27; $p = 0.99$) or OS (HR 1.03; 95% CI 0.83–1.34; $p = 0.80$) when compared with chemoradiation with bolus 5-FU/LV. In Europe, the strategy of adding postoperative radiation to the setting of perioperative chemotherapy (e.g. combining preoperative chemotherapy and postoperative chemoradiation) is being tested in an ongoing phase III trial (CRITICS; NCT00407186). A strategy of intensifying adjuvant chemotherapy has also been evaluated in East Asia and Europe. The ITACA-S trial conducted in Italy compared a more intensive adjuvant chemotherapy regimen (irinotecan plus 5-FU/LV followed by docetaxel plus cisplatin) with a less intensive regimen (5-FU/LV) in 1,100 patients who had curative resection (at least D1 dissection) for pN+ or pN-/pT2b-4 localized gastric cancer.[41] However, the more intensive regimen failed to show any benefit in DFS (HR 1.00; 95% CI 0.85–1.17; p = 0.974) or OS (HR 0.98; 95% CI 0.82–1.18; p = 0.865). The Korean AMC 0201 study randomized 855 patients with stage II–IV(M0) gastric cancer after D2 gastrectomy to mitomycin-C/short-term doxifluridine (three months) (Mf) or mitomycin-C/long-term doxifluridine (12 months)/cisplatin (MFP).[42] The intensifying adjuvant chemotherapy by increasing the duration of oral fluoropyrimidine and adding cisplatin did not show survival improvements either with a five-year RFS of 61.1% for Mf *vs.* 57.9% for MFP (HR 1.10; 95% CI 0.89–1.35; p = 0.39) and a five-year OS of 66.5% for Mf and 65.0% for MFP (HR 1.11; 95% CI 0.89–1.39; p = 0.33). These results suggest that simply intensifying adjuvant chemotherapy (with or without radiation) by adding more cytotoxic agents or prolonging treatment duration does not seem to enhance treatment efficacy in patients with localized gastric cancer. More novel approaches should be considered. The Korean AMC 0101 evaluated the efficacy of intraoperative intraperitoneal chemotherapy using cisplatin plus early initiation (day after surgery) of systemic chemotherapy with the same control arm of AMC 0201. The results demonstrated the significantly improved RFS (HR 0.70; 95% CI 0.54–0.90; p = 0.006) and OS (HR 0.71; 95% CI 0.53–0.95; p = 0.02).[43] The positive results of the AMC 0101 trial, in combination with the negative outcome of the AMC 0201 trial, suggest that early commencement of adjuvant chemotherapy and/or additional intraperitoneal chemotherapy may be effective strategies to further improve the effect of adjuvant chemotherapy.

Currently, another approach of adding preoperative chemotherapy to standard adjuvant chemotherapy in the setting of D2 surgery is being evaluated in East Asia (PRODIGY, NCT01515748; NCT00182611). In the Korean PRODIGY study, patients with resectable cT2-3/N+ or T4/any N gastric or GEJ adenocarcinoma were randomized to preoperative docetaxel/oxaliplatin/S-1 followed by surgery and then postoperative S-1 versus surgery followed by postoperative S-1. Since the neoadjuvant chemotherapy regimen should be highly active to increase the R0 resection rate and downstage tumors, the triplet regimen was selected as preoperative therapy in the PRODIGY study. The Japanese study (NCT00182611) is comparing neoadjuvant S-1/cisplatin followed by surgery and adjuvant S-1 with primary surgery followed by adjuvant S-1. These studies will help to clarify the role of neoadjuvant chemotherapy in Eastern patients who have standard D2 dissection with potentially excellent surgery.

Another potential way to improve perioperative therapy in the era of targeted oncology therapy is to include molecular targeted agents. A randomized phase II/III MAGIC-B/MRC ST03 trial in the United Kingdom evaluated the addition of beva-cizumab, a monoclonal antibody that inhibits vascular endothelial growth factor, to perioperative chemotherapy with epirubicin/cisplatin/capecitabine (ECX) in 1,063 patients with resectable stage Ib-IV(M0) adenocarcinoma of the lower esophagus (14%), GEJ (51%) or stomach (36%) (Reference: Cunningham D, Smyth E, Stenning S, Stevenson L, Robb C, Allum W, Grabsch H, Alderson D, Riddell A, Chua S, Crosby T, Mason R, Griffin M, Mansoor W, Coxon F, Falk S, Rowley S, Sumpter K, Blazeby J, Langley R. Peri-operative chemotherapy ± bevacizumab for resectable gastro-oesophageal adenocarcinoma: Results from the UK Medical Research Council randomised ST03 trial (ISRCTN 46020948) Presented at the Annual Meeting of European Cancer Congress/European Society for Medical Oncology, Vienna, Austria, 25–29 September 2015 (abstract 2201)). ECX plus beva-cizumab (ECX-B) did not improve OS (median, 33.97 months with ECX vs. 34.46 months with ECX-B; HR 1.067; p = 0.4784), DFS (HR 1.006; p = 0.9425), PFS (HR 1.026; p = 0.7683), R0 resection rate (75% vs. 76%, respectively), or pathologic complete response rate (8% vs. 10%, respectively). Other targeted agents, trastu-zumab and pertuzumab, which are monoclonal antibodies inhibiting human epider-mal growth factor receptor 2 (HER2), are being evaluated as perioperative treatment in a randomized phase II study for stage Ib-III resectable HER2-positive gastric or GEJ adenocarcinoma (INNOVATION; NCT02205047).

4 Unresectable or Metastatic Gastric Cancer

4.1 *First-line cytotoxic chemotherapy*

Palliative chemotherapy has been established as the standard of care since the 1990s several clinical trials demonstrated a significant improvement in OS and quality of life with chemotherapy over best supportive care for patients with unresectable or meta-static gastric cancer.[44–46] A meta-analysis also showed efficacy of chemotherapy com-pared with best supportive care, with an overall HR of 0.39 (95% CI 0.28–0.52), which translates to a benefit in the weighted mean average survival of about six months.[47]

One of the differences in first-line chemotherapy between the East and West is the preference for a doublet regimen in the East and a triplet regimen in several Western countries. Since it was common practice to offer second-line chemother-apy after failure of first-line chemotherapy in Asian countries before its survival benefit was even verified in prospective clinical trials, Asian countries preferred doublet first-line chemotherapy followed by sequential second-line therapy with other available active cytotoxic agents. In contrast, many Western countries where second-line chemotherapy has not been routinely performed preferred a triplet regimen as first-line therapy to administer the most active agents upfront.

The platinum plus fluoropyrimidine doublet regimen is current standard practice as first-line chemotherapy in many Asian countries. Whereas cisplatin plus infusional 5-FU has been the most commonly used regimen until recently, oral fluoropyrimidines such as capecitabine and S-1 have been replacing infusional 5-FU since recent clinical trials demonstrated that oral fluoropyrimidines are noninferior to infusional 5-FU in terms of efficacy, with favorable safety profiles and convenient administration.[48–51] In particular, S-1, which consists of tegafur (a prodrug of 5-FU) and two modulators, 5-chloro-2,4-dihydroxypyridine (an inhibitor of dihydropyrimidine dehydrogenase) and potassium oxonate (an inhibitor of orotate phosphoribosyltransferase), has been investigated mainly in Asia because it showed poor tolerability in Western populations.[52,53] The regional differences in S-1 tolerability are suggested to be attributed to differences in *CYP2A6* polymorphisms between Asians and Caucasians, affecting the conversion of tegafur to 5-FU, although a recent study did not show significant differences in 5-FU exposure after S-1 administration between Asians and Caucasians.[54]

In the Japanese JCOG 9912 study, S1 was found to be noninferior to 5-FU alone in terms of OS (HR 0.83; 95% CI 0.68–1.01; $p = 0.0005$ for noninferiority), with similar toxicity profiles.[48] In the subsequent SPIRITS trial, S1 plus cisplatin resulted in a significantly longer OS (median 13.0 *vs.* 11.0 months; HR 0.77; 95% CI 0.61–0.98; $p = 0.04$) and PFS (median 6.0 *vs.* 4.0 months; HR 0.57; 95% CI 0.44–0.73; $p < 0.0001$) compared with S1 alone.[55] Based on these results, S-1 is widely used as backbone chemotherapy in both clinical study and practice in Asian countries. Notably, S-1 plus cisplatin has different treatment schedules and dose intensity not only globally, but also within Asia. Japan uses the lower dose intensity of cisplatin (12 mg/m^2/week) in a five-weekly regimen (S-1 80–120 mg/body/day on days 1–21 and cisplatin 60 mg/m^2 on day 8 in a five-week cycle [SP5]) and South Korea uses a three-weekly regimen with cisplatin dose intensity of 20 mg/m^2/week (S-1 80 mg/m^2/day on days 1–14 and cisplatin 60 mg/m^2 on day 1 in a three-week cycle [SP3]). Although a recent phase III trial (SOS) performed in South Korea and Japan showed that SP3 was superior to SP5 in terms of PFS (the primary endpoint) (median 5.5 *vs.* 4.9 months; HR 0.82; 95% CI 0.68–0.99; $p = 0.0418$), both SP3 and SP5 are recommended for the first-line treatment of advanced gastric cancer because of the small benefit in PFS and no difference in OS (median 14.1 *vs.* 13.9 months; HR 0.99; 95% CI 0.81–1.21; $p = 0.9068$).[56]

S-1 has also been evaluated in Western populations in a phase III trial (FLAGS) that randomized patients to S-1/cisplatin versus 5-FU/cisplatin and used a much lower S-1 dosage (50 mg/m^2/day on days 1–21 in a four-week cycle) compared with Asian studies, based on the maximum tolerated dose in Western patients.[49,52] The dose intensity of cisplatin was similar to that of a Korean regimen (19 mg/m^2/week). There were no significant differences between the S-1/cisplatin and the 5-FU/cisplatin groups in OS (median 8.6 *vs.* 7.9 months; HR 0.92; 95% CI 0.80–1.05) (the primary endpoint), PFS, or overall response rate. Although S-1 is not approved in the United States, based on noninferiority of S-1/cisplatin to 5-FU/cisplatin in a *post hoc* noninferiority analysis for OS and a better safety profile, S-1/cisplatin has been approved in the EU for the treatment of advanced gastric cancer. However, these differences in treatment schedule and dose intensity among regions present a critical obstacle to the use of S-1 as the global standard cytotoxic chemotherapy regimen.

Capecitabine has also been demonstrated to be noninferior to 5-FU when both were combined with cisplatin in the ML17032 trial conducted in Asia, Europe, and Latin America.[50] The median PFS (the primary endpoint) was 5.6 months in the capecitabine/cisplatin group and 5.0 months in the 5-FU/cisplatin group (HR 0.81; 95% CI 0.63–1.04; $p < 0.001$ for noninferiority), and the median OS was 10.5 *vs* 9.3 months, respectively (HR 0.85; 95% CI 0.64–1.13; $p = 0.008$ for noninferiority). In contrast to S-1, because capecitabine did not show marked differences in a toxicity profile between Eastern and Western populations, capecitabine has been widely used as backbone chemotherapy worldwide in both clinical trials and practice.

Unlike in Asia, in Europe, a triplet cytotoxic chemotherapy regimen consisting of ECF has been preferred as first-line chemotherapy, based on a randomized trial by Webb *et al.* by comparing an unpopular regimen with high toxicity, 5-FU/doxorubicin/methotrexate (FAMTX).[57] The REAL-2 trial performed in the United Kingdom evaluated capecitabine and oxaliplatin as alternatives to 5-FU and cisplatin in the ECF backbone regimen for advanced esophagogastric cancer in two-by-two comparisons. The study demonstrated noninferiority for capecitabine to 5-FU (HR 0.86; 95% CI 0.80–0.99) and oxaliplatin to cisplatin (HR 0.92; 95% CI 0.80–1.10).[51] The median survival times in the ECF, ECX, EOF (epirubicin/oxaliplatin/5-FU), and EOX, ECX groups were 9.9, 9.9, 9.3, and 11.2 months, respectively. While the toxic effects of capecitabine and 5-FU were similar, oxaliplatin was associated with a more favorable safety profile compared with cisplatin. Similar findings were shown in the German Arbeitsgemeinschaft Internistische Onkologie (AIO) randomized phase III trial comparing 5-FU/LV/cisplatin (FLP) versus 5-FU/LV/oxaliplatin (FLO); there were no significant differences in PFS and OS between the two groups while FLO was better tolerated. There with a trend toward improved median PFS with FLO versus FLP (5.8 vs. 3.9 months, respectively; $p = 0.077$) and similar median OS (10.7 *vs.* 8.8 months, respectively).[58] Based on these results, ECF and its variant regimens with substitutions for 5-FU and/or cisplatin with capecitabine and/or oxaliplatin are widely used as first-line chemotherapy in European countries. However, there is still some debate regarding the role of epirubicin in the combination.

In North America, similar to Asia, platinum plus fluoropyrimidine-based doublet combination regimens are commonly used backbone chemotherapy. However, a triplet regimen consisting of docetaxel plus cisplatin/5-FU (DCF) had been an alternative regimen, based on the V325 study where DCF was superior to cisplatin/5-FU in the response rate (37% *vs.* 25%; $p = 0.01$), time to progression (median 5.6 *vs.* 3.7 months; HR 1.47; 95% CI 1.19–1.82; $p < 0.001$), and OS (median 9.2 *vs.* 8.6 months; HR 1.29; 95% CI 1.0–1.6; $p = 0.02$).[59] Since DCF was, however, associated with higher hematologic (grade 3/4 neutropenia, 82% *vs.* 57%; febrile neutropenia, 29% *vs.* 12%) and non-hematologic toxicities, this regimen has not gained wide acceptance and is only recommended for medically fit patients with good performance status and access to frequent toxicity evaluation. Instead, various modifications of the DCF regimen, such as dose reduction and/or replacement of cisplatin with oxaliplatin are used to reduce toxicity in North America and Europe.[60,61]

4.2 *Second-line or further cytotoxic chemotherapy*

Recently, the survival benefit of second-line chemotherapy after failure of first-line chemotherapy in advanced gastric cancer has been demonstrated in both Eastern and Western populations in phase III trials.[62,63] The first study conducted by AIO stopped prematurely after accruing only 40 patients who failed first-line chemotherapy; however, a significant survival improvement (median OS 4.0 *vs.* 2.4 months) was demonstrated with second-line irinotecan chemotherapy over best supportive care alone with a HR of 0.48 (95% CI 0.25–0.92; $p = 0.012$). The phase III COUGAR-02 trial performed in the United Kingdom randomized 168 patients who had failure of a platinum–fluoropyrimidine combination to second-line chemotherapy (docetaxel) or active symptom control alone, which demonstrated the improvement of median OS with second-line chemotherapy (5.2 *vs.* 3.6 months; HR 0.67; 95% CI 0.49–0.92; $p = 0.01$) and disease-specific health-related quality of life.[63] Similarly, in a Korean study, 202 patients pretreated with one or two prior chemotherapy regimens involving both fluoropyrimidines and platinum were randomized to salvage chemotherapy (docetaxel or irinotecan) or best supportive care.[62] Salvage chemotherapy was associated with a significant improvement in OS compared with best supportive care (median 5.3 *vs.* 3.8 months; HR 0.657; 95% CI 0.485–0.891; $p = 0.007$).

A difference noticed between East and West regarding salvage therapy is the proportion of patients who receive subsequent therapy after failure of first-line chemotherapy. In clinical trials of the first-line setting, about 70% of Asians received second-line chemotherapy, whereas it was administered in only about 15–30% of patients in Europe and America.[48,49,51,55,64] A Korean phase III trial showed that 40% of patients received subsequent therapy after second- or third-line chemotherapy.[62] Similar data was collected from a Japanese phase III trial with 81% of patients received subsequent therapy after second-line therapy. Since subsequent therapy affects survival after failure of first-line chemotherapy,[65] these marked regional differences in the use of salvage therapy might partly contribute to the differences in OS for first-line chemotherapy observed between the East and West.

4.3 *Molecular-targeted agents*

Targeted agents have emerged as a new treatment strategy for improving outcomes in cancer. The most successful molecular-targeted agent in gastric cancer is trastuzumab, a monoclonal antibody inhibiting human epidermal growth factor receptor-2 (HER2). The global phase III ToGA trial demonstrated that trastuzumab in combination with first-line platinum–fluoropyrimidine chemotherapy (cisplatin plus capecitabine or 5-FU) improved OS (median 13.8 *vs.* 11.1 months; HR 0.74; 95% CI 0.60–0.91; $p = 0.0046$) and PFS (median 6.7 *vs.* 5.5 months; HR 0.71; 95% CI 0.59–0.85; $p = 0.0002$) compared with chemotherapy alone in HER2-positive (immunohistochemistry staining [IHC] 3+ or fluorescence *in situ* hybridization [FISH]+) advanced gastric or GEJ cancer patients.[66] In exploratory subgroup analyses, the survival benefit from trastuzumab was more prominent in patients with IHC 3+ or IHC 2+/FISH+: a median survival of 16.0 *vs.* 11.8 months with a HR of 0.65 (95% CI 0.51–0.83). The trastuzumab treatment effect was not apparent in the subgroup with IHC 0 or 1+/FISH+ tumors (HR 1.07; 95% CI 0.70–1.62). These results led to a variation of the definition of HER2-positive gastric cancer for trastuzumab approval in different geographical regions: IHC 3+ or FISH positive with any IHC result in the United States and Japan or IHC 3+ or IHC 2+ plus FISH+ in Europe and Korea. The National Comprehensive Cancer Network (NCCN) guidelines panel recommends that cases showing IHC 2+ should be additionally examined by FISH (http://www.nccn.org). The different HER2 levels of expression according to the site of the primary tumor (32.2% in GEJ *vs.* 21.4% in stomach) and histological type (31.8% in the intestinal type *vs.* 6.1%/20.0% in the diffuse/mixed type) mostly contribute to the difference in HER2-positivity rates between countries.[67]

Lapatinib, another anti-HER2 agent that is a dual tyrosine kinase inhibitor against HER2 and epidermal growth factor receptor (EGFR), has also been investigated in HER2-positive advanced gastric and GEJ cancer patients. The global LOGiC phase III trial investigated the efficacy of lapatinib with capecitabine and oxaliplatin in HER2-positive (FISH+) gastric, esophageal, and GEJ adenocarcinoma in the first-line setting.[68] In contrast to the ToGA trial, prolongation of OS with the addition of lapatinib to chemotherapy was not statistically significant (median 12.2 *vs.* 10.5 months; HR 0.91; 95% CI 0.73–1.12; $p = 0.3492$). There were also no differences in OS according to the HER2 protein expression: a HR of 0.91 (95% CI 0.55–1.51) in HER2 IHC 0-1+ *vs.* 0.86 (95% CI 0.68–1.09) in HER2 IHC 2-3+. The Asian TyTAN phase III trial compared lapatinib plus paclitaxel to paclitaxel alone in patients with HER2-positive (FISH+) gastric cancer in the second-line setting.[69] The addition of lapatinib did not significantly improve OS (median 11.0 *vs.* 8.9 months; HR 0.84; 95% CI 0.64–1.11; $p = 0.2088$), although better efficacy was shown in the subgroup with HER2 IHC 3+ (median OS 14.0 *vs.* 7.6 months; HR 0.59; 95% CI 0.37–0.93; $p = 0.0176$).

Another recent successful approach in targeted therapy is represented by agents that inhibit tumor angoigenesis. The global AVAGAST phase III trial evaluated the efficacy of the addition of bevacizumab to chemotherapy (cisplatin and capecitabine or 5-FU) in the first-line treatment of advanced gastric cancer.[64] Although the addition of bevacizumab to chemotherapy did not significantly increase OS (median 12.1 *vs.* 10.1 months; HR 0.87; 95% CI 0.73–1.03; $p = 0.1002$), there were significant improvements in the overall response rate (46.0% vs. 37.4%; $p = 0.0315$) and PFS (median 6.7 *vs.* 5.3 months; HR 0.80; 95% CI 0.68–0.93; $p = 0.0037$), indicating clinical activity of bevacizumab plus chemotherapy. The global phase III trial REGARD showed that ramucirumab, a monoclonal antibody that inhibits vascular endothelial growth factor receptor-2 (VEGFR2), improved survival compared with best supportive care alone in patients advanced gastric or GEJ cancer progressing after first-line platinum- or fluoropyrimidine-containing chemotherapy (median 5.2 *vs.* 3.8 months; HR 0.776; 95% CI 0.603–0.998; $p = 0.047$).[70] In addition, in a global phase III trial (RAINBOW), ramucirumab improved OS (HR 0.807; 95% CI 0.678–0.962; $p = 0.0169$) and PFS (HR 0.635; 95% CI 0.536–0.752; $p < 0.0001$) when combined with paclitaxel compared with paclitaxel alone in the second-line setting.[71] Based on the results of the REGARD and RAINBOW studies, ramucirumab was recently approved for use as a single agent or in combination with paclitaxel for advanced or metastatic gastric or GEJ adenocarcinoma after failure of fluoropyrimidine- or platinum-containing chemotherapy in the United States, EU, and some Asian countries. In a recent Chinese randomized phase III study of apatinib, a VEGFR2 tyrosine kinase inhibitor versus placebo in patients with advanced gastric cancer who progressed after second-line chemotherapy showed a significant improvement of OS (median 195 vs. 140 days; HR 0.71; 95% CI 0.54–0.94; $p < 0.016$) and PFS (median 78 vs. 53 days; HR 0.44; 95% CI 0.33–0.61; $p < 0.0001$) with apatinib. Based on these results, apatinib has been approved by the Chinese Food and Drug Administration recently.[72]

The regional differences in treatment effects have been increasingly recognized in global clinical trials incorporating molecular targeted therapy. In the ToGA trial, in which Asian patients accounted for more than 50% of the subjects, OS benefits seemed larger in non-Asian subgroups than in Asian subgroups, with a HR of 0.82 in Asia, 0.44 in Central or South America, and 0.63 in Europe.[65] However, in the LOGiC trial, in which Asian patients accounted for 40% of the subjects, OS benefits seemed larger in Asian subgroups than in non-Asian subgroups, with a HR of 0.68 in the Asian population and 1.04 in the non-Asian population.[67] In the AVAGAST trial, in which about 50% of subjects consisted of Asia-Pacific patients, while the Asian population showed a better survival regardless of the treatment received, European and American populations displayed a shorter OS but obtained more benefit from addition of bevacizumab to chemotherapy; the HR was 0.97 in Asia (median OS 13.9 *vs.* 12.1 months), 0.85 in Europe (median OS 11.1 *vs.* 8.6 months), and 0.63 in Pan-America (median OS 11.5 *vs.* 6.8 months).[64] Although differences in the use of second-line therapy between regions — Asia (67%), Europe (29%), and Pan-America (15%) — might have in part influenced the different survival outcomes, a similar trend was still shown in terms of PFS; the HR was 0.92 in Asia (median PFS 6.7 *vs.* 5.6 months), 0.71 in Europe (median PFS 6.9 *vs.* 4.4 months), and 0.65 in Pan-America (median PFS 5.9 *vs.* 4.4 months). A reduced bevacizumab effect in the Asian subgroup might be associated with a low plasma VEGF-A level in Asian than non-Asian populations, given that a high VEGF-A level has been suggested as a predictive biomarker for bevacizumab.[73] On the other hand, in the RAINBOW trial, in which Asian patients accounted for 34% of the subjects, the benefit of the addition of ramucirumab to chemotherapy was similar in terms of PFS between regions (a HR of 0.63 in Asia with a median PFS of 5.5 *vs.* 2.8 months and a HR of 0.64 in non-Asian regions with a median of PFS 4.2 *vs.* 2.9 months). However, the effects on OS seemed to differ between regions (a HR of 0.99 in Asia with a median OS of 12.1 *vs.* 10.5 months and a HR of 0.73 in non-Asian regions with a median OS of 8.5 *vs.* 5.9 months).[71]

Taken together, there seem to be regional differences in the efficacy of targeted agents, with the pattern varying according to the targeted agent. Whether these discrepancies are related to differences in tumor biology, tumor burden, or practice pattern remains a matter of debate. In particular, possible survival prolongation by the more popular use of second-line therapy in Western populations, since it has also been recently established as the standard of care in the West, should be considered in the design and conduct of future clinical trials.

5 Conclusions

Although a multidisciplinary approach has been established as the standard of care in resectable gastric cancer, differences in epidemiology, clinical features, surgical outcomes, and prognosis have led to a different evolution in multimodality treatments from region to region. Postoperative adjuvant chemoradiation has been commonly conducted in North America, perioperative chemotherapy in Europe, and postoperative adjuvant chemotherapy in East Asia. Recently, long-standing controversies about optimal surgery have been resolved with D2 lymphadenectomy being adopted as the standard of surgery in both the East and West. However, there are still differences in surgical techniques in both clinical trials and practice between regions.

Similarly, treatment patterns and types of chemotherapy regimens used in unresectable or metastatic gastric cancer have differed somewhat between geographical regions. Although the fluoropyrimidine (5-FU, oral fluoropyrimidines such as S-1 and capecitabine)- and platinum (cisplatin, oxaliplatin)-based combinations are the most widely accepted backbone regimen in the first-line setting worldwide, moderate differences exist; a doublet regimen with fluoropyrimidine plus platinum is preferred in East Asia, a triplet regimen with epirubicin combined with fluoropyrimidine plus platinum predominates in Europe, and docetaxel combined with fluoropyrimidine plus platinum is often used, as well as a doublet regimen, in North America. A difference in chemotherapy involves in the use of salvage chemotherapy after failure of first-line chemotherapy, with a much higher proportion of patients undergoing salvage therapy in East Asia, which is increasingly recognized as a critical factor influencing survival outcomes. Lastly, in the molecular-targeted era, one of the challenges in the development of molecular targeted agents is to identify whether there are any differences in the molecular heterogeneity of the disease and, consequently, treatment outcomes among ethnicities.

References

1. Jemal A, *et al.* Global cancer statistics. *CA Cancer J Clin* 2011;**61**:69–90.
2. Jung KW, *et al.* Survival of Korean adult cancer patients by stage at diagnosis, 2006–2010: National cancer registry study. *Cancer Res Treat* 2013;**45**:162–171.
3. Nashimoto A, *et al.* Gastric cancer treated in 2002 in Japan: 2009 annual report of the JGCA nationwide registry. *Gastric Cancer*, 2013;**16**:1–27.
4. Strong VE, *et al.* Comparison of gastric cancer survival following R0 resection in the United States and Korea using an internationally validated nomogram. *Ann Surg* 2010;**251**:640–646.
5. Ferro A, *et al.* Worldwide trends in gastric cancer mortality (1980–2011), with predictions to 2015, and incidence by subtype. *Eur J Cancer* 2014;**50**:1330–1344.
6. Dubecz A, *et al.* Does the Incidence of adenocarcinoma of the esophagus and gastric cardia continue to rise in the twenty-first century? A SEER database analysis. *J Gastrointest Surg* 2014;**18**:124–129.
7. Orengo MA, *et al.* Trends in incidence rates of oesophagus and gastric cancer in Italy by subsite and histology, 1986–1997. *Eur J Gastroenterol Hepatol* 2006;**18**:739–746.
8. Han DS, *et al.* Nomogram predicting long-term survival after D2 gastrectomy for gastric cancer. *J Clin Oncol* 2012;**30**:3834–3840.
9. Kattan MW, *et al.* Postoperative nomogram for disease-specific survival after an R0 resection for gastric carcinoma. *J Clin Oncol* 2013;**21**:3647–3650.
10. Kim SY, *et al.* The predictors and clinical impact of positive resection margins on frozen section in gastric cancer surgery. *J Gastric Cancer* 2012;**12**:113–119.
11. Kamangar F, *et al.* Patterns of cancer incidence, mortality, and prevalence across five continents: Defining priorities to reduce cancer disparities in different geographic regions of the world. *J Clin Oncol* 2006;**24**:2137–2150.
12. Verdecchia A, *et al.* EUROCARE-4 Working Group. Recent cancer survival in Europe: A 2000–02 period analysis of EUROCARE-4 data. *Lancet Oncol* 2007;**8**:784–796.

13. Markar SR, *et al*. Long-term survival after gastrectomy for cancer in randomized, controlled oncological trials: Comparison between West and East. *Ann Surg Oncol* 2013;**20**:2328–2338.

14. Japanese Gastric Cancer Association. Japanese Classification of Gastric Carcinoma (2nd English Edition). *Gastric Cancer* 1998;**1**:10–24.

15. Cuschieri A, *et al*. Postoperative morbidity and mortality after D1 and D2 resections for gastric cancer: Preliminary results of the MRC randomised controlled surgical trial. The Surgical Cooperative Group. *Lancet* 1996;**347**:995–999.

16. Cuschieri A, *et al*. Patient survival after D1 and D2 resections for gastric cancer: Long-term results of the MRC randomized surgical trial. Surgical Co-operative Group. *Br J Cancer* 1999;**79**:1522–1530.

17. Bonenkamp JJ, *et al*, Dutch Gastric Cancer Group. Extended lymph-node dissection for gastric cancer. *N Engl J Med* 1999;**340**:908–914.

18. Bonenkamp JJ, *et al*. Randomised comparison of morbidity after D1 and D2 dissection for gastric cancer in 996 Dutch patients. *Lancet* 1995;**345**:745–748.

19. Sano T, *et al*. Gastric cancer surgery: Morbidity and mortality results from a prospective randomized controlled trial comparing D2 and extended para-aortic lymphadenectomy — Japan Clinical Oncology Group study 9501. *J Clin Oncol* 2004;**22**:2767–2773.

20. Park DJ, *et al*. Predictors of operative morbidity and mortality in gastric cancer surgery. *Br J Surg* 2005;**92**:1099–1102.

21. Songun I, *et al*. Surgical treatment of gastric cancer: 15-year follow-up results of the randomised nationwide Dutch D1D2 trial. *Lancet Oncol* 2010;**11**:439–449.

22. Degiuli M, *et al*. Italian Gastric Cancer Study Group. Morbidity and mortality in the Italian Gastric Cancer Study Group randomized clinical trial of D1 versus D2 resection for gastric cancer. *Br J Surg* 2010;**97**:643–649.

23. Coupland VH, *et al*. Hospital volume, proportion resected and mortality from oesophageal and gastric cancer: A population-based study in England, 2004–2008. *Gut* 2013;**62**:961–966.

24. Yun YH, *et al*. The influence of hospital volume and surgical treatment delay on long-term survival after cancer surgery. *Ann Oncol* 2012;**23**:2731–2737.

25. Wu CW, *et al*. Nodal dissection for patients with gastric cancer: A randomised controlled trial. *Lancet Oncol* 2006;**7**:309–315.

26. Sasako M, *et al*. Japan Clinical Oncology Group. D2 lymphadenectomy alone or with para-aortic nodal dissection for gastric cancer. *N Engl J Med* 2008;**359**:453–462.

27. Macdonald JS, *et al*. Chemoradiotherapy after surgery compared with surgery alone for adenocarcinoma of the stomach or gastroesophageal junction. *N Engl J Med* 2001;**345**:725–730.

28. Smalley SR, *et al*. Updated analysis of SWOG-directed intergroup study 0116: A phase III trial of adjuvant radiochemotherapy versus observation after curative gastric cancer resection. *J Clin Oncol* 2012;**30**:2327–2333.

29. Cunningham D, *et al*. Perioperative chemotherapy versus surgery alone for resectable gastroesophageal cancer. *N Engl J Med* 2006;**355**:11–20.

30. Ychou M, *et al*. Perioperative chemotherapy compared with surgery alone for resectable gastroesophageal adenocarcinoma: An FNCLCC and FFCD multicenter phase III trial. *J Clin Oncol* 2011;**29**:1715–1721.

31. Sasako M, *et al.* Five-year outcomes of a randomized phase III trial comparing adjuvant chemotherapy with S-1 versus surgery alone in stage II or III gastric cancer. *J Clin Oncol* 2011;**29**:4387–4393.

32. Noh SH, *et al.* Adjuvant capecitabine plus oxaliplatin for gastric cancer after D2 gastrectomy (CLASSIC): 5-year follow-up of an open-label, randomised phase 3 trial. *Lancet Oncol* 2014;**15**:1389–1396.

33. Miyashiro I, *et al.* Gastric Cancer Surgical Study Group in the Japan Clinical Oncology Group. Randomized clinical trial of adjuvant chemotherapy with intraperitoneal and intravenous cisplatin followed by oral fluorouracil (UFT) in serosa-positive gastric cancer versus curative resection alone: Final results of the Japan Clinical Oncology Group trial JCOG9206-2. *Gastric Cancer* 2011;**14**:212–218.

34. Park SR, *et al.* Prognostic value of preoperative clinical staging assessed by computed tomography in resectable gastric cancer patients: A viewpoint in the era of preoperative treatment. *Ann Surg* 2010;**251**:428–435.

35. Hyung WJ, *et al.* Changes in treatment outcomes of gastric cancer surgery over 45 years at a single institution. *Yonsei Med J* 2008;**49**:409–415.

36. Lee J, *et al.* Phase III trial comparing capecitabine plus cisplatin versus capecitabine plus cisplatin with concurrent capecitabine radiotherapy in completely resected gastric cancer with D2 lymph node dissection: The ARTIST trial, *J. Clin. Oncol* 2012;**30**: 268–273.

37. GASTRIC Group, Paoletti X, *et al.* Benefit of adjuvant chemotherapy for resectable gastric cancer: A meta-analysis. *JAMA* 2010;**303**:1729–1737.

38. Sakuramoto S, *et al.* ACTS-GC Group. Adjuvant chemotherapy for gastric cancer with S-1, an oral fluoropyrimidine. *N Engl J Med* 2007;**357**:1810–1820.

39. Bang YJ, *et al.* CLASSIC trial investigators. Adjuvant capecitabine and oxaliplatin for gastric cancer after D2 gastrectomy (CLASSIC): A phase 3 open-label, randomised controlled trial. *Lancet* 2012;**379**:315–321.

40. Fuchs CS, *et al.* Postoperative adjuvant chemoradiation for gastric or gastroesophageal junction (GEJ) adenocarcinoma using epirubicin, cisplatin, and infusional (CI) 5-FU (ECF) before and after CI 5-FU and radiotherapy (CRT) compared with bolus 5-FU/LV before and after CRT: Intergroup trial CALGB 80101. *J Clin Oncol* 2011;**29**(Suppl.; Abstr. 4003).

41. Bajetta E, *et al.* ITACA-S (Intergroup Trial of Adjuvant Chemotherapy in Adenocarcinoma of the Stomach Trial) Study Group. Randomized trial on adjuvant treatment with FOLFIRI followed by docetaxel and cisplatin versus 5-fluorouracil and folinic acid for radically resected gastric cancer. *Ann Oncol* 2014;**25**:1373–1378.

42. Kang YK, *et al.* Adjuvant chemotherapy for gastric cancer: A randomised phase 3 trial of mitomycin-C plus either short-term doxifluridine or long-term doxifluridine plus cisplatin after curative D2 gastrectomy (AMC0201). *Br J Cancer* 2013;**108**: 1245–1251.

43. Kang YK, *et al.* Enhanced efficacy of postoperative adjuvant chemotherapy in advanced gastric cancer: Results from a phase 3 randomized trial (AMC0101). *Cancer Chemother Pharmacol* 2014;**73**:139–149.

44. Glimelius B, *et al.* Randomized comparison between chemotherapy plus best supportive care with best supportive care in advanced gastric cancer. *Ann Oncol* 1997;**8**:163–168.

45. Murad AM, *et al.* Modified therapy with 5-fluorouracil, doxorubicin, and methotrexate in advanced gastric cancer. *Cancer* 1993;**72**:37–41.

46. Pyrhonen S, *et al.* Randomised comparison of fluorouracil, epidoxorubicin and methotrexate (FEMTX) plus supportive care with supportive care alone in patients with non-resectable gastric cancer. *Br J Cancer* 1995;**71**:587–591.

47. Wagner AD, *et al.* Chemotherapy in advanced gastric cancer: A systematic review and meta-analysis based on aggregate data. *J Clin Oncol* 2006;**24**:2903–2909.

48. Boku N, *et al.* Gastrointestinal Oncology Study Group of the Japan Clinical Oncology Group. Fluorouracil versus combination of irinotecan plus cisplatin versus S-1 in metastatic gastric cancer: A randomised phase 3 study. *Lancet Oncol* 2009;**10**:1063–1069.

49. Ajani JA, *et al.* Multicenter phase III comparison of cisplatin/S-1 with cisplatin/infusional fluorouracil in advanced gastric or gastroesophageal adenocarcinoma study: The FLAGS trial. *J Clin Oncol* 2010;**28**:1547–1553.

50. Kang YK, *et al.* Capecitabine/cisplatin versus 5-fluorouracil/cisplatin as first-line therapy in patients with advanced gastric cancer: A randomised phase III noninferiority trial. *Ann Oncol* 2009;**20**:666–673.

51. Cunningham D, *et al.* Upper Gastrointestinal Clinical Studies Group of the National Cancer Research Institute of the United Kingdom. Capecitabine and oxaliplatin for advanced esophagogastric cancer. *N Engl J Med* 2008;**358**:36–46.

52. Ajani JA, *et al.* Phase I pharmacokinetic study of S-1 plus cisplatin in patients with advanced gastric carcinoma. *J Clin Oncol* 2005;**23**:6957–6965.

53. Lee JL, *et al.* Phase I/II study of 3-week combination of S-1 and cisplatin chemotherapy for metastatic or recurrent gastric cancer. *Cancer Chemother Pharmacol* 2008;**61**:837–845.

54. Chuah B, *et al.* Comparison of the pharmacokinetics and pharmacodynamics of S-1 between Caucasian and East Asian patients. *Cancer Sci* 2011;**102**:478–483.

55. Koizumi W, *et al.* S-1 plus cisplatin versus S-1 alone for first-line treatment of advanced gastric cancer (SPIRITS trial): A phase III trial. *Lancet Oncol* 2008;**9**:215–221.

56. Ryu MH, *et al.* Comparison of two different S-1 plus cisplatin dosing schedules as first-line chemotherapy for metastatic and/or recurrent gastric cancer: A multicenter, randomized phase III trial (SOS). *Ann Oncol* 2015;**26**:2097–2101.

57. Webb A, *et al.* Randomized trial comparing epirubicin, cisplatin, and fluorouracil versus fluorouracil, doxorubicin, and methotrexate in advanced esophagogastric cancer. *J Clin Oncol* 1997;**15**:261–267.

58. Al-Batran SE, *et al.* Arbeitsgemeinschaft Internistische Onkologie. Phase III trial in metastatic gastroesophageal adenocarcinoma with fluorouracil, leucovorin plus either oxaliplatin or cisplatin: A study of the Arbeitsgemeinschaft Internistische Onkologie, *J Clin Oncol* 2008;**26**:1435–1442.

59. Van Cutsem E, *et al.* V325 Study Group. Phase III study of docetaxel and cisplatin plus fluorouracil compared with cisplatin and fluorouracil as first-line therapy for advanced gastric cancer: A report of the V325 Study Group. *J Clin Oncol* 2006;**24**:4991–4997.

60. Shah MA, *et al.* Randomized Multicenter phase II study of modified docetaxel, cisplatin, and fluorouracil (DCF) versus DCF plus growth factor support in patients with

metastatic gastric adenocarcinoma: A study of the US Gastric Cancer Consortium. *J Clin Oncol* 2015;**33**:3874–3879.

61. Al-Batran SE, *et al*. Biweekly fluorouracil, leucovorin, oxaliplatin, and docetaxel (FLOT) for patients with metastatic adenocarcinoma of the stomach or esophagogastric junction: A phase II trial of the Arbeitsgemeinschaft Internistische Onkologie. *Ann Oncol* 2008;**19**:1882–1887.

62. Kang JH, *et al*. Salvage chemotherapy for pretreated gastric cancer: A randomized phase III trial comparing chemotherapy plus best supportive care with best supportive care alone. *J Clin Oncol* 2012;**30**:1513–1518.

63. Ford HE, *et al*. COUGAR-02 Investigators. Docetaxel versus active symptom control for refractory oesophagogastric adenocarcinoma (COUGAR-02): An open-label, phase 3 randomised controlled trial. *Lancet Oncol* 2014;**15**:78–86.

64. Ohtsu A, *et al*. Bevacizumab in combination with chemotherapy as first-line therapy in advanced gastric cancer: A randomized, double-blind, placebo-controlled phase III study. *J Clin Oncol* 2011;**29**:3968–3976.

65 Hironaka, S., *et al*. (2013). Randomized, open-label, phase III study comparing irinotecan with paclitaxel in patients with advanced gastric cancer without severe peritoneal metastasis after failure of prior combination chemotherapy using fluoropyrimidine plus platinum: WJOG 4007 trial, *J. Clin. Oncol.*, 31, pp. 4438–4444.

66. Bang YJ, *et al*. ToGA Trial Investigators. Trastuzumab in combination with chemotherapy versus chemotherapy alone for treatment of HER2-positive advanced gastric or gastro-oesophageal junction cancer (ToGA): A phase 3, open-label, randomised controlled trial. *Lancet* 2010;**376**:687–697.

67. Van Cutsem E, *et al*. HER2 screening data from ToGA: Targeting HER2 in gastric and gastroesophageal junction cancer. *Gastric Cancer* 2015;**18**:476–484.

68. Hecht JR, *et al*. Lapatinib in combination with capecitabine plus oxaliplatin in human epidermal growth factor receptor 2-positive advanced or metastatic gastric, esophageal, or gastroesophageal adenocarcinoma: TRIO-013/LOGiC—a randomized phase III trial. *J Clin Oncol* 2016;34:443-451.

69. Satoh T, *et al*. Lapatinib plus paclitaxel versus paclitaxel alone in the second-line treatment of HER2-amplified advanced gastric cancer in Asian populations: TYTAN — a randomized, phase III study. *J Clin Oncol* 2014;**32**:2039–2049.

70. Fuchs CS, *et al*. REGARD Trial Investigators. Ramucirumab monotherapy for previously treated advanced gastric or gastro-oesophageal junction adenocarcinoma (REGARD): An international, randomised, multicentre, placebo-controlled, phase 3 trial. *Lancet* 2014;**383**:31–39.

71. Wilke H, *et al*. Ramucirumab plus paclitaxel versus placebo plus paclitaxel in patients with previously treated advanced gastric or gastro-oesophageal junction adenocarcinoma (RAINBOW): A double-blind, randomised phase 3 trial. *Lancet Oncol* 2014;**15**:1224–1235.

72. Van Cutsem E, *et al*. Bevacizumab in combination with chemotherapy as first-line therapy in advanced gastric cancer: A biomarker evaluation from the AVAGAST randomized phase III trial. *J Clin Oncol* 2012;**30**:2119–2127.

73. Qin S. Phase III study of apatinib in advanced gastric cancer: A randomized, double-blind, placebo-controlled trial. *J Clin Oncol* 2014;32:5s (suppl; abstr 4003).

Chapter 7

The Development
of Systemic Therapies for Esophageal
and Gastric Cancers

Tong Dai and Manish A. Shah

1 Introduction

Esophageal and gastric cancers are the eighth and fifth most common cancers in the world, respectively.[1,2] While these cancers are less common in the United States, they are associated with a five-year survival rate of less than 40%, even when diagnosed at an early stage.[3] Gastric cancer ranks fourth in global incidence, yet is second in cancer-related mortality.[4] During the recent years, sub-classification of gastric cancer using genetic profiling has not only provided prognostic value, but also guided selection of systemic chemotherapy. Accumulating data of the molecular mechanisms has led to identification of new therapeutic targets and development of novel small-molecule inhibitors and monoclonal antibodies which have demonstrated clinical efficacy.

2 Risk Factors

A meta-analysis of 132 studies showed an increased risk of esophageal squamous carcinoma in patients with human papilloma virus (HPV) infection.[5] Barrett's esophagus, cigarette smoking, Caucasian ethnicity, male gender, increased age, and poor diet are predominant risk factors for adenocarcinoma of esophagus.[6–8] *H. pylori* infection, while implicated in gastric cancer, may lower the risk of

153

esophageal disease development.[9] The majority of gastric cancer cases are related to *H. pylori* infection, with a conservative estimate of 74.7% of all the non-cardia gastric cancers.[10,11] It is well established that *H. pylori* causes premalignant lesions including atrophy, intestinal metaplasia, and dysplasia of the gastric mucosa.[12]

3 Genetics of Esophageal and Gastric Cancer

Genomic studies in squamous carcinoma of the esophagus revealed somatic copy number variations (SCNVs) involving several loci, as well as somatic mutations in *PIK3CA*, *TP53*, and *NOTCH1*.[13,14] A recently reported whole-exome/targeted deep sequencing of 139 paired squamous cell carcinoma (SCC) cases, and analysis of SCNV in over 180 esophageal squamous carcinoma patients identified additional mutated genes including *FAT1*, *FAT2*, *ZNF750*, and *KMT2D*.[15] Dysregulation of the receptor tyrosine kinase (RTK)–MAPK–PI3K pathway, cell cycle progression, and epigenetic regulation of gene expression appear to be the most common molecular alterations. In contrast, whole-exome sequencing of 149 esophageal adenocarcinoma identified 26 significantly mutated genes, including five previously described adenocarcinoma-associated genes (*TP53*, *CDKN2A*, *SMAD4*, *ARID1A*, and *PIK3CA*). In addition, chromatin-modifying factors and candidate contributors *SPG20*, *TLR4*, *ELMO1*, and *DOCK2* were significantly mutated.[16] Functional analyses of adenocarcinoma-derived mutations in *ELMO1* identifies increased cellular invasion, suggesting the potential activation of the RAC1 pathway as a molecular mechanism of esophageal adenocarcinoma.

4 Cytotoxic Chemotherapy

Traditionally, treatment of advanced esophageal and gastric cancer is systemic chemotherapy. The combination of cisplatin and 5-FU given by continuous infusion for 4–5 days has been studied extensively in advanced esophageal cancer.[17] A phase II study in locally advanced or metastatic SCC was the only trial which compared single-agent cisplatin with combination of cisplatin and 5-FU. This study showed that the cisplatin/5-FU arm had a higher response rate (35%) and better median survival (33 weeks) compared to the cisplatin arm (19% and 28 weeks, respectively), but these findings were not statistically significant.[18] Cisplatin plus paclitaxel or docetaxel also demonstrated increased activity in both advanced esophageal or gastroesophageal junction (GEJ) cancers.[19,20] Similarly, a combination of cisplatin and irinotecan was proven to be active in a phase II trial in metastatic or recurrent esophageal cancer, particularly in esophageal squamous carcinoma.[21] Patients treated with combination therapy had improved progression-free survival (PFS) and overall survival (OS) rates of 4.4 and 9.6 months, respectively.[22]

In a phase III trial in gastric and GEJ adenocarcinoma, the ECF regimen (epirubicin, cisplatin, and 5-FU) resulted in a superior response rate (45% *vs.* 21%), failure-free survival (7.4 *vs.* 3.4 months), and median survival (8.9 *vs.* 5.7 months) compared to FAMTX (5-FU, doxorubicin, and methotrexate).[23] The ECF regimen had a favorable toxicity profile, with less than 10% grade 3 or 4 toxicity. Another phase III study showed the DCF regimen (docetaxel, cisplatin, and 5-FU) resulted in a higher response rate (36%) and longer time to progression (5.6 months) compared to CF alone (cisplatin and 5-FU) (26% and 3.7 months, respectively), but the improvement in median survival (9.2 *vs.* 8.6 months) was minimal.[24] A randomized phase II trial comparing ECF to DCF in gastric and GEJ cancer showed superior response rate and time to progression (TTP) with DCF when compared to ECF, but increased toxicity mainly neutropenia and neutropenic fever.[25] The phase III REAL-2 study demonstrated capecitabine and oxaliplatin are as effective as fluorouracil and cisplatin when combined with epirubicine, respectively, in patients with previously untreated gastroesophageal cancer.[26] Median survival in the ECF, ECX, EOF, and EOX groups were 9.9 months, 9.9 months, 9.3 months, and 11.2 months, respectively.

Irinotecan is another commonly used chemotherapy agent.[27] A phase III French Intergroup trial recently showed first-line FOLFIRI (5-FU, leucovorin, and irinotecan) was well tolerated in advanced gastric and GEJ cancer, and prolonged median TTP compared to ECX (5.1 *vs.* 4.2 months), although there was no significant difference between the two groups in median PFS (5.3 *vs.* 5.8 months) and median OS (9.5 *vs.* 9.7 months).[28]

Irinotecan has also been evaluated extensively in the second-line setting. For example, it was compared to paclitaxel in advanced gastric cancer after failure of 5-FU-based therapy, and there was no significant difference in OS (9.5 *vs.* 8.4 months) or PFS (3.6 *vs.* 2.3 months).[29] Gastric/GEJ cancer patients who were given FOLFIRI as a second-line therapy after experiencing disease progression on or after first-line docetaxel-containing chemotherapy achieved PFS and OS of 3.8 and 6.2 months, respectively.[30] Recently, modified EOX and FOLFIRI were shown to have similar efficacy as second-line therapy in patients with metastatic gastric cancer who progressed on modified DCF regimen. Median PFS was 5.5 and 6.3 months, and median OS was 6.9 and 7.0 months in mEOX and FOLFIRI arms, respectively.[31]

4.1 *Treatment of gastric cancer by subtype*

Gastric cancers were traditionally classified into either Lauren's diffuse or intestinal subtypes based on histopathologic features.[32] A recent study identified two major genomic subtypes (G-INT and G-DIF) based on distinct patterns of gene expression.[33] In addition, the intrinsic subtypes, not subtypes based on Lauren's classification, were prognostic of survival. The G-INT cell lines were significantly more sensitive to 5-FU and oxaliplatin, whereas G-DIF cells were more sensitive to cisplatin. There was a trend of stage-adjusted survival benefit in patients with G-INT subtype from 5-FU adjuvant therapy. This data is consistent with data from the INT-0116 study, where a 10-year follow-up revealed that all gastric cancer subsets benefited from 5-FU therapy except for cases with diffuse histology.[34] Consistent with *in vitro* data, JCOG9912 showed the benefit of irinotecan/cisplatin over 5-FU-based monotherapy in diffuse but not intestinal subtypes.[35] A recent study suggested a combination of well-differentiated intestinal-type and microsatellite instability are markers of 5-FU-sensitive gastric adenocarcinomas.[36] By examining differentially expressed genes using microarray, Lei *et al.* classified gastric cancer into three novel subtypes: mesenchymal, proliferative, and metabolic.[37] The mesenchymal and proliferative subtypes largely coincide with Lauren's diffuse and intestinal subtypes, respectively. Tumors of the proliferative subtype had high levels of genomic instability, *TP53* mutations, and DNA hypomethylation. In contrast, tumors of the mesenchymal subtype contain cells with features of cancer stem cells, and cell lines of this subtype are particularly sensitive to PI3K-AKT-mTOR inhibitors *in vitro*. The newly designated metabolic subtype has elevated expression of genes associated with metabolic pathways. Cancer cells of the metabolic subtype were more sensitive to 5-FU than the other subtypes, and patients with this subtype appeared to have greater benefit with 5-FU treatment. Thus, molecular subtyping may guide selection of chemotherapy for gastric cancer.

5 Targeted Therapy

In the past decades, several genetic alterations have been found to be the drivers of human cancers. For example, *bcr-abl* translocation, *EGFR* mutation or deletion, and *ErbB2* amplification are the underlying molecular events for chronic myelogenic leukemia, a proportion of non-small cell lung cancer, and a subset of breast cancer, respectively.[38–40] More importantly, therapeutics specifically targeting these oncogenic pathways are effective in treating respective diseases and prolonging survival.[41–43] With the understanding of genetics of esophageal and gastric cancer, trastuzumab became the first targeted therapy developed for gastric cancer.[44,45]

5.1 *ErbB receptor family*

The ErbB (erythroblastic leukemia viral oncogen homolog) family of membrane-associated proteins consists of four members, including HER1 or

EGFR and HER2–HER4 proteins (ErbB2–ErbB4). These proteins are all involved in transmembrane signaling essential to cellular survival and replication. They have been shown to sustain malignant behavior of cells of various origins including breast, head and neck, and gastrointestinal sites. Ligand stimulation causes homo- and heterodimerization of these receptors with subsequent activation of tyrosine kinase and downstream major intracellular pathways such as Ras–Raf–MEK/MAPK and PI3K/AKT. Overexpression and amplification of HER2 have been described in 10–30% of GEJ adenocarcinomas with lower rates of expression on non-GEJ gastric cancers.[46] Interestingly, HER2 upregulation is reported less commonly in diffuse gastric cancer (2%) as opposed to intestinal type gastric cancer (20%). HER2 amplification has been variably shown to be associated with worse survival. In breast cancer, HER2 upregulation portends inferior 10-year survival rates for resectable disease.[47] In contrast, a recent analysis of 49 studies published up until January 2011 reporting on both resectable and metastatic gastric cancer failed to find a statistically significant difference in outcomes based on HER2 expression, with a median five-year survival rate of 42% and 52% in patients with and without HER2 overexpression, respectively.[48] A prospective tissue correlation study in 381 stage IV gastric cancer patients, none of whom received trastuzumab, a humanized anti-HER2 monoclonal antibody, noted that patients with HER2-positive disease had increased OS rates than HER2-negative patients (13.9 months *vs.* 11.4 months; $p = 0.047$).[49] A retrospective study of over 800 patients confirmed this finding with a hazard ratio (HR) of 0.58 ($p = 0.03$), favoring HER2-positive patients treated with trastuzumab. The MAGIC trial sought to determine the efficacy of perioperative chemotherapy in resectable gastric cancer. In localized disease, a post-hoc analysis of HER2 status of the patients treated on the MAGIC trial, where the prevalence of HER2 positivity was 10%, showed no difference in survival (HER2-positive HR 0.74; HER2-negative HR 0.58; $p = 0.7$).[50] Interestingly, in a retrospective review of localized esophageal adenocarcinomas, HER2 positivity conferred improved survival.[51]

Nevertheless, the ToGA study showed median OS was improved significantly with the addition of trastuzumab compared with chemotherapy (fluoropyrimidine and platinum) alone (13.5 *vs.* 11.1 months; $p = 0.0048$; HR 0.74) in advanced gastroesophageal adenocarcinoma.[45] Importantly, the benefit was most evident in patients with HER2-overexpressing tumors as defined as HER2 IHC 2+ or 3+ and FISH positive (OS 16.0 *vs.* 11.8 months; $p = 0.0046$). Based on this landmark study, trastuzumab in combination with chemotherapy is now the standard for HER2-positive gastric/GEJ adenocarcinoma globally.

Lapatinib is a dual inhibitor of the tyrosine kinase domains of EGFR and HER2. The TyTAN trial compared lapatinib/paclitaxel with paclitaxel alone in patients with HER2-positive gastric cancer, determined by FISH, who had progressed on platinum-based first-line therapy.[52] Median overall survival was 11.0 months for lapatinib/paclitaxel compared with 8.9 months with paclitaxel alone but did not reach statistical significance (HR 0.84; $p = 0.1044$). The benefit of lapatinib might be restricted to patients with higher HER2 expression, as in a preplanned subgroup analysis, median OS among patients in the HER2 IHC 3+ subgroup was 14.0 months *vs.* 7.6 months, in favor of the addition of lapatinib (HR 0.59; $p = 0.0176$). The LOGiC trial compared first-line therapy with capecitabine and oxaliplatin with or without lapatinib. Disappointingly, addition of lapatinib to CapeOx did not prolong media OS (12.2 *vs.* 10.6 months, HR 0.91), and instead increased toxicities, particularly diarrhea.[53]

Novel strategies to exploit the presence of HER2 on the cell membrane include the use of antibody–drug conjugates in order to deliver cytotoxic agents with a high degree of specificity. One such molecule is trastuzumab emtansine, or T-DM1. This construct links trastuzumab to mertansine, a cytotoxic anti-microtubule macrolide. T-DM1's mechanism of action is that it retains the effect of PI3K/AKT disruption due to targeted binding leading to HER2 receptor internalization, followed by lysosomal degradation. However, once internalized, T-DM1 catabolites bind to tubulin, preventing polymerization and suppressing microtubule dynamic instability.[54] In two randomized trials examining T-DM1 in metastatic breast cancer, trastuzumab emtansine showed efficacy in both first and second-line settings. This supports the theory that an alternate mechanism exists in the HER2 pathway which may target resistance mechanisms.[54–56] However, phase II/III GATSBY trial, an international registration study examining T-DM1 compared with single-agent taxane in previously treated metastatic gastric cancer patients, showed median OS of 7.9 months for the weekly T-DM1 group vs. 8.6 months for the taxane group (HR = 1.15). Moreover, median PFS was 2.7 months and 2.9 months, respectively.[57]

It is known that a minimum serum trough concentration (C_{min}) of trastuzumab of approximately 20 μg/mL causes maximal tumor growth inhibition in preclinical models.[58] In gastric cancer patients, it was observed that non-linear elimination pharmacokinetics govern serum levels of the drug, resulting in higher clearance rates. This is believed to be secondary to a target-mediated clearance process due to binding to the extracellular domain of the HER2 protein. Based on predicted concentrations, at standard FDA-approved dosing of 8 mg/kg on cycle 1 followed by 6 mg/kg maintenance doses every three weeks, the total clearance was found to be stable within the first three days but then increased by 48% over the subsequent days. There is evidence that patients in the lowest C_{min} quartile subgroup test had poorer outcomes. The HELOISE study compared two dose levels of trastuzumab along with standard fluoropyrimidine and platinum therapy in the front-line treatment of metastatic gastric cancer but failed to show that higher maintenance dosing regimen of trastuzumab improves overall survival compared to the standard dosing regimen (NCT01450696).

5.2 *HGF–MET*

MET (c-Met), also known as hepatocyte growth factor (HGF) receptor, is a tyrosine kinase receptor (RTK) with multiple downstream effects including regulation of cell survival and migration of epithelial and myogenic precursor cells.[59] Aberrant MET activation in gastric cancer occurs through receptor overexpression, upregulation of stromal HGF ligand production as well as gene amplification.[60] MET is also involved in resistance to therapies targeting other growth factor pathways.[61] Gene amplification, mutation of the *MET* gene, or increased MET expression is known to occur in gastric, hepatocellular, and pancreatic cancers, respectively.[62] Preclinical data shows that similar MET-mediated resistance mechanisms are occurring with anti-HER2 (ERbB2) in breast cancer and gastric cancer cell lines.[63]

Onartuzumab (MetMAb) is a monovalent, humanized anti-MET antibody, specifically designed to avoid agonistic activity that may occur when a bivalent antibody binds two MET molecules. MetMAb blocks HGF-induced MET dimerization and activation of the intracellular kinase domain. A complete response of two years has been reported in a patient with metastatic gastric cancer when treated with onartuzumab on a phase I study.[64] The phase III MET gastric study randomized patients with metastatic HER2-negative and Met-positive adenocarcinoma of stomach or GEJ to receive either onartuzumab or placebo in combination with mFOLFOX6 (NCT01662869). The addition of onartuzumab to mFOLFOX6 was ineffective in prolonging OS in ITT (11.0 vs. 11.3 months) or MET 2+/3+ (11.0 vs. 9.7 months) patients, although subgroup analysis suggests non-Asian patients and those without prior gastrectomy may benefit.[65]

Rilotumumab is a new fully humanized monoclonal antibody against HGF that prevents its binding to the MET receptor. A recently reported double-blind phase II study randomly assigned 121 previously untreated patients (1:1:1) with advanced gastric or GEJ cancer to receive rilotumumab 15 mg/kg, rilotumumab 7.5 mg/kg, or placebo, plus ECX (epirubicin, cisplatin, and capecitabine).[66] Median PFS was 5.1 months ($p = 0.164$ *vs.* placebo group) in the rilotumumab 15 mg/kg group, 6.8 months ($p = 0.009$) in the rilotumumab 7.5 mg/kg group, 5.7 months ($p = 0.016$) in both rilotumumab groups combined, and 4.2 months in the placebo group. Median OS were longer in the combined rilotumumab groups than in the placebo group, although it is not statistically significant. In addition, in patients with MET-positive tumor (IHC or FISH confirmed), median OS was prolonged when treated with combined rilotumumab *vs.* ECX alone (10.6 *vs.* 5.7 months). This is the first randomized study of an agent targeting the HGF–MET pathway in gastric and GEJ adenocarcinoma which prolong PFS when combined with chemotherapy in MET-high tumors. However, the phase III study RILOMET-1 comparing ECX plus rilotumumab (15 mg/kg) *vs.* placebo was recently halted due to increased deaths in the rilotumumab arm with significantly worse median OS compared to placebo arm (9.6 vs. 11.5 months, HR 1.37; NCT01697072).[67]

5.3 *Vascular endothelial growth factor*

Targeting tumor angiogenesis has been one of the most active areas of research for several decades. Over 30 years ago, vascular endothelial growth factor A (VEGF-A) was implicated as a central mediator of endothelial cell survival and vascular development, and subsequently its role in tumor angiogenesis was recognized.[68,69] Despite the ensuing improvement in OS in colorectal cancer with the angiogenesis inhibitor bevacizumab, a monoclonal antibody directed against VEGF-A, similar success has not been approved so far with upper gastrointestinal malignancies. The five VEGF ligands, VEGF-A through VEGF-D and placental growth factor (PGF) are the result of alternative splicing and proteolytic processing depending on the developmental and cellular context.[70] These ligands modulate various normal processes including cell proliferation, migration, maturation, vasculogenesis as well as the control of vessel permeability. The ligands interact with one or several of three transmembrane receptors (VEGFR1 through -3). VEGF family receptors belong to class V receptor tyrosine kinases (RTKs) carrying seven immunoglobulin-like domains in the extracellular domain (ECD). Similar to other RTK groups, VEGFR hetero- or homodimerization causes intracellular kinase activation and leads to downstream signaling via Src homology-2 (SH2) mediators with modulation of MAPK, AKT, and Ras/Raf pathways.

Bevacizumab is a recombinant, humanized monoclonal antibody that targets VEGF-A, forming a complex that prevents binding of the ligand on the receptor. Phase II studies which combined bevacizumab with standard chemotherapy showed promising median OS when compared to historical controls. In 47 patients with metastatic gastric carcinoma, the combination of cisplatin, irinotecan, and bevacizumab achieved a median survival of 12.3 months, while another study adding bevacizumab to docetaxel and oxaliplatin similarly reported a median survival of 11.1 months (95% CI 8.2–15.3).[71,72] Subsequently, the AVAGAST study randomized 700 metastatic gastric cancer patients to receive standard platinum/fluoropyrimidine with or without bevacizumab.[73] The study failed to show improvement in OS with the addition of bevacizumab (10.1 *vs.* 12.1 months, $p = 0.1002$) though statistically significant improvements in response rate (RR) and PFS were observed. However, in a subsequent subset analysis observed that patients with high baseline plasma VEGF-A levels had a trend toward improved OS (HR 0.72) *vs.* patients with low VEGF-A levels (HR, 1.01; interaction $p = 0.07$).[74]

Ramucirumab (IMC-1121B) is a fully human IgG1 monoclonal antibody targeting VEGF2. The REGARD study, a placebo-controlled, double-blind, phase III international trial, was conducted in the second-line setting in patients with metastatic gastric or GEJ adenocarcinoma.[52] Median OS was 5.2 months for ramucirumab and 3.8 months for placebo (HR 0.776). The RAINBOW study, a randomized phase III trial of ramucirumab in combination with paclitaxel *vs.* paclitaxel monotherapy in the second-line treatment of metastatic gastric cancer showed OS was significantly longer in the ramucirumab plus paclitaxel group than in the placebo plus paclitaxel group (9.6 *vs.* 7.4 months, HR 0.807).[75] These two studies demonstrated that VEGF pathways are valid targets for the treatment of advanced gastric or GEJ adenocarcinoma, and established ramucirumab as an important therapeutic for these diseases.

The ongoing anti-angiogenic therapy trial, ST-03, or MAGIC-B, is examining the impact of perioperative bevacizumab when added to ECX in a phase III setting (NCT00450203).

5.4 *JAK/STAT*

Signal transducers and activators of transcription (STATs) comprise a family of cytoplasmic transcription factors that mediate intracellular signaling from cell-surface receptors to the nucleus. Numerous studies have demonstrated constitutive activation of STAT3 in a wide variety of human tumors, including gastric cancer. STAT3 can be activated by the entire IL-6 family of cytokines and growth factors such as epidermal growth factor (EGF).[76,77] Binding of ligand to receptor results in dimerization of a signal transducer protein, gp130 in the cytoplasm,[78] followed by induction of Janus kinase (JAK) phosphorylation and subsequently STAT3 phosphorylation.[79] Phosphorylated STAT3 form dimers and translocate into the nucleus, leading to transcription of genes involved in cell survival and proliferation.[80] Persistent activation of STAT3 has been reported in a variety of primary human tumors, and the mechanisms include enhanced proliferation, cell survival, inflammation, invasion, and angiogenesis.[81–83] The broad function of STAT3 suggests it is a promising target for anti-cancer therapy.

BBI608 is an oral first-in-class cancer stemness inhibitor which inhibits the Stat3, β-catenin, and Nanog pathways. Preclinically, potent broad-spectrum anti-tumor and anti-metastatic activity was observed *in vitro* and *in vivo*, alone and in combination with other agents.[84] In addition, BBI608 and paclitaxel showed marked synergy *in vivo*. In a phase Ib dose-escalation study in 24 patients, BBI608 was given in combination with paclitaxel in full dose.[84] The most common adverse events included grades 1 and 2 toxicities such as diarrhea, abdominal cramps, nausea, and vomiting. Disease control (CR+PR+SD) was observed in 10 of 15 (67%) evaluable patients. Of five patients with refractory gastric/GEJ adenocarcinoma, two had partial responses (48% and 45% regressions), one had stable disease with 25% regression, and two (who failed prior taxane) had prolonged stable disease for more than or equal to 24 weeks. Given the encouraging anti-tumor activity of BBI608 plus paclitaxel, BRIGHTER trial, the phase III randomized, double-blind study comparing BBI608 plus weekly paclitaxel *vs.* placebo plus weekly paclitaxel is currently recruiting patients with advanced, previously treated gastric and GEJ adenocarcinoma (NCT02178956).

5.5 *Notch signaling*

The evolutionarily conserved Notch are transmembrane receptors (Notch 1–4) for five ligands, two of the Jagged family (Jagged 1–2) and three of the Delta-like family (DLL1, DLL3, and DLL4).[85] Notch is cleaved by γ-secretase complex upon binding to ligands, releasing the intracellular domain of the Notch receptor (NICD). NICD translocates into the nucleus and regulates the transcription of target genes, including the hairy enhancer of split (Hes) and Hes-related (Hey) family. Notch signaling pathway plays a pivotal role in self-renewal of stem cells and cell-fate determination of progenitors.[86] A meta-analysis of 15 studies examined Notch expression in 1,547 gastric cancer cases and 450 controls.[87] Overall, the expression of Notch1, Notch2, Delta-like 4, and Hes1 was significantly higher in tumor tissues compared to normal tissues. Specifically, stratified analyses showed that significantly increased expression of Notch1 was associated with non-cardia location, > 5 cm size, diffuse type, positive lymphovascular invasion, and distal metastasis. Statistically significantly higher expression of Notch3 was found in diffuse type. Jagged1 was also significantly over expressed in diffuse type and poor differentiation type of gastric cancer. DLL4 was significantly overexpressed in advanced T stage, N stage, and TNM stage in gastric cancer. In gastric cancer cell lines, DAPT, a potent γ-secretase inhibitor (GSI), has been shown to inhibit gastric cancer cell growth and epithelial–mesenchymal transition.[88] However, DAPT has limited ability to induce apoptosis, partly due to activation of ERK1/2 upon DAPT treatment.[89] This hypothesis is supported by the observation that selective inhibition of ERK1/2 activation dramatically sensitized gastric cancer cells to apoptosis via downregulating β-catenin signaling.[90] In addition, combination therapy with ERK inhibitor PD98059 and DAPT yielded additive antitumor effects when compared with either agent alone in a xenograft mouse model, providing proof-of-principle for a new strategy in treating gastric cancer. Several trials targeting Notch pathway in solid tumors are ongoing.

5.6 *Immune checkpoints*

Perhaps one of the most exciting findings in cancer research in the last decade is the realization that adaptive immunity plays an important role in host–tumor interaction, and the identification of immune checkpoints as a therapeutic target. Cytotoxic T-lymphocyte antigen 4 (CTLA-4), is a potent inhibitor of T-cell activation that helps to maintain self-tolerance, and was thought to confer evasion of cancer cells from immune-mediated killing.[91] Ipilimumab, an anti-CTAL-4 monoclonal antibody, with or without a gp100 peptide vaccine, as compared with gp100 alone, improved OS in patients with previously treated metastatic melanoma.[92] Addition of ipilimumab to dacarbazine also improved OS in this setting.[93]

A study of 101 advanced gastric cancer patients showed post-operative overall and disease-free survival (DFS) were significantly improved with high expression of tumor-infiltrating memory T cell, CD45RO compared to those of patients with low CD45RO expression.[94] Similarly, a study of 243 patients with curatively resected gastric cancer demonstrated better survival outcomes in patients with higher density of CD3(+) cells within the tumor microenvironment than in those with lower density of CD3(+) cells (five-year DFS rate, 80.9% *vs.* 67.0%; five-year OS rate, 82.5% *vs.* 68.0%; *p* values < 0.05).[92] However, expression of CTLA-4 and PD-L1, another T-cell co-inhibitory receptor, was related to less advanced stage, intestinal type, and well/moderately differentiated adenocarcinoma ($p < 0.05$),[95] which may reflect tumor response to the enhanced immune surveillance by host. A randomized phase II trial is comparing ipilimumab with standard of care immediately following first-line chemotherapy in gastric and GEJ cancer (NCT01585987).

Programmed cell death-1 (PD-1, Pdcd1), a member of the CD28/CTLA-4 family,[96] negatively regulates antigen receptor signaling by recruiting protein tyrosine phosphatase SHP2 upon interacting with either of two ligands, PD-L1 (B7-H1) and PD-L2 (B7-DC).[97–99] In contrast to CTLA4 ligands, CD80 (B7-1) and CD86 (B7-2), PD-L1 is selectively expressed on many tumors and on cells within the tumor microenvironment in response to inflammatory stimuli.[100] Blockade of the interaction between PD-1 and PD-L1 potentiates immune responses *in vitro* and mediates preclinical antitumor activity. Anti-PD-L1 antibody Nivolumab (BMS-936559) induced durable tumor regression (objective response rate of 6–17%) and prolonged stabilization of disease (rates of 12–41% at 24 weeks) in patients with advanced cancers, including non-small-cell lung cancer (NSCLC), melanoma, and renal cell cancer.[101] Dual blockade of PD-1 and CTAL-4 seems to feasible and enhance anti-tumor activity, as concurrent therapy with nivolumab and ipilimumab had a manageable safety profile and induced rapid and deep tumor regression in a substantial proportion of advanced melanoma patients.[102]

Similar to melanoma and NSCLC, upregulation of PD-1 on both CD4+ and CD8+ T cells may be responsible for immune evasion in gastric cancer.[103] Seven patients with gastric cancer were enrolled in the phase I trial of nivolumab, but were not included in efficacy analysis.[101] The phase I/II trial NCT01928394 is evaluating nivolumab alone or in combination with ipilimumab in advanced solid tumor, including gastric cancer. In a recently presented phase Ib study, anti-PD-1 antibody pembrolizumab was generally well tolerated and provided antitumor activity in patients with advanced gastric cancer that expressed PD-L1 evaluated by IHC.[104] Overall response rate (ORR; confirmed and unconfirmed) was 31.6% in Asia-Pacific and 30% in the rest of world, there was association between PD-L1 expression and PFS ($p = 0.032$) and ORR ($p = 0.071$). This study suggests that targeting immune checkpoints is a promising strategy treating advanced gastric cancer.

6 Summary

In advanced esophageal and gastric cancers, combination chemotherapy delivers superior efficacy compared to single-agent chemotherapy. Either combination or a single-agent regimen can be used in later-line treatment, depending on patient comorbidities and performance status. Recent studies have started to reveal the molecular pathogenesis of these diseases. Significant progress has been made with the development of therapeutics which target HER2 and VEGF pathways. Additional study is required to identify the patient population who may benefit from MET inhibition. Therapy incorporating agents that target STAT3 and Notch pathways also holds promise in eradicating cancer stems cells which may be the ultimate source of disease relapse and metastasis. In the near future, data from recent trials studying immune checkpoint inhibition are likely to dramatically change the paradigm of cancer treatment including advanced esophageal and gastric cancers.

References

1. Pennathur A, *et al*. Oesophageal carcinoma. *Lancet* 2013;**381**(9864):400–412.
2. Ferlay J, *et al*. Cancer incidence and mortality worldwide: Sources, methods and major patterns in GLOBOCAN 2012. *Int J Cancer* 2014;**136**(5):E359–E386.
3. Peery AF, *et al*. Burden of gastrointestinal disease in the United States: 2012 update. *Gastroenterology* 2012;**143**(5):1179–1187; e1–3.
4. Siegel R, *et al*. Cancer statistics, 2012. *CA Cancer J Clin* 2012;**62**(1):10–29.
5. Hardefeldt HA, *et al*. Association between human papillomavirus (HPV) and oesophageal squamous cell carcinoma: A meta-analysis. *Epidemiol Infect* 2014; **142**(6):1119–1137.
6. Cook MB, *et al*. Cigarette smoking increases risk of Barrett's esophagus: An analysis of the Barrett's and Esophageal Adenocarcinoma Consortium. *Gastroenterology* 2012;**142**(4):744–753.
7. Estores D, Velanovich V. Barrett's esophagus: Epidemiology, pathogenesis, diagnosis, and management. *Curr Probl Surg* 2013;**50**(5):192–226.
8. Kendall BJ, *et al*. The risk of Barrett's esophagus associated with abdominal obesity in males and females. *Int J Cancer* 2013;**132**(9):2192–2199.

9. Thrift AP, *et al. Helicobacter pylori* infection and the risks of Barrett's oesophagus: a population-based case-control study. *Int J Cancer* 2012;**130**(10):2407–2416.

10. Gonzalez CA, *et al. Helicobacter pylori* infection assessed by ELISA and by immunoblot and noncardia gastric cancer risk in a prospective study: The Eurgast-EPIC project. *Ann Oncol* 2012;**23**(5):1320–1324.

11. Jemal A, *et al. Global cancer statistics. CA Cancer J Clin* 2011;**61**(2):69–90.

12. Correa P. A human model of gastric carcinogenesis. *Cancer Res* 1988;**48**(13): 3554–3560.

13. Agrawal N, *et al.* Comparative genomic analysis of esophageal adenocarcinoma and squamous cell carcinoma. *Cancer Discov* 2012;**2**(10):899–905.

14. Shigaki H, *et al. PIK3CA* mutation is associated with a favorable prognosis among patients with curatively resected esophageal squamous cell carcinoma. *Clin Cancer Res* 2013;**19**(9):2451–2459.

15. Lin D-C, *et al.* Genomic and molecular characterization of esophageal squamous cell carcinoma. *Nat Genet* 2014;**46**(5):467–473.

16. Dulak AM, *et al.* Exome and whole-genome sequencing of esophageal adenocarcinoma identifies recurrent driver events and mutational complexity. *Nat Genet* 2013;**45**(5):478–486.

17. Ilson DH. Esophageal cancer chemotherapy: Recent advances. *Gastrointest Cancer Res* 2008;**2**(2):85–92.

18. Bleiberg H, *et al.* Randomised phase II study of cisplatin and 5-fluorouracil (5-FU) versus cisplatin alone in advanced squamous cell oesophageal cancer. *Eur J Cancer* 1997;**33**(8):1216–1220.

19. Ilson DH, *et al.* A phase II trial of paclitaxel and cisplatin in patients with advanced carcinoma of the esophagus. *Cancer J* 2000;**6**(5):316–323.

20. Kim JY, *et al.* A multi-center phase II study of docetaxel plus cisplatin as first-line therapy in patients with metastatic squamous cell esophageal cancer. *Cancer Chemother Pharmacol* 2010;**66**(1):31–36.

21. Ilson DH. Phase II trial of weekly irinotecan/cisplatin in advanced esophageal cancer. *Oncology (Williston Park)* 2004;**18**(14 Suppl. 14):22–25.

22. Lee DH, *et al.* A phase II trial of modified weekly irinotecan and cisplatin for chemotherapy-naive patients with metastatic or recurrent squamous cell carcinoma of the esophagus. *Cancer Chemother Pharmacol* 2008;**61**(1):83–88.

23. Webb A, *et al.* Randomized trial comparing epirubicin, cisplatin, and fluorouracil versus fluorouracil, doxorubicin, and methotrexate in advanced esophagogastric cancer. *J Clin Oncol* 1997;**15**(1):261–267.

24. Van Cutsem E, *et al.* Phase III study of docetaxel and cisplatin plus fluorouracil compared with cisplatin and fluorouracil as first-line therapy for advanced gastric cancer: a report of the V325 Study Group. *J Clin Oncol* 2006;**24**(31):4991–4997.

25. Roth AD, *et al.* Docetaxel-cisplatin-5FU (TCF) versus docetaxel-cisplatin (TC) versus epirubicin-cisplatin-5FU (ECF) as systemic treatment for advanced gastric carcinoma (AGC): A randomized phase II trial of the Swiss Group for Clinical Cancer Research (SAKK). *J Clin Oncol* 2004;**22**(317):Abstr. 4020.

26. Cunningham D, *et al.* Capecitabine and oxaliplatin for advanced esophagogastric cancer. *N Engl J Med* 2008;**358**(1):36–46.

27. Pozzo C, *et al.* Irinotecan in combination with 5-fluorouracil and folinic acid or with cisplatin in patients with advanced gastric or esophageal-gastric junction adenocarcinoma: results of a randomized phase II study. *Ann Oncol* 2004;**15**(12):1773–1781.

28. Guimbaud R, *et al.* Prospective, randomized, multicenter, phase III study of fluorouracil, leucovorin, and irinotecan versus Epirubicin, cisplatin, and capecitabine in advanced gastric adenocarcinoma: A French Intergroup (*Fédération Francophone de Cancérologie Digestive, Fédération Nationale des Centres de Lutte Contre le Cancer, and Groupe Coopérateur Multidisciplinaire en Oncologie*) Study. *J Clin Oncol* 2014;**32**(31):3520–3526.

29. Hironaka S, *et al.* Randomized, open-label, phase III study comparing irinotecan with paclitaxel in patients with advanced gastric cancer without severe peritoneal metastasis after failure of prior combination chemotherapy using fluoropyrimidine plus platinum: WJOG 4007 trial. *J Clin Oncol* 2013;**31**(35):4438–4444.

30. Maugeri-Sacca M, *et al.* FOLFIRI as a second-line therapy in patients with docetaxel-pretreated gastric cancer: a historical cohort. *J Exp Clin Cancer Res* 2013;**32**:67.

31. Sendur MA, *et al.* Comparison the efficacy of second-line modified EOX (epirubicin, oxaliplatin, and capecitabine) and irinotecan, 5-fluorouracil, and leucovorin (FOLFIRI) regimens in metastatic gastric cancer patients that progressed on first-line modified docetaxel and cisplatin plus fluorouracil (DCF) regimen. *Med Oncol* 2014;**31**(9):153.

32. Lauren P. The two histological main types of gastric carcinoma: Diffuse and so-called intestinal-type carcinoma an attempt at a histo-clinical classification. *Acta Pathol Microbiol Scand* 1965;**64**:31–49.

33. Tan IB, *et al.* Intrinsic subtypes of gastric cancer, based on gene expression pattern, predict survival and respond differently to chemotherapy. *Gastroenterology* 2011;**141**(2):476–485, 485, e1–e11.

34. Macdonald J. Chemoradiation of resected gastric cancer: A 10-year follow-up of the phase III trial INT0116 (SWOG 9008). *J Clin Oncol* 2009;**27**:Abstr. 4515.

35. Boku N, *et al.* Fluorouracil versus combination of irinotecan plus cisplatin versus S-1 in metastatic gastric cancer: A randomised phase 3 study. *Lancet Oncol* 2009;**10**(11):1063–1069.

36. An JY, *et al.* Microsatellite instability in sporadic gastric cancer: Its prognostic role and guidance for 5-FU based chemotherapy after R0 resection. *Int J Cancer* 2012;**131**(2):505–511.

37. Lei Z, *et al.* Identification of molecular subtypes of gastric cancer with different responses to PI3-kinase inhibitors and 5-fluorouracil. *Gastroenterology* 2013;**145**(3):554–565.

38. Heisterkamp N, *et al.* Structural organization of the bcr gene and its role in the Ph' translocation. *Nature* 1985;**315**(6022):758–761.

39. Lynch TJ, *et al.* Activating mutations in the epidermal growth factor receptor underlying responsiveness of non-small-cell lung cancer to gefitinib. *N Engl J Med* 2004;**350**(21):2129–2139.

40. Borg A, *et al.* HER2/neu amplification and comedo type breast carcinoma. *Lancet* 1989;**1**(8649):1268–1269.

41. Druker BJ, *et al*. Activity of a specific inhibitor of the BCR-ABL tyrosine kinase in the blast crisis of chronic myeloid leukemia and acute lymphoblastic leukemia with the Philadelphia chromosome. *N Engl J Med* 2001;**344**(14):1038–1042.

42. Paez JG, *et al*. EGFR mutations in lung cancer: Correlation with clinical response to gefitinib therapy. *Science* 2004;**304**(5676):1497–1500.

43. Pegram MD, *et al*. Phase II study of receptor-enhanced chemosensitivity using recombinant humanized anti-p185HER2/neu monoclonal antibody plus cisplatin in patients with HER2/neu-overexpressing metastatic breast cancer refractory to chemotherapy treatment. *J Clin Oncol* 1998;**16**(8):2659–2671.

44. Rebischung C, *et al*. The effectiveness of trastuzumab (Herceptin) combined with chemotherapy for gastric carcinoma with overexpression of the c-erbB-2 protein. *Gastric Cancer* 2005;**8**(4):249–252.

45. Bang Y-J, *et al*. Trastuzumab in combination with chemotherapy versus chemotherapy alone for treatment of HER2-positive advanced gastric or gastro-oesophageal junction cancer (ToGA): A phase 3, open-label, randomised controlled trial. *Lancet* 2010;**376**(9742):687–697.

46. Tanner M, *et al*. Amplification of HER-2 in gastric carcinoma: association with Topoisomerase IIalpha gene amplification, intestinal type, poor prognosis and sensitivity to trastuzumab. *Ann Oncol* 2005;**16**(2):273–278.

47. Pritchard KI, *et al*. HER2 and responsiveness of breast cancer to adjuvant chemo-therapy. *N Engl J Med* 2006;**354**(20):2103–2111.

48. Chua TC, Merrett ND. Clinicopathologic factors associated with HER2-positive gastric cancer and its impact on survival outcomes — a systematic review. *Int J Cancer* 2012;**130**(12):2845–2856.

49. Janjigian YY, *et al*. Prognosis of metastatic gastric and gastroesophageal junction cancer by HER2 status: A European and USA International collaborative analysis. *Ann Oncol* 2012;**23**(10):2656–2662.

50. Okines AF, *et al*. Effect of HER2 on prognosis and benefit from peri-operative chemo-therapy in early oesophago-gastric adenocarcinoma in the MAGIC trial. *Ann Oncol* 2013;**24**(5):1253–1261.

51. Yoon HH, *et al*. Association of HER2/ErbB2 expression and gene amplification with pathologic features and prognosis in esophageal adenocarcinomas. *Clin Cancer Res* 2012;**18**(2):546–554.

52. Satoh T, *et al*. Lapatinib plus paclitaxel versus paclitaxel alone in the second-line treatment of HER2-amplified advanced gastric cancer in Asian populations: TyTAN — a randomized, phase III study. *J Clin Oncol* 2014;**32**(19):2039–2049.

53. Hecht JR, *et al*. Lapatinib in combination with capecitabine plus oxaliplatin in human epidermal growth factor receptor 2-positive advanced or metastatic gastric, esopha-geal, or gastroesophageal adenocarcinoma: TRIO-013/LOGiC-a randomized phase III trial. *J Clin Oncol.* 2016 Feb 10;**34**(5):443–451.

54. LoRusso PM, *et al*. Trastuzumab emtansine: A unique antibody-drug conjugate in development for human epidermal growth factor receptor 2-positive cancer. *Clin Cancer Res* 2011;**17**(20):6437–6447.

55. Hurvitz SA, *et al*. Phase II randomized study of trastuzumab emtansine versus trastuzumab plus docetaxel in patients with human epidermal growth factor receptor 2-positive metastatic breast cancer. *J Clin Oncol* 2013;**31**(9):1157–1163.

56. Verma S, *et al*. Trastuzumab emtansine for HER2-positive advanced breast cancer. *N Engl J Med* 2012;**367**(19):1783–1791.

57. Yoon-Koo Kang, *et al*. A randomized, open-label, multicenter, adaptive phase 2/3 study of trastuzumab emtansine (T-DM1) versus a taxane (TAX) in patients (pts) with previously treated HER2-positive locally advanced or metastatic gastric/gastroesophageal junction adenocarcinoma (LA/MGC/GEJC). *J Clin Oncol* 2016;**34** (suppl 4S; abstr 5).

58. Hofmann M, *et al*. Assessment of a HER2 scoring system for gastric cancer: results from a validation study. *Histopathology* 2008;**52**(7):797–805.

59. Cooper CS, *et al*. Molecular cloning of a new transforming gene from a chemically transformed human cell line. *Nature* 1984;**311**(5981):29–33.

60. Konturek PC, *et al*. Expression of hepatocyte growth factor, transforming growth factor alpha, apoptosis related proteins Bax and Bcl-2, and gastrin in human gastric cancer. *Aliment Pharmacol Ther* 2001;**15**(7):989–999.

61. Engelman JA, *et al*. MET amplification leads to gefitinib resistance in lung cancer by activating ERBB3 signaling. *Science* 2007;**316**(5827):1039–1043.

62. Scagliotti GV, Novello, S, von Pawel J. The emerging role of MET/HGF inhibitors in oncology. *Cancer Treat Rev* 2013;**39**(7):793–801.

63. Liu L, *et al*. Synergistic effects of foretinib with HER-targeted agents in MET and HER1- or HER2-coactivated tumor cells. *Mol Cancer Ther* 2011;**10**(3):518–530.

64. Catenacci DV, *et al*. Durable complete response of metastatic gastric cancer with anti-Met therapy followed by resistance at recurrence. *Cancer Discov* 2011;**1**(7):573–579.

65. Shah MA, *et al*. METGastric: A phase III study of onartuzumab plus mFOLFOX6 in patients with metastatic HER2-negative (HER2-) and MET-positive (MET+) adenocarcinoma of the stomach or gastroesophageal junction (GEC). *J Clin Oncol* 2015;**33** (suppl; abstr 4012).

66. Iveson T, *et al*. Rilotumumab in combination with epirubicin, cisplatin, and capecitabine as first-line treatment for gastric or oesophagogastric junction adenocarcinoma: An open-label, dose de-escalation phase 1b study and a double-blind, randomised phase 2 study. *Lancet Oncol* 2014;**15**(9):1007–1018.

67. Cunningham D, *et al*. Phase III, randomized, double-blind, multicenter, placebo (P)-controlled trial of rilotumumab (R) plus epirubicin, cisplatin and capecitabine (ECX) as first-line therapy in patients (pts) with advanced MET-positive (pos) gastric or gastroesophageal junction (G/GEJ) cancer: RILOMET-1 study. *J Clin Oncol* 2015;**33** (suppl; abstr 4000).

68. Ferrara N, Henzel WJ. Pituitary follicular cells secrete a novel heparin-binding growth factor specific for vascular endothelial cells. *Biochem Biophys Res Commun* 1989; **161**(2):851–858.

69. Folkman J. Angiogenesis in cancer, vascular, rheumatoid and other disease. *Nat Med* 1995;**1**(1):27–31.

70. Stuttfeld E, Ballmer-Hofer K. Structure and function of VEGF receptors. *IUBMB Life* 2009;**61**(9):915–922.

71. Shah MA, *et al.* Multicenter phase II study of irinotecan, cisplatin, and bevacizumab in patients with metastatic gastric or gastroesophageal junction adenocarcinoma. *J Clin Oncol* 2006;**24**(33):5201–5206.

72. El-Rayes BF, *et al.* A phase II study of bevacizumab, oxaliplatin, and docetaxel in locally advanced and metastatic gastric and gastroesophageal junction cancers. *Ann Oncol* 2010;**21**(10):1999–2004.

73. Ohtsu A, *et al.* Bevacizumab in combination with chemotherapy as first-line therapy in advanced gastric cancer: A randomized, double-blind, placebo-controlled phase III study. *J Clin Oncol* 2011;**29**(30):3968–3976.

74. Van Cutsem E, *et al.* Bevacizumab in combination with chemotherapy as first-line therapy in advanced gastric cancer: A biomarker evaluation from the AVAGAST randomized phase III trial. *J Clin Oncol* 2012;**30**(17):2119–2127.

75. Wilke H, *et al.* Ramucirumab plus paclitaxel versus placebo plus paclitaxel in patients with previously treated advanced gastric or gastro-oesophageal junction adenocarcinoma (RAINBOW): a double-blind, randomised phase 3 trial. *Lancet Oncol* 2014;**15**(11): 1224–1235.

76. Yu H, *et al.* STATs in cancer inflammation and immunity: A leading role for STAT3. *Nat Rev Cancer* 2009;**9**(11):798–809.

77. Siveen KS, *et al.* Targeting the STAT3 signaling pathway in cancer: Role of synthetic and natural inhibitors. *Biochimt Biophys Acta* 2014;**1845**(2):136–154.

78. Calvisi DF, *et al.* Ubiquitous activation of Ras and Jak/Stat pathways in human HCC. *Gastroenterology* 2006;**130**(4):1117–1128.

79. Hirano T, *et al.* Roles of STAT3 in mediating the cell growth, differentiation and survival signals relayed through the IL-6 family of cytokine receptors. *Oncogene* 2000;**19**(21):2548–2556.

80. Chen RJ, *et al.* Rapid activation of Stat3 and ERK1/2 by nicotine modulates cell proliferation in human bladder cancer cells. *Toxicol Sci* 2008;**104**(2):283–293.

81. Azare J, *et al.* Constitutively activated Stat3 induces tumorigenesis and enhances cell motility of prostate epithelial cells through integrin $\beta6$. *Mol Cell Biol* 2007;**27**(12): 4444–4453.

82. Kanda N, *et al.* STAT3 is constitutively activated and supports cell survival in association with survivin expression in gastric cancer cells. *Oncogene* 2004;**23**(28):4921–4929.

83. Laird AD, *et al.* Src family kinase activity is required for signal tranducer and activator of transcription 3 and focal adhesion kinase phosphorylation and vascular endothelial growth factor signaling *in vivo* and for anchorage-dependent and -independent growth of human tumor cells. *Mol Cancer Ther* 2003;**2**(5):461–469.

84. Hitron M. A phase 1b study of the cancer stem cell inhibitor BBI608 administered with paclitaxel in patients with advanced malignancies. *J Clin Oncol* 2014;**32**(5s, Suppl.):Abstr. 2530.

85. Ranganathan P, *et al.* Notch signalling in solid tumours: A little bit of everything but not all the time. *Nat Rev Cancer* 2011;**11**(5):338–351.

86. Artavanis-Tsakonas S, *et al.* Notch signaling: Cell fate control and signal integration in development. *Science* 1999;**284**(5415):770–776.

87. Du X, *et al.* Role of Notch signaling pathway in gastric cancer: A meta-analysis of the literature. *World J Gastroenterol* 2014;**20**(27):9191–9199.

88. Li LC, *et al.* Gastric cancer cell growth and epithelial-mesenchymal transition are inhibited by gamma-secretase inhibitor DAPT. *Oncol Lett* 2014;**7**(6):2160–2164.

89. Yao J, *et al.* Combination treatment of PD98059 and DAPT in gastric cancer through induction of apoptosis and downregulation of WNT/beta-catenin. *Cancer Biol Ther* 2013;**14**(9):833–839.

90. Andersson ER, Lendahl U. Therapeutic modulation of Notch signalling — are we there yet? *Nat Rev Drug Discov* 2014;**13**(5):357–378.

91. Melero I, *et al.* Immunostimulatory monoclonal antibodies for cancer therapy. *Nat Rev Cancer* 2007;**7**(2):95–106.

92. Hodi FS, *et al.* Improved survival with ipilimumab in patients with metastatic melanoma. *N Engl J Med* 2010;**363**(8):711–723.

93. Robert C, *et al.* Ipilimumab plus dacarbazine for previously untreated metastatic melanoma. *N Engl J Med* 2011;**364**(26):2517–2526.

94. Wakatsuki K, *et al.* Clinical impact of tumor-infiltrating CD45RO(+) memory T cells on human gastric cancer. *Oncol Rep* 2013;**29**(5):1756–1762.

95. Kim JW, *et al.* Prognostic implications of immunosuppressive protein expression in tumors as well as immune cell infiltration within the tumor microenvironment in gastric cancer. *Gastric Cancer* 2014. [Epub ahead of print]

96. Okazaki T, Honjo T. PD-1 and PD-1 ligands: From discovery to clinical application. *Int Immunol* 2007;**19**(7):813–824.

97. Iwai Y, *et al.* Involvement of PD-L1 on tumor cells in the escape from host immune system and tumor immunotherapy by PD-L1 blockade. *Proc Natl Acad Sci U S A* 2002;**99**(19):12293–12297.

98. Dong H, *et al.* Tumor-associated B7-H1 promotes T-cell apoptosis: A potential mechanism of immune evasion. *Nat Med* 2002;**8**(8):793–800.

99. Latchman Y, *et al.* PD-L2, a novel B7 homologue, is a second ligand for PD-1 and inhibits T cell activation. *FASEB J* 2001;**15**(4):A345.

100. Zou W, Chen L. Inhibitory B7-family molecules in the tumour microenvironment. *Nat Rev Immunol* 2008;**8**(6):467–477.

101. Brahmer JR, *et al.* Safety and activity of anti-PD-L1 antibody in patients with advanced cancer. *N Engl J Med* 2012;**366**(26):2455–2465.

102. Wolchok JD, *et al.* Nivolumab plus ipilimumab in advanced melanoma. *N Engl J Med* 2013;**369**(2):122–133.

103. Saito H, *et al.* Increased PD-1 expression on CD4+and CD8+T cells is involved in immune evasion in gastric cancer. *J Surg Oncol* 2013;**107**(5):517–522.

104. Muro K, *et al.* A phase 1b study of pembrolizumab (Pembro; MK-3475) in patients (Pts) with advanced gastric cancer. *Eur Soc Med Oncol* 2014; Retrieved from http://www.esmo.org/Conferences/Past-Conferences/ESMO-2014-Congress/News-Articles/Pembrolizumab-Shows-Promise-in-Several-Solid-Tumours.

Chapter 8

Intraperitoneal Therapy of Gastrointestinal Cancers

Jonathon C. King and James F. Pingpank, Jr.

1 Background/Introduction

Traditionally thought to be a relative contraindication to curative surgery, peritoneal carcinomatosis (PC) from a variety of gastrointestinal (GI) malignancies is now regarded as a potentially salvageable surgical disease in properly selected patients. Advances in surgical technique, delivery of intraperitoneal chemotherapeutics, and systemic chemotherapeutics have allowed for the development of safe and effective means of treatment with proven clinical benefit for disseminated peritoneal surface malignancies.

2 Anatomy/Pathophysiology

More than a simple coating of the parietal and visceral structures, the peritoneum is a dynamic and complex organ system. The peritoneal cavity is covered with a layer of mesothelial cells (mesothelium) with underlying loose connective tissue and a basement membrane that serves as a barrier to cellular and large-molecule translocation. The peritoneum itself secretes fluid that is continually renewed, circulated and resorbed.[1] The balance of production and re-absorption is in-part governed by Starling forces (hydrostatic and oncotic pressures of capillary and peritoneal compartments). Disorders in production, such as elevated visceral hydrostatic pressure (portal hypertension) and resorption, as in lymphatic obstruction from tumor infiltration, lead to imbalance of homeostasis resulting in ascites.

Additionally, disruption of the basement membrane causing "leaky" capillaries may allow accumulation of protein-rich fluid in the peritoneal cavity, thus raising the oncotic pressure and contributing to the formation of ascites. This may be seen in inflammatory states causing exudative effusions as well as with tumors which typically have under-developed lymphatics and incomplete barrier function of the basement membrane. There is also an important component of active transport across the peritoneum that utilizes various protein/enzyme pores and transporters that influence protein, fluid, and small-molecule/drug distribution between the peritoneum and bloodstream.

Circulation of peritoneal fluid is influenced by posture, gravity respiratory rate, and hydrostatic pressure. Lymphatic stomata on the undersurface of the diaphragm drain excess peritoneal fluid along with solubilized proteins and cells (bacteria, lymphocytes, mesothelial cells, tumor cells). The omentum also performs a considerable role in reabsorption of peritoneal fluid via transcellular vacuolization. There is a characteristic flow of peritoneal fluid within the abdomen and as a result, patterns of peritoneal metastasis emerge with the most common sites for tumor implants being the undersurfaces of the diaphragms (right greater than left), lesser omentum, right lower quadrant, and pelvis. These represent areas of net reabsorption of peritoneal fluid or regions of relative stasis due to gravity and pooling of peritoneal fluid.[2]

Mechanisms of peritoneal dissemination also differ between tumor types with benign and low-grade mucinous lesions spreading after a prolonged localized growth phase prior to tumor rupture and intraperitoneal contamination. In high-grade malignancy tumor cell shedding into the peritoneum occurs after invasion through the wall of the viscera. Less commonly, hematogenous metastasis leads to PC as in breast cancer and melanoma. Primary peritoneal malignancy such as peritoneal mesothelioma and primary peritoneal carcinoma occur as primary sites of disease.[3] Finally, iatrogenic tumor rupture as may occur during attempted surgical resection of hepatocellular carcinoma, gastrointestinal stromal tumor (GIST), and gallbladder carcinoma are recognized routes of peritoneal tumor spread.

The mere presence of free-floating tumor cells within the peritoneal cavity does not universally correlate with PC. Attachment, implantation, and proliferation are all necessary steps in the establishment and growth of intraperitoneal disease.[4] Characteristics favoring the establishment of lymphatic and/or hematogenous metastases do not always favor intraperitoneal tumor seeding. Upregulation of adhesion molecules correlate with a "sticky" tumor phenotype and low immunogenicity of these tumor cells may allow escape from immune surveillance. In order to establish tumors once successful implantation has occurred, induction of new vessel growth must be possible, or tumors need to be capable of obtaining nutrients from ascitic fluid. Traditionally, these characteristics are present in slow-growing, low-grade tumors.

3 Appendiceal Neoplasms

Appendiceal neoplasms span a broad spectrum of disease ranging from indolent mucinous lesions to highly aggressive high-grade carcinoma.[5] As such, the primary prognostic factor determining the course of disease is usually the histologic grade of the tumor and factors heavily on decisions for systemic and local/regional therapies. This section will primarily address low and intermediate grade mucinous appendiceal lesions; for high-grade mucinous carcinomas and neuroendocrine tumors (previously carcinoid), see the corresponding sections later in this chapter.

3.1 *Pseudomyxoma peritonei*

Mucinous neoplasms of the appendix are hypothesized to arise as appendiceal mucoceles, which if discovered prior to rupture may be removed and cured by simple appendectomy. Adenomatous tissue in the appendiceal lumen produces acellular mucin which distends the appendix and eventually leads to rupture and subsequent peritoneal seeding with neoplastic cells. These cells then continue to secrete mucinous material which gives rise to the clinical syndrome pseudomyxoma peritonei (PMP), which is further classified as either disseminated peritoneal adenomucinosis (DPAM) or peritoneal mucinous carcinomatosis (PMCA). The differentiation between DPAM and PMCA is based on the cellularity and grade of tumor with DPAM appearing as an acellular/hypocellular neoplasm with low-grade histologic features and lacking invasive components.[6] Conversely, PMCA is associated with mucinous tumor that has higher cellularity and higher-grade histology. These tumors tend to be more invasive locally and may have the capability to metastasize to lymph nodes and visceral organs. Many clinicians recognize an intermediate-grade tumor that has features of DPAM but behave more aggressively and are termed PMCA-ID (intermediate/borderline). As mentioned previously, the prognosis of DPAM differs significantly from that of PMCA, making clinical differentiation of the two entities critically important. High-grade appendiceal neoplasms exhibit biology more closely resembling colorectal carcinoma and their treatment will be discussed later in this chapter.

3.2 *Clinical presentation and diagnosis*

PMP is more common in females given the occurrence of mucinous ascites with gynecologic malignancies and typically presents as increasing abdominal girth, abdominal pain, and sometimes changes in bowel habits, such as early satiety. In a significant proportion of male patients, presentation may include a new inguinal hernia. Mucinosis as an incidental finding on laparotomy/laparoscopy, or elective hernia repair may also occur and mandates tissue sampling as well as documentation of extent of disease whenever possible. The differentiation of PMP resulting from ovarian malignancy and that of appendiceal and colorectal neoplasms may be difficult given the considerable overlap in peritoneal distribution of disease, pathologic/histologic similarities, and inconsistent expression of tumor markers. Nonetheless, it is an important distinction to make given the differing prognostic and treatment implications. Management of disseminated ovarian malignancy is beyond the scope of this chapter and will not be addressed.

Serologic assays of tumor markers such as carcinoembryonic antigen (CEA), CA125, CA19-9, and CA15-3 are helpful for monitoring progression of disease and should generally be assessed prior to treatment and, if elevated, periodically during treatment and surveillance. Unfortunately, there is no universal tumor marker though most patients will have elevation of at least one tumor marker.[7] In one study, CEA was elevated in 75% of patients at diagnosis and CA19-9 in 58%. CA19-9 was more useful as both a prognostic and predictive indicator than CEA.[8] The absolute level of CA19-9 may have prognostic implications as well with levels >1,000 U/mL associated with worse five-year survival.[7,9] Similarly CA125 elevation portends a poorer prognosis.[9]

Computed tomography (CT) and magnetic resonance imaging (MRI) are often instrumental in diagnosis, longitudinal surveillance, and treatment planning for appendiceal mucoceles and DPAM. In the case of mucocele, the appendix will appear dilated and filled with homogenous low-density fluid, often without surrounding tissue stranding/inflammation that is typical of infectious appendicitis. Differentiating between appendiceal mucocele, cystadenoma, and cystadenocarcinoma based on imaging findings is difficult, but may be suggested by increased appendiceal wall thickness and serosal irregularity.[10] DPAM presents radiographically as similar low-attenuation mucinous ascites with varying degrees of dissemination throughout the abdominal cavity and pelvis. A hallmark that distinguishes mucinous ascites from simple ascites is visceral scalloping, particularly on the surface of the liver. There is a recognized pattern of disease progression that follows the normal circulatory pattern of fluid in the peritoneal cavity; mucin first accumulates in areas of stasis such as the right lower quadrant and pelvis and progressively involves the right paracolic gutter, right upper quadrant/diaphragms, and finally the central abdomen.[11] Another imaging hallmark of DPAM is a lack of discrete peritoneal based mass(es) and/or lymphadenopathy, consistent with the non-invasive biology of DPAM. Hematogenous spread of low-grade appendiceal malignancies is extraordinarily unusual.

MRI using diffusion-weighted sequences and gadolinium contrast has shown promise for accurate detection of peritoneal disease, particularly in the postoperative surveillance phase which avoids the cumulative effects of repeated irradiation associated with CT.[12] Positron emission tomography (PET/CT) is not generally useful in evaluation of DPAM due to the low metabolic rate and low volume of cellular tumor. However, 18-FDG uptake may indicate a high-grade component to an otherwise low-grade mucinous neoplasm signaling a more aggressive tumor phenotype.

Diagnostic laparoscopy remains the preferred diagnostic method when cross-sectional imaging and serologic testing is inconclusive or equivocal. At the time of laparoscopy, biopsies may be performed allowing histologic diagnosis and survey of the peritoneal cavity can accurately determine disease extent. The PC index (PCI), a staging system that divides the abdominal cavity into nine segments and the small bowel into four additional regions, has been developed as a tool to standardize the staging of peritoneal surface malignancies. Each region is scored based on the volume of disease from 0 to 3. These scores are added to create a composite score from 0 to 39 (Figure 1).[13] The PCI allows direct comparison of pathologic and

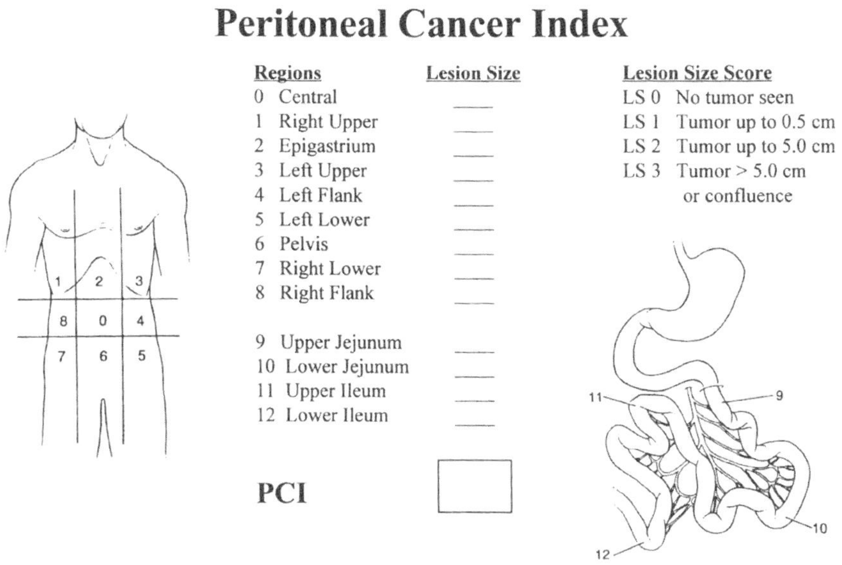

Peritoneal Cancer Index

Regions	Lesion Size	Lesion Size Score
0 Central	___	LS 0 No tumor seen
1 Right Upper	___	LS 1 Tumor up to 0.5 cm
2 Epigastrium	___	LS 2 Tumor up to 5.0 cm
3 Left Upper	___	LS 3 Tumor > 5.0 cm
4 Left Flank	___	or confluence
5 Left Lower	___	
6 Pelvis	___	
7 Right Lower	___	
8 Right Flank	___	
9 Upper Jejunum	___	
10 Lower Jejunum	___	
11 Upper Ileum	___	
12 Lower Ileum	___	

PCI ☐

Score	Cytoreduction	Size of largest residual tumour nodule
0	*En bloc* resection	Nodules not visible
1	Complete cytoreduction	Nodules < 0.25 cm
2	Incomplete cytoreduction, moderate residual disease	Nodules 0.25–2.5 cm
3	Incomplete cytoreduction, gross residual disease	Nodules > 2.5 cm

Figure 1   (a) Peritoneal carcinomatosis index (PCI) and (b) completeness of cytoreduction (CC) scoring. *Adapted from*: Sugarbaker PH. Peritonectomy procedures. *Surg Oncol Clin N Am* 2003;**12**:703–727.

operative data between institutions and also correlates to overall prognosis and response to treatment when combined with completeness of cytoreduction (CC) score and histolopathologic subtype.

3.3 *Therapy*

DPAM is generally unresponsive to systemic chemotherapy, most likely as a result of the low mitotic rate of the adenomatous cells, and is thus a surgical disease. The preferred approach is maximal cytoreductive surgery (CRS) followed by hyperthermic intraperitoneal chemotherapy (HIPEC). This is a labor-intensive procedure in which all visible and palpable tumor is excised and the peritoneal cavity is perfused with heated chemotherapy intraoperatively (various agents, see below; Table 1). Operation begins with a midline incision followed by detailed inspection of the abdomen with documentation of disease extent and volume (laparoscopic CRS/HIPEC techniques have been developed but are generally more appropriate for low-volume or limited disease). Tumor extent is assessed using the PCI (see above) and intraoperative biopsies with frozen section analysis may be useful at this time to confirm the histologic grade of the tumor. Excision for DPAM is usually able to be performed without extensive visceral resection as the tumor is generally able to be debrided from the surface of hollow viscus and solid organs such as the liver. When areas of invasive tumor are encountered (as in PMCA) bowel resection, (partial) gastrectomy, splenectomy, cholecystectomy, hysterectomy, bladder resection, and

Table 1   Chemotherapeutic agents used most commonly for hyperthermic intraperitoneal chemotherapy (HIPEC).

	Class	**Indication**	**Cost**	**+ / –**
Mitomycin C (MMC)	Alkylating agent	DPAM/PMP, colorectal cancer, mesothelioma	+	Extensive experience; neutropenia
Oxaliplatin	Alkylating agent	Colorectal cancer	+++	Possibly more effective for colorectal cancer; costly
Cisplatin	Alkylating agent	Mesothelioma	+	Possibly more effective for mesothelioma; nephrotoxicity
Doxorubicin	Topoisomerase-II inhibitor	Colorectal cancer	+	Limited experience
Irinotecan	Topoisomerase-I inhibitor	Colorectal cancer	+	Limited experience

DPAM: disseminated peritoneal adenomucinosis; PMP: pseudomyxoma peritoneii; CRC: colorectal carcinoma.

peritonectomies are performed as indicated to achieve a complete cytoreduction (termed CC 0). Omentectomy is performed routinely in contrast to other visceral resections which are performed on an as-needed basis. In cases where complete cytoreduction is not accomplished, the resection is graded CC 1–3 depending on the volume of disease remaining *in situ* (Figure 1). HIPEC is performed in a standardized fashion once resection is complete; intraperitoneal inflow and outflow catheters are placed along with temperature monitors and the abdomen is closed temporarily (Figure 2).[14] Perfusion is performed with mitomycin C (30 mg at time 0 followed by re-dosing of 10 mg at 60 min) at 42°C while continually agitating the abdomen. At the end of perfusion, the inflow/outflow and temperature probes are removed, the abdomen is irrigated, bowel anastomosis and diverting ostomy (as indicated) are created, and the abdomen is closed.

The rationale for HIPEC is based on extensive basic and translational science investigations. The agents used most commonly are mitomycin C, cisplatin, and oxaliplatin; all of which have poor penetration of the peritoneal layer when given systemically, yet this same property makes regional delivery at high concentration safe due to the fact that there is very little systemic absorption during the procedure.[15] Hyperthermia exerts a direct tumor-killing effect, enhances the cytotoxicity of chemotherapy, and increases penetration of drug in the peritoneal layer, maximizing tumoricidal effect of the drug.[16] The duration of perfusion varies between

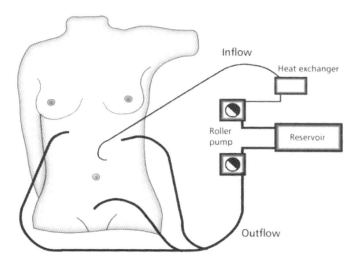

Figure 2 Schematic representation of hyperthermic intraperitoneal chemotherapy (HIPEC) setup. *Adapted from*: Glockzin G, Schlitt HJ, Piso P. Peritoneal carcinomatosis: Patient selection, perioperative complications and quality of life related to cytoreductive surgery and hyperthermic intraperitoneal chemotherapy. *World J Surg Oncol* 2009;**7**:5.

protocols and is typically 60–120 min. It is done immediately following resection (as opposed to perioperatively) to prevent attachment of cells shed into the peritoneum during the resection. Finally, agitation of the abdomen/perfusate prevents occlusion of the catheters by bowel and eliminates areas of abdominal "dead-space."

A variation on this approach employs intraperitoneal chemotherapeutic infusions without hyperthermia in the postoperative period via surgically placed catheters (early postoperative intraperitoneal chemotherapy; EPIC). Infusions are performed in the first postoperative week and may be done following HIPEC or cytoreductive surgery alone. EPIC has not been studied alongside HIPEC in a prospective fashion, limiting the ability to assess comparative efficacy in terms of progression-free and overall survival. A retrospective analysis of HIPEC alone versus HIPEC followed by EPIC did find a higher rate of complications in the EPIC group (44.7% *vs.* 31% morbidity), leading the authors to conclude that HIPEC should be performed without concomitant EPIC.[17]

The utilization of HIPEC for appendiceal DPAM/PMP has been studied extensively with retrospective clinical trials which have demonstrated the technique to be efficacious and safe (Table 2); however, randomized controlled trial (RCT) data are lacking. Retrospective studies evaluating cytoreductive surgery without HIPEC show 5- and 10-year survival rates of 53% and 21–32%, respectively;[18,19] contrasting with modern series of CRS/HIPEC in which 5- and 10-year survival rates are 74% and 63%, respectively.[20] Recurrences are still the norm for patients with DPAM, even in the HIPEC-era with median recurrence-/progression-free survival of 98 months (8.2 years) reported in the largest series to date.[20]

3.4 *Follow-up/surveillance*

The propensity to recur despite HIPEC highlights the importance of ongoing surveillance following surgery. Despite its importance, active surveillance has not been well studied and protocols are based on expert opinion and clinical judgement. For truly low-grade mucinous lesions/DPAM, we perform a staging CT scan at three months postoperatively and yearly thereafter in conjunction with serum assay of tumor markers (CEA, CA19-9, and CA125). For intermediate- and high-grade tumors or patients with low-grade tumors who are more likely to recur early (rapid pre-treatment disease progression, high PCI, CC >0, marked elevation of preoperative tumor markers), the schedule of follow-up imaging and laboratory assessment is accelerated, generally every 3–4 months for two years followed by every six months through year 5 and annually thereafter. Serum tumor markers (discussed above), when elevated preoperatively, may be helpful as they may rise prior to changes seen CT/MRI. Imaging with MRI may be superior to CT based on earlier

Table 2 Retrospective studies of cytoreductive surgery and regional chemotherapy for disseminated peritoneal adenomucinosis (DPAM) and peritoneal mucinous carcinomatosis (PMCA).

Study	n	Technique	Histology	Morbidity/Mortality	Five-Year OS	10-Year OS	MS (months)
Chua, 2012	2,298	HIPEC + EPIC, MMC	DPAM 62% PMCA 30%	24% / 2%	NR	63%	196
Wagner, 2012	50	EPIC, 5-FU / Leucovorin	DPAM 10% PMCA 74%	34% / 0%	70%	NR	118
Sorensen, 2012	93	HIPEC, MMC EPIC MMC / 5-FU	DPAM 61% PMCA 23%	24% / 2%	NR	69%	Not reached
Jimenez, 2014	202	HIPEC, MMC	DPAM 38% PMCA 62%	16% (grade III/IV only)/0%	56%	47%	90
Austin, 2012	282	HIPEC, MMC	DPAM 25% PMCA 75%	25% / 1%	53%	NR	81
Baratti, 2007	95	HIPEC, MMC/Cisplatin	DPAM 74% PMCA 26%	19% / 1%	78%	NR	NR

MMC: mitomycin C; HIPEC: hyperthermic intraperitoneal chemotherapy; EPIC: early postoperative intraperitoneal chemotherapy; OS: overall survival; MS: median survival; NR: not reported.

detection of recurrent carcinomatosis allowing earlier surgical intervention at a time when repeat cytoreduction is able to be performed more completely. One study found median survival was 50 months for 11 patients with earlier MRI detection of recurrence *vs.* 33 months for the 19 patients with recurrence documented by CT scanning, though only 22% of patients in this cohort were classified as having DPAM with the rest having PMCA.[12]

For those patients who experience recurrence (roughly 25% in one large study[21]), repeat CRS/HIPEC is generally indicated, provided their performance status and operative risk are acceptable. Particularly for DPAM, where effective non-surgical treatment options do not exist, it is likely that patients will need repeated surgical interventions over their lifetime. Fortunately, repeat HIPEC can be performed safely with morbidity and mortality that approximates the index operation.[21]

4 Colorectal Carcinoma

The pathophysiology of carcinomatosis in colorectal cancer is fundamentally different than that of low-grade appendiceal neoplasms. While direct peritoneal seeding can be a mode of spread in cases of ruptured (AJCC T4b) colon tumors, hematogenous and lymphatic dissemination accounts for a greater proportion of cases as shown by studies of peritoneal fluid cytology at the time of laparotomy for elective colon resection and also accounts for metachronous carcinomatosis occurring in the absence of locoregional recurrence.[22] In one large study of over 3,000 colorectal cancer patients, PC occurred in 13% of patients with an approximately even distribution of colon and rectal primaries. Close to two-thirds of these were recognized at the time of diagnosis while in one-third, PC was diagnosed during postoperative follow-up. Synchronous PC metastases were localized to the peritoneal cavity 58% of the time while 42% had concomitant liver metastases (Figure 3).[23] In another retrospective study of 27,632 patients from a national cancer registry, 10.3% of patients with M1 disease had isolated peritoneal metastases.[24] For many patients, the peritoneal cavity is the only site of metastatic disease throughout their disease course representing a distinct tumor biology; locoregional therapies such as CRS/HIPEC are designed to treat these patients.

4.1 *Clinical presentation and diagnosis*

Signs and symptoms of peritoneal disease in colorectal cancer are most commonly absent and symptoms, if present, are attributable to the primary colon tumor. Bleeding, pain, or colonic obstruction typically signal the presence of disease

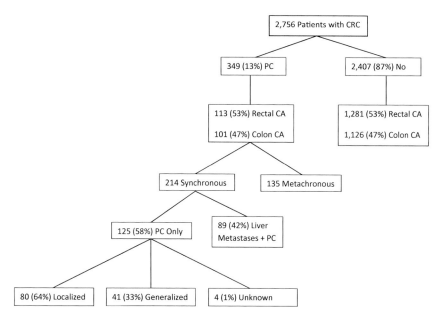

Figure 3   Incidence and distribution of peritoneal carcinomatosis (PC) in patients with colorectal cancer (CRC). *Adapted from*: Jayne DG, Fook S, Loi C, Seow-Cohen F. Peritoneal carcinomatosis from colorectal cancer. *Br J Surg* 2002;**89**:1545–1550.

CRC: colorectal cancer; PC: peritoneal carcinomatosis.

before progressive abdominal distention/ascites or *small bowel* obstruction become apparent. Most commonly, peritoneal dissemination is found at the time of laparotomy or on follow-up imaging. Symptomatic carcinomatosis at presentation carries an ominous prognosis.

Colonoscopy is an essential component of the preoperative work up not only for localization of the primary tumor and operative planning, but also to provide tissue diagnosis and histologic grade of the tumor. As in appendiceal carcinomas, tumor grade correlates highly with overall prognosis with low- to moderate-grade tumors faring better than high-grade or signet-ring cell histologies. Another important consideration is the mutational status of the *Kras* gene as this has implications for biologic therapy in conjunction with neoadjuvant cytotoxic chemotherapy (see below).

Abdominal MRI and CT scans are necessary to define the extent of disease and document extra-peritoneal metastases if present. CT with fluorodeoxyglucose (FDG)-PET is helpful to assess for the presence of extra-peritoneal metastatic disease. Thoracic and bony metastases, if present, represent a contraindication to CRC/HIPEC. Multiple bilobar liver metastases are a relative contraindication to attempts at curative surgery, particularly if they are progressive or unresponsive to chemotherapy. Lower-volume metastatic disease in the liver may be treated with non-anatomic wedge resection or ablative therapy (radiofrequency ablation [RFA], cryotherapy, op microwave ablation) at the time of CRS/HIPEC with minimal impact on overall perioperative morbidity and mortality.[25] Even anatomic lobectomy may be performed safely; however, this should be approached with caution as there may be significant increased risk of major morbidity, especially in the face of bulky peritoneal disease requiring other major visceral resections.[26] Oncologic outcome appears to favor hepatic resection when combined with CRS/HIPEC versus systemic chemotherapy alone or systemic chemotherapy following CRS/HIPEC without hepatic resection though prospective data is lacking.[27] CT/MRI images may be misleading in the case of lesions at the surface of the liver; often, tumor deposits on the undersurface of the diaphragm may indent the liver parenchyma and appear to originate from the liver. Diagnostic laparoscopy can help to differentiate peritoneal-based diaphragm disease from liver surface disease, and should be performed prior to the initiation of preoperative intravenous chemotherapy whenever possible.

Serum tumor markers are often helpful for monitoring disease progression through (neo-)adjuvant chemotherapy and during postoperative surveillance. CEA is most commonly a useful tumor marker, though CA19-9 and CA125 are also routinely checked, and if elevated, examined serially. These biomarkers also provide prognostic information in some cases as described above in the previous section on appendiceal neoplasms.

4.2 *Therapy*

Patients presenting with obstruction, intestinal perforation, or significant gastrointestinal bleeding in conjunction with peritoneal disease require surgical intervention to correct the problem. This is done without specific regard to peritoneal metastatic disease other than to perform the minimal extent of surgical procedure that will correct the immediate problem, thus avoiding creating difficulty for subsequent surgical procedures. Whenever possible, endoscopic means (i.e. stents for rectal cancers, endoscopic hemostasis, ureteral stent for hydronephrosis, etc.) or minimally invasive/laparoscopic procedures for diversion of obstruction or resection of bleeding or perforated colon tumors should be employed. There is no role for "limited debulking: at the time of palliative surgery unless performed to palliate a specific symptom or impending symptom.

All patients with effectively palliated disease and those with manageable symptoms should be considered for neoadjuvant chemotherapy. The rationale for preoperative treatment is to (1) "down-stage" the disease to minimize the extent of eventual surgical resection; (2) allow assessment of chemotherapeutic efficacy by monitoring response of tumor markers and/or imaging; and (3) provide an *in vivo* estimation of tumor biology through a period of non-operative treatment — patients who progress while receiving chemotherapy are often unlikely to benefit from aggressive CRS/ HIPEC. We typically treat with three months of neoadjuvant chemotherapy (six cycles of FOLFOX+/-cetuximab/bevicizumab or similar) followed by reimaging and surgery four weeks after last dose of chemotherapy. Of note, care must be taken to withhold bevicizumab (if given) from the last cycle so that there is at least six weeks from date of last administration until the planned surgery date.[28]

Patient selection for CRS/HIPEC is a major consideration and response to neoadjuvant therapy is a major component of the decision to proceed with surgery. This may be assessed by improvement/progression of symptoms, tumor marker response, and imaging. Additionally a preoperative scoring system (Peritoneal Surface Disease Severity Score; PSDSS) designed to predict prognosis more completely than American Joint Committee on Cancer (AJCC) staging may be helpful to determine which patients are likely to benefit from CRS/HIPEC.[29]

As with low-grade appendiceal neoplasms/PMP, the most important surgical factors impacting disease-free survival and overall survival are the PCI score and completeness of cytoreduction (CC). Those patients who achieve a CC 0 are significantly more likely to experience long-term survival.[30] This has been studied in a RCT of CRS/HIPEC versus systemic chemotherapy alone (5-FU with leukovorin) or with palliative surgery as needed and median survival was significantly improved in the CRS/HIPEC group (12.6 months *vs.* 22.4; $p = 0.032$). Furthermore, the best survival was observed in patients with limited extent of disease (i.e. lower PCI) and with complete cytoreduction (median survival 20.0 *vs.* 5.0 months for CC 1 *vs.* CC 0; $p < 0.0001$).[30] Significant questions remain regarding the comparative efficacy of HIPEC versus systemic chemotherapy, particularly in the era of oxaliplatin- and irinotecan-based chemotherapy and, more recently, biologic agents (bevicizumab, cetuximab) which offer median survival close to that which was achieved in the HIPEC arm of the RCT (20 months). A retrospective study performed with 48 patients undergoing HIPEC and 48 historical controls who received oxaliplatin- and irinotecan-based chemotherapies found median survival of 23.9 *vs.* 62.7 months in the systemic chemotherapy and CRS/HIPEC groups, respectively.[31] Unfortunately, due to its retrospective nature, there are still questions regarding the optimal treatment strategy that will not be answered until another RCT is reported.

4.3 *Follow-up/surveillance*

Serial CT scans and tumor markers should be followed postoperatively as described above for high-grade appendiceal neoplasms. Most patients with an acceptable performance status will require adjuvant chemotherapy; usually another three months (six cycles) of FOLFOX/FOLFIRI+/-cetuximab/bevicizumab to complete a full six-month (12-cycle) course. If there was a lack of response or progression of disease pre-operatively, switching to second-line chemotherapy may be indicated. For those patients with exceedingly high risk of recurrence or those with persistent disease, maintenance chemotherapy may be indicated as well.

Given colon cancer has a propensity for multifocality and metachronous recurrence, colonoscopy is indicated one year following operation for surveillance of the remaining colon. This should be performed serially at prescribed intervals based on surveillance protocols developed for colon cancer.[32]

As described above for appendiceal neoplasms, peritoneal recurrences in patients with acceptable performance status may be treated with repeat CRS/HIPEC as long as the tumor biology and disease-free interval are compatible with aggressive local therapy. We prefer to avoid repeat CRS/HIPEC prior to at least one year from prior operation though this benchmark is somewhat arbitrary.

5 Gastric Carcinoma

Patients with metastatic gastric carcinoma are regarded by most surgeons as relatively poor candidates for CRS/HIPEC. This is in a large part due to the comparatively poor responsiveness of gastric carcinoma to systemic chemotherapy. In the absence of effective systemic chemotherapy options, patients are particularly susceptible to liver and extra-abdominal metastases that make regional therapy to the peritoneum ultimately ineffective in prolonging survival. Nevertheless, there is a subset of patients in whom CRS/HIPEC is effective and research is ongoing to identify this cohort and better define the indications for HIPEC in gastric cancer.

In one phase III RCT of 68 patients with stage IV gastric cancer, median survival was improved from 6.5 to 11.0 months when CRS/HIPEC was compared to maximal tumor debulking alone. For this study the median PCI was 15, indicating a moderate disease burden, and most underwent adequate cytoreduction (CC 0–1 58.8%). Factors influencing survival were addition of HIPEC (HR 2.6), CC 1–2 (*vs.* 3; HR 2.7) and synchronous versus metachronous carcinomatosis (HR 2.2). The occurrence of serious adverse events (14.7% in HIPEC group *vs.* 11.7% in CRS alone) were strongly associated with poorer survival (HR 4.3).[33]

A more recent RCT compared CRS/HIPEC combined with adjuvant chemotherapy with FOLFOXIRI to maximal systemic chemotherapy with FOLFOXIRI alone. Despite being underpowered to show a statistically significant survival benefit (report is an interim analysis, accrual is ongoing), overall survival was 4.3 months in the chemotherapy-only arm versus 11.3 months with HIPEC. The authors observed several long-term survivors in the HIPEC arm all of whom had PCI scores of <15.[34]

While HIPEC does appear to afford some survival benefit when applied to populations, on the individual level, there are clearly some patients who have durable remissions (12–24 months), while others tend to progress regionally or distantly despite surgery. Retrospective analyses have investigated factors associated with poorer prognosis after HIPEC and identified presence of numerous lymph node metastases, CC score, and the extent of resection as significant predictors.[35]

Some have argued for "prophylactic" intraperitoneal chemotherapy (either via HIPEC or EPIC) as a means of reducing the occurrence of metachronous PC. This practice is based on the observation that up to 4–6.5% of T1–2 tumors and up to 10–20% of patients with T3 tumors will have positive peritoneal cytology.[36,37] Using immunocytochemical methods increases the sensitivity further with 43% of patients having immuno-cytologically detectable cancer cells on peritoneal washings in one study.[38] The clinical significance of positive peritoneal cytology is highlighted by the finding that the overall survival of patients with positive peritoneal cytology has been reported to be similar to that of patients who have macroscopic carcinomatosis (M1).[37] A meta-analysis of RCTs investigating HIPEC and EPIC for gastric carcinoma found six studies reporting outcomes following gastrectomy and lymphadenectomy and prophylactic HIPEC/EPIC in stage I–IV gastric cancer patients without carcinomatosis. Intraperitoneal chemotherapy was associated with an increased overall survival (HR 0.34 for death at three years).[39] There are no randomized studies comparing prophylactic intraperitoneal chemotherapy versus adjuvant systemic chemotherapy alone and so it is impossible to determine whether HIPEC or EPIC improves upon standard therapy at this time.

Taken together, these data indicate that patients with synchronous or metachronous PC may be considered for aggressive cytoreductive surgery in cases where disease has been stable on preoperative chemotherapy, the extent of disease is limited, PCI score is low, and a complete surgical cytoreduction is expected. For patients with metachronous carcinomatosis, there should have been a significant disease-free interval (>12 months). Prophylactic intraperitoneal chemotherapy also requires further study to determine which patients are most likely to benefit from an aggressive surgical approach.

6 Conclusions

Significant progress has been made in the treatment of disseminated peritoneal metastases from gastrointestinal primaries. While PMP and peritoneal carcinomatosis still present formidable management challenges, we can now offer multimodality care that has proven efficacy in terms of disease control, symptom palliation, and improved survival. Further developments will allow better ability to identify patients who are most likely to benefit from surgical therapy, and with continually improving systemic chemotherapeutics, increase the number of patients who are candidates for cytoreductive surgery and regional chemotherapy. Challenges remain, particularly in the realm of validating clinical efficacy of surgical approaches with RCTs.

References

1. Pingpank JF, Jr. Surgical management of metastases. In Bartlett DL, Thirunavukarasu P, Neal MD, eds. *Surgical Oncology: Fundamentals, Evidence-Based Approaches and New Technology*. St Louis: Jaypee Brothers; 2011: pp. 593–609.
2. Carmignani CP, *et al*. Intraperitoneal cancer dissemination: Mechanisms of the patterns of spread. *Cancer Metastasis Rev* 2003;**22**(4):465–472.
3. Yamamura S, *et al*. Two types of peritoneal dissemination of pancreatic cancer cells in a hamster model. *J Nippon Med Sch* 1999;**66**(4):253–261.
4. Jayne DG, *et al*. A three-dimensional *in-vitro* model for the study of peritoneal tumour metastasis. *Clin Exp Metastasis* 1999;**17**(6):515–523.
5. McCusker ME, *et al*. Primary malignant neoplasms of the appendix: A population based study from the Surveillance, Epidemiology and End-Results program, 1973–1998. *Cancer* 2002;**94**:3307.
6. Ronnett BM, *et al*. Disseminated peritoneal adenomucinosis and peritoneal mucinous carcinomatosis. A clinicopathologic analysis of 109 cases with emphasis on distinguishing pathologic features, site of origin, prognosis, and relationship to "pseudomyxoma peritonei." *Am J Surg Pathol* 1995;**19**(12):1390–1408.
7. Wagner PL, *et al*. Significance of serum tumor marker levels in peritoneal carcinomatosis of appendiceal origin. *Ann Surg Oncol* 2013;**20**(2):506–514.
8. Van Ruth S, *et al*. Prognostic value of baseline and serial carcinoembryonic antigen and carbohydrate antigen 19.9 measurements in patients with pseudomyxoma peritonei treated with cytoreduction and hyperthermic intraperitoneal chemotherapy. *Ann Surg Oncol* 2002;**9**(10):961–967.
9. Koh JL, *et al*. Carbohydrate antigen 19-9 (CA19-9) is an independent prognostic indicator in pseudomyxoma peritonei post-cytoreductive surgery and perioperative intraperitnoeal chemotherapy. *J Gastrointest Oncol* 2013;**4**(2):173–181.
10. Wang H, *et al*. Appendiceal mucocele: A diagnostic dilemma in differentiating malignant from benign lesions with CT. *Am J Roentgenol* 2013;**201**(4):W590–W595.
11. Sulkin TV, *et al*. CT in pseudomyxoma peritonei: A review of 17 cases. *Clin Radiol* 2002;**57**(7):608–613.
12. Low RN, *et al*. Surveillance MR imaging is superior to serum tumor markers for detecting early tumor recurrence in patients with appendiceal cancer treated with surgical cytoreduction and HIPEC. *Ann Surg Oncol* 2013;**20**(4):1074–1081.
13. Jacquet P, *et al*. Clinical research methodologies in diagnosis and staging of patients with peritoneal carcinomatosis. In Sugarbaker PH, ed. *Peritoneal Carcinomatosis: Principles of Management*. Boston: Kluwer; 1996: pp. 359–374.

14. Turaga K, *et al.* Consensus guidelines from the American Society of Peritoneal Surface Malignancies on standardize the delivery of hyperthermic intraperitoneal chemotherapy (HIPEC) in colorectal cancer patients in the United States. *Ann Surg Oncol* 2014; **21**(5):1501–1505.

15. Dedrick RL, *et al.* Pharmacokinetic rationale for peritoneal drug administration in the treatment of ovarian cancer. *Cancer Treat Rep* 1978;**62**(1):1–11.

16. Los G, *et al.* Optimisation of intraperitoneal cisplatin therapy with regional hyperthermia in rats. *Eur J Cancer* 1991;**27**(4):472–477.

17. McConnell YJ, *et al.* HIPEC + EPIC versus HIPEC-alone: Differences in major complications following cytoreductive surgery for peritoneal malignancy. *J Surg Oncol* 2013;**107**(6):591–596.

18. Gough DB, *et al.* Pseudomyxoma peritonei. Long-term patient survival with an aggressive regional approach. *Ann Surg* 1994;**219**(2):112–119.

19. Miner TJ, *et al.* Long-term survival following treatment of pseudomyxoma peritonei: An analysis of surgical therapy. *Ann Surg* 2005;**241**(2):300–308.

20. Chua TC, *et al.* Early- and long-term outcome data of patients with pseudomyxoma peritonei from appendiceal origin treated by a strategy of cytoreductive surgery and hyperthermic intraperitoneal chemotherapy. *J Clin Oncol* 2012;**30**(20):2449–2456.

21. Lord AC, *et al.* Recurrence and outcome after complete tumour removal and hyperthermic intraperitoneal chemotherapy in 512 patients with pseudomyxoma peritonei from perforated appendiceal mucinous tumours. *Eur J Surg Oncol* 2014; doi: 10.1016/j. ejso.2014.08.476; Accessed Oct 2, 2014.

22. Koppe MJ, *et al.* Peritoneal carcinomatosis of colorectal origin: Incidence and current treatment strategies. *Ann Surg* 2006;**243**(2):212–222.

23. Jayne DG, *et al.* Peritoneal carcinomatosis from colorectal cancer. *Br J Surg* 2002;**89**:1545–1550.

24. Thomassen I, *et al.* Incidence, prognosis, and treatment options for patients with synchronous peritoneal carcinomatosis and liver metastases from colorectal origin. *Dis Colon Rectum* 2013;**56**(12):1373–1380.

25. Randle RW, *et al.* Peritoneal surface disease with synchronous hepatic involvement treated with cytoreductive surgery (CRS) and hyperthermic intraperitoneal chemotherapy (HIPEC). *Ann Surg Oncol* 2014; doi: 10.1245/s10434-014-3987-9; Accessed Oct 2, 2014.

26. Glockzin G, *et al.* Hepatobiliary procedures in patients undergoing cytoreductive surgery and hyperthermic intraperitoneal chemotherapy. *Ann Surg Oncol* 2011; **18**(4):1052–1059.

27. De Cuba EM, *et al.* Cytoreductive surgery and HIPEC for peritoneal metastases combined with curative treatment of colorectal liver metastases: Systematic review of all literature and meta-analysis of observational studies. *Cancer Treat Rev* 2013;**39**:321–327.

28. Ceelen W, *et al.* Neoadjuvant chemotherapy with bevacizumab may improve outcome after cytoreduction and hyperthermic intraperitoneal chemoperfusion (HIPEC) for colorectal carcinomatosis. *Ann Surg Oncol* 2014;**21**(9):3023–3028.

29. Esquivel J, *et al.* The American Society of Peritoneal Surface Malignancies (ASPSM) multiinstitution evaluation of the Peritoneal Surface Disease Severity Score (PSDSS) in

1,013 patients with colorectal cancer with peritoneal carcinomatosis. *Ann Surg Oncol* 2014; doi: 10.1245/s10434-014-3798-z; Accessed Oct 2, 2014.

30. Verwaal VJ, *et al*. Randomized trial of cytoreduction and hyperthermic intraperitoneal chemotherapy versus systemic chemotherapy and palliative surgery in patients with peritoneal carcinomatosis of colorectal cancer. *J Clin Oncol* 2003;**21**(20):3737–3743.

31. Elias D, *et al*. Complete cytoreductive surgery plus intraperitoneal chemohyperthermia with oxaliplatin for peritoneal carcinomatosis of colorectal origin. *J Clin Oncol* 2009;**27**(5):681–685.

32. Meyerhardt JA, *et al*. Follow-up care, surveillance protocol, and secondary prevention measures for survivors of colorectal cancer: American Society of Clinical Oncology Clinical Practice Guideline Endorsement. *J Clin Oncol* 2013;**31**:4465–4470.

33. Yang XJ, *et al*. Cytoreductive surgery and hyperthermic intraperitoneal chemotherapy improves survival of patients with peritoneal carcinomatosis from gastric cancer: Final results of a phase III randomized clinical trial. *Ann Surg Oncol* 2011;**18**:1575–1581.

34. Rudloff U, *et al*. Impact of maximal cytoreductive surgery plus regional heated intraperitoneal chemotherapy (HIPEC) on outcome of patients with peritoneal carcinomatosis of gastric origin: Results of the GYMSSA trial. *J Surg Oncol* 2014;**110**(3):275–284.

35. Magge D, *et al*. Aggressive locoregional surgical therapy for gastric peritoneal carcinomatosis. *Ann Surg Oncol* 2014;**21**(5):1448–1455.

36. Bentrem D, *et al*. The value of peritoneal cytology as a preoperative predictor in patients with gastric carcinoma undergoing a curative resection. *Ann Surg Oncol* 2005;**12**(5):347–353.

37. Burke EC, *et al*. Peritoneal lavage cytology in gastric cancer: An independent predictor of outcome. *Ann Surg Oncol* 1998;**5**(5):411–415.

38. Juhl H, *et al*. Immunocytological detection of micrometastatic cells: Comparative evaluation of findings in the peritoneal cavity and the bone marrow of gastric, colorectal and pancreatic cancer patients. *Int J Cancer* 1994;**57**(3):330–335.

39. Coccolini F, *et al*. Intraperitoneal chemotherapy in advanced gastric cancer. Meta-analysis of randomized trials. *Eur J Surg Oncol* 2014;**40**(1):12–26.

Chapter 9

The Role of Diagnostic Radiology in Pancreatic Cancer Management

Benjamin L. Yam and Evan S. Siegelman

1 Introduction

Pancreatic cancer is the 10th leading cause of cancer in the United States but the fourth most common cause of cancer death, accounting for nearly 40,000 deaths per year.[1] Despite progress in the detection and management of pancreatic cancer, the overall prognosis for patients with this disease remains poor, with one- and five-year survival rates of 27% and 6%, respectively.[1,2] Of note, recent advancements in genetic mapping and understanding of the molecular basis of pancreatic cancer may permit future screening for curable precursor lesions in individuals at risk.[3] Still, the only curative treatment for pancreatic cancer is complete surgical resection. However, only 20% of patients with pancreatic cancer have potentially resectable disease at presentation.[4] Even in patients who have successfully undergone surgical resection with negative margins, five-year survival rates range from 3–16%.[5] Nonetheless, complete surgical resection remains the only treatment shown to improve survival, prolonging mean survival to 24 months as compared to 12 months in patients with unresectable disease.[6] Therefore, early detection and appropriate selection of surgical candidates is critical in the management of these patients. Imaging plays a central role in determining the extent and initial stage of disease, thereby allowing selection of either medical or surgical therapy for patients depending on the likelihood of resectability. In addition to the initial staging of pancreatic cancer, imaging can aid in the characterization of incidentally detected pancreatic lesions, guiding surgical and radiotherapeutic planning, assessment of treatment response, and surveillance for residual or recurrent disease following therapy. This chapter focuses on the role of radiology in the management of pancreatic ductal adenocarcinoma (PDAC), which accounts for 85% of pancreatic cancers, and emphasizes techniques and imaging findings that aid in characterization and determination of resectability.

2 Clinical Findings

Pancreatic cancer is more common in males and most commonly presents in the sixth decade. The most common risk factor for PDAC is cigarette smoking, with greater than twice the risk of developing PDAC in smokers than non-smokers.[7] Other risk factors include long-standing diabetes mellitus, heavy alcohol consumption, and chronic pancreatitis. Most patients with localized PDAC are initially asymptomatic and consequently often remain undiagnosed until late in the disease course, when curative resection is often impossible. When present, clinical signs and symptoms are often nonspecific. More common symptoms are secondary to the complications caused by invasion into adjacent organs and/or structures and include abdominal pain (typically epigastric radiating to the back), weight loss, jaundice, clay-colored stools, nausea, or a combination of these. Patients may also present with new-onset diabetes or findings of chronic pancreatitis. Migratory thrombophlebitis, a paraneoplastic syndrome, is observed in approximately 10% of patients.[8]

3 Multimodality Imaging and Diagnosis

The main goals of imaging in patients with pancreatic lesions are to diagnose and characterize malignancies, assist in staging and determination of resectability, and assist in treatment planning. Imaging assessment of suspected pancreatic pathology may be accomplished using several modalities, including transabdominal ultrasound (US), computed tomography (CT), magnetic resonance imaging (MRI)-magnetic resonance cholangiopancreatography (MRCP), positron emission tomography (PET), and endoscopic US (EUS). In general, CT is the preferred modality for imaging the patient with pancreatic cancer due to its availability, non-invasiveness, and superior spatial resolution, which is helpful for determining the local extent of tumor, delineating the relationship of tumor to surroundings structures, and staging.[9] The National Comprehensive Cancer Network (NCCN) guidelines recommend imaging with CT or MRI in patients with suspected pancreatic cancer or ductal dilation.[10] EUS is useful when CT or MRI reveals ductal stricture without identifiable tumor, in evaluating for lymph node involvement, and for tissue sampling.

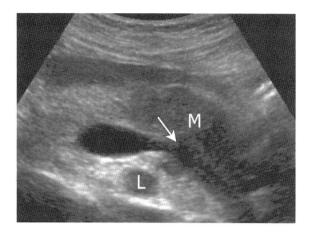

Figure 1 Ultrasound (US) illustration of pancreatic adenocarcinoma in a 65-year-old man with hyperbilirubinemia. Transverse gray-scale US image demonstrates a hypoechoic mass (M) within the pancreatic neck and body abutting the splenic vein (arrow). An enlarged peripancreatic lymph node (L) is present.

US is often the first imaging study obtained in patients presenting with abdominal pain or painless jaundice, and has an overall sensitivity of 76% and specificity of 75% in the detection of pancreatic cancers.[11] Advantages of US include the ability to image in real time, availability, cost, and lack of ionizing radiation. However, US evaluation of the pancreas is often technically challenging due to adjacent bowel gas and/or large body habitus. Ingestion of water prior to scanning and positional maneuvers may help diminish obscuration of the pancreas by bowel gas and improve visualization of the pancreaticobiliary ducts.

When visualized on US, PDAC typically appears as a poorly circumscribed hypoechoic mass (Figure 1). US can identify the presence and level of biliary obstruction with >90% sensitivity.[12] Color and power Doppler US are used to aid in distinguishing dilated ducts from adjacent vasculature (Figure 2). Dilatation of both the common bile duct (CBD) and pancreatic duct, also termed the "double duct sign," is very suggestive of ductal carcinoma of the pancreatic head, even in the absence of a sonographically discernable mass. While US remains a useful modality in the evaluation of pancreatic cancers, limiting technical factors make it a relatively less optimal study for diagnosis and staging. Therefore, patients with sonographic findings of pancreatic cancer are usually then staged with cross-sectional imaging, typically CT. Although EUS with tissue sampling is typically necessary, CT is usually obtained first to avoid post procedural artifacts and complications which can decrease the diagnostic accuracy of CT.

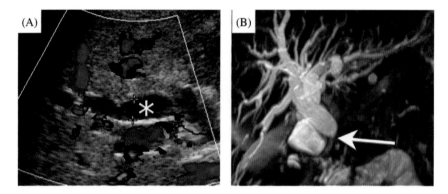

Figure 2   Biliary ductal dilation secondary to an occult obstructing pancreatic adenocarcinoma in a 57-year-old woman with new-onset jaundice. (A) Sagittal color Doppler image shows dilation of the extrahepatic bile duct (asterisk). (B) Coronal magnetic resonance cholangiopancreatography (MRCP) image shows intra- and extrahepatic biliary ductal dilation with abrupt transition distally (arrow). No pancreatic dilation is seen due to obstruction above the level of the pancreaticobiliary junction.

CT is the most widely utilized and best validated modality for the imaging evaluation of pancreatic cancer. A pancreatic protocol CT, as discussed below, is typically the study of choice, with thin-section post-contrast imaging providing optimal tumor detection, depiction of vascular involvement, and ductal obstruction.[13] Multidetector CT has a sensitivity of 86–97% for the detection of all pancreatic tumors, although sensitivity for detection of tumors less than 2 cm decreases to 77%.[14–16]

Routine CT consists of a single-phase post-contrast acquisition in the portal venous phase. Although pancreatic cancers may be detected on routine CT, these routine studies are often suboptimal for accurate assessment of local invasion. Consequently, a dedicated pancreatic protocol CT should be performed to improve the accuracy of local staging. A dedicated pancreatic protocol CT consists of multiphasic thin-section abdominal CT acquisitions following the oral administration of negative contrast, such as water, and the rapid bolus intravenous injection of iodinated contrast (120–150 mL at 4–5 mL/sec).[17,18] Distension of the stomach and duodenum with negative contrast allows improved depiction of invasion of these structures and accentuates the region of the ampulla of Vater, while optimized post-contrast imaging allows for improved tumor conspicuity and better evaluation of extrapancreatic tumor extension along blood vessels and peripancreatic tissues. Biphasic post-contrast imaging is performed first in the late arterial phase (35–50 s after the start of contrast injection) and during the portal venous phase (50–80 s after injection).[15] Multiplanar post-processing is performed to view the pancreas in multiple projections, which can add confidence to diagnosis. Limitations of CT

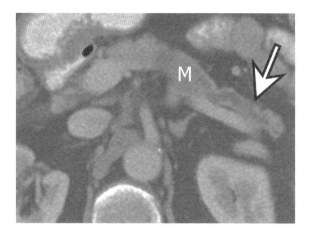

Figure 3   Isodense pancreatic adenocarcinoma in a 63-year-old man with presenting with right upper quadrant abdominal pain. Axial contrast-enhanced computed tomography (CT) image shows an isodense tumor (M) within the pancreatic body causing obstruction of the main pancreatic duct with upstream pancreatic ductal dilation and atrophy (arrow).

include exposure to ionizing radiation and contrast exposure and limited detection of small metastases.

Most PDACs (60%) are located within the pancreatic head, while 15% are within the body, 5% are within the tail, and 20% demonstrate diffuse pancreatic involvement.[19] In 90–95% of patients with PDAC, a hypoattenuating mass is identified on images acquired during the late arterial phase.[20] However, 5–10% of PDACs will not show significant attenuation differences on late arterial phase images and are referred to as "isodense" tumors.[20] These isodense tumors are most often < 2 cm in size, and in such cases, the only suggestion of an underlying pancreatic mass may be dilatation of the upstream pancreatic duct.[16] Therefore, attention to secondary findings such as CBD and/or pancreatic ductal dilation, upstream pancreatic atrophy, and focal contour deformity are important findings particularly for isodense tumors (Figure 3). Notably, duct dilatation and cutoff may be the first finding to suggest PDAC, observed in up to 50% of cases 2 to 18 months prior to establishing the diagnosis of pancreatic cancer.[21]

On CT, pancreatic cancer typically appears as a poorly defined hypoattenuating mass on late arterial phase owing to its relative hypovascularity (Figure 4).[15] Conspicuity of PDAC is most pronounced during peak pancreatic parenchymal enhancement in the late arterial phase.[15] The splanchnic arterial vasculature, particularly the celiac axis and superior mesenteric artery (SMA), is best opacified during the late arterial phase, facilitating detection of subtle perivascular tumor infiltration.[22] In addition, late arterial phase images of the liver may show

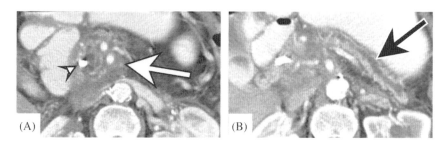

Figure 4   CT demonstration of unresectable pancreatic adenocarcinoma in a 71-year-old woman. (A) Axial contrast-enhanced CT image demonstrates circumferential (360°) encasement of the SMA by a hypoattenuating pancreatic head adenocarcinoma (arrow). A cross-section of radio-opaque common bile duct (CBD) stent is present (arrowhead). (B) Axial contrast-enhanced CT image shows upstream dilation of the main pancreatic duct and parenchymal atrophy (arrow) due to the obstructing pancreatic head mass.

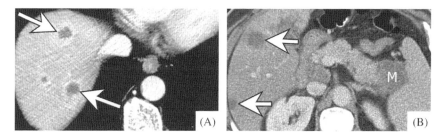

Figure 5   CT examples of metastatic pancreatic adenocarcinoma of the liver. (A) Axial contrast-enhanced CT image obtained in the late arterial phase in a 59-year-old man with pancreatic adenocarcinoma demonstrates multiple rim-enhancing hepatic metastases (arrows). (B) Axial contrast-enhanced CT image obtained in the portal venous phase in a 60-year-old man shows a hypoenhancing pancreatic tail mass (M) and multiple hypoattenuating hepatic metastases (arrows).

rim-enhancing hepatic metastases or abnormal perfusional phenomena such as transient hepatic attenuation differences peripheral to a metastatic lesion (Figure 5).[23]

Portal venous phase images are useful for the detection of liver metastases during peak liver enhancement (Figure 6). Because liver metastases from PDAC are not supplied by the portal vein, these metastases typically appear hypoattenuating, reflecting their hypovascularity relative to the surrounding liver. In addition, the portal venous system is optimally opacified during the portal venous phase, allowing for assessment of venous encasement or obstruction by pancreatic tumor. If present, peripancreatic and perisplenic varices opacify during the portal venous phase and may be seen in the setting of portal or splenic venous narrowing or occlusion. Lymph nodes metastases and peritoneal implants may also be evident on this phase.

MRI is an alternative to CT for pancreatic imaging and provides comparable accuracy for staging PDAC.[24,25] Although MRI demonstrates lower spatial

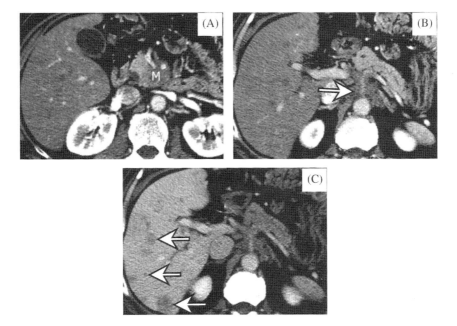

Figure 6 Metastatic pancreatic adenocarcinoma in a 57-year-old man. (A,B) Axial contrast-enhanced CT image obtained in the late arterial phase shows a hypoenhancing tumor within the uncinate process (M) with superior mesenteric artery (SMA), superior mesenteric vein (SMV), and celiac artery encasement (arrow). (C) Axial portal phase CT image depicts multiple hypoattenuating hepatic metastases (arrows) to better advantage compared to (B).

resolution as compared to CT, it provides superior contrast resolution and excellent depiction of the pancreaticobiliary system without the use of ionizing radiation. The high intrinsic contrast resolution makes MRI a reasonable alternative in patients who cannot tolerate iodinated contrast due to allergy or renal insufficiency. In addition, MRI can be helpful for detecting and characterizing isoattenuating pancreatic lesions seen on CT.[20] Limitations of the MRI include cost and availability. In addition, MRI is contraindicated in patients with some metallic implants such as pacemakers and brain aneurysm clips.

A standard pancreatic MRI examination includes fat-suppressed T1-weighted, T2-weighted, and dynamic post-gadolinium enhanced fat-suppressed T1-weighted sequences. MRI is often combined with heavily T2-weighted MRCP to optimize visualization of pancreaticobiliary ductal anatomy. Diffusion-weighted imaging (DWI) is an additional sequence that is often added, aiding in the differentiation between benign and malignant disease with sensitivity and specificity of 96.2% and 98.6%, respectively (Figure 7).[26] DWI may also improve detection of solid liver metastases, which often have restricted diffusion.[27]

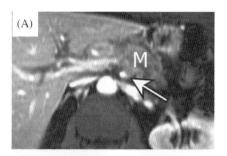

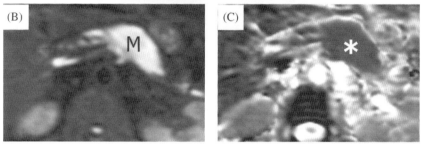

Figure 7 Pancreatic adenocarcinoma in a 73-year-old woman presenting with loss of appetite. (A) Axial postcontrast fat-suppressed T1-weighted magnetic resonance (MR) image shows a heterogeneous hypoenhancing tumor (M) within the pancreatic body with SMA abutment by 180° (arrow). (B) Axial diffusion-weighted image with a b-value of 500 s/mm^2 shows the hyperintense tumor (M) with SMA abutment. (C) Corresponding apparent diffusion coefficient map depicts restricted diffusion (asterisk) within the pancreatic mass.

On MRI, PDAC typically appear hypointense relative to adjacent pancreas on fat-suppressed T1-weighted sequences (Figure 8).[28] Although tumors may not be as easily discernable on T2-weighted images due to similarity in contrast of tumors to underlying pancreatic parenchyma, T2-weighted sequences may be useful in depicting dilated ducts and relatively hyperintense hepatic metastases. The most useful sequences for depicting the pancreatic mass are usually the dynamic gadolinium-enhanced fat-suppressed T1-weighted images.[29] Similar to the enhancement kinetics seen on CT, PDAC is typically hypointense relative to normal pancreas in the arterial phase and hypointense or isointense in the portal venous phase.[29] Rim enhancement may be observed in smaller pancreatic tumors.[28] If pancreatic ductal obstruction is present, pancreatic parenchyma upstream from the tumor may appear hypointense on T1-weighted images secondary to changes from pancreatitis, possibly limiting tumor conspicuity.[30] MRCP images are particularly useful in the assessment for obstruction of the pancreatic duct and CBD. Identification of pancreatic duct and/or CBD obstruction can help detect small isointense tumors that do not exhibit mass effect. Similar to findings seen on other modalities, concurrent

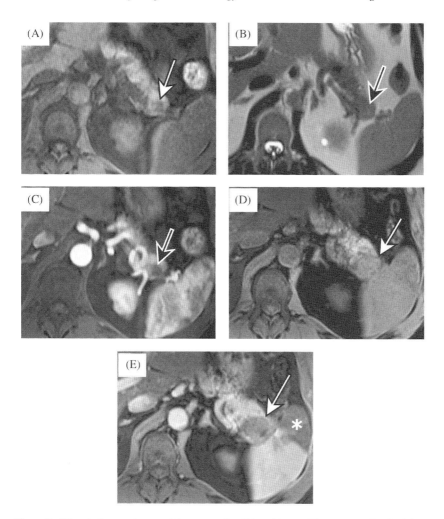

Figure 8   Missed adenocarcinoma of the pancreatic tail in a 66-year-old man presenting for follow-up imaging of non-aggressive cystic pancreatic lesions. (A) Axial fat-saturated T1-weighted image demonstrates a hypointense lesion within the pancreatic tail (arrow). This lesion is hypointense on the axial T2-weighted MR image (B) and hypoenhancing on the axial postcontrast fat-saturated T1-weighted image (C), suggestive of pancreatic adenocarcinoma (arrows). Follow-up MRI 13 months later demonstrates interval enlargement of the adenocarcinoma on axial precontrast (D) and postcontrast (E) fat-saturated T1-weighted images with invasion of the splenic hilum (arrows) and associated splenic infarct (asterisk). A hepatic metastasis present on follow-up rendered the patient unresectable (not shown).

obstruction of both the pancreatic and CBD strongly suggests an underlying neoplasm (Figure 9).[28]

Relative to normal hepatic parenchyma, liver metastases are typically hypointense on T1-weighted and slightly hyperintense on T2-weighted images, with signal characteristics similar to spleen. Metastatic PDAC demonstrates variable enhancement on the arterial phases of dynamic gadolinium enhancement and appear as hypointense masses with poorly defined margins on portal venous phase images (Figures 9A and 10).

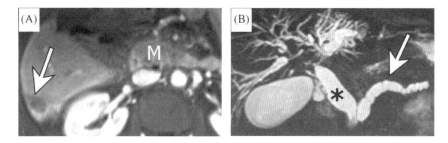

Figure 9   Metastatic pancreatic adenocarcinoma in a 60-year-old man. (A) Axial postcontrast fat-suppressed T1-weighted image in the late arterial phase shows a hypoenhancing pancreatic head mass (M) and a hypoenhancing hepatic metastasis (arrow). (B) Coronal magnetic resonance cholangiopancreatography (MRCP) maximum intensity projection (MIP) image depicts the "double-duct" sign with dilation of both the CBD (asterisk) and main pancreatic duct (arrow). There is also dilation of the left and right intrahepatic bile ducts with abrupt transition at the level of the hepatic hilum related to additional infiltrative hepatic metastases (not shown).

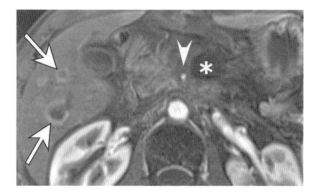

Figure 10   Metastatic pancreatic adenocarcinoma in a 41-year-old woman. (A) Axial post-contrast fat-suppressed T1-weighted MR image obtained in the late arterial phase demonstrates multiple rim-enhancing hepatic metastases (arrows). Ill-defined hypoenhancing tumor is seen within the pancreatic body with circumferential SMA encasement (arrowhead). Susceptibility artifact (asterisk) related to fiducial markers is present adjacent to the tumor.

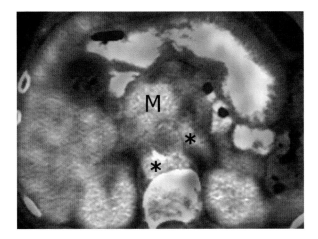

Figure 11 Metastatic pancreatic adenocarcinoma in a 74-year-old man. Axial fused positron emission tomography (PET)-CT image shows an 18F-fluorodeoxyglucose (FDG)-avid pancreatic head adenocarcinoma (M). PET-CT characterized indeterminate left paraaortic and retroaortic lymph nodes seen on CT as metastatic (asterisks).

Although not a first line imaging modality, PET may be utilized as an ancillary study in selected instances. The NCCN does not provide specific recommendations regarding PET, except to note that it is not currently a substitute for high quality contrast-enhanced CT, as its imaging role is still under establishment. Nonetheless, PET has high sensitivity and specificity for the detection of pancreatic cancer, with reported sensitivities and specificities of 71–100% and 64–90%, respectively.[31] In a meta-analysis that evaluated PET-CT and EUS for usefulness in the diagnosis of all pancreatic carcinomas, overall pooled sensitivities were 90% and 81% and specificities were 80% and 93%, respectively.[32] Advantages of PET-CT include depiction of metastatic disease and clarification of equivocal CT findings (Figure 11). PET-CT may also help differentiate pancreatic cancer from autoimmune pancreatitis.[33] Limitations of PET-CT include radiation exposure and cost. PET is acquired following the administration of 18F-fluorodeoxyglucose (FDG) and is typically combined with CT. Pancreatic cancer and its metastases typically demonstrate increased FDG uptake on PET imaging (Figure 12).

EUS has an established role in the diagnosis and staging of pancreatic cancer. Whereas the pancreas may be obscured by bowel gas on US, EUS allows for placement of the transducer within close proximity to the pancreas, eliminating the problem of gas from adjacent bowel contents. EUS has a high sensitivity for the detection of small pancreatic head tumors, even when <2 cm in size.[34] Similar to US, PDAC typically appears as a poorly defined hypoechoic mass on EUS (Figure 13). When

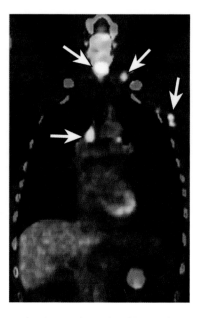

Figure 12   Metastatic pancreatic adenocarcinoma in a 55-year-old woman with history of pancreatic adenocarcinoma post Whipple procedure. Coronal fused PET-CT image shows FDG-avid left axillary, left supraclavicular, mediastinal, and C7 vertebral body metastases (arrows) despite no locally recurrent disease.

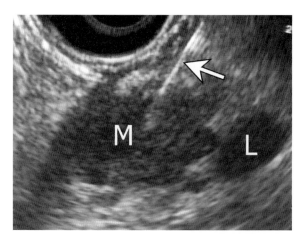

Figure 13   Pancreatic adenocarcinoma in a 65-year-old man. Endoscopic US (EUS) view of a pancreatic body mass (M) during fine needle aspiration (arrow). An adjacent enlarged peripancreatic lymph node is present (L).

performed with color Doppler, EUS permits tissue sampling by fine-needle aspiration (FNA) while minimizing vascular injury. Limitations of this technique include availability, operator experience, sedation requirements, and procedure time. EUS with FNA has a complication rate of 3%, including acute pancreatitis, abdominal pain, fever, and oversedation.[35] When a pancreatic mass is found on cross-sectional imaging, the patient is often referred to EUS with FNA for histopathologic diagnosis and to aid in local tumor staging. In addition, EUS may be performed with endoscopic retrograde cholangiopancreatography to guide biliary stent placement in patients with obstructive jaundice.

4 Staging

Sensitivity and specificity of US for determining resectability of pancreatic cancer is only 63% and 83%, respectively.[11] As a result, staging is typically accomplished with cross-sectional imaging. A staging pancreatic-protocol CT often is used to determine resectability and guide therapeutic approach.[36] The staging of PDAC is based on the determination of tumor size, location within the pancreas, local extent of tumor (including arterial and venous involvement), and the presence of metastases. In general, staging guidelines tend to favor specificity over sensitivity during preoperative staging to avoid denying potentially resectable patients the chance for curative surgery.

Two commonly used staging systems for pancreatic cancer in the United States are outlined by the NCCN and the American Joint Committee on Cancer (AJCC). The NCCN staging system is based on the relationship of the tumor to adjacent major vascular structures and is used to define resectability in the absence of metastatic disease.[37] NCCN criteria classify pancreatic cancer into the three main categories: resectable, borderline resectable, and unresectable disease.

Since the pancreas does not have a capsule, PDAC spreads relatively easily into adjacent structures. Local tumor spread is determined by its site of origin, with a tendency for perineural invasion and spread along neurovascular bundles.[38] Cancers located in the region of the pancreatic head, uncinate process, and neck often involve adjacent vessels, including the celiac, common hepatic, proper hepatic, and superior mesenteric arteries (SMAs). Anterior pancreatic head lesions tend to involve the gastroduodenal and common hepatic arteries, while posterior head lesions tend to involve the portal and superior mesenteric veins (SMVs) and later, the SMA. Uncinate tumors often grow along the inferior pancreaticoduodenal artery towards the SMA. PDACs within the pancreatic body typically involve the celiac artery and/or portal vein, while pancreatic tail lesions commonly grow along the splenic artery and vein into adjacent organs. These relationships are important,

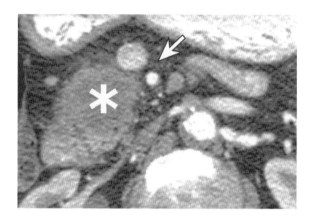

Figure 14   Resectable pancreatic adenocarcinoma in a 72-year-old woman. Axial contrast-enhanced CT image demonstrates a hypoenhancing tumor within the pancreatic head (asterisk) without vascular encasement or abutment. Preserved fat-planes surrounding the SMA and SMV are present (arrow).

as they impact surgical management. Tumors of the pancreatic head, uncinate process, and proximal neck are typically resected via pancreaticoduodenectomy (Whipple procedure), whereas tumors of the distal pancreatic neck, body, and tail are removed via distal pancreatectomy with splenectomy.[39]

Per NCCN criteria, PDACs categorized as resectable are localized to the pancreas and demonstrate no imaging findings of either distant metastasis or extrapancreatic organ invasion.[40] A clear intervening fat plane between the tumor and adjacent peripancreatic vessels, specifically the celiac, common hepatic, proper hepatic, and superior mesenteric arteries, should be present (Figure 14). In addition, no portal vein involvement, tumor thrombus, or venous encasement should be present. Limited extension of tumor into the peripancreatic fat, duodenum or gastroduodenal artery does not render a tumor unresectable, as these structures are resected with the tumor *en bloc*.[10]

Borderline resectable lesions include PDACs that are potentially resectable if certain criteria regarding the degree of arterial and venous involvement are met, in the absence of metastases. Per NCCN guidelines, tumor contacting ≤180° of a vessel circumference is termed "abutment" and tumor contacting >180° of a vessel is referred to as "encasement".[41] In cases of arterial involvement, borderline resectability refers to tumor abutting the celiac axis (celiac, common hepatic, or proper hepatic arteries), replaced hepatic artery, or SMA (Figure 15).[42]

In contrast to the arterial involvement, resectability in cases of venous involvement depends on the feasibility of resecting and reconstructing the involved vein.[43] Tumor invasion or encasement of the portal vein, SMV, or splenic vein is managed differently from arteries. Both abutment and encasement of these veins is

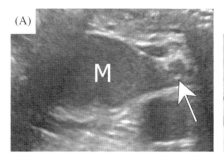
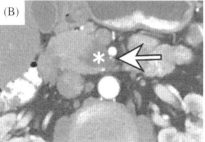

Figure 15 Borderline resectable pancreatic adenocarcinoma in a 54-year-old man presenting with abdominal pain. (A) Transverse gray-scale US image shows a hypoechoic mass (M) within the uncinate process abutting the SMA (arrow). (B) Corresponding axial contrast-enhanced CT image demonstrates SMA abutment by the hypoattenuating adenocarcinoma (asterisk) within the uncinate process with ≤180° loss of the intervening fat plane (arrow). The patient subsequently underwent successful resection.

considered borderline resectable as long as the SMV–portal vein confluence can be reconstructed following tumor resection. Tumors involving the SMV–portal vein confluence can be reconstructed because the portal vein and SMV can be re-anastomosed. The negative-margin resection and survival benefit are higher in patients with either smooth or focal unilateral narrowing of the SMV and/or portal vein compared to patients with bilateral SMV and/or portal vein narrowing and mass effect on these vessels due to the high probability of achieving positive margins in the latter.[43]

Although surgery for borderline resectable tumors is technically feasible, the probability of a positive margin at resection remains high and therefore neoadjuvant chemotherapy and radiation therapy should be considered. Neoadjuvant therapy allows selection of patients who are more likely to benefit from surgical resection and increases likelihood of a negative resection margin.[44] Patients may proceed to resection if the tumor remains stable or regresses following neoadjuvant therapy.

The accuracy of imaging is particularly poor for vascular involvement following neoadjuvant therapy. Cross-sectional imaging to determine extent of vascular involvement following neoadjuvant treatment can be misleading; false-positives are common, with sensitivity of 71% and specificity of 58% for detecting vascular involvement after chemoradiation.[45,46] Therefore, when a favorable response to neoadjuvant therapy is achieved, preoperative planning for vascular resection and reconstruction should be based on pretherapy imaging.

Unresectable tumors include those with distant metastasis, usually to the liver or peritoneal cavity, or vascular encasement (>180° circumferential involvement) of the celiac axis or SMA (Figure 16).[40] Using a threshold of 180° of

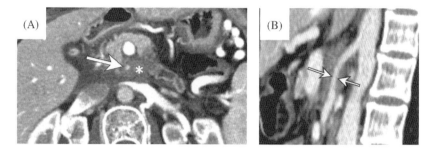

Figure 16 Unresectable pancreatic adenocarcinoma in a 40-year-old woman. (A) Axial contrast-enhanced CT image demonstrates circumferential (360°) encasement of the SMA (arrow) by a hypoattenuating adenocarcinoma involving the pancreatic head and uncinate process (asterisk). (B) Contrast-enhanced sagittal reformatted CT image shows segmental narrowing of the SMA (arrows) due to tumor encasement.

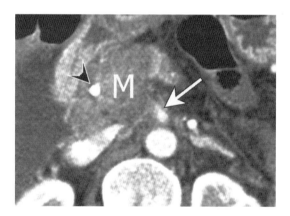

Figure 17 Pancreatic adenocarcinoma with SMA invasion in a 64-year-old woman. (A) Axial post-contrast CT image shows a hypoenhancing pancreatic head mass (M) with tethering of the SMA, resulting in a teardrop configuration of the vessel (arrow). A radio-opaque CBD stent is present (arrowhead).

vascular involvement on CT yields a sensitivity of 84% and specificity of 98% for unresectable disease.[40] Encasement of the celiac axis or SMA always renders the tumor unresectable. Additional imaging findings that suggest vascular encasement include dilation of the gastrocolic trunk (a tributary of the SMV), the mesenteric teardrop sign (teardrop-shaped configuration of the SMV due to tethering by PDAC), and flattening of the vessel, although these signs are less sensitive and specific NCCN criteria for vascular abutment and encasement (Figure 17).[47,48] Other criteria of unresectable disease include portal vein occlusion or direct tumor invasion and circumferential encasement of proximal jejunal vessels.[40] Tumors involving longer segments of portal vein high in the porta hepatis or SMV where there are multiple draining tributaries are not technically reconstructable and therefore considered unresectable disease.

The NCCN staging criteria do not include assessment of overall nodal status because of the low sensitivity and specificity of cross-sectional imaging in detecting or excluding microscopic metastasis to normal sized lymph nodes, as the commonly used short-axis size criteria of >1 cm utilized to differentiate normal from abnormal nodes is not accurate.[49] Although the presence of peripancreatic lymph node metastases is associated with poorer prognosis, this finding does not constitute a contraindication to resection. However, if there is obvious lymphadenopathy beyond the extent of Whipple resection, these cases are generally considered unresectable.

Additional imaging findings not specifically addressed in the NCCN guidelines but nonetheless important for surgical planning included presence of bland or tumor thrombus, tumor contact with the proper hepatic artery to the level of the bifurcation into the right and left hepatic arteries, extension of tumor contact to the first SMA branch, and presence of hazy attenuation contacting the vessel, particularity post radiation therapy.[41]

The AJCC staging system is another widely utilized system to stage PDAC based on the TNM (Tumor, Node, Metastases) staging system, which has undergone revisions to emphasize the importance of resectability, provide assessment of immediate and long-term clinical prognosis, and generate survival data for patients based on disease stage.[42]

T stage is based on tumor size and whether the tumor extends beyond the pancreas, with or without contact with adjacent vessels. The presence of regional lymphadenopathy and distant metastases form the basis of the N and M stages, respectively. Importantly, only regional lymph nodes located along the lymphatic drainage pathways that would be included in the field surgical resection are included in the N categories. Lymph node metastases outside of these drainage pathways are classified as M1 stage. Under the AJCC staging system, stages I and II are considered resectable, and a subset of stage III is considered borderline resectable. The remaining subset of stage III defined as locally advanced and stage IV constitute unresectable disease.

CT is most reliable for staging in patients with extensive locally advanced disease or metastasis, typically to the liver (Figure 18). The sensitivity of thin-section CT in predicting resectability of pancreatic carcinoma ranges from 88–93%, based predominantly on NCCN criteria.[48]

MRI is comparable to CT in accuracy of staging PDAC (Figure 19).[24,25] A comparison of MR with MR angiography and CT with CT angiography, using >180° of tumor contact with vessels and effect on vascular contour as the criteria

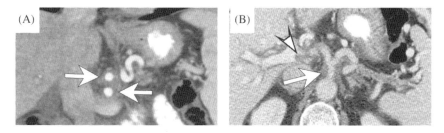

Figure 18   Unresectable pancreatic adenocarcinoma in a 53-year-old man. (A) Contrast-enhanced coronal reformatted CT image shows ill-defined hypoattenuating soft tissue contacting >180° of the circumference of both the celiac artery and the SMA (arrows), consistent with tumor encasement. (B) Axial contrast-enhanced CT image shows ill-defined hypoattenuating soft tissue surrounding celiac artery (arrow). Splenic vein occlusion (not shown) and portal vein thrombosis (arrowhead) is present, with development of perigastric and perisplenic varices. Atrophy of the pancreatic body and tail due to the obstructing pancreatic tumor is also present.

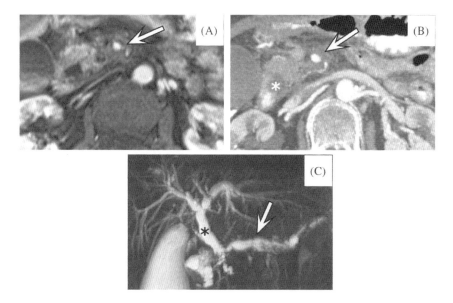

Figure 19   Unresectable pancreatic adenocarcinoma in a 79-year-old woman. (A) Axial postcontrast fat-saturated T1-weighted MR image shows ill-defined hypoenhancing soft tissue circumferentially encasing the SMA (arrow). (B) Corresponding axial contrast-enhanced CT image depicts ill-defined soft tissue circumferentially encasing the SMA (arrow) and CBD dilation (asterisk). (C) Coronal MRCP MIP image shows dilation of both the CBD (asterisk) and main pancreatic duct (arrow) due to a distally obstructing pancreatic tumor ("double-duct" sign).

for unresectability, showed no statistically significant difference in staging.[50] On MRI, the assessment of vascular involvement by tumor is best evaluated on T1-weighted and dynamic post-contrast fat-suppressed T1-weighted images to visualize the integrity of fat planes surrounding vessels and the degree of circumferential involvement by tumor.

EUS can aid in staging by evaluating tumor size, location, and potential vascular or lymph node involvement. The utility of EUS with FNA for diagnosing pancreatic cancer is well established, with reported accuracy of EUS with FNA of 88%, sensitivity of 86%, specificity of 94%, positive-predictive value of 100%, and negative-predictive value of 86%.[51] CT appears to be more accurate than EUS for T-staging and equivalent for N-staging.[52] However, EUS is more sensitive than CT for detection of pancreatic masses <3 cm in size, with sensitivities as high as 97%.[53] EUS can also detect vascular invasion with sensitivities >90% in some studies.[34] Visualization of the portal and splenic veins is excellent on EUS, but it may be more difficult to visualize the SMA and SMV.[54] Nonetheless, in patients with high suspicion of pancreatic cancer despite negative cross-sectional imaging, EUS should be considered. Restaging post-neoadjuvant therapy is limited, as EUS cannot reliably distinguish viable tumor from sterile post-treatment changes.

5 Surveillance

Following surgical resection of pancreatic cancer, follow-up cross-sectional imaging is typically performed at three-month intervals to evaluate for residual or recurrent tumor. CT is the most commonly utilized modality, with accuracy of 94% for detecting recurrence.[55] The most common sites of tumor recurrence are within the pancreatic bed and liver. Although it may be difficult to distinguish recurrent tumor from post-treatment changes, increasing soft tissue at the surgical resection site, sites of nodal drainage, or adjacent to the main peripancreatic arteries should raise suspicion for recurrence (Figure 20). Secondary signs such as increasing pancreaticobiliary ductal dilation should also raise suspicion for recurrence.

6 Differential Diagnosis

It is important to be aware of lesions that may mimic PDAC on imaging, as management can differ. The differential diagnosis for PDAC includes chronic focal pancreatitis, mass-forming autoimmune pancreatitis, lymphoma, and metastases (Figure 21).[56] As a result, pathologic confirmation by biopsy is often necessary prior to treatment. Focal and autoimmune pancreatitis, particularly when involving the pancreatic head, may appear as discrete mass lesions that can mimic PDAC and

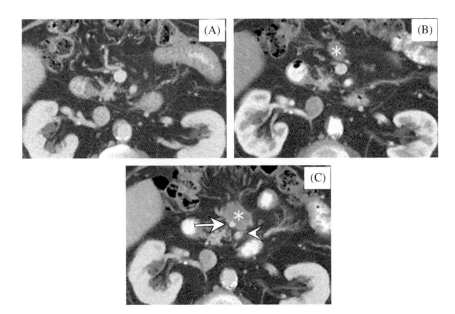

Figure 20 Recurrent pancreatic adenocarcinoma in a 74-year-old man post distal pancreatectomy and splenectomy. (A) Satisfactory initial axial contrast-enhanced CT image without findings of recurrent tumor. (B) 6-month follow-up axial contrast-enhanced CT image shows a new hypoenhancing soft tissue mass anterior to the SMV (asterisk), representing recurrent pancreatic adenocarcinoma. (C) One-year follow up axial contrast-enhanced CT image shows interval enlargement of the recurrent tumor (asterisk) with SMV encasement (arrow) and focal tethering of the SMA (arrowhead).

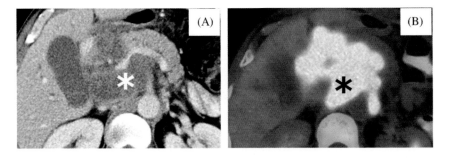

Figure 21 Lymphoma involving the pancreatic head in a 58-year-old man presenting with abdominal pain and abnormal liver function tests. (A) Axial contrast-enhanced CT image demonstrates a hypoenhancing pancreatic head mass (asterisk) encasing the SMV, splenic vein, and SMA. No pancreatic duct dilation is present. This mass demonstrates marked FDG avidity (asterisk) on the axial fused PET-CT image (B). Diffuse large B-cell lymphoma was proven on biopsy.

cause secondary changes, such as upstream dilatation of the pancreatic duct or extrahepatic bile duct (Figure 22).[57] Smooth narrowing of the traversing duct within the area of the mass may support underlying focal chronic pancreatitis.[57] The "duct-penetrating sign," the visualization of an unobstructed main pancreatic duct

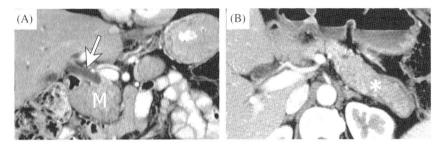

Figure 22 Mass-like autoimmune pancreatitis in a 71-year-old man presenting with weight loss. (A) Contrast-enhanced coronal reformatted CT image shows a heterogeneously enhancing pancreatic head mass (M) with associated CBD obstruction and dilation (arrow). (B) Axial contrast-enhanced CT image shows a heterogeneous sausage-shaped pancreatic body and tail surrounded by a hypoattenuating halo (asterisk). The pancreas demonstrates sharp margins with loss of lobular contour and absence of pancreatic clefts.

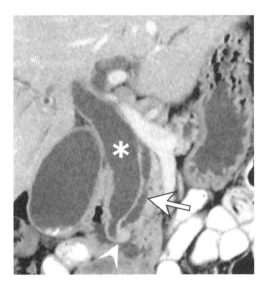

Figure 23 Obstructing ampullary carcinoma with "double-duct" sign in a 61-year-old woman presenting with painless jaundice and pruritis. Contrast-enhanced coronal reformatted CT image shows a hyperenhancing ampullary mass (arrowhead) causing obstruction and resultant dilation of both the CBD (asterisk) and main pancreatic duct (arrow).

penetrating a pancreatic mass, can help distinguish chronic pancreatitis from cancer, as it has been observed in 85% of patients with chronic pancreatitis but only 4% of patients with cancer.[28] The presence of calcifications within the pancreatic duct or parenchyma can also support the diagnosis of chronic pancreatitis. In addition, chronic pancreatitis more often causes a long, smooth narrowing of both the pancreatic and CBD. Although autoimmune pancreatitis may also present as a focal mass, it more often involves a large segment of the gland. Serum IgG4 is typically elevated in the most common type of autoimmune pancreatitis and may be helpful in distinguishing this diagnosis from PDAC.[58] In addition, it is essential to distinguish PDAC from an ampullary tumor, given the far better prognosis associated with the latter, which has a 40% five-year survival (Figure 23).[59,60]

7 Conclusion

Radiologic imaging plays a crucial role in the management of PDAC by facilitating accurate staging, assessment of resectability, tissue sampling, and surveillance. While CT is currently the most widely utilized imaging modality, several modalities play complementary roles for evaluating pancreatic cancer and determining the extent of tumor, relationship to major vascular structures, and presence of metastases. The prognosis for PDAC remains poor, and margin-negative surgery remains the only treatment shown to prolong survival. One must be familiar with the critical imaging findings that determine resectability in order to guide optimal patient management.

References

1. Cancer Facts & Figures 2014. http://www.cancer.org/acs/groups/content/@research/documents/webcontent/acspc-042151.pdf. Accessed 14 March 2016.
2. Wolfgang CL, *et al.* Recent progress in pancreatic cancer. *CA Cancer J Clin* 2013; **63**:318–348.
3. Lennon AM, *et al.* The early detection of pancreatic cancer: What will it take to diagnose and treat curable pancreatic neoplasia? *Cancer Res* 2014;**74**:3381–3389.
4. Michl P, *et al.* Evidence-based diagnosis and staging of pancreatic cancer. Best practice & research. *Clin Gastroenterol* 2006;**20**:227–251.
5. Geer RJ, Brennan MF. Prognostic indicators for survival after resection of pancreatic adenocarcinoma. *Am J Surg* 1993;**165**:68–72; discussion 72–63.
6. Howard TJ, *et al.* A margin-negative R0 resection accomplished with minimal postoperative complications is the surgeon's contribution to long-term survival in pancreatic cancer. *J Gastrointest Surg* 2006;**10**:1338–1345; discussion 1345–1336.

7. Bosetti C, *et al.* Cigarette smoking and pancreatic cancer: An analysis from the International Pancreatic Cancer Case-Control Consortium (Panc4). *Ann Oncol* 2012;**23**:1880–1888.

8. Goad KE, Gralnick HR. Coagulation disorders in cancer. *Hematol Oncol Clin North Am* 1996;**10**:457–484.

9. Hidalgo M. Pancreatic cancer. *N Engl J Med* 2010;**362**:1605–1617.

10. NCCN practice guidelines for pancreatic cancer, version 2. http://www.nccn.org/professionals/physician_gls/pdf/pancreatic.pdf. Accessed 1 November 2015.

11. Bipat S, *et al.* Ultrasonography, computed tomography and magnetic resonance imaging for diagnosis and determining resectability of pancreatic adenocarcinoma: A meta-analysis. *J Comput Assist Tomogr* 2005;**29**:438–445.

12. Laing FC, *et al.* Biliary dilatation: defining the level and cause by real-time US. *Radiology* 1986;**160**:39–42.

13. Vargas R, *et al.* MDCT in Pancreatic adenocarcinoma: Prediction of vascular invasion and resectability using a multiphasic technique with curved planar reformations. *Am J Roentgenol* 2004;**182**:419–425.

14. Agarwal B, *et al.* Endoscopic ultrasound-guided fine needle aspiration and multidetector spiral CT in the diagnosis of pancreatic cancer. *Am J Gastroenterol* 2004;**99**: 844–850.

15. Fletcher JG, *et al.* Pancreatic malignancy: Value of arterial, pancreatic, and hepatic phase imaging with multi-detector row CT. *Radiology* 2003;**229**:81–90.

16. Yoon SH, *et al.* Small (</= 20 mm) pancreatic adenocarcinomas: Analysis of enhancement patterns and secondary signs with multiphasic multidetector CT. *Radiology* 2011;**259**:442–452.

17. Schueller G, *et al.* Multidetector CT of pancreas: Effects of contrast material flow rate and individualized scan delay on enhancement of pancreas and tumor contrast. *Radiology* 2006;**241**:441–448.

18. Tublin ME, *et al.* Effect of injection rate of contrast medium on pancreatic and hepatic helical CT. *Radiology* 1999;**210**:97–101.

19. Ichikawa T, *et al.* MDCT of pancreatic adenocarcinoma: Optimal imaging phases and multiplanar reformatted imaging. *Am J Roentgenol* 2006;**187**:1513–1520.

20. Kim JH, *et al.* Visually isoattenuating pancreatic adenocarcinoma at dynamic-enhanced CT: Frequency, clinical and pathologic characteristics, and diagnosis at imaging examinations. *Radiology* 2010;**257**:87–96.

21. Gangi S, *et al.* Time interval between abnormalities seen on CT and the clinical diagnosis of pancreatic cancer: Retrospective review of CT scans obtained before diagnosis. *Am J Roentgenol* 2004;**182**:897–903.

22. Boland GW, *et al.* Pancreatic-phase versus portal vein-phase helical CT of the pancreas: Optimal temporal window for evaluation of pancreatic adenocarcinoma. *Am J Roentgenology* 1999;**172**:605–608.

23. Desser TS. Understanding transient hepatic attenuation differences. *Semin Ultrasound CT MR* 2009;**30**:408–417.

24. Lee JK, *et al*. Prediction of vascular involvement and resectability by multidetector-row CT versus MR imaging with MR angiography in patients who underwent surgery for resection of pancreatic ductal adenocarcinoma. *Eur J Radiol* 2010;**73**:310–316.

25. Mehmet Erturk S, *et al*. Pancreatic adenocarcinoma: MDCT versus MRI in the detection and assessment of locoregional extension. *J Comput Assist Tomogr* 2006;**30**:583 –590.

26. Muhi A, *et al*. High-b-value diffusion-weighted MR imaging of hepatocellular lesions: Estimation of grade of malignancy of hepatocellular carcinoma. *J Magn Reson Imaging* 2009;**30**:1005–1011.

27. Galea N, *et al*. Liver lesion detection and characterization: Role of diffusion-weighted imaging. *J Magn Reson Imaging* 2013;**37**:1260–1276.

28. Fayad LM, Mitchell DG. Magnetic resonance imaging of pancreatic adenocarcinoma. *Int J Gastrointest Cancer* 2001;**30**:19–25.

29. O'Neill E, *et al*. MR imaging of the pancreas. *Radiol Clinics North Am* 2014;**52**: 757–777.

30. Pamuklar E, Semelka RC. MR imaging of the pancreas. *Magn Reson Imaging Clin North Am* 2005;**13**:313–330.

31. Dibble EH, *et al*. PET/CT of cancer patients: Part 1, pancreatic neoplasms. *Am J Roentgenol* 2012;**199**:952–967.

32. Tang S, *et al*. (Usefulness of 18F-FDG PET, combined FDG-PET/CT and EUS in diagnosing primary pancreatic carcinoma: A meta-analysis. *Eur J Radiol* 2011;**78**:142–150.

33. Lee TY, *et al*. Utility of 18F-FDG PET/CT for differentiation of autoimmune pancreatitis with atypical pancreatic imaging findings from pancreatic cancer. *Am J Roentgenol* 2009;**193**:343–348.

34. Wiersema MJ. Accuracy of endoscopic ultrasound in diagnosing and staging pancreatic carcinoma. *Pancreatology* 2001;**1**:625–632.

35. Eloubeidi MA, *et al*. Endoscopic ultrasound-guided fine needle aspiration biopsy of patients with suspected pancreatic cancer: Diagnostic accuracy and acute and 30-day complications. *Am J Gastroenterol* 2003;**98**:2663–2668.

36. Brennan DD, *et al*. Comprehensive preoperative assessment of pancreatic adenocarcinoma with 64-section volumetric CT. *Radiographics* 2007;**27**:1653–1666.

37. Tempero MA, *et al*. Pancreatic adenocarcinoma, version 2.2012: featured updates to the NCCN Guidelines. *J Natl Compr Canc Netw* 2012;**10**:703–713.

38. Yi SQ, *et al*. Innervation of the pancreas from the perspective of perineural invasion of pancreatic cancer. *Pancreas* 2003;**27**:225–229.

39. Wolfgang CL, *et al*. Pancreatic surgery for the radiologist, 2011: An illustrated review of classic and newer surgical techniques for pancreatic tumor resection. *Am J Roentgenol* 2011;**197**:1343–1350.

40. Callery MP, *et al*. Pretreatment assessment of resectable and borderline resectable pancreatic cancer: Rxpert consensus statement. *Ann Surg Oncol* 2009;**16**:1727–1733.

41. Al-Hawary MM, *et al*. Pancreatic ductal adenocarcinoma radiology reporting template: Consensus statement of the Society of Abdominal Radiology and the American Pancreatic Association. *Radiology* 2014;**270**:248–260.

42. Tamm EP, *et al*. Imaging of pancreatic adenocarcinoma: Update on staging/resectability. *Radiol Clin North Am* 2012;**50**:407–428.

43. Chun YS, *et al*. Defining venous involvement in borderline resectable pancreatic cancer. *Ann Surg Oncol* 2010;**17**:2832–2838.

44. Pingpank JF, *et al*. Effect of preoperative chemoradiotherapy on surgical margin status of resected adenocarcinoma of the head of the pancreas. *J Gastrointest Surg* 2001;**5**:121–130.

45. Katz MH, *et al*. Response of borderline resectable pancreatic cancer to neoadjuvant therapy is not reflected by radiographic indicators. *Cancer* 2012;**118**:574 –5756.

46. Donahue TR, *et al*. Downstaging chemotherapy and alteration in the classic computed tomography/magnetic resonance imaging signs of vascular involvement in patients with pancreaticobiliary malignant tumors: Influence on patient selection for surgery. *Arch Surg* 2011;**146**:836–843.

47. Hough TJ, *et al*. Teardrop superior mesenteric vein: CT sign for unresectable carcinoma of the pancreas. *Am J Roentgenol* 1999;**173**:1509–1512.

48. Li H, *et al*. Pancreatic adenocarcinoma: The different CT criteria for peripancreatic major arterial and venous invasion. *J Comput Assist Tomogr* 2005;**29**:170–175.

49. Sai M, *et al*. Peripancreatic lymphatic invasion by pancreatic carcinoma: Rvaluation with multi-detector row CT. *Abdom Imaging* 2010;**35**:154–162.

50. Schima W, *et al*. State-of-the-art magnetic resonance imaging of pancreatic cancer. *Topics Magn Reson Imaging* 2007;**18**:421–429.

51. Wiersema MJ, *et al*. Endosonography-guided fine-needle aspiration biopsy: Diagnostic accuracy and complication assessment. *Gastroenterology* 1997;**112**:1087–1095.

52. DeWitt J, *et al*. Comparison of endoscopic ultrasonography and multidetector computed tomography for detecting and staging pancreatic cancer. *Ann Intern Med* 2004;**141**: 753–763.

53. Volmar KE, *et al*. Pancreatic and bile duct brushing cytology in 1000 cases: Review of findings and comparison of preparation methods. *Cancer* 2006;**108**:231–238.

54. Brugge WR, *et al*. The use of EUS to diagnose malignant portal venous system invasion by pancreatic cancer. *Gastrointest Rndosc* 1996;**43**:561–567.

55. Mortele KJ, *et al*. Postoperative findings following the Whipple procedure: Determination of prevalence and morphologic abdominal CT features. *Eur Radiol* 2000;**10**: 123–128.

56. Kim T, *et al*. Pancreatic mass due to chronic pancreatitis: Correlation of CT and MR imaging features with pathologic findings. *Am J Roentgenol* 2001;**177**:367–371.

57. Lee H, *et al*. Is there any clinical or radiologic feature as a preoperative marker for differentiating mass-forming pancreatitis from early-stage pancreatic adenocarcinoma? *Hepatogastroenterology* 2007;**54**:2134–2140.

58. Khandelwal A, *et al*. Recent advances in the diagnosis and management of autoimmune pancreatitis. *Am J Roentgenol* 2014;**202**:1007–1021.

59. Allema JH, *et al*. Results of pancreaticoduodenectomy for ampullary carcinoma and analysis of prognostic factors for survival. *Surgery* 1995;**117**:247–253.

60. Raman SP, Fishman EK. Abnormalities of the distal common bile duct and ampulla: Diagnostic approach and differential diagnosis using multiplanar reformations and 3D Imaging. *Am J Roentgenol* 2014;**203**:17–28.

Chapter 10

Radiotherapy for Pancreatic Cancer

Brian C. Baumann and Edgar Ben-Josef

1 Introduction

In spite of widespread use, the role for radiation therapy in the management of non-metastatic adenocarcinoma of the pancreas is not clearly established. Radiation, often coupled with concurrent sensitizing chemotherapy, is frequently employed as adjuvant treatment following resection because of the high propensity for local recurrence after surgery. Radiation has also been utilized as neoadjuvant therapy for resectable or marginally resectable disease, as definitive treatment for unresectable lesions, or as palliative treatment for locally advanced or metastatic tumors. In this chapter, we will discuss each of these potential roles for radiation therapy.

2 Rationale for Adjuvant Therapy for Resectable or Borderline Resectable Disease

Definitive resection with negative margins is the only curative treatment option for adenocarcinoma of the pancreas. However, local–regional and distant failures are common even with seemingly complete surgical resection.

Adjuvant chemotherapy has been utilized to address the high risk of distant failure since ~42% of patients will develop peritoneal metastases and 60% of patients will relapse with hepatic metastases after resection.[1,2] There is compelling evidence that the addition of adjuvant chemotherapy is superior to surgery alone, with the (CONKO-001) trial and ESPAC-3 trial showing a significant improvement in overall survival with adjuvant chemotherapy.[3,4]

Local failure following surgery has also been recognized as a serious problem that occurs in ~50% of patients following resection.[1,2] Local failures cause considerable morbidity and mortality. A recent autopsy series from Johns Hopkins demonstrated that uncontrolled local progression was implicated as the cause of death in up to 30% of patients with overt metastatic disease.[5]

Radiation therapy, given either adjuvantly or neoadjuvantly, has been explored for patients with resectable or marginally resectable pancreas lesions in an attempt to improve local control. Such radiation is typically combined with sensitizing chemotherapy such as 5-FU, capecitabine, or gemcitabine.

The optimal strategy for the adjuvant treatment of patients with resectable or borderline resectable disease, particularly the role of radiation in addition to chemotherapy, remains controversial because of a paucity of high-quality prospective randomized studies, the frequent use of suboptimal radiation regimens in the literature, and the widespread failure to report the effect of various treatment regimens on local control rates.

3 Resectable Patients

3.1 *Retrospective series of adjuvant radiation therapy after resection*

Retrospective series suggest that adjuvant radiation after resection, when used in conjunction with adjuvant chemotherapy, can improve local control and overall survival.

One of the early studies from the University of Pennsylvania reported on 72 consecutive patients with resectable pancreas cancer.[6] By institutional preference, the cohort treated from 1981–1984 received surgery alone, the next 11 patients received adjuvant radiation without chemotherapy, the next eight patients received adjuvant radiation plus bolus 5-FU and the next 20 patients received post-operative radiation plus infusional 5-FU and a single dose of mitomycin C. All patients received a feeding jejunostomy at the time of surgery. Patients received a continuous course of radiation to doses of 45–48.6 Gy with a boost to 54–63 Gy for positive margins or residual disease. All patients were followed with regularly scheduled surveillance CT (computed tomography) scans. Local control was improved with the addition of radiation or chemoradiation compared to surgery alone. Of the evaluable patients, 85% receiving surgery alone had a component of local recurrence, while 55% of those receiving adjuvant radiation without chemotherapy had local failures, but only 28% of patients receiving adjuvant radiation with sensitizing chemotherapy failed locally. This data suggest that radiation, especially when combined with chemotherapy, can reduce local recurrences after resection.

A pooled analysis of the Hopkins/Mayo Clinic experience included 1,045 patients treated with resection from 1985–2005 who were either observed following surgery or treated with concurrent chemoradiation therapy with 5-FU (51%).[7] Radiation was delivered to a median dose of 50.4 Gy without a scheduled treatment interruption. Chemoradiation was associated with a significantly improved median survival (22.5 months *vs.* 16.3 months; $p < 0.001$). In their multivariate analysis, adjuvant chemoradiation significantly improved survival after resection regardless of tumor size, margin status, node status, tumor differentiation, or age.

On the controversial issue of whether adjuvant chemoradiation is superior to adjuvant chemotherapy alone, the National Cancer Database's population-based assessment of 11,526 patients resected from 1998–2002 included 46% who received adjuvant chemoradiation, 9% who received adjuvant chemotherapy, and 45% who received no adjuvant treatments.[8] Patients were matched by propensity scores in an attempt to minimize bias. The analysis concluded that chemoradiation was associated with improved overall survival compared to adjuvant chemotherapy alone when both were matched to surgery alone with a hazard ratio (HR) of 0.70 for chemoradiation (95% CI 0.61–0.80) versus an HR of 1.04 for chemotherapy alone (95% CI 0.93–1.18).

These retrospective, non-randomized studies suggest that radiation in doses adequate to control microscopic residual disease may play a useful role in the adjuvant management of resected pancreas cancers.

3.2 *Randomized clinical trials utilizing adjuvant radiation therapy following resection*

There have been a limited number of prospective randomized clinical trials investigating the potential benefit of adjuvant radiation. The three most important trials are the GITSG experience, the EORTC 40891 study, and the ESPAC-1 trial. Each has methodological problems that limit their applicability to current practice.

The Gastrointestinal Study Group (GITSG)'s small randomized trial from the 1980s was the first to show a statistically significant survival advantage for patients who received adjuvant chemoradiation following curative resection for pancreatic cancer.[9] Forty-three patients underwent complete gross (R0) resection for adenocarcinoma of the pancreas and were randomized to observation alone following surgery or split-course radiation to 40 Gy in 2-Gy daily fractions with a two-week treatment interruption after 20 Gy. The radiation was given with concurrent 5-FU (500 mg/m^2 daily for three days each with 20 Gy course of treatment). After completion of chemoradiation, patients in the treatment arm received weekly maintenance 5-FU for two years. The two-year actuarial survival was 42% for patients treated with chemoradiation versus 15% in the observation group

($p < 0.05$). The GITSG enrolled an additional 30 patients who received the identical adjuvant chemoradiation treatment and found this cohort had a comparable two-year actuarial survival of 46%.[10] While these results were encouraging, a survival benefit of this magnitude for adjuvant therapy has never been observed in subsequent prospective clinical trials. This study raised more questions than it answered. It was unclear how much, if any, of the survival advantage observed in the trial was due to the radiation component compared to the chemotherapy. The 40-Gy split course regimen is considered suboptimal by modern standards because of the prolongation of the treatment time and the reduced biological effectiveness of split course compared to continuous course treatments. Unlike the University of Pennsylvania study in which higher doses of radiation were given in a continuous course, there was no observed reduction in local recurrences in the treatment arm compared to the observation arm (7/15 local failures *vs.* 7/21), suggesting that low-dose radiation is ineffective at reducing the high risk of local recurrence after resection.

The European EORTC 40891 trial also addressed the question of whether adjuvant chemoradiotherapy provided benefit following surgical resection. In this study, 218 patients with T1/T2 periampullary cancers treated with gross resection, including pancreatic adenocarcinomas, were randomized to concurrent 5-FU with split course radiotherapy to 40 Gy versus observation.[11] Unlike the GITSG study, 5-FU was delivered as a continuous infusion, and no maintenance chemotherapy was given following completion of radiation. In the subgroup with pancreatic adenocarcinoma ($n = 114$), chemoradiation ($n = 60$) was associated with a marginally significant improved median survival of 17.1 *vs.* 12.6 months in the surgery alone arm with two-year overall survival of 37% *vs.* 23% and five-year overall survival of 20% *vs.* 10% in favor of chemoradiation. The updated results after 11.7 years of follow-up reported no long-term difference in overall survival or progression-free survival with chemoradiation.[12] There are several caveats to this study. The trial, which was powered to detect a 20% benefit at two years, was underpowered to detect a smaller but still potentially meaningful benefit from adjuvant therapy. Because 42% of the enrolled subjects had non-pancreatic periampullary tumors that have a significantly better prognosis than adenocarcinoma of the pancreas, the study was especially underpowered to detect a benefit for adjuvant chemoradiation in the subgroup with pancreatic adenocarcinoma. Twenty percent of the patients assigned to the chemoradiation arm did not receive the prescribed treatment for a variety of reasons, so the results of the analysis, which used an intent-to-treat approach, may underestimate the potential benefit of adjuvant chemoradiation for patients who can complete therapy. By not mandating a CT scan prior to surgery or radiation, the study did not effectively screen out patients with metastatic disease who would be very unlikely to benefit from chemoradiation therapy. This study utilized the same suboptimal radiation regiment as the GITSG study and did not report local recurrence rates by treatment and primary site, merely stating that local recurrence as the first site of failure was the same in both study arms. This raises the question of whether radiation in higher, more appropriate doses might have had an impact on outcomes.

ESPAC-1, a large, multi-center European phase III trial enrolling 541 patients, examined post-operative chemotherapy and chemoradiotherapy following R0/R1 resection for pancreas cancer.[13,14] One of its goals was to determine if the survival benefit seen in the GITSG trial was secondary to adjuvant chemotherapy, chemoradiotherapy, or both. The study demonstrated a survival benefit for adjuvant chemotherapy but reported a deleterious effect for chemoradiotherapy. ESPAC-1 is frequently criticized for a lack of attention to quality control for the radiation therapy as there was no centralized review or protocol directives for how the radiation treatments should be planned or delivered. The study also allowed "background" therapy, where patients could receive treatments other than those to which they had been randomized at the discretion of the treating physician.[15] There was also a poor degree of patient compliance with the protocol as only 70% of patients in the cohort randomized to receive chemoradiation actually received the prescribed dose of radiation and only 50% of the patients randomized to receive chemotherapy alone received the full course of chemotherapy. This study also prescribed the same low-dose, radiobiologically suboptimal 40-Gy split course radiation regimen as the GITSG study, but the actual dose delivered was very heterogeneous with 30% of patients receiving doses that were more or less than the protocol prescription. No information was reported on the impact of this radiation on local failure rates. The patients in the chemoradiation arm experienced an average delay of 11 days before starting their chemotherapy compared to the cohort in the chemotherapy alone arm, and this may also have biased the results in favor of chemotherapy alone.

In addition to the three randomized studies just mentioned, there have been other, smaller randomized studies. The phase II GERCOR study compared adjuvant gemcitabine to gemcitabine radiation and found no differences in disease-free survival (10.9 months *vs.* 11.8 months) or in overall survival (24.4 months *vs.* 24.3 months) between the two study arms, each of which incorporated only 45 patients.[16] The multicenter phase III CapRI study reported similar outcomes between adjuvant 5-FU alone versus adjuvant radiation given with 5-FU, cisplatin, and interferon alfa-2b followed by additional 5-FU.[17]

A recent meta-analysis of prospective randomized studies that relies heavily on the ESPAC and EORTC databases also concluded that there was a deleterious effect from adjuvant chemoradiation compared to chemotherapy alone when comparing the HRs for death between these two groups compared to observation alone following resection.[18] The HR for adjuvant 5-FU alone was 0.62 (95% CI 0.42–0.88) and 0.68 for gemcitabine alone (95% CI 0.44–1.07) compared to an HR of 0.91 for chemoradiation (95% CI 0.55–1.46). There did not appear to be an advantage to chemoradiation followed by additional 5-FU chemotherapy compared to chemotherapy alone, but there was a small benefit for chemoradiation followed by additional gemcitabine compared to chemotherapy alone with a HR of 0.88 (95% CI 0.29–2.52) compared to gemcitabine alone and a HR of 0.80 (95% CI 0.30–2.04) compared to 5-FU alone. There was increased toxicity associated with the use of chemoradiation followed by additional chemotherapy compared to chemotherapy alone. The very wide confidence intervals reported in this meta-analysis reflect the relative paucity of data available to settle the question about the value of chemoradiation in the adjuvant setting.

The available randomized clinical trials on adjuvant chemoradiation therapy have reported conflicting and inconclusive results on the value of adjuvant chemoradiotherapy. All have methodological flaws that render them incapable of determining whether modern adjuvant radiation therapy offers any benefit either in terms of local control or survival.

A more definitive answer on the role of adjuvant radiation is expected when the currently accruing RTOG 0848 trial is published. This is a phase III study of patients with resected head of the pancreas tumors treated with adjuvant gemcitabine for five cycles +/– erlotinib. Patients without evidence of progressive disease are then secondarily randomized to receive either one additional cycle of chemotherapy or one additional cycle of chemotherapy followed by concurrent chemoradiation with 5-FU or capecitabine to a total dose of 50.4 Gy. This study is well designed, has a centralized review of the radiation plans, and utilizes relatively modern techniques.

It is clear that more research is needed to determine the optimal role for adjuvant chemoradiation therapy and to better select patients who are most likely to benefit from such adjuvant treatment. Until such time, our approach to treating patients following resection is adjuvant chemotherapy followed by concurrent chemoradiotherapy, an approach that is commonly used in the United States. Several prognostic factors have been identified which confer a higher risk of relapse following resection, including margin status (R0 vs. R1/R2), tumor stage, tumor grade (1 or 2 vs. 3), CA19-9 level (higher than 90 U/mL), node status, number of nodes removed, lymph node density, and perineural/perivascular invasion.[19–21] Patients with these high-risk features would be candidates who are likely to benefit from adjuvant therapy. For patients with positive resection margins (R1/R2 resection), upfront chemoradiation therapy to the area of residual disease may be a good option. For patients with elevated CA19-9 levels following an R0 resection, there is a higher likelihood of metastatic disease, and initial treatment with adjuvant chemotherapy may be the most prudent course followed by concurrent chemoradiation. In general, we prefer gemcitabine-based chemotherapy followed by concurrent chemoradiotherapy with 5-FU or capecitabine if the patient has no evidence of distant metastases on restaging following adjuvant chemotherapy. Concurrent chemoradiation with gemcitabine is also an option. Full-dose gemcitabine with an attenuated dose of radiation (36 Gy) or full-dose radiation (50–54 Gy) with attenuated gemcitabine are both tolerable for patients and had comparable survival.[19] RTOG 9704 investigated gemcitabine or fluorouracil for three weeks before and 12 weeks after 5-FU based chemoradiotherapy and reported no difference in overall survival between the two groups, although patients with pancreatic head tumors showed a trend toward better overall survival with gemcitabine.[22] Adjuvant chemotherapy is under investigation in randomized trials (RTOG 0848). An alternative approach is to deliver adjuvant chemotherapy alone, which is the preferred approach in parts of Europe. Neoadjuvant chemoradiation for resectable disease may also be a good option, although data is more limited.

4 Borderline Resectable Patients

Tumors considered to be marginally resectable have vascular invasion of adjacent veins and arteries that is sufficiently limited to permit tumor excision and vascular reconstruction but do not extend to the celiac axis and have no evidence of distant metastases.[23] No randomized, prospective data exist to guide treatment decisions in patients with borderline resectable disease. A common approach for these patients is neoadjuvant chemotherapy +/– radiation therapy prior to restaging and surgical re-evaluation.

4.1 *Neoadjuvant chemoradiation for borderline resectable or resectable patients*

There are several potential advantages to neoadjuvant treatment for either resectable or borderline resectable disease.

1) Neoadjuvant therapy could potentially downstage and thereby improve the resectability of >10% of patients who are thought to be resectable by imaging but who are found at exploratory laparotomy to have locally advanced unresectable disease.[24]
2) The delay in surgery associated with neoadjuvant treatment will allow patients with rapidly progressive micrometastatic disease to declare themselves as having overt metastases and thus potentially avoid a needless surgical

intervention. Based on the results of the GERCOR trials, this could apply to 10–15% of patients who undergo surgery without neoadjuvant treatment.

3) Because ~20% of patients are unable to tolerate adjuvant treatment following surgical resection,[25] neoadjuvant treatment might increase the percentage of patients who are able to receive multi-modality therapy with chemoradiation in addition to surgery.

Several studies of borderline resectable disease using neoadjuvant chemoradiation have shown promising results. A retrospective series from the University of Texas MD Anderson Cancer Center looking at patients with marginally resectable disease treated between 1999 and 2006 found that a large proportion of patients (41%) became resectable following induction chemoradiation therapy.[26] MD Anderson investigators analyzed neoadjuvant chemoradiation in a series of prospective trials that included 5-FU in combination with standard fractionation radiation to 50.4 Gy[27] or rapid-fractionation radiation (30 Gy in 10 fractions),[28] and paclitaxel-based chemoradiation.[29] Paclitaxel did not improve outcomes compared to 5-FU. Based on results that showed that gemcitabine was superior to bolus 5-FU for the treatment of advanced pancreas cancer,[30] gemcitabine-based neoadjuvant chemoradiation was investigated in phase I and phase II clinical trials at MD Anderson.[31,32] In the phase II study, 86 patients with potentially resectable disease received seven weekly infusions of gemcitabine plus radiation therapy (30 Gy in 10 fractions).[31] Patients underwent restaging after chemoradiation, and 85% were taken to surgery with 74% successfully undergoing pancreaticoduodenectomy. Median survival was 34 months for the patients who underwent resection *vs.* seven months for unresected patients. Five-year survival was 36% and 0%, respectively. The study reported encouraging survival for gemcitabine-based neoadjuvant chemoradiation followed by surgery and suggested that neoadjuvant chemoradiation could be used to identify the patients most likely to benefit from resection.

Additional data in support of neoadjuvant chemoradiation therapy comes from a multi-institutional phase II study led by the University of Michigan. The regimen consisted of neoadjuvant full-dose gemcitabine and oxaliplatin with concurrent radiation therapy to 30 Gy in 15 fractions.[33] Twenty-three of the 68 patients (34%) had resectable disease; 39 (57%) were judged to have borderline resectable disease; and six had unresectable tumors. Following neoadjuvant chemoradiation, 30 of the 39 borderline resectable patients were judged to be resectable based on restaging imaging and underwent exploratory laparotomy. Twenty-four of these patients (62%) were able to undergo definitive surgical resection. Overall, neoadjuvant chemoradiation therapy with oxaliplatin and gemcitabine was associated with a high percentage of R0 resections in the entire cohort, and the treatment had acceptable toxicity.

Additional prospective data on the benefit of neoadjuvant treatment will be available once the results of the ACOSOG Z5041 phase II trial are published, which looks at neoadjuvant and adjuvant gemcitabine and erlotinib.

Our current treatment recommendation for marginally resectable disease is to offer upfront concurrent chemoradiation therapy +/– additional chemotherapy followed by restaging to assess for resectability of the primary site and to rule out metastatic disease. Enrollment of these patients on clinical trials is encouraged.

5 Unresectable Disease

Chemoradiation therapy is a commonly used treatment option for unresectable disease, although the benefit of chemoradiation compared to chemotherapy alone is still a matter of debate as is the timing of chemoradiation relative to chemotherapy. Radiation therapy alone is not a preferred option for unresectable disease as the GITSG prospective study ($n = 194$) published in 1981 revealed significantly worse median survival for the RT only group treated to 60 Gy than the cohorts receiving chemoradiation to either 60 Gy or 40 Gy (22.9 *vs.* 40.3 *vs.* 42.2 weeks, respectively).[34]

5.1 *Upfront chemoradiation therapy for unresectable disease*

The available data is conflicting regarding the merits of initial chemoradiation versus chemotherapy alone. In the ECOG 4201 trial, 74 patients with localized, unresectable adenocarcinoma of the pancreas were randomized to receive gemcitabine versus gemcitabine plus concurrent radiation therapy to a dose of 50.4 Gy in 1.8 Gy fractions.[35] The study closed early because of slow accrual; however, local failures were less frequent in the chemoradiation arm (4 of 34 patients *vs.* 11 of 37 patients in the chemotherapy alone arm) although the differences were not reported as statistically significant. Median survival was significantly improved for chemoradiotherapy (11.1 *vs.* 9.2 months; $p = 0.017$). Chemoradiotherapy was associated with more treatment-related deaths, but grades 3–4 toxicities were similar for the two study arms (77% *vs.* 79%) as were quality of life measurements at six, 15, and 36 weeks.

In the phase III FFCD-SFRO trial from France, 119 patients with unresectable pancreas cancer were randomized to gemcitabine alone versus chemoradiation with 5-FU and cisplatin to a dose of 60 Gy in 2 Gy fractions.[36] Both arms received maintenance gemcitabine until disease progression or toxicity. Local control was not reported, although fewer patients in the chemoradiation arm had evidence of tumor progression on CT scans (64% *vs.* 73%). Overall survival was worse for chemoradiation (median survival of 8.6 months *vs.* 13 months for chemotherapy alone; $p = 0.03$). The intensive chemotherapy used in the chemoradiation arm, more aggressive than what was used in the ECOG 4201 study, was associated with significantly worse grades 3–4 toxicity (36% *vs.* 22% during induction and 32% *vs.* 18% during maintenance gemcitabine treatment) and may explain the lower survival in the chemoradiation arm.

5.2 *Chemoradiation after induction chemotherapy for unresectable disease*

The more common approach is to use chemoradiation following an induction course of chemotherapy. Typically, patients with locally advanced, unresectable cancer are treated with 2–6 cycles of chemotherapy followed by concurrent chemoradiation therapy if they have no evidence of distant metastases on restaging imaging and have a good performance status. According to the National Comprehensive Cancer Network (NCCN), this approach is particularly appropriate for patients who are highly unlikely to become resectable and therefore would not benefit from upfront local therapy to improve their chances of resection, patients who are suspected of having distant metastases, and patients with borderline performance status who may not be able to tolerate chemoradiotherapy.

There are several studies that have investigated initial chemotherapy followed either by chemoradiotherapy or additional chemotherapy alone for locally advanced, unresectable disease. As with so many other studies of pancreas cancer therapy, the results are contradictory.

A retrospective analysis of four phase II and III GERCOR studies reported the outcomes of 128 patients with unresectable disease who received three months of upfront chemotherapy (either gemcitabine alone, leucovorin/5-FU/ gemcitabine (FOLFUGEM), or gemcitabine/oxaliplatin) and had no evidence of progression on restaging.[37] Of these 128 patients, 56 (44%) continued with additional chemotherapy while 72 (56%) were treated with concurrent chemoradiation to 55 Gy. The two groups were balanced based on initial characteristics (performance status, age, sex, and type of chemotherapy). Chemoradiation was associated with significantly improved median progression-free survival (10.8 *vs.* 7.4 months, $p < 0.01$) and median overall survival (15.0 *vs.* 11.7 months; $p < 0.01$).

The LAP 07 phase III trial investigated the use of induction gemcitabine +/– erlotinib in 442 patients with locally advanced cancers. The 269 patients with localized disease after induction chemotherapy were then randomized to two additional months of chemotherapy or to chemoradiation delivering 54 Gy in 1.8 Gy fractions with sensitizing capecitabine.[38] The results reported at ASCO 2013 did not show any improvement in overall survival with chemoradiation. The median survival was 16.5 months with chemotherapy alone compared to 15.3 months in the chemoradiation arm. Gemcitabine monotherapy used in this trial is increasingly being replaced by more active chemotherapeutic regimens such as FOLFORINOX, gemcitabine plus albumin-bound paclitaxel, and other gemcitabine-based combination chemotherapy. Clinical trials of chemoradiation combined with these more active chemotherapies are in process.

In an effort to improve the outcomes in patients with unresectable disease, radiation dose escalation has been evaluated using IMRT (intensity-modulated radiation therapy) to reduce the dose to the adjacent organs at risk to minimize complications while simultaneously increasing the dose delivered to the pancreatic lesion to enhance tumor response. A phase I dose escalation study from MD Anderson using concurrent gemcitabine and IMRT delivered to portals that encompassed not only gross disease but also electively covered the regional lymph nodes had to be closed due to excessive toxicity.[39] A phase I/II trial of 50 patients at the University of Michigan escalated IMRT dose from 50 Gy in 2 Gy fractions to 60 Gy in 2.4 Gy fractions (median dose 55 Gy) given concurrently with the same full-dose gemcitabine.[40] Elective radiation to the clinically uninvolved regional lymph nodes was omitted. The rate of severe toxicity (24%) compared favorably with toxicities reported with other regimens. This approach resulted in a median survival of 14.8 months and a two-year survival rate of 30% that was superior to the median survival of 11.2 months and two-year survival rate of 13% for historical controls treated at Michigan with full-dose gemcitabine to 36 Gy in 15 fractions (the maximum dose that was feasible with 3D conformal techniques).[41] In this study, 25% underwent curative surgery after completion of chemoradiation, even though all had been deemed unresectable prior to radiation. The University of Michigan experience with dose escalation has informed the design of RTOG 1201 that investigates whether intensified chemoradiation to 63 Gy in 28 fractions using IMRT plus concurrent capecitabine or standard dose chemoradiation to 50.4 Gy in 28 fractions using IMRT or 3D conformal radiation with capecitabine following upfront treatment with gemcitabine plus albumin-bound paclitaxel is better than chemotherapy alone with gemcitabine plus albumin-bound paclitaxel. The study will also test whether SMAD4 is a useful biomarker to predict patients at higher risk for local *vs.* distant failure and identify patients who may be more or less likely to benefit from chemoradiation *vs.* chemotherapy alone.

6 Metastatic Pancreatic Cancer

Radiation therapy is frequently used with much success as part of a multidisciplinary approach for palliation of locally advanced disease and/or metastatic disease. Palliative radiation therapy to the primary site should be considered for patients with localized back pain refractory to narcotic therapy even in the presence of metastatic disease. In these cases, radiation can be given with or without concurrent chemotherapy with doses ranging from 25–36 Gy in 2.4–5 Gy fractions per the NCCN 2015 guidelines.[42]

7 Radiation Treatment Planning and Techniques

Patients are simulated with CT scan images obtained in the supine position using appropriate immobilization. Because of the significant motion of the pancreas associated with the breathing cycle, 4D CT scans to capture respiratory motion or breath-hold techniques are recommended.[40] MRI (magnetic resonance imaging) or PET (positron emission tomography)/CT scans can be fused with the CT imaging acquired at the time of simulation to assist in delineating targets and organs of interest. For resected disease, an RTOG contouring atlas is available to guide clinical target volume (CTV) delineation.[43] The CTV covers the pre-operative tumor site and includes a 1.0–1.5 cm margin around the post-operative surgical bed and the anastomoses (pancreaticojejunostomy and choledochal or hepaticojunostomy), as well as the nodal regions at risk of harboring subclinical metastasis (peripancreatic, celiac, superior mesenteric, porta hepatitis, and para-aortic regions). Clinicians must exercise judgment in the design of the CTV with respect to the regional lymph nodes so as to avoid exposing an excessive volume of normal tissue to radiation. The CTV is then expanded by approximately 0.5 cm to create a planning target volume (PTV) that accounts for motion and daily errors in treatment setup. Important normal structures to contour include the duodenum, liver, kidneys, bowel, stomach, and spinal cord. The dose to the regional lymphatics is typically 45 Gy in 1.8 Gy daily fractions and the dose to the tumor bed is in the range of 50.4 Gy to 60 Gy.

Treatment for unresectable disease includes the gross tumor volume (GTV) (primary tumor and involved nodes) plus a margin to encompass residual microscopic disease to create a CTV. There is no broad consensus on whether to treat clinically uninvolved nodes electively when there is unresectable disease. At our institution, we favor omitting the elective nodes from our treatment volume because including these nodes increases treatment toxicity and does not add to local control.[40,44] A representative volumetric modulated arc therapy (VMAT) plan for a patient with unresectable cancer is shown in Figure 1.

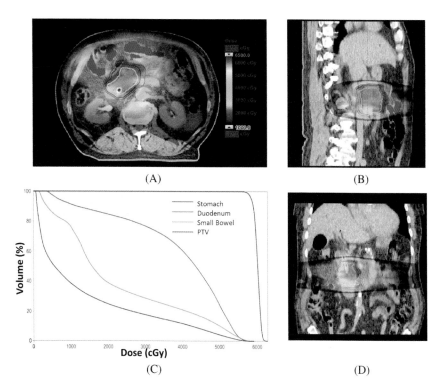

(A)   (B)

(C)   (D)

Figure 1 Axial (A), sagittal (B), and coronal (D) views of a volumetric modulated arc therapy (VMAT) treatment plan for a patient with locally advanced, unresectable pancreatic cancer. A dose color wash displays the prescribed dose delivered to each region. The light blue contour represents the gross tumor volume (GTV). The dark blue contour represents the clinical target volume (CTV) and the red contour represents the planning target volume (PTV). A representative dose volume histogram (DVH) is shown (C).

8 Radiation Therapy Treatment Modalities

The radiation modality typically used for pancreas cancer is photon-based, 3D conformal radiation therapy. The more advanced IMRT technique allows for even greater dose conformality that limits the high-dose coverage to the target volume while minimizing radiation dose to neighboring normal tissues. IMRT has been explored with favorable results. Several dosimetric analyses have been performed that have demonstrated that IMRT results in lower radiation dose to normal tissues compared to 3D conformal treatment plans, and this has facilitated the escalation of dose, which may be particularly helpful in treating unresectable pancreatic cancers where the limited tolerance of the adjacent bowel constrains the dose that can be delivered to the tumor using conventional techniques.[45] The University of Maryland compared the acute toxicity from the RTOG 9704 trial, which used concurrent chemotherapy and 3D conformal radiation, to patients treated at their institution with concurrent chemoradiation using IMRT. They reported significantly lower grade 3–4 gastrointestinal toxicity (nausea, vomiting, and diarrhea) for patients treated with IMRT versus 3D conformal radiation.[46] The Michigan experience with dose escalation also demonstrated the value of IMRT for successfully dose-escalating treatment with acceptable toxicity[40,44]

Proton radiation therapy for unresectable pancreatic cancer was explored, but protons did not result in a reduction in the volume of normal tissue receiving high-dose radiation compared to IMRT, although the volume receiving low-to-intermediate doses was reduced by protons.[47] The clinical significance of these observations remains to be determined.

Stereotactic body radiation therapy, a technique that involves high dose per fraction treatments delivered conformally to a target volume that includes only a small margin of normal tissue around the tumor, has also been explored for pancreas cancer with mixed results. Stanford reported on their experience with 16 patients with unresectable disease who were treated with gemcitabine followed by stereotactic body radiation therapy (SBRT) to deliver 25 Gy in a single fraction.[48] SBRT was associated with comparable-to-inferior survival compared to conventional chemoradiotherapy (median survival 6.7 months). Acute toxicities were limited; however, 7 of 16 patients developed duodenal ulceration (grade 2–4) as a delayed complication. The high dose per fraction used in this study raises serious concerns about delayed toxicity. A more fractionated approach to SBRT was adopted at Johns Hopkins where 84 patients were treated with SBRT to 20–33 Gy in five fractions. Early results suggest comparable outcomes to standard-dose conventionally fractionated radiotherapy, but more data is needed, particularly on delayed toxicity.[49]

Intraoperative radiation therapy is another option that has been used in a limited number of highly selected patients. This technique permits dose to be delivered to the target volume while limiting dose to the adjacent bowel that is packed away from the pancreas during the treatment.[50] Similarly, a limited number of highly selected patients have been treated in the past with interstitial radioactive implants in an attempt to deliver a higher dose to regions of gross tumor that could not be resected. With the widespread availability of highly conformal treatment techniques such as IMRT, these other options are now rarely considered.

9 Conclusions

Pancreatic adenocarcinoma has a very poor prognosis in spite of various advances in care. Surgery remains the mainstay of treatment for patients with resectable disease. Adjuvant chemotherapy has been shown to be an effective treatment following surgery in multiple clinical trials. The role of adjuvant or neoadjuvant chemoradiation therapy remains controversial for resectable patients, borderline resectable patients, and patients with unresectable disease. Trials are currently in development to better define the role of radiation therapy for the treatment of adenocarcinoma of the pancreas.

References

1. Griffin JF, *et al*. Patterns of failure after curative resection of pancreatic carcinoma. *Cancer* 1990;**66**(1):56–61.
2. Van den Broeck A, *et al*. Patterns of recurrence after curative resection of pancreatic ductal adenocarcinoma. *Eur J Oncol* 2009;**35**(6):600–604.
3. Oettle H, *et al*. Adjuvant chemotherapy with gemcitabine and long-term outcomes among patients with resected pancreatic cancer: The CONKO-001 randomized trial. *JAMA* 2013;**310**(14):1473–1481.
4. Neoptolemos JP, *et al*. Effect of adjuvant chemotherapy with fluorouracil plus folinic acid or gemcitabine *vs*. observation on survival in patients with resected periampullary adenocarcinoma: The ESPAC-3 periampullary cancer randomized trial. *JAMA* 2012;**308**(2):147–156.
5. Iacobuzio-Donahue CA, *et al*. *DPC4* gene status of the primary carcinoma correlates with patterns of failure in patients with pancreatic cancer. *J Clin Oncol* 2009;**27**(11):1806–1813.
6. Whittington R, *et al*. Adjuvant therapy of resected adenocarcinoma of the pancreas. *Int J Radiat Oncol Biol Phys* 1991;**21**(5):1137–1143.
7. Hsu CC, *et al*. Adjuvant chemoradiation for pancreatic adenocarcinoma: The Johns Hopkins Hospital–Mayo Clinic collaborative study. *Ann Surg Oncol* 2010;**17**(4): 981–990.
8. Kooby DA, *et al*. Impact of adjuvant radiotherapy on survival after pancreatic cancer resection: An appraisal of data from the national cancer data base. *Ann Surg Oncol* 2013;**20**(11):3634–3642.
9. Kalser MH, Ellenberg SS. Pancreatic cancer. Adjuvant combined radiation and chemotherapy following curative resection. *Arch Surg* 1985;**120**(8):899–903.
10. Gastrointestinal Tumor Study Group. Further evidence of effective adjuvant combined radiation and chemotherapy following curative resection of pancreatic cancer. *Cancer* 1987;**59**(12):2006–2010.
11. Klinkenbijl JH, *et al*. Adjuvant radiotherapy and 5-fluorouracil after curative resection of cancer of the pancreas and periampullary region: phase III trial of the EORTC gastrointestinal tract cancer cooperative group. *Ann Surg* 1999;**230**(6):776–782; discussion 782–774.
12. Smeenk HG, *et al*. Long-term survival and metastatic pattern of pancreatic and periampullary cancer after adjuvant chemoradiation or observation: Long-term results of EORTC trial 40891. *Ann Surg* 2007;**246**(5):734–740.
13. Neoptolemos JP, *et al*. Adjuvant chemoradiotherapy and chemotherapy in resectable pancreatic cancer: A randomised controlled trial. *Lancet* 2001;**358**(9293):1576–1585.

14. Neoptolemos JP, *et al*. A randomized trial of chemoradiotherapy and chemotherapy after resection of pancreatic cancer. *N Engl J Med* 2004;**350**(12):1200–1210.
15. Abrams RA, *et al*. Continuing controversy over adjuvant therapy of pancreatic cancer. *Lancet* 2001;**358**(9293):1565–1566.
16. Van Laethem JL, *et al*. Adjuvant gemcitabine alone versus gemcitabine-based chemoradiotherapy after curative resection for pancreatic cancer: A randomized EORTC-40013-22012/FFCD-9203/GERCOR phase II study. *J Clin Oncol* 2010;**28**(29): 4450–4456.
17. Schmidt J, *et al*. Open-label, multicenter, randomized phase III trial of adjuvant chemoradiation plus interferon alfa-2b versus fluorouracil and folinic acid for patients with resected pancreatic adenocarcinoma. *J Clin Oncol* 2012;**30**(33):4077–4083.
18. Liao WC, *et al*. Adjuvant treatments for resected pancreatic adenocarcinoma: A systematic review and network meta-analysis. *Lancet Oncol* 2013;**14**(11):1095–1103.
19. Small W, *et al*. *Radiation Oncology: Difficult Cases and Practical Management*. New York: Demos Medical, 2013.
20. Gunderson LL, *et al*. *Clinical Radiation Oncology*. Philadelphia: Elsevier Saunders, 2012.
21. Showalter TN, *et al*. The influence of total nodes examined, number of positive nodes, and lymph node ratio on survival after surgical resection and adjuvant chemoradiation for pancreatic cancer: A secondary analysis of RTOG 9704. *Int J Radiat Oncol Biol Phys* 2011;**81**(5):1328–1335.
22. Regine WF, *et al*. Fluorouracil-based chemoradiation with either gemcitabine or fluorouracil chemotherapy after resection of pancreatic adenocarcinoma: 5-year analysis of the U.S. Intergroup/RTOG 9704 phase III trial. *Ann Surg Oncol* 2011;**18**(5):1319–1326.
23. Callery MP, *et al*. Pretreatment assessment of resectable and borderline resectable pancreatic cancer: expert consensus statement. *Ann Surg Oncol* 2009;**16**(7):1727–1733.
24. Stefanidis D, *et al*. The current role of staging laparoscopy for adenocarcinoma of the pancreas: A review. *Ann Oncol* 2006;**17**(2):189–199.
25. Meszoely IM, *et al*. Preoperative chemoradiation therapy for adenocarcinoma of the pancreas: The Fox Chase Cancer Center experience, 1986–2003. *Surg Oncol Clin North Am* 2004;**13**(4):685–696, x.
26. Katz MH, *et al*. Borderline resectable pancreatic cancer: The importance of this emerging stage of disease. *J Am Coll Surg* 2008;**206**(5):833–846; discussion 838–846.
27. Evans DB, *et al*. Preoperative chemoradiation and pancreaticoduodenectomy for adenocarcinoma of the pancreas. *Arch Surg* 1992;**127**(11):1335–1339.
28. Pisters PW, *et al*. Rapid-fractionation preoperative chemoradiation, pancreaticoduodenectomy, and intraoperative radiation therapy for resectable pancreatic adenocarcinoma. *J Clin Oncol* 1998;**16**(12):3843–3850.
29. Pisters PW, *et al*. Preoperative paclitaxel and concurrent rapid-fractionation radiation for resectable pancreatic adenocarcinoma: Toxicities, histologic response rates, and event-free outcome. *J Clin Oncol* 2002;**20**(10):2537–2544.
30. Burris HA, *et al*. Improvements in survival and clinical benefit with gemcitabine as first-line therapy for patients with advanced pancreas cancer: A randomized trial. *J Clin Oncol* 1997;**15**(6):2403–2413.

31. Evans DB, *et al.* Preoperative gemcitabine-based chemoradiation for patients with resectable adenocarcinoma of the pancreatic head. *J Clin Oncol* 2008;**26**(21): 3496–3502.

32. Wolff RA, *et al.* Phase I trial of gemcitabine combined with radiation for the treatment of locally advanced pancreatic adenocarcinoma. *Clin Cancer Res* 2001;**7**(8): 2246–2253.

33. Kim EJ, *et al.* A multi-institutional phase 2 study of neoadjuvant gemcitabine and oxali-platin with radiation therapy in patients with pancreatic cancer. *Cancer* 2013; **119**(15):2692–2700.

34. Moertel CG, *et al.* Therapy of locally unresectable pancreatic carcinoma: A randomized comparison of high dose (6000 rads) radiation alone, moderate dose radiation (4000 rads + 5-fluorouracil), and high dose radiation + 5-fluorouracil: The Gastrointestinal Tumor Study Group. *Cancer* 1981;**48**(8):1705–1710.

35. Loehrer PJ, Sr., *et al.* Gemcitabine alone versus gemcitabine plus radiotherapy in patients with locally advanced pancreatic cancer: An Eastern Cooperative Oncology Group trial. *J Clin Oncol* 2011;**29**(31):4105–4112.

36. Chauffert B, *et al.* Phase III trial comparing intensive induction chemoradiotherapy (60 Gy, infusional 5-FU and intermittent cisplatin) followed by maintenance gemcitabine with gemcitabine alone for locally advanced unresectable pancreatic cancer. Definitive results of the 2000-01 FFCD/SFRO study. *Ann Oncol* 2008; **19**(9):1592–1599.

37. Huguet F, *et al.* Impact of chemoradiotherapy after disease control with chemotherapy in locally advanced pancreatic adenocarcinoma in GERCOR phase II and III studies. *J Clin Oncol* 2007;**25**(3):326–331.

38. Hammel P, *et al.* Comparison of chemoradiotherapy (CRT) and chemotherapy (CT) in patients with a locally advanced pancreatic cancer (LAPC) controlled after 4 months of gemcitabine with or without erlotinib: Final results of the international phase III LAP 07 study [abstract]. *J Clin Oncol* 2013;**31**:LBA4003.

39. Crane CH, *et al.* Phase I study of concomitant gemcitabine and IMRT for patients with unresectable adenocarcinoma of the pancreatic head. *Int J Gastrointest Cancer* 2001;**30**(3):123–132.

40. Ben-Josef E, *et al.* A phase I/II trial of intensity modulated radiation (IMRT) dose escalation with concurrent fixed-dose rate gemcitabine (FDR-G) in patients with unresectable pancreatic cancer. *Int J Radiat Oncol Biol Phys* 2012;**84**(5):1166–1171.

41. Murphy JD, *et al.* Full-dose gemcitabine and concurrent radiotherapy for unresectable pancreatic cancer. *Int J Radiat Oncol Biol Phys* 2007;**68**(3):801–808.

42. Zimmermann FB, *et al.* Dose escalation of concurrent hypofractionated radiotherapy and continuous infusion 5-FU-chemotherapy in advanced adenocarcinoma of the pancreas. *Hepatogastroenterology* 2005;**52**(61):246–250.

43. Goodman KA, *et al.* Radiation Therapy Oncology Group consensus panel guidelines for the delineation of the clinical target volume in the postoperative treatment of pancreatic head cancer. *Int J Radiat Oncol Biol Phys* 2012;**83**(3):901–908.

44. Hunter KU, *et al.* Radiation therapy with full-dose gemcitabine and oxaliplatin for unresectable pancreatic cancer. *Int J Radiat Oncol Biol Phys* 2012;**83**(3):921–926.

45. Spalding AC, *et al*. Potential for dose-escalation and reduction of risk in pancreatic cancer using IMRT optimization with lexicographic ordering and gEUD-based cost functions. *Med Phys* 2007;**34**(2):521–529.

46. Yovino S, *et al*. Intensity-modulated radiation therapy significantly improves acute gastrointestinal toxicity in pancreatic and ampullary cancers. *Int J Radiat Oncol Biol Phys* 2011;**79**(1):158–162.

47. Thompson RF, *et al*. A dosimetric comparison of proton and photon therapy in unresectable cancers of the head of pancreas. *Med Phys* 2014;**41**(8):081711.

48. Schellenberg D, *et al*. Gemcitabine chemotherapy and single-fraction stereotactic body radiotherapy for locally advanced pancreatic cancer. *Int J Radiat Oncol Biol Phys* 2008;**72**(3):678–686.

49. Moningi S, *et al*. Stereotactic body radiation therapy for pancreatic cancer: Single institutional experience. *ASCO Meeting Abstr* 2014;**32**(3 Suppl.):328.

50. Crane CH, *et al*. The role of intraoperative radiotherapy in pancreatic cancer. *Surg Oncol Clin North Am* 2003;**12**(4):965–977.

Chapter 11

Advances in the Surgical Approach to Pancreatic Cancer

Jennifer Miller, Herbert Zeh and Amer H. Zureikat

1 Introduction

With advanced understanding of pancreatic disease and improved diagnostic imaging, the frequency of pancreatic procedures has rapidly increased over the past several decades. The indications for pancreatic surgery have expanded to include a larger spectrum of conditions. Pancreaticoduodenectomy (PD) is increasingly utilized for premalignant lesions, such as pancreatic cysts and cystic neoplasm; endocrine tumors; pancreatitis and its sequelae; biliary ductal cancers; and others cancers of the gastrointestinal tract.[1]

As the application of pancreatic surgery has expanded, so have the available technologies utilized by surgeons. Platforms for performing minimally invasive surgery, such as laparoscopy and robotic surgery, afford improvements in patient metrics such as decreased blood loss, surgical site infections, and postoperative pain with equivalent or superior outcomes in comparison to open surgery.

2 Evolution of Pancreatic Cancer Surgery

The field of pancreatic surgery has dramatically evolved since its inception nearly two centuries ago. In 1841, Friedrich Wilhelm Wandesleben (1800–1868) performed the first reported human pancreatic operation; the small town German physician is credited with surgical drainage of a traumatic pancreatic pseudocyst.[2]

Allen O. Whipple, described the pancreaticoduodenectomy in 1935.[3] His innovation laid the foundation for American pancreatic surgery. Initially described to the American Surgical Association as a two-stage procedure, the Whipple procedure was refined to a one-stage operation five years later.[4] In 1978, Traverso and Longmire described the pylorus sparing modification.[5] PD remains one of the most complex abdominal operations owing to the anatomic relationship of the pancreas to major vascular structures as well as the construction of three complex anastomoses: pancreaticojejunostomy, hepaticojejunostomy, and gastrojejunostomy in order to restore enteric continuity.[6] Early widespread implementation of pancreatic resection — most commonly PD for pancreatic carcinoma — during the 1960s and 1970s was stifled by the high morbidity and mortality; the latter exceeding 20%.[7]

3 Evolution of Minimally Invasive Pancreas Surgery

It was not until 1985 when the first laparoscopic cholecystectomy was performed that interest in minimally invasive surgery began to emerge.[8] Laparoscopy affords patient advantages such as smaller incisions, decreased postoperative pain, faster recovery, and decreased morbidity. Despite the advantages conferred by laparoscopy, its application has been more limited in complex resections, such as pancreatic surgery due to the technical difficulty associated with the retroperitoneal location, vicinity to major vasculature, and challenging composition of the gland.[6]

In 1994, Gagner and Pomp introduced the laparoscopic PD (LPD).[9] However, its broad application was initially met with skepticism and consequently only a few small series were reported during the decade following its debut.[9,10] Laparoscopic surgery for complex resection is limited by technical constraints including: restricted range of motion, poor ergonomics, two-dimensional visualization, and difficulty in complex suturing.[11] The limitations of traditional laparoscopic instruments necessitate modification of technical principles required for open pancreatic surgery particularly for complex resections and reconstruction. Its utility has been limited to experienced surgeons at high volume tertiary centers.

As literature investigating LPD versus open PD(OPD) expanded, the safety of the procedure was confirmed but only by a few skilled surgeons. For example, a review in 2011 described an overall mortality of 2% and morbidity of 48% in LPD, similar to that of OPD.[10]

4 Robotic Surgery

Robotic surgery, a computer-assisted surgical platform, has evolved over the past three decades.[12] The first described surgical robots were used to improve accuracy and precision. The earliest described surgical robot, the Arthrobot, assisted total hip arthroplasty while the later developed Puma 560 improved neurosurgical biopsies.[13] These early innovations paved the way for technologies, which would revolutionize all fields of surgery. In the 1990s, a robotic system named telerobics was introduced; this was followed by the introduction of the da Vinci® system (Intuitive Surgical, Sunnyvale, CA, USA) in 1990. Intuitive Surgical has become the sole producer of surgical robotic devices since its merger with other robotic developers in 2003.[14]

Although robot-assisted surgery initially found application in cardiothoracic surgery with the first robotic-assisted cardiac bypass performed in Germany, the widespread use of robotic-assisted surgery is most closely linked to urology.[14] Following the initial robotic-assisted radical prostatectomy described in 2000, the technology experienced widespread popularity such that 80% of prostatectomies in the United States estimated to have been performed robotically.[15]

Robotic surgery confers technological advantages over laparoscopy such as three-dimensional binocular vision, improved surgeon ergonomics, and increased degrees of freedom. These additional parameters enable the surgeon to perform the complex maneuvers such of delicate retroperitoneal dissections and meticulous suturing required in pancreatic surgery.[6] Guilianotti *et al.* are credited with the first reported robotic PD (RPD) in 2010.[34] Since then, reports of minimally invasive pancreatic resections have continued to increase.

4.1 *Robotic pancreaticoduodenectomy*

As with any surgical platform, patient selection remains key to implementation of RPD. At our institution, preoperative planning includes a triphasic CT (computed tomography) scan and EUS (endoscopic ultrasound) as these modalities have proven important in predicting the probability of margin-negative (R0) resection.[17] Borderline resectable tumors — those with SMV/PV (superior Mesenteric vein/ portal vein) vascular abutment or encasement — currently present a contraindication to PD at our institution. RPD should be performed by surgeons experienced in open PD and venous reconstruction if necessary (Figures 1 and 2).

Our technique begins laparoscopically with six trocars. Following insufflation, the abdomen is inspected for metastatic disease. If the abdomen is free of metastases, a Kocher maneuver and a Cattell–Braasch maneuver are performed in order to mobilize the duodenum and right colon. Dissection continues laparoscopically until the stomach and jejunum are transected; at this point the robot is docked. Next, the portal structures and retropancreatic tunnel are dissected. The pancreas is transected with electrocautery; "cold" transection is reserved for the duct, which affords the surgeon the ability to identify even the smallest duct in a soft (normal) gland. The robotic platform confers the advantage of high magnification and high degrees of

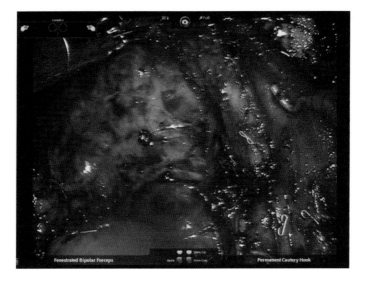

Figure 1   Shown here is the resection bed following a robotic pancreaticoduodenectomy (RPD) for pancreatic adenocarcinoma. Note the superior mesenteric vein/portal vein overlying the superior mesenteric artery (SMA). The robotic platform allows meticulous dissection of all pancreatic and lymphatic tissue on the right side of the SMA in order to maximize the rate of negative margin resections.

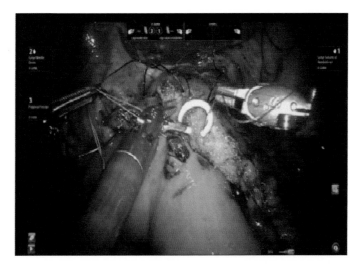

Figure 2   Shown here is the pancreaticojejunostomy reconstruction in end to-side, duct-to-mucosa fashion for a soft pancreatic gland with a non-dilated (normal) 2-mm duct, after RPD. The robotic platform allows precise placement of these sutures with favorable ergonomics, under direct magnification. Also shown is a 4 French internal pancreatic stent (white) used to ensure patency of the anastomosis.

instrument articulation for meticulous dissection around major vasculature such as the gastroduodenal artery as well as superior and inferior pancreaticoduodenal arteries thereby potentially reducing bleeding. After the pancreas is divided, attention is turned to dissecting the retroperitoneal margin and unicinate process. The robotic platform facilitates precision in removal of all peripancreatic and perivascular tissue along the plane of Leriche. The enteric reconstruction is then carried out. First, a duct-to-mucosa pancreaticojejunostomy is performed using fine 5-0 suture. Second, the hepaticojejunostomy is constructed, either by interrupted or continuous suture depending on duct size. Third, the gastrojejunostomy (or duodenojejunostomy) is performed in a two-layered anastomosis.[18]

In 2006, one of the largest series of OPD was reported by Johns Hopkins with 1,432 cases for pancreatic malignancies. Winter *et al.* report a mean operative time of 380 min, a mean blood loss of 800 mL, mean length of stay of nine days, 58% R0 resections, 5% pancreatic fistula rate (pre-ISPFG criteria), and a 2% mortality rate.[19] This study provides a useful benchmark for comparing outcomes of a new technology against OPD.

The University of Pittsburgh recently reported the institution's first 250 consecutive robotic resections; 132 of these were RPD. With a conversion rate of 8% (4.5 in the last 112 cases), the review demonstrated a median estimated blood loss of 300 mL, mean length of stay of 10 days, 7.4% pancreatic leak (grades B and C) by ISGPF criteria, and a 1.5% and 3.8% 30- and 90-day mortality rate, respectively.[20]

There remains a paucity of literature comparing minimally invasive PD to OPD. Nonetheless, the available literature suggests that outcomes of both LPD and RPD are not inferior to OPD (Table 1). Minimally invasive platforms demonstrate advantages in decreasing blood loss if performed by high volume surgeons who have surpassed their learning curves for PD. Importantly, there is no increase in operative mortality with RPD. It must be noted that case control comparisons between robotic and open PD suffer from lack of numbers since these are all single institutional series; the largest robotic case control study boasts only 44 cases.[21–24]

4.2 Robotic distal pancreatectomy

Laparoscopic distal pancreatectomy (LDP) was first performed for chronic pancreatitis in 1994, the same year that Gagner introduced the LPD.[25] This procedure witnessed increased greater appeal as compared to PD, likely secondary to the lack of anastomoses and greater ability to control bleeding if encountered. There have been a number of series reporting minimally invasive DP (Table 2).

Our institution utilizes a hybrid approach for the robotic distal pancreatectomy, similar to the RPD technique. Initially, the dissection is performed laparoscopically. The lesser sac is entered, short gastric arteries transected, and anterior surface of the

Table 1.   Laparoscopic pancreaticoduodenectomy (LPD) and Robotic pancreaticoduodenectomy (RPD).

Series	Type	Patients (n)	Conversion to Open (%)	Time (min)	EBL (mL)	LOS (days)	30-Day Mortality (%)	Pancreatic Fistula (%)	R0 Resection (%)	Lymph Node (n)
Asburn, Stauffer[39]	LPD	53	17	541	195	8	5.7	16.7	94.9	23
Corcione[40]	LPD	22	9.1	392	NR	NR	4.5	27.2	100	NR
Dulucq[41]	LPD	25	12	287	107	16.2	4	4	100	18
Kendrick[42]	LPD	65	5	368	240	7	1.5	18	89	15
Palanivelu[43]	LPD	75	0	357	74	8.2	1.3	7	97.4	14
Pugliese[44]	LPD	19	32	461	180	18	0	16	100	12
Zureikat[33]	LPD	14	14	456	300	8	7	36	100	19
Bao[22]	RPD	28	14	431	100	7.4	7	29	63	15
Buchs[23]	RPD	44	4.5	444	387	13	4.5	18	90.9	16.8
Chalikonda[21]	RPD*	30	10	476	485	9.8	3	7	100	13
Giulianotti	RPD	50	22	568	394	22	8	38	90	18
Lia[24]	RPD	20	5	492	247	13.7	0	35	73	10
Zureikat[20]	RPD	132	8	527	300	10	1.5	17	88	19

EBL: expected blood loss; LOS: length of stay

Table 2   Laparoscopic distal pancreatectomy (LDP) and robotic distal pancreatectomy (RDP).

Series	Type	Patients (n)	Conversion to Open (%)	Time (min)	EBL (mL)	LOS (days)	30-Day Mortality (%)	Pancreatic Fistula (%)	R0 Resection (%)	Lymph Node (n)	Splenic Preservation (%)
Fernandez Cruz[45]	LDP	82	NR	222	370	6.5	0	7	77	14.5	63.4
Jayarman[46]	LDP	107	32	193	150	5	NR	16	97	6	21
Kooby[26]	LDP	142	13	230	357	5.9	0	26	93	NR	3
Daouadi[28]	RDP	30	0	293	212	6.1	0	13	100	18.6	7
Giulianotti[34]	RDP	46	3	NR	NR	NR	0	9	NR	NR	50
Kang[47,48]	RDP	20	NR	348	372	7.1	0	NR	18.6	NR	95
Waters[49]	RDP	17	2	298	279	4	0	0	100	5	65
Zureikat[20]	RDP	83	2	256	150	6	0	43	97	16	NR

EBL: expected blood loss; LOS: length of stay

pancreas cleared laparoscopically. At this point, the robot is docked. The superior and inferior borders of the pancreas are then meticulously dissected. Attention then turns to vascular control through visualization of the splenic vessels. The retropancreatic tunnel is then carefully dissected to visualize and divide the neck of the gland. Additionally, the robotic platform affords the ability to then perform complete lymphadenectomy.[6]

In 2008, a large multi-institutional study by Kooby *et al.* evaluated LPD and open distal pancreatectomy (ODP) in a 3:1 matched comparison. The study demonstrated decreased blood loss, shorter length of stay, increased splenic preservation, and decreased overall morbidity without an increase in pancreatic fistula rates in the laparoscopic group as compared to open.[26] This study suggests superiority of the minimally invasive technique when applied to appropriately selected patients.

The University of Pittsburgh demonstrated similar results in retrospective study published in 2013. Magge *et al.* compared ODP to the minimally invasive approach (both LDP and RPD) and demonstrated equivalent outcomes. Short-term oncologic outcomes, R0 status, and lymph node clearance were equivalent across the groups. Furthermore, decreased length of hospital stay, reduced blood loss, and similar frequency of postoperative complications were demonstrated by the minimally invasive group, with equivalent median overall survival.[27]

The University of Pittsburgh group also analyzed outcomes of LDP and RDP for pancreatic adenocarcinoma in a retrospective matched comparison. The authors concluded that RDP confers numerous advantages such as fewer conversions to open surgery, lower estimated blood loss, and improved oncologic outcomes versus LDP. The study demonstrated a statistically significant decrease in the open conversion rate in the RDP group (0%) compared to the LDP (16%). Additionally, no positive margins were incurred in the RDP group as compared to 35 %in the LPD group. The study mitigated selection bias by relegating the LDP cohort to a period of time when robotic technology was unavailable. It was thus concluded that RDP was superior to LDP for resection of pancreatic adenocarcinoma.[28]

4.3 *Robotic central pancreatectomy*

Central pancreatectomy (CP), or medial pancreatectomy, is a technique applicable to benign or low-grade malignant neoplasms located to the left of the gastroduodenal artery in the region of the splenomesenteric confluence.[29] This procedure is indicated infrequently as few pancreatic neck lesions are amenable to less than distal pancreatectomy. As such, CP is less frequently described in the literature. Open CP (OCP) confers a high degree of risk due to the dissection around splenic vessels as well as risk of fistula associated with pancreatic transection at two sites.[30]

The procedure remains an attractive option due to the potential for avoiding diabetes or exocrine insufficiency when resecting low-grade or benign lesions.

At our institution, RCP is carried out in a technique similar to RDP. The initial dissection is performed laparoscopically before the robot is docked. After docking, the lesion is resected proximally with an endoscopic stapler. The distal margin is resected with electrocautery, with great attention to avoiding thermal injury to the duct. The reconstruction is then created via pancreaticogastrostomy or pancreatico-jejunostomy using a modified Blumgart technique.[6]

Several case series have demonstrated safety of RCP with similar oncologic outcomes as compared to open CP. In a nine-patient case series by Abood from the University of Pittsburgh, median estimated blood loss was 190 mL, operative time was 425 min, and length of stay was 10 days. The ISGPF defined fistula rate was 78% overall; however, only 22% were clinically significant, i.e. grades B or C. Both of the clinically significant fistulas resolved nonoperatively.[31] Another series of 10 patients by Zhan showed similar outcomes with estimated blood loss of 158 mL, operative time of 219 min, and length of stay of 26.3 days. They reported a 70% pancreatic fistula rate; all of these were grade A and managed conservatively.[32]

4.4 *Other robotic-assisted pancreatic procedures*

The robotic platform serves a role in pancreatic enucleations for small neuroendocrine tumors (NETs) and premalignant lesions such as intraductal papillary mucinous neoplasm (IPMN). The robotic platform enables careful dissection of small pancreatic lesions through high visual resolution and improved dexterity to spare pancreatic parenchyma and associated morbidity.[18] Additional complex pancreatic resections for malignant lesions, such as the Appleby procedure and total pancreatectomy with auto islet transplantation have also been described.

For benign lesions, the robotic platform may also be safely applied. Robotic lateral pancreaticojejunostomy has been described in small numbers at both the University of Pittsburgh and other institutions with minimal complication.[33,34] Furthermore, the robotic platform has been implemented for cystgastrostomy and cystjejunostomy for complications associated with pancreatitis.[34]

4.5 *Benefits of the robotic platform*

Like laparoscopic surgery, robotic-assisted surgery may confer advantages such as reduced surgical site infections and decreased blood loss. Data from the University of Pittsburgh suggest that RPD patients are more likely to receive adjuvant chemotherapy than OPD patients (data presented in abstract from at AHPBA in 2014);

Table 3   Laparoscopic central pancreatectomy (LCP) and robotic central pancreatectomy (RCP).

Series	Type	Patients (n)	Conversion to Open (%)	Time (min)	EBL (mL)	LOS (days)	30-Day Mortality (%)	Pancreatic Fistula (%)	R0 Resection (%)	Lymph Node (n)	Pancreatic Insufficiency (%)
Dokmak[30]	LCP	13	8	190	100	24	0	30.8	NR	NR	8
Rotellar[50]	LCP	9	11.1	435	100	13.5	0	22	NR	NR	NR
SaCunha[51]	LCP	6	16.7	225	125	18	0	12.5	NR	NR	0
Zhang[52]	LCP	8	0	286	57	10	0	33	NR	NR	0
Abood[31]	RCP	9	11.1	425	190	10	0	70	100	NR	0
Giulianotti[34]	RCP	3	0	320	233	9 to 27	0	78	NR	NR	0
Kang[48]	RCP	5	0	432	275	14.6	0	20	NR	NR	NR
Zhan[53]	RCP	10	0	219	158	26.3	0	33.3	NR	NR	NR

EBL: expected blood loss; LOS: length of stay

since pancreatic cancer survival is increased with adjuvant therapy, the robotic platform may prove to have an oncologic benefit.

Robotic surgery may also find a niche in "prophylactic surgery." As imaging technologies advance, the ability to identify precursors of pancreatic cancer expands. A minimally invasive approach may shift the risk-benefit ratio toward early intervention, including prophylactic resection of premalignant lesions.[37]

Surgeon ergonomic factors may play an important role in favoring robotic platforms. A 2005 study investigated the physical and mental stress of simulated surgical tasks by medical students and residents on a robotic system versus a laparoscopic system. Although mental stress was similar, physical stress was increased with laparoscopy. The potential risk of musculoskeletal was therefore increased compared to robotic surgery.[38]

4.6 *Limitations of the robotic platform*

One significant limitation of the robotic platform is the inability to access multiple quadrants of the abdomen. Additionally, once the robot is docked the operating table cannot be moved. This limiting factor can be alleviated by performing the initial dissection and mobilization steps laparoscopically during robotic-assisted surgery.[18]

The lack of haptic feedback remains a criticism of the robotic platform. This greatly improved magnification leads the surgeon to rely on visual clues that — with sufficient experience — compensate for the lack of tactile feedback. There is a steep learning curve, which may be rapidly overcome for the surgeon to acquire skills such as complex dissection and meticulous suturing.[38]

Cost remains perhaps the greatest criticisms of robotic surgery due to the expense of the console, equipment, maintenance fees, and operating room fees. Overall costs however will likely decrease due to potential for decreased length of stay, complications, and readmissions, once the learning curve is attained.

5 Conclusions

Pancreatic surgery has greatly evolved since its inception. The advent of minimally invasive techniques will likely improve outcomes further. In a very short period of time, the robotic platform has already been established as a safe and feasible alternative to open pancreatic surgery. As learning curves are overcome, robotic pancreatic surgery may afford pancreatic cancer patients improved morbidity and possibly improved survival.

References

1. Mohammed S, Fisher WE. Quality metrics in pancreas surgery. *Surg Clin North Am* 2013;**93**:693–709.
2. Schnelldorfer T. The birth of pancreatic surgery: A tribute to Friedrich Wilhelm Wandesleben. *World J Surg* 2010;**34**(1):190–193.
3. Whipple AO, *et al.* Treatment of carcinoma of the ampulla of Vater. *Ann Surg* 1935; **102**:763–779.
4. Fernandez-del Castillo C, *et al.* Evolution of the Whipple procedure at the Massachusetts General Hospital. *Surgery* 2012;**152**(3 Suppl. 1):S56–S63.
5. Traverso LW, Longmire WP, Jr. Preservation of the pylorus in pancreaticuoduodenectomy. *Surg Gynecol Obstet* 1978;**146**;959–962.
6. Winer J, *et al.* The current state of robotic-assisted pancreatic surgery. *Nat Rev Gastroenterol Hepatol* 2012;**9**(8):468–476.
7. Lieberman MD, *et al.* Relation of perioperative deaths to hospital volume among patients undergoing pancreatic resections for malignancy. *Ann Surg* 1995;**222**:638–645.
8. Reynolds W, Jr. The first laparoscopic cholecystectomy. *JSLS* 2001;**5**:89–94.
9. Gagner M, Pomp A. Laparoscopic pylorus — preserving pancreatoduodenectomy. *Surg Endosc* 1994;**8**:408–410.
10. Gumbs AA, *et al.* Laparoscopic pancreatoduodenectomy: A review of 285 published cases. *Ann Surg Oncol* 2011;**18**(5):1335–1341.
11. McDougall EM, *et al.* Comparison of three-dimensional and two-dimensional laparoscopic video systems. *J Endourol* 1996;**10**:371–374.
12. Zureikat AH, *et al.* Can laparoscopic pancreaticoduodenectomy be safely implemented? *J Gastrointest Surg* 2011;**15**:1151–1157.
13. Kwoh YS, *et al.* A robot with improved absolute positioning accuracy for CT guided stereotactic brain surgery. *IEEE Trans Biomed Eng* 1988;**35**(2):153–160.
14. Yates DR, *et al.* From Leonardo to da Vinco: The history of robot-assisted surgery in urology. *BJU Int* 2011;**108**(11):1708–1713.
15. Jacobs EF, *et al.* Advances in robotic-assisted radical prostatectomy over time. *Prostate Cancer* 2013;**2013**:902686.
16. Barbash GI, Glied SA. New technology and health care costs — the case of robot-assisted surgery. *N Engl J Med* 2010;**363**:701–704.
17. Bao P, *et al.* Validation of a prediction rule to maximize curative (R0) resection of early-stage pancreatic adenocarcinoma. *HPB (Oxford)* 2009;**11**(7):606–611.
18. Ongchin M, *et al.* Essentials and future directions of pancreatic surgery. In Kroh M, Chalikonda S, eds. *Essentials of Robotic Surgery.* New York: Springer, 2015, pp. 131–148.
19. Winter JM, *et al.* 1423 pancreaticoduodenectomies for pancreatic cancer: A single-institution experience. *J Gastrointest Surg* 2006;**10**(9):1199–1210; discussion 1210–1211.
20. Zureikat AH, *et al.* 250 robotic pancreatic resections: safety and feasibility. *Ann Surg* 2013;**258**(4):554–559; discussion 559–562.
21. Chalikonda S, *et al.* Laparoscopic robotic-assisted pancreaticoduodenectomy: A case-matched comparison with open resection. *Surg Endosc* 2012;**26**:2397–2402.

22. Bao PQ, *et al.* Retrospective comparison of robot-assisted minimally invasive versus open pancreaticoduodenectomy for periampullary neoplasms. *J Gastrointest Surg* 2013;**18**(4):682–689.

23. Buchs NC, *et al.* Robotic versus open pancreaticoduodenectomy: A comparative study at a single institution. *World J Surg* 2011;**35**(12):2739–2746.

24. Lai EC, *et al.* Robot-assisted laparoscopic pancreaticoduodenectomy versus open pancreaticoduodenectomy-a comparative study. *Int J Surg* 2012;**10**(9):475–479.

25. Cuschieri A, *et al.* Laparoscopic distal 70% pancreatectomy and splenectomy for chronic pancreatitis. *Ann Surg* 1996;**223**:280–285.

26. Kooby DA, *et al.* Left-sided pancreatectomy: A multicenter comparison of laparoscopic and open approaches. *Ann Surg* 2008;**248**(3):438–446.

27. Magge D, *et al.* Comparative effectiveness of minimally invasive and open distal pancreatectomy for ductal adenocarcinoma. *JAMA Surg* 2013;**148**(6):525–531.

28. Daouadi M, *et al.* Robot-assisted minimally invasive distal pancreatectomy is superior to the laparoscopic technique. *Ann Surg* 2013;**257**(1):128–132.

29. Sauvanet A, *et al.* Medial pancreatectomy: A multi-institutional retrospective study of 53 patients by the French Pancreas Club. *Surgery* 2002;**132**(5):836–843.

30. Dokmak S, *et al.* Pure laparoscopic middle pancreatectomy: Single-center experience with 13 cases. *Surg Endosc* 2014;**28**(5):1601–1606.

31. Abood GJ, *et al.* Robotic-assisted minimally invasive central pancreatectomy: Technique and outcomes. *J Gastrointest Surg* 2013;**17**(5):1002–1008.

32. Zhou NX, *et al.* Outcomes of pancreatoduodenectomy with robotic surgery versus open surgery. *Int J Med Robot* 2011;**7**:131–137.

33. Zureikat AH, *et al.* Can laparoscopic pancreaticoduodenectomy be safely implemented? *J Gastrointest Surg* 2011;**15**(7):1151–1157.

34. Giulianotti PC, *et al.* Robot-assisted laparoscopic pancreatic surgery: Single-surgeon experience. *Surg Endosc* 2010;**24**(7):1646–1657.

35. Lee GC, *et al.* High-performing Whipple patients: Factors associated with short length of stay after open pancreaticoduodenectomy. *J Gastrointest Surg* 2014;**18**(10): 1760–1769.

36. Sinn M, *et al.* Does long-term survival in patients with pancreatic cancer really exist? Results from the CONKO-001 study. *J Surg Oncol* 2013;**108**(6):398–402.

37. Lee EC, *et al.* Ergonomics and human factors in endoscopic surgery: A comparison of manual *vs.* telerobotic simulation systems. *Surg Endosc* 2005;**19**(8):1064–1070.

38. Zeh HJ, *et al.* Robotic-assisted major pancreatic resection. *Adv Surg* 2011;**45**(1): 323–340.

39. Asbun HJ, Stauffer JA. Laparoscopic *vs.* open pancreaticoduodenectomy: Overall outcomes and severity of complications using the Accordion Severity Grading System. *J Am Coll Surg* 2012;**215**(6):810819.

40. Corcione F, *et al.* Laparoscopic pancreaticoduodenectomy: Rxperience of 22 cases. *Surg Endosc* 2013;**27**(6):2131–2136.

41. Dulucq JL, *et al.* Laparoscopic pancreaticoduodenectomy for benign and malignant diseases. *Surg Endosc* 2006;**20**(7):1045–1050.

42. Kendrick M, Cusanti D. Total laparoscopic pancreaticoduodenectomy: Feasibility and outcome in an early expereince. *Arch Surg* 2010;**145**(1):19–23.

43. Palanivelu C, *et al.* Laparoscopic lateral pancreaticojejunostomy: A new remedy for an old ailment. *Surg Endosc* 2006;**20**(3):458–461.

44. Pugliese R, *et al.* Laparoscopic pancreaticoduodenectomy: A retrospective review of 19 cases. *Surg Laparosc Endoscs Percutan Tech* 2008;**18**:13–18.

45. Fernandez-Cruz L, *et al.* Curative laparoscopic resection for pancreatic neoplasms: A critical analysis from a single institution. *J Gastrointest Surg* 2007;**11**(12): 1607–1621; discussion 1621–1622.

46. Jayaraman S, *et al.* Laparoscopic distal pancreatectomy: Evolution of a technique at a single institution. *J Am Coll Surg* 2010;**211**(4):503–509.

47. Kang CM, *et al.* Conventional laparoscopic and robot-assisted spleen-preserving pancreatectomy: Does da Vinci have clinical advantages? *Surg Endosc* 2011;**25**(6): 2004–2009.

48. Kang CM, *et al.* Initial experiences using robot-assisted central pancreatectomy with pancreaticogastrostomy: A potential way to advanced laparoscopic pancreatectomy. *Surg Endosc* 2011;**25**(4):1101–1106.

49. Waters JA, *et al.* Robotic distal pancreatectomy: Cost effective? *Surgery* 2010;**148**(4): 814–823.

50. Rotellar F, *et al.* Totally laparoscopic Roux-en-Y duct-to-mucosa pancreaticojejunostomy after middle pancreatectomy: A consecutive nine-case series at a single institution. *Ann Surg* 2008;**247**(6):938–944.

51. Sa Cunha A, *et al.* Laparoscopic central pancreatectomy: Single institution experience of 6 patients. *Surgery* 2007;**142**(3):405–409.

52. Zhang R, *et al.* Laparoscopic central pancreatectomy with pancreaticojejunostomy: Preliminary experience with 8 cases. *J Laparoendosc Adv Surg Tech A* 2013;**23**(11): 912–918.

53. Zhan Q, *et al.* Robotic-assisted pancreatic resection: A report of 47 cases. *Int J Med Robot* 2013;**9**(1):44–51.

Chapter 12

Systemic Therapy in Pancreatic Cancer

Aju Mathew and Nathan Bahary

1 Introduction

Pancreatic cancer is the most fatal malignancy in adult humans with only a 6% survival rate at the five-year mark.[1] In the year 2014, it is estimated that 46,420 men and women will be diagnosed with pancreatic cancer. The mortality to incidence ratio is nearly 85%, as compared to 17% for breast cancer, signifying the tremendous burden of this disease. Pancreatic cancer is projected to be the second leading cause of cancer-related death with an estimated 88,000 new diagnosis and 63,000 deaths by the year 2030.[2] Surgical resection is the only curative treatment option in pancreatic cancer. Unfortunately, less than 20% of patients have resectable diseases at the time of presentation. The majority of patients have either locally advanced cancer or distant metastatic disease at the time of diagnosis. Even in patients who undergo resection of the pancreatic mass followed by adjuvant systemic therapy, the five-year survival rate is around 23%.[3]

Despite these numbers, recent developments in combination cytotoxic therapy are finally leading to improved outcomes.[4,5] More importantly, advances in genomics and sequencing technologies promise a new era in targeted agents including immunomodulatory therapies. This chapter reviews the current understanding of the etiology, diagnosis, and management of pancreatic cancer, principally focusing on the latest research in systemic therapy.

2 Pathology

Pancreatic cancer can arise from either the exocrine (95%) or the endocrine (5%) parenchyma. Ductal adenocarcinoma is the main histologic subtype of exocrine malignancy, while other rare forms such as acinar cell carcinoma, adenosquamous, mucinous, and anaplastic carcinoma have a cumulative incidence rate of less than 5%. For the purpose of this chapter, pancreatic cancer refers to ductal adenocarcinoma.

3 Etiology

Any attempt to decrease the burden of cancer must begin with prevention strategies. Identifying the risk factors and understanding the etiology of pancreatic cancer is crucial to developing early interventional strategies. Although germline mutation of PRSS1 (hereditary pancreatitis) and STK11 (Peutz–Jeghers syndrome) convey the highest risk for development of pancreatic cancer, tobacco exposure is likely the contributor that has the greatest public health significance.[6–8] Various epidemiologic cohort studies have found a 50% increased risk for pancreatic cancer with tobacco abuse.[9] In fact, the purported association of alcohol with pancreatic cancer may have been confounded by tobacco, given the conflicting evidence from epidemiologic studies.[10–12]

Environmental toxin exposure is another etiology factor. Epidemiologic studies have consistently found an elevated risk for persons with exposure to chlorinated hydrocarbon solvents and pesticides. However, the most debated risk factor for pancreatic cancer is diabetes mellitus and glucose intolerance. Although a meta-analysis of 35 cohort studies observed a higher risk for pancreatic cancer in patients with diabetes, reverse causality (pancreatic cancer causes diabetes) contributing to this putative association cannot be overlooked.[13,14] Nevertheless, new onset diabetes in adults can rarely be a harbinger of pancreatic cancer.[15] Obesity has also been associated with an increased risk for pancreatic cancer.[16] Several nutritional epidemiologic studies have investigated dietary factors as an etiology of pancreatic cancer. Although a meta-analysis of cohort studies suggested a causal link between pancreatic cancer and increased consumption of processed meat and high-fat diet, there are a number of cohort studies that have observed otherwise.[17–19]

Whereas the link between nutritional factors or alcohol and pancreatic cancer is weak, chronic pancreatitis is a strong risk factor for pancreatic cancer. A meta-analysis of six cohort studies and one case-control study reports a 13-fold increased risk for pancreatic cancer among patients with chronic pancreatitis.[20] The delay in time between onset of chronic pancreatitis changes and development of cancer may run as long as 10–20 years, with only 5% of patients with chronic pancreatitis eventually developing cancer over a 20-year period.[20] Additionally, hereditary pancreatitis, a rare autosomal dominant inherited disorder with high penetrance, significantly increases the risk for pancreatic cancer. A literature-based meta-analysis of three cohort studies found a 69-fold increased risk for pancreatic cancer in patients with hereditary pancreatitis.[20] The most common germline mutation seen in patients with hereditary pancreatitis is in the *PRSS1* gene encoding cationic trypsinogen.[6] It results in premature activation of trypsin within the pancreas and autodigestion of the pancreatic tissue. Recurrent episodes of acute pancreatitis causes irreversible damage characteristic of chronic pancreatitis and thereby, increases the risk for pancreatic cancer.

Several gene mutations have been identified as an etiologic factor of pancreatic cancer.[21,22] Tumor suppressor genes encoding proteins essential for DNA repair, such as *BRCA2*, *ATM*, and *PALB2*, when mutated can result in an increased risk for familial pancreatic cancer.[23–26] This increased risk for cancer is mediated by defective DNA repair resulting in genomic instability and accumulated DNA damage and unregulated tumor growth. A rare autosomal dominant inherited disorder called familial atypical multiple mole melanoma (FAMMM) syndrome is seen in patients with a germline mutation in the *CDKN2A* gene regulating the cell cycle via the p16 protein.[27] A recent study observed that the prevalence of CDKN2A mutation in unselected pancreatic cancer patients was 0.6%, which increased to 3.3% when restricted to patients with a family history of pancreatic cancer or melanoma.[28] Peutz–Jeghers syndrome is another rare autosomal dominant condition that increases a person's risk for pancreatic cancer. It is characterized by germline mutations in the *STK11* (LKB1) gene and is associated with small intestinal and colonic polyps as well as mucocutaneous hyperpigmentation.[7,8] Lynch syndrome is a genetic condition associated with colon polyps, colon cancer, and a rare, but significantly increased risk for pancreatic cancer.[29] It is characterized by germline mutations in the mismatch repair genes (*MLH1*, *MSH2*, *MSH6*, *PMS2*), resulting in microsatellite instability in tumors.

Despite having made strides in understanding the etiology of pancreatic cancer, an appropriate screening strategy is lacking. Persons with significant family history of pancreatic cancer and those who have known germline mutations should be offered genetic counseling. Routine imaging studies to identify early pancreatic cancer could be considered in such patients, albeit with careful discussion of risks and benefits of intervention such as biopsy and surgery. Regardless, smoking cessation will unequivocally decrease the risk for pancreatic malignancies.

4 Genomics of Pancreatic Cancer

Germline mutations account for only 5–10% of the incidence of pancreatic cancer.[21] Somatic alterations and non-mutational changes through epigenetic mechanism or deregulated microRNA expression account for a vast majority of pancreatic cancer cases.[22,30–32] One such mechanism, telomere shortening, is an early step in pancreatic carcinogenesis and predisposes to chromosomal instability. Activating mutations in *KRAS* are seen in more than 90% of cancers.[33,34] Inactivating mutations in tumor suppressor genes such as *CDKN2A* (p16), *TP53* (p53), and *SMAD4* (DPC4) are also high-frequency mutations in pancreatic cancer.[33,34] In addition to these highly prevalent somatic mutations, low-frequency mutations in *TGFBR1*, *TGFBR2*, *ACVR1B*, and *MAPK4* genes have also been described.[35]

Whereas the *KRAS* mutation appears to be an early event in pancreatic tumorigenesis, mutations in *TP53* and *SMAD4* are noted to occur at later stages. Interestingly, a study of 89 patients who underwent pancreaticoduodenectomy found *SMAD4* inactivation as a poor prognostic marker for overall survival as compared to patients with intact *SMAD4*.[36] *CDKN2A* or *TP53* were not found to be associated with survival.[36] In a rapid autopsy series of 76 patients with pancreatic cancer, loss of *SMAD4* (DPC4), as measured by DPC4 immunohistochemistry, was found to correlate with the presence of more widely metastatic disease rather than with locally advanced disease.[34,37]

In order to explore the process of tumorigenesis, Jones *et al.* performed comprehensive genetic analysis of 24 pancreatic cancers.[38] Through whole-exome sequencing analyses, they defined a core set of 12 cellular signaling pathways that were altered in pancreatic adenocarcinomas, including dysregulation of apoptosis, TGF-β signaling, *KRAS* oncogenic signaling, invasion, DNA repair, and control of G1/S phase transition. Another comprehensive whole-exome sequencing and copy-number analysis of 99 early-stage pancreatic cancers confirmed the findings of Jones *et al.*, and noted that genetic changes in axon guidance factors appeared to be altered in oncogenesis.[33]

There are several implications of these findings relating to the therapy of advanced pancreatic cancer. First, with newer next-generation sequencing techniques, it is possible to understand specific genetic changes in tumor tissue, or non-mutational epigenetic alterations in DNA methylation or aberrant expression of microRNA's that have also been implicated in the pathogenesis of pancreatic cancer.[30–32] Such a detailed understanding of dysregulated genes and cellular signaling processes may help in developing novel therapeutics. Second, pancreatic cancer exhibits considerable genetic heterogeneity. Therefore, a targeted approach to a single genetic alteration may not be effective in curtailing tumor growth and invasion.[35] Finally, understanding the pathways of tumorigenesis may aid in selecting therapeutic strategies that inhibit downstream signaling and provide an avenue for personalized management of the disease.

5 Clinical Presentation

Most cases of pancreatic cancer present with symptoms of abdominal pain and/or jaundice. Symptoms are often related to the location of the tumor within the gland. For instance, a pancreatic mass in the head or uncinate process may cause obstruction of the biliary duct resulting in jaundice. If the mass invades neural structures, it may cause severe abdominal pain. Weight loss, anorexia, and venous thromboses are commonly seen in patients with metastatic disease. Occasionally, pancreatic cancer can also present with symptoms due to gland dysfunction — both exocrine and endocrine, manifesting with steatorrhea or new diagnosis of adult-onset diabetes with unintentional progressive weight loss. Infrequently, acute pancreatitis can be a presenting symptom of pancreatic cancer.

6 Diagnostic Work-Up

The majority of patients with pancreatic cancer do not have any specific physical examination findings. Laboratory studies may demonstrate abnormal liver function tests and hyperbilirubinemia. Various imaging modalities may be pursued alone or in combination, in the diagnostic work-up of pancreatic cancer. A multiphase CT (computed tomography) scan of abdomen (pancreatic mass protocol) is the most common modality used in the work-up of pancreatic cancer. Imaging of the pancreas and surrounding structures are obtained in arterial, pancreatic parenchymal, and portal venous phases of contrast administration. Such an imaging modality assists determining the resectability of the pancreatic mass by evaluating for abutment or invasion of the portal vein (PV), superior mesenteric vein (SMV), celiac axis, or the superior mesenteric artery (SMA). Furthermore, a multiphase MRI (magnetic resonance image) can also be used in place of CT imaging, but without clear superiority to CT scan. PET (positron emission tomography) scan alone or in combination with CT scan is not currently recommended in the work-up of pancreatic cancer. The role of endoscopic retrograde cholangiopancreatography (ERCP) is limited to the management of cholestasis associated with biliary obstruction and for placement of biliary stent. An endoscopic ultra sonogram (EUS) should be performed in combination with an appropriate CT or MRI scan to improve the accuracy of determining resectability of the mass. Tissue diagnosis of pancreatic cancer can be obtained through either EUS-guided fine needle aspiration (FNA) biopsy or CT-guided FNA biopsy. The latter technique is less preferable due to the potential risk for seeding of the peritoneum. Another method of obtaining tissue diagnosis of pancreatic cancer is through ERCP-guided ductal brushing or cytology; however, the yield of cytology is only around 20%.

6.1 *Tumor markers*

Carbohydrate antigen 19-9 (CA19-9) is the only well-validated biomarker in pancreatic cancer. However, carcinoembryonic antigen (CEA) and cancer antigen 125 (CA125) may also be elevated in patients with the disease. CA19-9 is a sialylated red cell Lewis antigen secreted by exocrine epithelial cells.[39] The sensitivity of CA19-9 is around 70–80% and specificity is 80–90%.[40,41] Due to the low incidence of pancreatic cancer in general population, the positive predictive value of elevated CA19-9 is around 60%, making it a poor screening biomarker.[40] However, highly elevated CA19-9 level at the time of diagnosis or following surgical resection, is a poor prognostic marker and is associated with low resectability and reduced survival.[42–45] An elevated CA19-9 level is a prognostic factor in advanced pancreatic cancer as well.[46,47] Serial monitoring of CA19-9 can help in the management of metastatic disease, and its rise or fall may predict the response to therapy in those patients who had an elevated CA19-9 level at the initiation of systemic chemotherapy.[46,48] In as much as CA19-9 is a useful biomarker for prognosis and prediction of treatment response in pancreatic cancer, the test result can be falsely elevated in the setting of biliary obstruction, which influence the clinical interpretation of an elevated value. Therefore, CA19-9 may be used for prognostication only after biliary decompression has been performed.[40] In addition, the CA19-9 level could be low or normal in patients who do not secrete Lewis antigen.[39]

7 Clinical Staging of Pancreatic Cancer

Recent advances in imaging techniques have altered the clinical staging of pancreatic cancer. Better visualization of the pancreas and mesenteric vessels permit accurate assessment of resectability. Since the only defined curative treatments for pancreatic cancer incorporate surgical resection, every attempt should be made to achieve that goal. However, around 80% of patients present with locally advanced or distant metastatic disease that precludes surgical resection. Several retrospective studies have showed that an R1 resection (surgical margins are microscopically involved by cancer) is a predictor of early recurrence and poor outcomes as compared to an R0 resection (surgical margins are uninvolved by cancer).[49] Vessel encasement (>180° circumferential involvement by cancer) and/or abutment (≤180° circumferential involvement) are the major limitations to achieving an R0 resection.

Therefore, accurate assessment of arterial and venous involvement of pancreatic cancer is vital in determining resectability of the mass. A multiphase CT scan of abdomen helps delineate the mass and the mesenteric vasculature. EUS is an important adjunct as well. Using both CT imaging and EUS, we can now classify pancreatic cancer into four categories: resectable, borderline resectable, locally advanced unresectable, and metastatic disease.

The definitions of the first and the last categories are straightforward. A resectable pancreatic tumor is defined as having no distant metastases and no radiographic evidence of SMV and portal vein abutment, encasement or tumor thrombus, and has clear fat planes around the celiac axis, hepatic artery, and SMA.[50] Detection of distant metastatic deposits obviates the need for pancreatectomy since it does not improve survival in the setting of incurable metastatic disease. Locally advanced disease is further broken down into unresectable and borderline disease. Unresectable disease occurs when the mass encases the major arteries in the area — SMA, celiac axis, or proximal hepatic artery.[50] The presence of extensive venous thromboses within portal vein or SMV also precludes resection of a pancreatic mass. Borderline resectable disease is essentially considered when there is a high likelihood of not achieving an R0 resection. In order to better define this category, objective assessment of vascular involvement must be performed. Tumor abutment of the SMA (≤180° circumferential involvement by cancer), short segment encasement of common hepatic artery (>180° circumferential involvement), or abutment of common hepatic artery with an uninvolved celiac axis, and a short segment occlusion of the SMV or portal vein from a tumor thrombus or from tumor encasement are considered to define borderline resectability.[49]

8 Systemic Therapy

8.1 *Systemic therapy for resectable disease (adjuvant therapy)*

Among those who undergo resection, the median disease-free survival (DFS) is 6.7 months and without adjuvant chemotherapy, and 90% of patients will succumb to pancreatic cancer within five years, and 93% in 10 years.[3] In this context, adjuvant chemotherapy or concurrent chemoradiation has been evaluated with an aim to improve outcomes in resectable pancreatic cancer.

The earliest study on the benefit of adjuvant therapy was from the Gastrointestinal Tumor Study Group (GITSG), which evaluated 43 patients who underwent resection. Patients were randomized into a chemoradiation or observation alone group.[51] The initial analyses as well as data from an extension phase of 30 patients recruited into the chemoradiation arm suggested a beneficial role for adjuvant chemoradiation with a two-year survival rate of 43% for the treatment arm as compared to 18% for the observation group.[52] Chemotherapy consisted of bolus doses of 5-fluorouracil (5-FU) along with concurrent radiation. Maintenance chemotherapy was continued for 2 years or until disease progression. In order to confirm these results, the EORTC group conducted a randomized trial of chemoradiation (infusional 5-FU given concurrently with radiation) compared to observation in 218 patients who underwent resection of pancreatic head and periampullary region.[53] There was no difference in median overall survival or two- and five-year survival rates between the two groups. However, subgroup analysis of patients who had resection of a pancreatic head cancer suggested a trend to improved outcomes in the treatment arm ($p = 0.09$). Both these studies had significant differences in study design and chemotherapy use. For instance, the GITSG trial used maintenance chemotherapy with 5-FU for an extended duration as compared to no such chemotherapy administration for patients in the EORTC study.

Subsequently, the European Study Group for Pancreatic Cancer (ESPAC) conducted a randomized trial (ESPAC 1) using a two-by-two factorial design to compare chemoradiation *vs.* no-chemoradiation and chemotherapy *vs.* no chemotherapy in 289 patients with resected disease.[54] Patients in the chemoradiation arm received 20-Gy dose over a two-week period along with an intravenous bolus dose of 5-FU (500 mg/m^2 for a total of six days during and after radiation). Chemotherapy consisted of folinic acid (20 mg/m^2 bolus) followed by bolus 5-FU (425 mg/m^2 for five days every 28 days for six cycles). The third group received both chemoradiation followed by chemotherapy for six cycles. The ESPAC 1 study found a significant survival benefit for adjuvant chemotherapy *vs.* no-chemotherapy (five-year estimated survival rates: 21% *vs.* 8%) and noted a harmful impact for chemoradiation *vs.* no-chemoradiation (five-year estimated survival rates: 10% *vs.* 20%).[54] Although the study had significant flaws due to a factorial study design resulting in uncontrolled confounding, and poor quality control for radiation therapy, it unequivocally confirmed a beneficial effect for adjuvant chemotherapy following pancreatic cancer resection. Furthermore, analysis of 458 patients (which included 144 patients from the original ESPAC 1 study) randomized to 5-FU or observation found a 30% risk reduction for death with adjuvant 5-FU chemotherapy (5-year survival rate: 24% *vs.* 14%; median survival: 23.2 months *vs.* 16.8 months).[55]

Coincident with the conduct of the ESPAC 1 trial, the German Study Group for Pancreatic cancer investigated the role of adjuvant chemotherapy with gemcitabine (CONKO-001 trial).[3] Patients were randomized to receive weekly doses of gemcitabine (1 g/m^2 on days 1, 8, and 15 every 28 days for six cycles) or observation alone. Out of the 354 evaluable patients, those who received gemcitabine had a median disease-free survival of 13.4 months *vs.* 6.7 months in the observation arm and a 24% risk reduction for death (median overall survival of 22.8 months in gemcitabine group *vs.* 20.2 months in observation group; $p = 0.01$). The 10-year survival rate for gemcitabine arm was 12.2% *vs.* 7.7% in observation group.

Based on the ESPAC 1 and CONKO-001 studies, both adjuvant 5-FU and gemcitabine have demonstrated similar improvement in outcomes when compared to observation alone. Subsequently, the European Study Group conducted a randomized trial in patients who underwent pancreatic resection comparing 5-FU and gemcitabine administered for duration of 6 months (ESPAC 3 version-2 study).[56] After a median follow-up of around three years, there was no difference in overall survival between the two chemotherapy regimens (median overall survival — 23 months in 5-FU group *vs.* 23.6 months in gemcitabine group). There were fewer serious adverse events with gemcitabine as compared to 5-FU use ($p < 0.001$). Another study compared 5-FU *vs.* gemcitabine as pre- and post-concurrent 5-FU based chemoradiation therapy, which did not observe survival differences (RTOG 9704 trial).[57]

In Japan, a cytotoxic drug called S-1, a combination of three compounds — tegafur (a prodrug of 5-FU), gimeracil (inhibitor of dihydropyrimidine dehydrogenase which degrades 5-FU in the blood), and oteracil (blocks orotate phosphoribosyltransferase and decreases gastrointestinal side effects of 5-FU) — was compared with gemcitabine in the adjuvant treatment of resected pancreatic cancer in a phase III trial.[58] The primary endpoint of the JASPAC-1 study was noninferiority of S-1 to gemcitabine in overall survival. At two years of follow-up, S-1 was found not only to be noninferior to gemcitabine, but may also be superior to the standard therapy in the primary endpoint of overall survival (S-1: 70%, gemcitabine: 53%; HR 0.54).[59] S-1 may be superior to gemcitabine in Japanese population, but multinational trials are necessary before these results can be extrapolated to other populations.

A recent literature-based meta-analysis of the adjuvant trials in pancreatic cancer confirmed the beneficial effect of chemotherapy using either 5-FU or gemcitabine and suggested a deleterious role for adjuvant chemoradiation or chemoradiation followed by chemotherapy.[60] Although there is conclusive evidence that adjuvant chemotherapy is beneficial in decreasing risk for pancreatic cancer recurrence, similar evidence is lacking for combined chemoradiation. There may still be a role for adjuvant radiation in patients with close surgical margins. In fact, a retrospective study suggested that a margin clearance of ≤1.5 mm had inferior outcomes compared to those with clearance of >1.5 mm.[61] Therefore, in a subset of patients with high risk for local recurrence, radiation could still be considered as part of adjuvant therapy. The results of the RTOG 0848 trial investigating the combination of gemcitabine and erlotinib *vs.* gemcitabine alone and fluoropyrimidine-based concurrent chemoradiation *vs.* chemotherapy alone may help clarify the role of adjuvant chemoradiation in resected pancreatic cancer.

Furthermore, efforts are underway to improve systemic therapy following resection of pancreatic cancer. One means of achieving this is to delineate predictive markers of therapy. A post-hoc analysis of RTOG 9704 trial has shown that post-operative serum CA19-9 level ≥90U/ml is predictive of poor overall survival in patients who received gemcitabine.[62] On a similar note, low expression of human equilibrative nucleoside transporter 1 (hENT1) was associated with decreased median survival of 17.1 months compared to 26.2 months for those with high expression of the biomarker ($p = 0.002$).[63] Another approach entails adding chemotherapy agents (capecitabine) or targeted therapy (erlotinib) to gemcitabine. Until the results from these clinical trials are available, the current standard of care for resectable pancreatic cancer involves adjuvant therapy with gemcitabine or 5-FU for six months. In the future, some of the chemotherapy regimens that are currently used in metastatic disease may improve control of micro-metastatic disease and may eventually improve the outcomes following adjuvant radiation therapy.

8.2 Systemic therapy for borderline resectable disease

As mentioned above, improved imaging techniques have identified a subset of localized pancreatic cancer, termed borderline resectable, that has involvement of mesenteric vessels precluding a successful completion of R0 resection. Borderline resectable disease would qualify for neoadjuvant systemic therapy with or without local radiation. There are several advantages to such an approach. First, patients may have micro-metastatic disease at presentation that could be systemically treated prior to a surgical resection of the primary cancer. Second, patients may develop metastatic disease while awaiting surgery, in which case an upfront surgery would only bring forth significant morbidity without any likely survival benefit. Other than this method of "biological selection," neoadjuvant systemic therapy may also help in assessing *in vitro* drug activity on the resected tissue.[64] Most importantly, neoadjuvant therapy for borderline resectable disease improves R0 resection rates and therefore helps decrease local recurrences.

The increased R0 resection rates in patients who have undergone successful completion of neoadjuvant therapy can be as high as 90%. A retrospective study from Katz *et al.* showed that 94% of patients who underwent pancreatectomy after successful completion of neoadjuvant therapy had R0 resection.[65] This series included 160 patients with borderline resectable disease, out of which 78% received neoadjuvant therapy and 66 patients (41%) eventually underwent pancreatectomy. The median survival among patients who underwent pancreatectomy was 40 months compared to 13 months for those who did not undergo resection of the pancreatic mass.[65] An improvement in survival of this magnitude may have a great impact. Interestingly, more than 50% of resected specimen had a partial or complete response to treatment (<50% remaining viable tumor cells).

Two recent retrospective studies described outcomes following an aggressive systemic chemotherapy regimen of FOLFIRINOX (5-FU, leucovorin, irinotecan, and oxaliplatin) with or without stereotactic body radiation therapy (SBRT) for the neoadjuvant management of borderline resectable and locally advanced unresectable pancreatic cancer.[66,67] Out of the 11 patients with borderline resectable disease treated with FOLFIRINOX with or without SBRT in the Boone *et al.* series, 55% had an R0 resection. Among four patients with borderline resectable disease in the Hosein *et al.* study treated with neoadjuvant FOLFIRINOX, three underwent surgical resection with an R0 resection rate of 100%. Cumulatively, out of the 15 patients in both studies treated with neoadjuvant systemic therapy, 11 underwent surgical resection of which nine had R0 resection (60%). Of note, in the retrospective cohort of patients described by Katz *et al.*, 50% of patients with borderline resectable disease who completed neoadjuvant treatment underwent an R0 resection.[33]

Based on these retrospective studies, neoadjuvant systemic therapy should be considered for patients with borderline resectable disease. It appears that using the more aggressive FOLFIRINOX with or without SBRT compared to single agent chemotherapy may have only increased the R0 resection rate by 10%.[65–67] Furthermore, several questions remain unanswered. Will such a difference in R0 resection rate translate to meaningful improvement in survival? What is the appropriate chemotherapeutic regimen for neoadjuvant use? What is the role of locoregional radiation therapy in the neoadjuvant setting? Much clinical research needs to be conducted in the area of borderline resectable disease before which a standard of care could be recommended. Until then, neoadjuvant systemic therapy is considered the standard of care for all patients diagnosed with borderline resectable pancreatic cancer under the careful watch of a multidisciplinary management team led by medical, surgical, and radiation oncologists.

8.3 *Systemic therapy for locally advanced disease*

Locally advanced pancreatic cancer is unresectable when the mass encases the major arteries or has venous thromboses within the portal vein or SMV. Systemic chemotherapy with or without radiation may convert this disease into a resectable condition. Induction chemotherapy with FOLFIRINOX followed by concurrent external beam chemoradiation with gemcitabine resulted in one-third of patients achieving an R0 resection in a retrospective single-institution study.[66] Another approach entails delivery of radiation guided by fiducial markers placed via EUS. SBRT ensures delivery of high doses of radiation into small volumes. Although the aim of using SBRT is to decrease radiation delivery to normal tissues in the vicinity of the pancreatic mass, it is not without adverse effects. Stereotactic radiation to pancreatic mass can result in late gastrointestinal toxicity, particularly causing duodenal ulcers, stenosis, and perforation.[68] Notwithstanding that, the benefit of SBRT remains uncertain. For instance, the R0 resection rate was only 10% in a retrospective single-institution study where FOLFIRINOX followed by stereotactic body radiation was utilized for the management of locally advanced unresectable disease.[67]

The recent SCALOP trial used induction chemotherapy with gemcitabine and capecitabine and randomized patients into two arms of concurrent chemoradiation with either of the two drugs.[69] Although the study did not find a statistically significant difference in the primary endpoint of progression-free survival, it noted a significant difference in median overall survival favoring the capecitabine group. Overall capecitabine-based radiation was found to be less toxic compared to gemcitabine group.[69]

Another approach that improves survival in patients with locally advanced unresectable disease involves induction chemotherapy followed by concurrent chemotherapy with external beam radiation. When compared to patients treated with upfront concurrent chemoradiation, those who received induction chemotherapy followed by concurrent chemoradiation had a significant improvement in overall survival (median overall survival 11.9 months vs. 8.5 months; $p < 0.001$).[70] Only 3% of patients in this study underwent R0 resection, although their median overall survival was 29.4 months. Such an approach also ensures that only patients with better outcomes will eventually need radiation therapy. Around 30% of patients who receive induction chemotherapy will become metastatic during the course of treatment.[71] Those patients who do not have disease progression during induction chemotherapy may benefit from a course of concurrent chemoradiation compared to chemotherapy alone.[71,72]

The LAP 07 trial prospectively investigated the role of concurrent chemoradiation versus chemotherapy alone following induction chemotherapy with gemcitabine with or without erlotinib.[73] Patients with locally advanced unresectable disease were randomly assigned to receive gemcitabine plus erlotinib or gemcitabine alone for four months. Those patients who had at least stable disease at the end of four months of therapy were further randomly assigned to either two more months of chemotherapy or chemoradiation with capecitabine. After a three-year follow-up, the study failed to find a difference in overall survival between chemoradiation and chemotherapy alone — the primary endpoint of the trial.[73] Based on the results of the LAP 07 study, following induction chemotherapy, administration of chemoradiation did not improve overall survival compared with chemotherapy alone.

In conclusion, induction chemotherapy is probably more effective than concurrent chemoradiation given upfront, in patients with locally advanced unresectable pancreatic cancer. The role of chemoradiation compared with chemotherapy alone, in patients who have stable disease after induction chemotherapy is unproven and of questionable benefit. More effective chemotherapy regimens given in the upfront setting may eventually define a role for chemoradiation in patients with stable disease, by achieving better local control.

8.4 *Systemic therapy for metastatic disease*

In contrast with locally advanced disease, there have been a number of randomized trials investigating systemic therapy options in metastatic disease. However, several of these clinical trials included patients with locally advanced disease in addition to those with distant metastatic pancreatic cancer. The early studies in the field used 5-FU alone or in combination with other chemotherapy agents. These trials were hampered by low response rates and lack of survival benefit. The first advance in pancreatic cancer systemic therapy occurred when a trial of gemcitabine given at a dose of 1,000 mg/m^2 weekly for seven weeks followed by a week of rest, followed by weekly for three weeks every four weeks versus 5-FU 600 mg/m^2 weekly noted a survival benefit for patients in gemcitabine arm compared to 5-FU arm.[74] The one-year survival rate for patients on gemcitabine was 18% compared to 2% for 5-FU group. Improvements in survival and clinical symptoms, in addition to its good tolerability, led to FDA approval for gemcitabine use in pancreatic cancer.

Despite this, the survival rates from pancreatic cancer remained grim. Further efforts to improve upon the clinical benefit derived from gemcitabine resulted in several clinical trials of gemcitabine-based combination chemotherapy. The first class of drugs that underwent extensive investigation were platinum analogs, supported by good *in vitro* synergy data and proven efficacy in gastrointestinal cancers. Gemcitabine and oxaliplatin combination therapy proved to be superior to gemcitabine with respect to response rate (26.8% *vs.* 17.3%) and progression-free survival (5.8 *vs.* 3.7 months), but failed to meet statistical significance for an overall survival advantage.[75] Similarly, gemcitabine and cisplatin combination therapy showed a favorable trend to improved overall survival and progression-free survival compared to gemcitabine monotherapy, but did not reach statistical significance.[76] Another study comparing gemcitabine and cisplatin combination therapy versus gemcitabine alone found no difference in outcomes of overall survival or progression-free survival, with more hematological toxicity noted in the cisplatin arm (GIP 1 study).[77]

Capecitabine, an oral fluoropyrimidine cytotoxic drug ensures a prolonged fluorouracil exposure closely mimicking continuous intravenous administration of 5-FU. With both gemcitabine and 5-FU known to be efficacious in pancreatic cancer, it was thought that the combination therapy may improve survival in patients with advanced disease. However, a European study of gemcitabine and capecitabine combination therapy failed to prolong survival compared to gemcitabine alone, except in a subgroup of patients with good performance status.[78] In contrast, another phase III study from Europe noted improvement in response rate and progression-free survival with combination therapy, and a trend toward improved overall survival.[79] Interestingly, pooled meta-analyses of three trials (included both phase III trials listed above and a phase II trial) noted a statistically significant survival benefit for patients who were treated with gemcitabine and capecitabine compared to gemcitabine monotherapy (HR 0.86; 95% CI 0.75–0.98; $p = 0.02$; $I^2 = 0\%$).[79] Unlike oxaliplatin or cisplatin-based therapy that had greater gastrointestinal and hematological toxicity, gemcitabine and capecitabine combination had a similar grade 3–4 toxicity profile compared to gemcitabine alone.[79]

With no combination chemotherapy showing a clear survival benefit in advanced pancreatic cancer, the concept of gemcitabine-based combination therapy was tested in a meta-analysis of 15 trials.[80] Although the results of the meta-analysis showed a significant survival benefit for gemcitabine-based cytotoxic therapy compared to gemcitabine alone in advanced pancreatic cancer, the most interesting observation from the analysis was obtained from five trials having information on baseline performance status. The meta-analysis noted a favorable survival benefit for the use of combination therapy in patients with good performance status compared to no such efficacy in those with poor performance status.

The largest innovation in chemotherapy for metastatic pancreatic cancer resulted when a four drug combination chemotherapy regimen (irinotecan 180 mg/m^2, oxaliplatin 85 mg/m^2, bolus 5-FU 400 mg/m^2, leucovorin 400 mg/m^2, and infusional 5-FU 2,400 mg/m^2 given over 46 h) was compared to single agent gemcitabine in patients with a good performance status.[4] This FOLFIRINOX regimen administered every two weeks was compared to gemcitabine monotherapy given weekly for seven weeks of eight weeks and then weekly for 3 of 4 weeks for up to six months. Patients with metastatic pancreatic cancer who were younger than 76 years and having an ECOG performance status of 0–1 were included. The trial noted a 43% risk reduction for death ($p < 0.001$) with a median overall survival of 11.1 months for patients on the FOLFIRINOX arm as compared to 6.8 months in the gemcitabine group. The combination therapy proved beneficial compared to gemcitabine with regard to improving quality of life as well.[81] However, there were more adverse events in FOLFIRINOX group with significantly more neutropenia (with 45.7 % of G3/4 neutropenia), febrile neutropenia, diarrhea and peripheral neuropathy.

Since patients with metastatic pancreatic cancer often have a poorer performance status than those who were studied in the FOLFIRINOX trial, the search for a less aggressive regimen led to trials using an albumin-bound nanoparticle formulation of paclitaxel (*nab*-paclitaxel). Molecular profiling of pancreatic tumor tissue found overexpression of albumin-binding SPARC protein (secreted protein acidic and rich in cysteine), which led to the hypothesis that *nab*-paclitaxel might bind SPARC and therefore have considerable activity in pancreatic tumors.[82] The combination therapy consisting of *nab*-paclitaxel and gemcitabine showed considerable antitumor activity in a phase I/II trial.[83] The phase III trial randomized patients (*n* = 861) with metastatic pancreatic cancer to nab-paclitaxel 125 mg/m^2 followed by gemcitabine 1,000 mg/m^2 on days 1, 8, and 15 every four weeks or gemcitabine monotherapy at standard dose (MPACT trial).[5] Patients who had a Karnofsky performance status of ≥ 70 were included in the study. Nearly 10% of patients were > 75 years of age and 8% had an ECOG performance status of 2. The trial noted a 28% risk reduction for death ($p < 0.001$) with a median overall survival of 8.5 months for patients on the *nab*-paclitaxel and gemcitabine combination therapy group as compared to 6.7 months in the gemcitabine group. The regimen was also noted to be tolerable, with grade 3 neutropenia rates of 38% in nab-paclitaxel-based arm *vs.* 27% in gemcitabine group. Fatigue and peripheral neuropathy were more common in the *nab*-paclitaxel and gemcitabine combination arm *vs.* gemcitabine alone. Although *nab*-paclitaxel demonstrated significant improvement in survival benefit, recent analysis of data from the MPACT trial found that SPARC expression level was neither prognostic nor predictive for treatment benefit.[84]

Another gemcitabine combination trial in the metastatic setting was conducted in Japan using the oral fluoropyrimidine drug — S-1. It was investigated alone or in combination with gemcitabine versus gemcitabine monotherapy in chemotherapy-naïve patients with locally advanced or metastatic pancreatic cancer (GEST study).[85] S-1 demonstrated noninferiority to gemcitabine monotherapy, but the combination of gemcitabine and S-1 was not shown to be superior to gemcitabine alone. Since the pharmacokinetics and pharmacodynamics of S-1 differ between Caucasian and Japanese patients with resultant higher gastrointestinal toxicities, it has not been approved for use in the United States.[86]

In addition to combination cytotoxic therapy, gemcitabine has also been used along with targeted agents such as cetuximab, erlotinib, and bevacizumab. The epidermal growth factor receptor (EGFR) mediates several key cellular processes such as proliferation, angiogenesis, metastasis, and inhibition of apoptosis. Targeted therapies aimed at inhibiting EGFR signaling are approved for use in colon and lung cancers. In addition, preclinical studies in pancreatic cancer animal models have suggested a beneficial antitumor role for gemcitabine and an anti-EGFR therapy using either a monoclonal antibody (cetuximab) or a tyrosine kinase inhibitor (erlotinib). Gemcitabine and erlotinib combination therapy was compared against gemcitabine and placebo in a phase III international trial of unresectable locally advanced or metastatic pancreatic cancer.[87] Around 20% of patients had an ECOG performance status of 2. Although the study met the criteria for statistically significant difference in overall survival, progression-free survival, and one-year survival, the difference in median survival was only about 10 days (6.24 months *vs.* 5.91 months; $p = 0.038$). The safety profile of the two groups was also similar except for an increased prevalence of skin rash noted with erlotinib use. Another anti-EGFR therapy, cetuximab, when used in combination with gemcitabine did not improve overall survival or progression-free survival when compared to gemcitabine alone.[88] Similarly, no survival benefit was seen when gemcitabine was combined with bevacizumab, a monoclonal antibody against vascular endothelial growth factor (VEGF) as compared to gemcitabine alone.[89] While combinations of targeted therapy with gemcitabine has not shown significant survival benefit in these trials, improved understanding of the pathways of pancreatic carcinogenesis may help design clinical trials with study populations who may particularly benefit from these agents.

The question of second-line chemotherapy for patients with advanced pancreatic cancer who progressed on gemcitabine therapy was investigated in a phase III trial comparing combination therapy using oxaliplatin, folinic acid, and 5-FU (OFF) with best supportive care.[90] The trial demonstrated a benefit for second-line chemotherapy over best supportive care with a median survival of 4.8 months for OFF versus 2.3 months for supportive care ($p = 0.008$). The OFF regimen was also noted to be well tolerated by patients with no differences in grade 3–4 toxicities when compared to those who did not receive second-line chemotherapy. Another phase III trial compared second-line use of OFF versus folinic acid and 5-FU combination (FF) in a similar patient population (CONKO-003 trial).[91] FF regimen consisted of folinic acid 200 mg/m^2 bolus followed by a continuous infusion of 5-FU 2,000 mg/m^2 over 24 h on days 1, 8, 15, and 22 every 42 days. Oxaliplatin 85 mg/m^2 was administered before FF on days 8 and 22 in the OFF regimen. The median survival in the OFF group was 5.9 months compared to 3.3 months in FF group ($p = 0.010$). Adverse events were similar between the two study arms. Based on these two trials, OFF demonstrated a clear survival benefit in the second-line setting for patients with advanced pancreatic cancer with a Karnofsky performance status of $\geq 70\%$.[90,91]

In addition to oxaliplatin based regimen, newer agents are being investigated in the second line setting. One such novel molecule is a nanoliposome-bound irinotecan (MM-398). Patients with metastatic pancreatic cancer who progressed through or following gemcitabine-based therapy was randomly assigned to one of three groups: MM-398 plus 5-FU/leucovorin or MM-398 alone or the control arms of 5-FU/leucovorin (NAPOLI-1).[92] The combination of MM-398 and 5-FU/leucovorin improved overall survival compared with 5-FU/leucovorin alone (median OS: 6.1 months versus 4.2 months; HR 0.67; $p = 0.012$). However, single-agent use of MM-398 did not demonstrate efficacy compared with control group. The major adverse effects of MM-398 combination therapy pertained to low white blood cell count and fatigue. The major limitation of the second-line trials arises due to the fact that these studies were designed before FOLFIRINOX and gemcitabine/*nab*-paclitaxel combination therapy demonstrated efficacy in the first-line setting.[4,5]

Furthermore, since FOLFIRINOX and gemcitabine/*nab*-paclitaxel were not investigated against each other in management of patients with metastatic pancreatic cancer who are chemotherapy naïve, the superiority of one regimen over the other cannot be established. Treatment decisions should be mainly guided by age and performance status of patients. Gemcitabine/*nab*-paclitaxel is likely to be a better choice for use in the elderly or those with poor functional status than the more aggressive FOLFIRINOX regimen.[4,5] In the future, combination chemotherapy and biological agents with a backbone of gemcitabine-based doublets may improve outcomes in advanced pancreatic cancer.

9 Future Directions in Systemic Therapy

Despite the recent advances in our understanding of the molecular pathways involved in oncogenesis in general, and pancreatic cancer in particular, progress toward novel agents to treat pancreatic cancer has been limited. Increasingly, a cellular pathway driven approach is used in oncology care. For instance, platinum analogs have shown improvement in clinical outcomes in patients with *BRCA* mutations. Similarly, DNA damaging agents such as mitomycin C demonstrated good tumor response in a patient with *PALB2* gene inactivation.[93,94] *KRAS* is the most common mutated gene in pancreatic cancer. However, no direct RAS inhibitors have been developed to date due to the difficulty in targeting the functional KRAS domains. Transfer of a farnesyl group to KRAS is a required post-translational modification, however in clinical trials the farnesyltransferase inhibitors tipifarnib and lonafarnib did not yield any clinical activity above that offered by gemcitabine alone.[95,96] KRAS activation leads to the activation of the MEK/ERK pathways. Early trials using the MEK inhibitor selumetinib did not show efficacy above that of capecitabine in a randomized phase II study.[97] The MEK inhibitor trametinib also failed to show utility in a phase II trial.[98] Recently research has suggested that combined inhibition of the MEK and PI3K, or the MEK and EGFR pathways may be key to targeting this pathway.[99] Clinical trials investigating these combinations are currently underway.

Other studies have defined HSP90 as a possible target for *KRAS*-mutated onco-genesis.[100] A different approach to target activated RAS is through GI-4000, a heat-killed recombinant *S. cerevisiae* that expresses a mutated RAS protein.[101] Clinical trials have demonstrated its safety and currently it is being investigated in combination with gemcitabine in the adjuvant setting.[101,102] Other pathway inhibitors, including those of the PI3K/AKT/mTOR, notch and the transforming growth factor beta (TGF-*β*) have also shown varying preclinical promise and are being pursued in clinical trials. Data from a phase II study of the JAK inhibitor ruxolitinib or placebo with capecitabine, also known as the RECAP study, recently suggested that the combination may improve survival in patients with refractory stage IV disease with an elevated c reactive protein (CRP), an established marker of generalized inflammation.[103] A larger study is currently underway to validate these preliminary results. These results also support the emerging paradigm that ongoing inflammation may either incite or promote carcinogenesis.[104,105] Further insights into this paradigm will hopefully translate to other agents as well. Recently, a molecule isolated in a screen for HSP70 inhibitors identified a compound triptolide from a plant, *Tripterygium wilfordii*, was found to have significant antitumor activity. A water-soluble analog called Minnelide, showed remarkable activity against multiple models of pancreatic cancer.[106] This agent was noted to be even more effective than gemcitabine *in vivo* studies and clinical trials are now underway.

The finding that autophagy is a critical mediator of DAMP-induced tumor cell survival has led multiple investigators to examine autophagy inhibitors in cancer. Chloroquine (CQ) and its derivatives such as hydroxychloroquine (HCQ) are synthetic 4-aminoquinolines that block acidification of the lysosome, thus inhibiting the last step in autophagy. Evidence in mouse models and human cancer cell lines suggest CQ may have significant anti-tumor activity by inhibiting autophagy induced by cancer therapy.[107–109] Early phase trials have shown evidence of activity of HCQ in particular, and autophagy in general as a target for treatment of cancer. Several studies are ongoing examining the role of autophagy inhibition in addition to chemotherapy in the treatment of pancreatic cancer.

Immunological targeted agents have shown great promise in a variety of cancers. Recently checkpoint modulation using agents targeting PDL-1, PD-1, and CTLA-4 have shown activity in a variety of cancers, but to date no significant activity has been found in pancreatic cancer.[110–112] Combinations with these agents are currently being developed and may hold promise as the immune milieu of pancreatic cancers is deciphered.[113] Recently a combination of GVAX, derived from a cell line modified to overexpress GM-CSF, and CRS207 a live-attenuated listeria that has been engineered to express the tumor-associated antigen mesothelin showed encouraging results in a phase II study.[114] Median overall survival in the group receiving GVAX plus CRS207 was 6.1 months compared with 3.9 months in

GVAX alone group. Granted breakthrough status by the FDA, an ongoing phase IIb trial (ECLIPSE) will evaluate the safety, immune response and efficacy of the combination immunotherapy of GVAX Pancreas (with low-dose cyclophosphamide) and CRS-207 compared to chemotherapy or to CRS-207 alone (NCT02004262). Algenpantucel-L (NewLinks Genetics) is a vaccine consisting of two pancreatic cancer cell lines (HAPa-1 and HAPa-2) that have been genetically modified to express alpha-gal carbohydrates on cell-surface molecules.[115] Once injected into a patient, the alpha-gal stimulates an immune response against pancreatic cancer-specific antigens in the tumor cell lines. A phase II study demonstrated that an increase in anti-mesothelin antibodies in patients receiving Algenpantucel-L correlated with improved survival.[116] A large phase III trial randomizing 722 patients to either gemcitabine alone or a combination of gemcitabine and Algenpantucel-L after resection of pancreatic cancer has completed enrollment and its results are pending (NCT01836432).

There has been an increased appreciation that the stroma surrounding the tumor as well as the tumor microenvironment plays a critical role in supporting pancreatic adenocarcinoma growth. This can take the form of either inhibiting entry of chemotherapeutic agents into the tumor proper, as well as altering the immune environment of the cancer. The interaction of the stroma and the immune system is a complicated one, with recent studies suggesting that parts of the stroma may actually restrain tumor growth and loss of fibroblast surrounding the tumor may promote tumor growth, yet its loss may facilitate treatment with immunological and targeted agents.[117,118] Hedgehog signaling is one pathway involved in the maintenance of the tumor microenvironment.[119] Preclinical data suggested that the addition of the hedgehog antagonist saridegib (IPI-926) facilitated access of gemcitabine to tumors in multiple animal models, and correlated with higher intracellular gemcitabine concentrations. Unfortunately, a double-blind placebo controlled trial in 122 patients with metastatic disease was associated with worse survival in patients receiving saridegib and halted in an interim analysis.[120] This clinical finding reflects the noted preclinical data suggesting multiple roles of the microenvironment in pancreatic carcinogenesis. Ongoing trials utilizing PEGylated hyaluronidase to directly degrade the stroma facilitating drug delivery to the cancer itself are underway. TH-302 is an agent activated in the hypoxic tumor microenviroment.[121] A phase II trial showing promising results of the combination is being investigated further in a large phase III trial.[122]

10 Conclusions

While multidisciplinary care of patients with pancreatic cancer is integral to achieving better outcomes, it is expected that improved drug delivery of cytotoxic agents and personalized management of cancer using genomic testing will revolutionize the management of all stages of the disease. While the basic science is being unraveled on multiple levels, the ongoing translation of improved outcomes in the metastatic setting using combination cytotoxic agents into the adjuvant setting will hopefully improve the cure rates following surgical resection. Similarly, the use of more aggressive regimens in the neoadjuvant setting may tackle the potential role of micro-metastatic disease in disease recurrence and thus improve outcomes as well. As the distance between the lab and the clinic becomes narrower, it is expected that a wide variety of improved systemic therapies with greater efficacy and lesser toxicity will reach patients in various stages of pancreatic cancer. Certainly, the future treatment of pancreatic cancer is one that involves multiple agents targeting specific pathways, the tumor microenvironment and alteration of the immune response to improve the survival of patients afflicted with pancreatic cancer.

References

1. Siegel R, *et al.* Cancer statistics, 2014. *CA Cancer J Clin* 2014;**64**:9–29.
2. Rahib L, *et al.* Projecting cancer incidence and deaths to 2030: The unexpected burden of thyroid, liver, and pancreas cancers in the United States. *Cancer Res* 2014;**74**:2913–2921.
3. Oettle H, *et al.* Adjuvant chemotherapy with gemcitabine and long-term outcomes among patients with resected pancreatic cancer: The CONKO-001 randomized trial. *JAMA* 2013;**310**:1473–1481.
4. Conroy T, *et al.* FOLFIRINOX versus gemcitabine for metastatic pancreatic cancer. *N Engl J Med* 2011;**364**:1817–1825.
5. Von Hoff DD, *et al.* Increased survival in pancreatic cancer with *nab*-paclitaxel plus gemcitabine. *N Engl J Med* 2013;**369**:16911703.
6. Whitcomb DC, *et al.* Hereditary pancreatitis is caused by a mutation in the cationic trypsinogen gene. *Nat Genet* 1996;**14**:141–145.
7. Giardiello FM, *et al.* Very high risk of cancer in familial Peutz-Jeghers syndrome. *Gastroenterology* 2000;**119**:1447–1453.
8. Korsse SE, *et al.* Pancreatic cancer risk in Peutz–Jeghers syndrome patients: A large cohort study and implications for surveillance. *J Med Genet* 2013;**50**:59–64.
9. Bosetti C, *et al.* Cigarette smoking and pancreatic cancer: an analysis from the International Pancreatic Cancer Case-Control Consortium (Panc4). *Ann Oncol* 2012;**23**:1880–1888.
10. Lucenteforte E, *et al.* Alcohol consumption and pancreatic cancer: a pooled analysis in the International Pancreatic Cancer Case-Control Consortium (PanC4). *Ann Oncol* 2012;**23**:374–382.
11. Ye W, *et al.* Alcohol abuse and the risk of pancreatic cancer. *Gut* 2002;**51**:236–239.

12. Rohrmann S, *et al*. Ethanol intake and the risk of pancreatic cancer in the European Prospective Investigation into Cancer and Nutrition (EPIC). *Cancer Causes Control* 2009;**20**:785–794.

13. Ben Q, *et al*. Diabetes mellitus and risk of pancreatic cancer: A meta-analysis of cohort studies. *Eur J Cancer* 2011;**47**:1928–1937.

14. Li D, *et al*. Diabetes and risk of pancreatic cancer: A pooled analysis of three large case-control studies. *Cancer Causes Control* 2011;**22**:189–197.

15. Ben Q, *et al*. The relationship between new-onset diabetes mellitus and pancreatic cancer risk: A case-control study. *Eur J Cancer* 2011;**47**:248–254.

16. Renehan AG, *et al*. Body-mass index and incidence of cancer: A systematic review and meta-analysis of prospective observational studies. *Lancet* 2008;**371**:569–578.

17. Larsson SC, Wolk A. Red and processed meat consumption and risk of pancreatic cancer: Meta-analysis of prospective studies. *Br J Cancer* 2012;**106**:603–607.

18. Arem H, *et al*. Dietary fat intake and risk of pancreatic cancer in the Prostate, Lung, Colorectal and Ovarian Cancer Screening Trial. *Ann Epidemiol* 2013;**23**:571–575.

19. Rohrmann S, *et al*. Meat and fish consumption and risk of pancreatic cancer: results from the European Prospective Investigation into Cancer and Nutrition. *Int J Cancer* 2013;**132**:617–624.

20. Raimondi S, *et al*. Pancreatic cancer in chronic pancreatitis: Aetiology, incidence, and early detection. *Best Pract Res Clin Gastroenterol* 2010;**24**:349–358.

21. Solomon S, *et al*. Inherited pancreatic cancer syndromes. *Cancer J* 2012;**18**:485–491.

22. Rustgi AK. Familial pancreatic cancer: Genetic advances. *Genes Dev* 2014;**28**:1–7.

23. Roberts NJ, *et al*. ATM mutations in patients with hereditary pancreatic cancer. *Cancer Discov* 2012;**2**:41–46.

24. Jones S, *et al*. Exomic sequencing identifies *PALB2* as a pancreatic cancer susceptibility gene. *Science* 2009;**324**:217.

25. Goggins M, *et al*. Germline *BRCA2* gene mutations in patients with apparently sporadic pancreatic carcinomas. *Cancer Res* 1996;**56**:5360–5364.

26. Breast Cancer Linkage Consortium. Cancer risks in BRCA2 mutation carriers. *J Natl Cancer Inst* 1999;**91**:1310–1316.

27. Lynch HT, *et al*. Phenotypic variation in eight extended CDKN2A germline mutation familial atypical multiple mole melanoma-pancreatic carcinoma-prone families: The familial atypical mole melanoma-pancreatic carcinoma syndrome. *Cancer* 2002; **94**:84–96.

28. McWilliams RR, *et al*. Prevalence of *CDKN2A* mutations in pancreatic cancer patients: Implications for genetic counseling. *Eur J Hum Genet* 2011;**19**:472–478.

29. Kastrinos F, *et al*. Risk of pancreatic cancer in families with Lynch syndrome. *JAMA* 2009;**302**:1790–1795.

30. Bloomston M, *et al*. MicroRNA expression patterns to differentiate pancreatic adenocarcinoma from normal pancreas and chronic pancreatitis. *JAMA* 2007;**297**: 1901–1908.

31. Drakaki A, Iliopoulos D. MicroRNA-gene signaling pathways in pancreatic cancer. *Biomed J* 2013;**36**:200–208.

32. Sato N, Goggins M. The role of epigenetic alterations in pancreatic cancer. *J Hepatobiliary Pancreat Surg* 2006;**13**:286–295.

33. Biankin AV, *et al.* Pancreatic cancer genomes reveal aberrations in axon guidance pathway genes. *Nature* 2012;**491**:399–405.

34. Iacobuzio-Donahue CA, *et al.* DPC4 gene status of the primary carcinoma correlates with patterns of failure in patients with pancreatic cancer. *J Clin Oncol* 2009;**27**: 1806–1813.

35. Makohon-Moore A, *et al.* Pancreatic cancer genomics: insights and opportunities for clinical translation. *Genome Med* 2013;**5**:26.

36. Blackford A, *et al. SMAD4* gene mutations are associated with poor prognosis in pancreatic cancer. *Clin Cancer Res* 2009;**15**:4674–4679.

37. Wilentz RE, *et al.* Immunohistochemical labeling for dpc4 mirrors genetic status in pancreatic adenocarcinomas: A new marker of *DPC4* inactivation. *Am J Pathol* 2000;**156**:37–43.

38. Jones S, *et al.* Core signaling pathways in human pancreatic cancers revealed by global genomic analyses. *Science* 2008;**321**:1801–1806.

39. Tempero MA, *et al.* Relationship of carbohydrate antigen 19-9 and Lewis antigens in pancreatic cancer. *Cancer Res* 1987;**47**:5501–5503.

40. Fong ZV, Winter JM. Biomarkers in pancreatic cancer: diagnostic, prognostic, and predictive. *Cancer J* 2012;**18**:530–538.

41. Ballehaninna UK, Chamberlain RS. The clinical utility of serum CA 19-9 in the diagnosis, prognosis and management of pancreatic adenocarcinoma: An evidence based appraisal. *J Gastrointest Oncol* 2012;**3**:105–119.

42. Hartwig W, *et al.* CA19-9 in potentially resectable pancreatic cancer: Perspective to adjust surgical and perioperative therapy. *Ann Surg Oncol* 2013;**20**:2188–2196.

43. Berger AC, *et al.* Postresection CA 19-9 predicts overall survival in patients with pancreatic cancer treated with adjuvant chemoradiation: A prospective validation by RTOG 9704. *J Clin Oncol* 2008;**26**:5918–5922.

44. Kondo N, *et al.* Prognostic impact of perioperative serum CA 19-9 levels in patients with resectable pancreatic cancer. *Ann Surg Oncol* 2010;**17**:2321–2329.

45. Ferrone CR, *et al.* Perioperative CA19-9 levels can predict stage and survival in patients with resectable pancreatic adenocarcinoma. *J Clin Oncol* 2006;**24**:2897–2902.

46. Bauer TM, *et al.* Carbohydrate antigen 19-9 is a prognostic and predictive biomarker in patients with advanced pancreatic cancer who receive gemcitabine-containing chemotherapy: A pooled analysis of 6 prospective trials. *Cancer* 2013;**119**:285–92.

47. Yang GY, *et al.* Change in CA 19-9 levels after chemoradiotherapy predicts survival in patients with locally advanced unresectable pancreatic cancer. *J Gastrointest Oncol* 2013;**4**:361–369.

48. Halm U, *et al.* Decrease of CA 19-9 during chemotherapy with gemcitabine predicts survival time in patients with advanced pancreatic cancer. *Br J Cancer* 2000;**82**: 1013–1016.

49. Varadhachary GR, *et al.* Borderline resectable pancreatic cancer: Definitions, management, and role of preoperative therapy. *Ann Surg Oncol* 2006;**13**:1035–1046.

50. Callery MP, *et al*. Pretreatment assessment of resectable and borderline resectable pancreatic cancer: Expert consensus statement. *Ann Surg Oncol* 2009;**16**:1727–1733.

51. Kalser MH, Ellenberg SS. Pancreatic cancer. Adjuvant combined radiation and chemotherapy following curative resection. *Arch Surg* 1985;**120**:899–903.

52. Further evidence of effective adjuvant combined radiation and chemotherapy following curative resection of pancreatic cancer. Gastrointestinal Tumor Study Group. *Cancer* 1987;**59**:2006–2010.

53. Klinkenbijl JH, *et al*. Adjuvant radiotherapy and 5-fluorouracil after curative resection of cancer of the pancreas and periampullary region: Phase III trial of the EORTC gastrointestinal tract cancer cooperative group. *Ann Surg* 1999;**230**:776–782; discussion 82–84.

54. Neoptolemos JP, *et al*. A randomized trial of chemoradiotherapy and chemotherapy after resection of pancreatic cancer. *N Engl J Med* 2004;**350**:1200–1210.

55. Neoptolemos JP, *et al*. Adjuvant 5-fluorouracil and folinic acid vs observation for pancreatic cancer: Composite data from the ESPAC-1 and -3(v1) trials. *Br J Cancer* 2009;**100**:246–250.

56. Neoptolemos JP, *et al*. Adjuvant chemotherapy with fluorouracil plus folinic acid vs gemcitabine following pancreatic cancer resection: A randomized controlled trial. *JAMA* 2010;**304**:1073–1081.

57. Regine WF, *et al*. Fluorouracil-based chemoradiation with either gemcitabine or fluorouracil chemotherapy after resection of pancreatic adenocarcinoma: 5-year analysis of the U.S. Intergroup/RTOG 9704 phase III trial. *Ann Surg Oncol* 2011; **18**:1319–1326.

58. Maeda A, *et al*. Randomized phase III trial of adjuvant chemotherapy with gemcitabine versus S-1 in patients with resected pancreatic cancer: Japan Adjuvant Study Group of Pancreatic Cancer (JASPAC-01). *Jpn J Clin Oncol* 2008;**38**:227–229.

59. Fukutomi U, *et al*. JASPAC 01: Randomized phase III trial of adjuvant chemotherapy with gemcitabine versus S-1 for patients with resected pancreatic cancer. *J Clin Oncol* 2013;**31**:(Suppl.; Abstr. 4008).

60. Liao WC, *et al*. Adjuvant treatments for resected pancreatic adenocarcinoma: A systematic review and network meta-analysis. *Lancet Oncol* 2013;**14**:1095–1103.

61. Chang DK, *et al*. Margin clearance and outcome in resected pancreatic cancer. *J Clin Oncol* 2009;**27**:2855–2862.

62. Berger AC, *et al*. Five year results of US intergroup/RTOG 9704 with postoperative CA 19-9 </=90 U/mL and comparison to the CONKO-001 trial. *Int J Radiat Oncol Biol Phys* 2012;**84**:e291–e297.

63. Greenhalf W, *et al*. Pancreatic cancer hENT1 expression and survival from gemcitabine in patients from the ESPAC-3 trial. *J Natl Cancer Inst* 2014;**106**:djt347.

64. Abrams RA, *et al*. Combined modality treatment of resectable and borderline resectable pancreas cancer: Expert consensus statement. *Ann Surg Oncol* 2009;**16**: 1751–1756.

65. Katz MH, *et al*. Borderline resectable pancreatic cancer: The importance of this emerging stage of disease. *J Am Coll Surg* 2008;**206**:833–846; discussion 46–48.

66. Hosein PJ, *et al*. A retrospective study of neoadjuvant FOLFIRINOX in unresectable or borderline-resectable locally advanced pancreatic adenocarcinoma. *BMC Cancer* 2012;**12**:199.
67. Boone BA, *et al*. Outcomes with FOLFIRINOX for borderline resectable and locally unresectable pancreatic cancer. *J Surg Oncol* 2013;**108**:236–241.
68. Schellenberg D, *et al*. Gemcitabine chemotherapy and single-fraction stereotactic body radiotherapy for locally advanced pancreatic cancer. *Int J Radiat Oncol Biol Phys* 2008;**72**:678–686.
69. Mukherjee S, *et al*. Gemcitabine-based or capecitabine-based chemoradiotherapy for locally advanced pancreatic cancer (SCALOP): A multicentre, randomised, phase 2 trial. *Lancet Oncol* 2013;**14**:317–326.
70. Krishnan S, *et al*. Induction chemotherapy selects patients with locally advanced, unresectable pancreatic cancer for optimal benefit from consolidative chemoradiation therapy. *Cancer* 2007;**110**:47–55.
71. Huguet F, *et al*. Impact of chemoradiotherapy after disease control with chemotherapy in locally advanced pancreatic adenocarcinoma in GERCOR phase II and III studies. *J Clin Oncol* 2007;**25**:326–31.
72. Loehrer PJ, Sr., *et al*. Gemcitabine alone versus gemcitabine plus radiotherapy in patients with locally advanced pancreatic cancer: An Eastern Cooperative Oncology Group trial. *J Clin Oncol* 2011;**29**:4105–4112.
73. Hammel P, *et al*. Comparison of chemoradiotherapy (CRT) and chemotherapy (CT) in patients with a locally advanced pancreatic cancer (LAPC) controlled after 4 months of gemcitabine with or without erlotinib: Final results of the international phase III LAP 07 study. *J Clin Oncol* 2013;**31**(Suppl.; Abstr. LBA4003).
74. Burris HA III, *et al*. Improvements in survival and clinical benefit with gemcitabine as first-line therapy for patients with advanced pancreas cancer: A randomized trial. *J Clin Oncol* 1997;**15**:2403–2413.
75. Louvet C, *et al*. Gemcitabine in combination with oxaliplatin compared with gemcitabine alone in locally advanced or metastatic pancreatic cancer: Results of a GERCOR and GISCAD phase III trial. *J Clin Oncol* 2005;**23**:3509–3516.
76. Heinemann V, *et al*. Randomized phase III trial of gemcitabine plus cisplatin compared with gemcitabine alone in advanced pancreatic cancer. *J Clin Oncol* 2006;**24**:3946–3952.
77. Colucci G, *et al*. Randomized phase III trial of gemcitabine plus cisplatin compared with single-agent gemcitabine as first-line treatment of patients with advanced pancreatic cancer: The GIP-1 study. *J Clin Oncol* 2010;**28**:1645–1651.
78. Herrmann R, *et al*. Gemcitabine plus capecitabine compared with gemcitabine alone in advanced pancreatic cancer: A randomized, multicenter, phase III trial of the Swiss Group for Clinical Cancer Research and the Central European Cooperative Oncology Group. *J Clin Oncol* 2007;**25**:2212–2217.
79. Cunningham D, *et al*. Phase III randomized comparison of gemcitabine versus gemcitabine plus capecitabine in patients with advanced pancreatic cancer. *J Clin Oncol* 2009;**27**:5513–5518.

80. Heinemann V, *et al*. Meta-analysis of randomized trials: evaluation of benefit from gemcitabine-based combination chemotherapy applied in advanced pancreatic cancer. *BMC Cancer* 2008;**8**:82.
81. Gourgou-Bourgade S, *et al*. Impact of FOLFIRINOX compared with gemcitabine on quality of life in patients with metastatic pancreatic cancer: Results from the PRODIGE 4/ACCORD 11 randomized trial. *J Clin Oncol* 2013;**31**:23–29.
82. Infante JR, *et al*. Peritumoral fibroblast SPARC expression and patient outcome with resectable pancreatic adenocarcinoma. *J Clin Oncol* 2007;**25**:319–325.
83. Von Hoff DD, *et al*. Gemcitabine plus nab-paclitaxel is an active regimen in patients with advanced pancreatic cancer: A phase I/II trial. *J Clin Oncol* 2011;**29**:4548–4554.
84. Hidalgo M, *et al*. SPARC analysis in the phase III MPACT trial of nab-paclitaxel plus gemcitabine versus gemcitabine alone for patients with metastatic pancreatic cancer. *Ann Oncol* 2014;**25**:ii106.
85. Ueno H, *et al*. Randomized phase III study of gemcitabine plus S-1, S-1 alone, or gemcitabine alone in patients with locally advanced and metastatic pancreatic cancer in Japan and Taiwan: GEST study. *J Clin Oncol* 2013;**31**:1640–1648.
86. Chuah B, *et al*. Comparison of the pharmacokinetics and pharmacodynamics of S-1 between Caucasian and East Asian patients. *Cancer Sci* 2011;**102**:478–483.
87. Moore MJ, *et al*. Erlotinib plus gemcitabine compared with gemcitabine alone in patients with advanced pancreatic cancer: A phase III trial of the National Cancer Institute of Canada Clinical Trials Group. *J Clin Oncol* 2007;**25**:1960–1966.
88. Philip PA, *et al*. Phase III study comparing gemcitabine plus cetuximab versus gemcitabine in patients with advanced pancreatic adenocarcinoma: Southwest Oncology Group-directed intergroup trial S0205. *J Clin Oncol* 2010;**28**:3605–3610.
89. Kindler HL, *et al*. Gemcitabine plus bevacizumab compared with gemcitabine plus placebo in patients with advanced pancreatic cancer: Phase III trial of the Cancer and Leukemia Group B (CALGB 80303). *J Clin Oncol* 2010;**28**:3617–3622.
90. Pelzer U, *et al*. Best supportive care (BSC) versus oxaliplatin, folinic acid and 5-fluorouracil (OFF) plus BSC in patients for second-line advanced pancreatic cancer: A phase III-study from the German CONKO-study group. *Eur J Cancer* 2011;**47**:1676–1681.
91. Oettle H, *et al*. Second-Line oxaliplatin, folinic acid, and fluorouracil versus folinic acid and fluorouracil alone for gemcitabine-refractory pancreatic cancer: Outcomes from the CONKO-003 trial. *J Clin Oncol* 2014; doi: 10.1200/JCO.2013.53.6995
92. Von Hoff D, *et al*. NAPOLI-1: Randomized phase 3 study of MM-398 (NAL-IRI) with or without 5-Fluorouracid and leucovorin, versus 5-Fluorouracid and leucovorin, in metastatic pancreatic cancer progressed on or following gemcitabine-based therapy. *Ann Oncol* 2014;**25**:ii105–ii6.
93. Lowery MA, *et al*. An emerging entity: pancreatic adenocarcinoma associated with a known *BRCA* mutation: Clinical descriptors, treatment implications, and future directions. *Oncologist* 2011;**16**:1397–1402.
94. Villarroel MC, *et al*. Personalizing cancer treatment in the age of global genomic analyses: *PALB2* gene mutations and the response to DNA damaging agents in pancreatic cancer. *Mol Cancer Ther* 2011;**10**:3–8.

95. Van Cutsem E, *et al*. Phase III trial of gemcitabine plus tipifarnib compared with gemcitabine plus placebo in advanced pancreatic cancer. *J Clin Oncol* 2004;**22**:1430–1438.

96. Lersch C, *et al*. Randomised Phase II study of SCH66336 and gemcitabine in the treatment of metastatic adenocarcinoma of the pancreas. *Proc Am Soc Clin Oncol* 2001 (Abstr. 608).

97. Bodoky G, *et al*. A phase II open-label randomized study to assess the efficacy and safety of selumetinib (AZD6244 [ARRY-142886]) versus capecitabine in patients with advanced or metastatic pancreatic cancer who have failed first-line gemcitabine therapy. *Invest New Drugs* 2012;**30**:1216–1223.

98. Infante JR SB, *et al*. A randomized, double-blind, placebo-controlled trial of trametinib, a mek inhibitor, in combination with gemcitabine for patients with untreated metastatic adenocarcinoma of the pancreas. *J Clin Oncol* 2013;**31**(Suppl. 4):291a.

99. Rexer BN, *et al*. Inhibition of PI3K and MEK: It is all about combinations and biomarkers. *Clin Cancer Res* 2009;**15**:4518–4520.

100. Acquaviva J, *et al*. Targeting KRAS-mutant non-small cell lung cancer with the Hsp90 inhibitor ganetespib. *Mol Cancer Ther* 2012;**11**:2633–2643.

101. D'Angelo SP, *et al*. Immunogenicity of GI-4000 vaccine in adjuvant consolidation therapy following definitive treatment in patients with stage I–III adenocarcinoma of the lung with *G12C, G12D*, or *G12V KRAS* mutations. *J Clin Oncol* 2011;**29**:7070a.

102. Muscarella P, *et al*. A randomized, placebo-controlled, double blind, mul- ticenter phase II adjuvant trial of the efficacy, immunogenicity, and safety of GI-4000 plus gem versus gem alone in patients with resected pancreas cancer with activating *RAS* mutations/ survival and immunology analysis of the R1 subgroup. *J Clin Oncol* 2012;**30**(Suppl.; Abstr. e14501).

103. Hurwitz H, *et al*. A randomized double-blind phase 2 study of ruxolitinib (RUX) or placebo (PBO) with capecitabine (CAPE) as second-line therapy in patients (pts) with metastatic pancreatic cancer (mPC). *J Clin Oncol* 2014;**32**:5s(Suppl.; Abstr. 4000).

104. Gukovsky I, *et al*. Inflammation, autophagy, and obesity: common features in the pathogenesis of pancreatitis and pancreatic cancer. *Gastroenterology* 2013;**144**:1199–1209; e4.

105. Hotchkiss RS, Moldawer LL. Parallels between cancer and infectious disease. *N Engl J Med* 2014;**371**:380–383.

106. Chugh R, *et al*. A preclinical evaluation of Minnelide as a therapeutic agent against pancreatic cancer. *Sci Transl Med* 2012;**4**:156ra39.

107. Hashimoto D, *et al*. Autophagy is needed for the growth of pancreatic adenocarcinoma and has a cytoprotective effect against anticancer drugs. *Eur J Cancer* 2014;**50**:1382–1390.

108. DiNorcia J, *et al*. RAGE gene deletion inhibits the development and progression of ductal neoplasia and prolongs survival in a murine model of pancreatic cancer. *J Gastrointest Surg* 2012;**16**:104–112; discussion 12.

109. Amaravadi RK, *et al*. Principles and current strategies for targeting autophagy for cancer treatment. *Clin Cancer Res* 2011;**17**:654–666.

110. Brahmer JR, *et al.* Safety and activity of anti-PD-L1 antibody in patients with advanced cancer. *N Engl J Med* 2012;**366**:2455–2465.

111. Topalian SL, *et al.* Safety, activity, and immune correlates of anti-PD-1 antibody in cancer. *N Engl J Med* 2012;**366**:2443–2454.

112. Royal RE, *et al.* Phase 2 trial of single agent ipilimumab (anti-CTLA-4) for locally advanced or metastatic pancreatic adenocarcinoma. *J Immunother* 2010;**33**:828–833.

113. Aglietta M, *et al.* A phase I dose escalation trial of tremelimumab (CP-675,206) in combination with gemcitabine in chemotherapy-naive patients with metastatic pancreatic cancer. *Ann Oncol* 2014;**25**(9):1750–1755.

114. Le DT, *et al.* A phase 2, randomized trial of GVAX pancreas and CRS-207 immunotherapy versus GVAX alone in patients with metastatic pancreatic adenocarcinoma: Updated results. *J Clin Oncol* 2014;**32**(Suppl. 3; Abstr. 177).

115. Springett GM. Novel pancreatic cancer vaccines could unleash the army within. *Cancer Control* 2014;**21**:242–246.

116. Hardacre JM, *et al.* Addition of algenpantucel-L immunotherapy to standard adjuvant therapy for pancreatic cancer: A phase 2 study. *J Gastrointest Surg* 2013;**17**:94–100; discussion p–1.

117. Ozdemir BC, *et al.* Depletion of carcinoma-associated fibroblasts and fibrosis induces immunosuppression and accelerates pancreas cancer with reduced survival. *Cancer Cell* 2014;**25**:719–734.

118. Rhim AD, *et al.* Stromal elements act to restrain, rather than support, pancreatic ductal adenocarcinoma. *Cancer Cell* 2014;**25**:735–747.

119. Olive KP, *et al.* Inhibition of Hedgehog signaling enhances delivery of chemotherapy in a mouse model of pancreatic cancer. *Science* 2009;**324**:1457–1461.

120. Catenacci DVT, *et al.* A phase IB/randomized phase II study of gemcitabine (G) plus placebo (P) or vismodegib (V), a hedgehog (Hh) pathway inhibitor, in patients (pts) with metastatic pancreatic cancer (PC): Interim analysis of a University of Chicago phase II consortium study. *J Clin Oncol* 2012;**30**(Suppl.; Abstr. 4022).

121. Sun JD, *et al.* Selective tumor hypoxia targeting by hypoxia-activated prodrug TH-302 inhibits tumor growth in preclinical models of cancer. *Clin Cancer Res* 2012;**18**: 758–770.

122. Weiss GJ, *et al.* Phase 1 study of the safety, tolerability, and pharmacokinetics of TH-302, a hypoxia-activated prodrug, in patients with advanced solid malignancies. *Clin Cancer Res* 2011;**17**:2997–3004.

Chapter 13

Systemic Therapy for Metastatic Colorectal Cancer

Mark H. O'Hara and Bruce J. Giantonio

1 Introduction

In the United States, colorectal cancer is the second leading cause of cancer-related death. Yet, with an increased use of screening, there has been a decrease in the incidence of both early- and late-stage colorectal cancer, an improvement in the age adjusted 5 year survival rates over the past three decades,[1–3] and it is anticipated by 2030 deaths from pancreatic cancer will outnumber those from colorectal cancer largely due to the increased use of colorectal cancer screening.[4] However, despite these improvements, the management of metastatic colorectal cancer represent a significant health concern: about 20% of patients have evidence of metastatic spread at the time of diagnosis of colorectal cancer and 30–50% of patients initially diagnosed with locally advanced disease will develop metastatic recurrence.[5–7] And while about 10–20% of patients with metastatic disease can undergo surgical resection of their disease, the only definitive potential therapy for cure in this population,[8,9] the vast majority of patients with metastatic colorectal cancer can experience an extended survival with the use of systemic therapy.

The treatment of metastatic colorectal cancer has significantly improved since the introduction of 5-fluorouracil (5-FU) in the 1960s. Modern therapy regimens currently employ combinations of cytotoxic chemotherapy — namely 5-FU, irinotecan, and oxaliplatin — and biologic therapies, including vascular endothelial growth factor inhibitors, and epidermal growth factor inhibitors. Continued advancements in the combinations of these therapies have extended the median overall survival to more than 2.5 years. With the number of cytotoxic and targeted drugs available for the treatment of metastatic colorectal cancer, and with patients living longer, it is necessary to approach the management of patient with metastatic colorectal cancer in a manner that employs strategic personalized planning.

In this chapter, we will outline the development of the cytotoxic chemotherapy regimens used currently in the treatment of metastatic colorectal cancer patients and discuss the addition of targeted agents, and the incorporation of treatment "breaks" or "holidays," maintenance therapy, and the use of genomic profiling for risk stratification and treatment selection.

2 Cytotoxic Chemotherapy

Cytotoxic therapy, namely 5-FU, irinotecan, and oxaliplatin, remains the mainstay of therapy for metastatic colorectal cancer. In most settings, optimal regimens employ a combination of at least two cytotoxic agents and a biologic agent.

2.1 *Antimetabolites*

2.1.1 *5-fluorouracil*

5-fluorouracil (5-FU) has been the principal chemotherapeutic agent for colorectal cancer for over 40 years. This fluoropyrimidine has multiple pharmacologic activities associated with cytotoxicity. The primary mode of action is as an irreversible inhibitor of thymidylate synthesis, an enzyme responsible for the reductive methylation of 2′-deoxyuridine-5′-monophosphate (dUMP) to 2′-deoxythymidine-5′-monophosphate (dTMP), the first step in the *de novo* synthesis of the essential DNA precursor 2′-deoxythymidine-5′-triphosphate (dTTP). In addition to decreased production of this DNA synthesis precursor, blocked conversion from dUMP to dTTP leads to accumulation of dUMP, which can be incorrectly incorporated into DNA resulting in single- and double-strand DNA breaks through DNA repair mechanisms. Furthermore, DNA synthesis and function can be interrupted by DNA incorporation of 5-fluoro-2′-deoxyuridine-5′-triphosphate (FdUTP), a nucleotide resulting from the conversion of 5-FU. 5-FU can also be converted to 5-FUTP, which can be incorporated into and inhibit the processing of normal RNA.[10–14] The underlying mechanism of cytotoxicity associated with 5-FU is dependent on the method of delivery. For example, 5-FU inhibition of RNA synthesis is related to high peak concentrations of 5-FU as can be obtained with bolus administration. Inhibition of thymidylate synthase, however, is not enhanced at high doses of 5-FU, and growth inhibition parallels thymidylate synthase inhibition at low doses of 5-FU obtained as a continuous infusion.[15–17]

The different mechanisms of 5-FU activity are important not only because 5-FU is effective as a continuous infusion and when given as a bolus injection, but also because the side effects associated with the two modes of delivery are different. For example, myelosuppression was a noted toxicity in even the earliest trials of bolus, single-agent 5-FU in patients with metastatic colorectal cancer.[18] When compared to bolus administration, however, continuous infusion single-agent 5-FU causes less myelosuppression, but more stomatitis, diarrhea, and palmar-plantar erythrodysesthesia.[19,20] In addition, outcomes can differ; several randomized controlled trials (RCTs) that have shown improvement in response rates with continuously infused 5-FU compared to bolus 5-FU (although with no significant difference in overall survival).[21–23] A meta-analysis of six RCTs found a statistically significant improvement in response rate (odds ratio, OR 0.55) and overall survival (hazard ratio, HR 0.88) with continuous infusion 5-FU.[20] For this reason, 5-FU is generally administered as a continuous infusion when given to patients with metastatic colorectal cancer.

Single agent 5-FU is associated with modest response rates of 10–15%.[24,25] Since the adoption of 5-FU as a treatment for metastatic colorectal cancer in the 1960s, combination therapy was attempted with drugs such as semustine, vincristine, methotrexate, interferon, and PALA, but these combinations either failed to show a substantial improvement in overall survival or worsened adverse events.[26–36] Biomodulation with leucovorin, however, was found to be beneficial. Leucovorin, also known as folinic acid or calcium folinate, is a mixture of two stereoisomers ([6R,S]-5-formyltetrahydrofolate), with the L-isomer representing the active compound, and potentiates the activity of 5-FU in preclinical models by increasing the intracellular concentration of 5-10-methylenetetrahydrofolate, a coenzyme in the biosynthesis of thymidine. 5-10-methylenetetrahydrofolate binds to thymidylate synthetase with the 5-FU byproduct FdUMP to augment inhibition of thymidylate synthetase.[37–40] A meta-analysis of published RCTs comparing 5-FU and leucovorin to 5-FU alone shows a response rate of 21% with the combination in comparison to 11% with 5-FU (HR 0.53). There is also a statistically significant improvement in overall survival, with an 11.7-month median overall survival with 5-FU and leucovorin and 10.5-month overall survival with 5-FU alone (HR 0.90),[25] with slightly increased rates of diarrhea, stomatitis, and nausea noted in the 5-FU and leucovorin arm compared to an equivalent 5-FU dose.[29,41,42] The higher response rate, modest increase in overall survival, and tolerable side effects led to the adoption of the combination of 5-FU and leucovorin as standard therapy for metastatic colorectal cancer.

Despite studies showing that both continuous infusion 5-FU and bolus 5-FU in combination with leucovorin are superior to bolus 5-fluorouracil alone, the data is limited on the role of leucovorin with continuous infusion 5-FU. One study suggests that daily leucovorin over the four days of continuous infusion 5-FU is nearly identical to daily bolus 5-FU and leucovorin over five days,[43] and another study suggests that weekly leucovorin in combination with continuous infusion 5-FU over 28 days was no better than the same continual infusion 5-FU regimen alone, 5-FU bolus over five days, or bolus 5-FU with leucovorin.[44] The conclusions from these studies is that leucovorin does not add any additional benefit when used in combination continuous infusion 5-FU.

Current practices commonly use a combination of both bolus and continuous infusion 5-FU based on preclinical studies indicating an additive inhibition of thymidylate synthase, perhaps by targeting the principal difference in 5-FU cytotoxic mechanism produced by the schedule of delivery.[45] These findings provided support for studies showing that combinations of leucovorin, bolus 5-FU and continuous infusion 5-FU is safe and allows for delivery of more 5-FU over a given month.[46] In addition, a phase III study comparing a bimonthly combination of leucovorin, bolus 5-FU, and continuous infusion 5-FU (LV5FU2) to the monthly Mayo bolus 5-FU and leucovorin regimen (regimens outlined in Table 1) found that the bimonthly combination regimen yielded a statistically significant superior response rate and progression free survival and a trend toward improved survival.[47] A simplified LV5FU2 was at least as effective as LV5FU2, has low toxicity, and is more convenient for patients,[48,49] and both LV5FU2 and simplified LV5FU2 have been commonly used as "backbones" to most of the commonly used chemotherapy regimens.

2.1.2 *Capecitabine*

Capecitabine, a prodrug to 5-FU, was developed to improve 5-FU delivery to tumor cells with predictable kinetics, reduced side effects and the convenience of oral administration. Capecitabine, a fluoropyrimidine carbonate, is converted to 5-FU through a series of three enzymatic steps that selectively occurs within tumor cells as the last enzyme in the conversion pathway — thymidine phosphorylase — is four times more concentrated in tumor cells compared with normal tissue.[67,68] Although cytotoxicity was enhanced when 5-FU was combined with leucovorin as noted above, leucovorin has no effect on capecitabine pharmacokinetics or activity.[69,70]

Two phase III clinical trials comparing capecitabine with the Mayo Clinic regimen of bolus 5-FU and leucovorin in treatment-naïve metastatic colorectal cancer patients found that capecitabine has a favorable response rate and side effect profile compared to 5-FU with no statistically significant difference in overall survival.[71,72] A meta-analysis of these two studies combined the 1,207 total patients and resulted

Table 1 Cytotoxic chemotherapy regimens.

Regimen Name	Regimen	Cycle Length
5-fluorouracil-containing regimens		
Mayo Regimen[50]	LV 20 mg/m^2 IV bolus D 1–5 5-FU 425 mg/m^2 IV bolus D 1–5	4 weeks
Roswell Park Regimen[51]	LV 500 mg/m^2 IV × 2 hours D 1, 8, 15, 22, 29, 36 5-FU 500 mg/m^2 IV bolus D 1, 8, 15, 22, 29, 36	8 weeks
LV5FU2[47]	LV 200 mg/m^2 IV over 2 h daily D 1, 2 5-FU 400 mg/m^2 IV bolus D 1, 2 5-FU 600 mg/m^2 CI × 22 h per day D 1, 2	2 weeks
sLV5FU2[49]	LV 400 mg/m^2 IV over 2 h D 1 5-FU 400 mg/m^2 IV bolus D 1 5-FU 2400 mg/m^2 CI × 46 h D 1, 2	2 weeks
Irinotecan-containing regimens		
IFL[52]	Irinotecan 125 mg/m^2 IV D 1, 8, 15, 22 5-FU 500 mg/m^2 IV bolus D 1, 8, 15, 22 Folinic acid 20 mg/m^2 IV bolus D 1, 8, 15, 22	6 weeks
mIFL[53]	Irinotecan 125 mg/m^2 IV D 1, 8 5-FU 500 mg/m^2 IV bolus D 1, 8 Folinic acid 20 mg/m^2 IV bolus D 1, 8, 15, 22	3 weeks
FOLFIRI[54]	Irinotecan 180 mg/m^2 IV D1 Leucovorin 200 mg/m^2 IV D 1, 2 5-FU 400 mg/m^2 IV bolus D 1, 2 5-FU 600 mg/m^2 CI × 22 h D 1, 2	2 weeks
sFOLFIRI[49]	Irinotecan 180 mg/m^2 IV D 1 Folinic acid 400 mg/m^2 IV D 1 5-FU 400 mg/m^2 IV bolus D 1 5-FU 2400 mg/m^2 IV CI × 46 h	2 weeks
CapeIRI[53]	250 mg/m^2 IV D 1 Capecitabine 1,000 mg/m^2 orally twice daily D 1–14	3 weeks
Oxaliplatin-containing regimens		
FOLFOX1[55]	Oxaliplatin 130 mg/m^2 IV × 2 h D 1* LV 500 mg/m^2 IV × 2 h D 1, 2 5-FU 1,500–2,000 mg/m^2 CI × 22 h D 1, 2**	2 weeks
FOLFOX2[56]	Oxaliplatin 100 mg/m^2 IV × 2 h D 1 LV 500 mg/m^2 IV × 2 h D 1 5-FU 1,500–2,000 mg/m^2 CI × 22 h D 1, 2**	2 weeks
FOLFOX3[57]	Oxaliplatin 85 mg/m^2 IV × 2 h D 1 LV 500 mg/m^2 IV × 2 h D 1, 2 5-FU 1,500 mg/m^2 CI × 22 h D 1, 2**	2 weeks

(*Continued*)

Table 1   (*Continued*)

Regimen Name	Regimen	Cycle Length
FOLFOX4[58]	Oxaliplatin 85 mg/m^2 IV × 2 h D 1 LV 200 mg/m^2 IV × 2 h D 1, 2 5-FU 400 mg/m^2 IV bolus D 1, 2 5-FU 600 mg/m^2 CI × 22 h D 1, 2	2 weeks
FOLFOX5[59]	Oxaliplatin 100 mg/m^2 IV × 2 h D 1 LV 200 mg/m^2 IV × 2 ho D 1, 2 5-FU 400 mg/m^2 IV bolus D 1, 2 5-FU 600 mg/m^2 CI × 22 h D 1, 2	2 weeks
FOLFOX6[59]	Oxaliplatin 100 mg/m^2 IV × 2 h D 1 LV 400 mg/m^2 IV × 2 h D 1 5-FU 400 mg/m^2 IV bolus D 1 5-FU 2400–3000 mg/m^2 CI × 46 h[**]	2 weeks
mFOLFOX6[60]	Oxaliplatin 85 mg/m^2 IV × 2 h D 1 LV 400 mg/m^2 IV × 2 h D 1 5-FU 400 mg/m^2 IV bolus D 1 5-FU 2,400 mg/m^2 CI × 46 h	2 weeks
FOLFOX7[61]	Oxaliplatin 130 mg/m^2 IV × 2 h D 1 LV 400 mg/m^2 IV × 2 h D 1 5-FU 400 mg/m^2 IV bolus D 1 5-FU 2,400 mg/m^2 CI × 46 h	2 weeks
Nordic FLOX[62]	Oxaliplatin 85 mg/m^2 IV × 2 h D 1 LV 60 mg/m^2 IV bolus D 1, 2 5-FU 500 mg/m^2 IV bolus D 1, 2	2 weeks
XELOX (CapeOx)[63]	Oxaliplatin 130 mg/m^2 IV × 2 h D 1 Capecitabine 1,000 mg/m^2 orally twice daily D 1–14	3 weeks
CAPOX[64]	Oxaliplatin 70 mg/m^2 D 1, 8 Capecitabine 1,000 mg/m^2 orally twice daily D 1–14	3 weeks
Triplet cytotoxic chemotherapy		
FOLFOXIRI (GONO)[65]	Irinotecan 165 mg/m^2 IV D 1 Oxaliplatin 85 mg/m^2 IV D 1 Leucovorin 200 mg/m^2 IV D 1 5-FU 3,200 mg/m^2 CI × 48 h	2 weeks
FOLFOXIRI (HORG)[66]	Irinotecan 150 mg/m^2 IV D 1 Leucovorin 200 mg/m^2 IV D 2, 3 5-FU 400 mg/m^2 IV bolus D 2, 3 5-FU 600 mg/m^2 CI x 22 hours D 2, 3 Oxaliplatin 65 mg/m^2 IV infusion D2	2 weeks

LV: leucovorin; 5-FU: 5-fluorouracil; IV: intravenous; D: day; CI: continuous infusion

*Oxaliplatin given every other cycle.

**5-FU started at the lower dose for first two cycles and increased to the higher dose if the maximum toxicity was less than grade 2.

in a 22% response rate with capecitabine compared to 13% with 5-FU/LV. The time to progression (HR 0.997) and median overall survival were not statistically different (HR 0.95).[73] Overall, compared to 5-FU, capecitabine is associated with less diarrhea, alopecia, and nausea with statistically significantly less grades 3 and 4 stomatitis, neutropenia, and neutropenic fever. The incidence of grades 3 and 4 palmar-plantar erythrodysesthesia (hand–foot syndrome), however, is increased in patients undergoing treatment with capecitabine and is often a dose-limiting toxicity in clinical practice requiring dose interruptions and reduction.[71–74] Given that the hand–foot syndrome is seen in a large population, many clinicians will choose to initiate therapy at a dose that is lower than the recommended 1,250 mg/m^2, taken orally twice daily for two continuous weeks on an every three-week schedule, with escalation to full dose if toxicity is manageable.

2.1.3 *Dihydropyrimidine dehydrogenase*

Dihydropyrimidine dehydrogenase (DPD) is a key enzyme responsible for catabolism of both intravenous 5-FU and capecitabine, and deficiency of the DPD enzyme is associated with significant drug toxicity due to the inability to degrade 5-FU.[75–79] DPD activity is dependent on circadian rhythm variation, drug–drug interactions, genetic polymorphisms, and epigenetic modulation, all resulting in potential partial or complete inability to detoxify 5-FU in patients. Studies evaluating genomic variation of the *DPYD* gene have used denaturing high-performance liquid chromatography, pyrosequencing, restricting fragment-length polymorphism, single-strand conformation polymorphisms, or detection of epigenetic modification through methylation patterns on the *DPYD* promoter. The most common and well-characterized genetic polymorphism, *DPYD*2A*, is found to be heterozygous in 1.8–3.5% of the population.[80,81] In addition, other genetic polymorphisms in the *DPYD* gene are well characterized with over 50 genetic variants reported, though not all variants are clearly associated with increased fluoropyrimidine-related toxicity.[82] Furthermore, some studies indicate that significant toxicity can occur in the absence of a distinct *DPYD* gene mutation.[83] Though hypermethylation of the *DPYD* promoter may in part explain this finding,[84] epigenetic modification of *DPYD* is not associated with severe 5-FU toxicity in all studies.[85,86]

Given an incomplete association between *DPYD* genomic variation and severe 5-FU toxicity, it would seem reasonable that a functional assay, including detection of DPD activity in peripheral mononuclear cells, the uracil breath test, detection of the plasma dihydrouracil:uracil ratio, and 5-FU drug monitoring after a 5-FU test dose, would best assess for DPD deficiency. These tests are simply surrogate markers for liver DPD activity and each are limited by cost, time, sensitivity, specificity, or lack of a consistent definition of DPD deficiency.[87]

Despite a lack of a clear gold standard test, studies show that DPD deficiency is likely a common cause of severe 5-FU toxicity, with an estimated 40–60% of patients with severe 5-FU toxicity who are DPD-deficient.[88,89] Furthermore, studies suggest that women have about 15% less DPD activity than do men,[90] and a study of non-cancer patients showed African American have about a 7.7% incidence of DPD deficiency compared to 2.3% in Caucasians.[91] Even with the relatively frequent finding of DPD deficiency, the lack of an optimized standardized test for screening patients undergoing treatment with 5-FU for DPD deficiency limits the use of evaluation for DPD deficiency to those patients who develop significant toxicity from a fluoropyrimidine.

2.2 Topoisomerase inhibitors

2.2.1 Irinotecan

Irinotecan hydrochloride (CPT-11), a camptothecin derivative, is an inhibitor of topoisomerase 1, a nuclear enzyme responsible for formation of single-strand breaks in DNA, permitting uncoiling of DNA and enabling replication and transcription to proceed. Irinotecan is metabolized in the liver and gut by carboxylesterase to a more active metabolite, 7-ethyl-10-hydroxycamptothecin (SN-38).[92] Irinotecan and SN-38 bind to topoisomerase 1, forming stable topoisomerase 1–DNA cleavable complexes that results in the accumulation of single-strand breaks, interference with the DNA replication fork, and cell death.[92–96] Common side effects associated with irinotecan include neutropenia, both acute and delayed diarrhea, fatigue, alopecia, nausea, vomiting, and acute cholinergic-like syndrome. The acute cholinergic-like syndrome can both be treated and prevented with administration of subcutaneous atropine.

Irinotecan monotherapy has been evaluated in both the first-line setting and after progression on 5-FU and leucovorin. Response rates are similar, with an 18.7–32% response rate in the first line setting[97–100] and 8–25% response rate after progression on 5-FU and leucovorin.[97,98,101–104] Randomized phase III studies of single agent irinotecan following progression on 5-FU and leucovorin demonstrated an improvement in overall survival compared to best supportive care alone,[105] and improved progression-free and overall survival when compared to continuous infusion 5-FU and leucovorin.[106] Although these studies indicate that single-agent irinotecan is an acceptable treatment in any line of therapy for patients with metastatic colorectal cancer, irinotecan is more commonly given in combination with a biologic therapy with or without 5-FU given results of several studies as outlined below.

Preclinical evidence of the combination of irinotecan with 5-FU and leucovorin suggested separate but synergistic activity of the combination, with increased

Table 2   Irinotecan-containing regimens.

Study	Phase	Regimens	Pt #	RR (%)	OR (p)	SD (%)	PFS (m)	HR (p)	mOS (m)	HR (p)
First line										
Pitot[98]	II	Weekly irinotecan	31	25.8	—	54.8	NR	—	11.8	—
Rougier[97]	II	Irinotecan 350 mg/m^2 Q3W	48	18.7	—	43.8	4.6	—	12.0	—
Conti[100]	II	Weekly irinotecan	41	32	—	44	4.2	—	12.1	—
Firvida[99]	II	Irinotecan 350 mg/m^2 Q3W	65	24.7	—	41.5	6.4	—	19.9	—
Douillard[110]	III	5-FU and irinotecan	199	34.8	(<0.005)	35.4	6.7	(<0.001)	17.4	(0.031)
		5-FU	188	21.9		46.0	4.4		14.1	
Saltz[109]	III	IFL	231	39	(<0.001)	NR	7.0	(0.004)	14.8	(0.04)
		5-FU Mayo regimen	226	21	(NS)		4.3	(NS)	12.6	(NS)
		Weekly irinotecan	226	18			4.2		12.0	
BICC-C	III	sFOLFIRI	144	47.2	—	—	7.6	1.51 (.004)	23.1	(0.09)
Fuchs[53,111]		mIFL	141	43.3			5.9	B–C(0.46)	17.6	(0.93)
		CapeIRI	145	38.6			5.8	A–C(1.36) (.015)	18.9	A–C (0.27)
Van Cutsem[112]	II	Irinotecan 350 mg/m^2 D1 + Mayo 5-FU/LV D22–26 Q6W	33	30	—	49	7.2	—	16	—
Glimelius[113]	II	Irinotecan 210 mg/m^2 + Nordic 5-FU/LV	74	39	—	22	6.4	—	15.6	—
Glimelius[114]	III	FLIRI	281	35	(0.001)	44	9.4	1.1	19.4	1.0
		LV5FU2-IRI	286	49		35	9.0		19.0	

(*Continued*)

Table 2 (*Continued*)

Study	Phase	Regimens	Pt #	RR (%)	OR (p)	SD (%)	PFS (m)	HR (p)	mOS (m)	HR (p)
Second line and beyond										
Shimada[101]	II	Irinotecan 100 mg/m²/W	31	22.6	—	29.0	NR	—	9.3 (total)	—
		Irinotecan 150 mg/m² Q2W	32	31.3		31.3				
Rothenberg[102]	II	Weekly irinotecan	43	23	—	31	NR	—	10.4	—
Pitot[98]	II	Weekly irinotecan	90	13.3	—	57.8	NR	—	8.3	—
Rougier[97]	II	Irinotecan 350 mg/m² Q3W	130	17.7	—	33.8	4.2	—	10	—
Van Cutsem[103]	II	Irinotecan 350 mg/m² Q3W	95	13.7	—	44.2	3.9	—	10.4	—
Rothenberg[104]	II	Weekly irinotecan	64	14.1	—	43.8	5.1	—	10.6	—
		Low-dose weekly irinotecan	102	8.8		38.2	3.3		9.3	
Cunningham[105]	III	Irinotecan 350 mg/m² Q3W	189	NR	—	NR	NR	—	9.2	(0.0001)
		Best supportive care	90						6.5	
Rougier[106]	III	Irinotecan 350 mg/m² Q3W	133	15.0	—	NR	4.2	(0.030)	10.8	(0.035)
		5-FU CI	134	5.2			2.9		8.5	
Fuchs[115]	III	Irinotecan 350 mg/m² Q3W	95	NR	—	NR	4.0	(0.54)	9.9	(0.43)
		Weekly irinotecan	196				3.0		9.9	
Andre[49] 3rd line	II	FOLFIRI	33	6	—	61	4.2	—	9.9	—

RR: response rate; SD: stable disease rate; PFS: median progression-free survival/time to progression; mOS: median overall survival; OR: odds ratio; HR: hazard ratio; p: p-value; m: months; W: week; Q: every (cycle length); CI: continual infusion; NR: not reported; NS: not statistically significant

Weekly irinotecan: irinotecan 125 mg/m²/W × 4W Q6W (low dose 100 mg/m²); CapeIRI: capecitabine 1,000 mg/m² BID D1–14, irinotecan 250 mg/m² Q3W; FLIRI: Nordic 5-FU/LV + irinotecan 180 mg/m² Q2W; LV5FU2-IRI: LV5FU2 with irinotecan 180 mg/m² Q2W cytotoxicity when irinotecan was administered prior to 5-FU.[107,108] As outlined in Table 2 and below, clinical evaluation of the combination also proved that the combination of 5-FU, leucovorin, and irinotecan is more effective than either irinotecan or 5-FU and leucovorin alone. First-line studies of the combination of 5-FU, leucovorin, and irinotecan evaluated both bolus administration and continuously infused 5-FU. The first phase III study evaluating IFL, a weekly irinotecan in combination with bolus 5-FU and leucovorin, demonstrated an improvement in response rate, progression-free survival, and overall survival when compared to both bolus 5-FU and leucovorin (using the Mayo regimen), and single-agent irinotecan, with the single-agent irinotecan arm and Mayo regimen arm showing comparable efficacy.[109] The combination of irinotecan with 5-FU and leucovorin increased treatment related toxicities over 5-FU and leucovorin alone, including grade 3/4 diarrhea and neutropenic infections,[109,110] and similar side effects were noted between single-agent irinotecan and the combination of 5-FU and leucovorin and irinotecan.[109] (See Table 2.) A parallel first-line study to the IFL study evaluated continuous infusion 5-FU and leucovorin in combination with irinotecan. In this study, patients randomized to the irinotecan arm were treated either with a once weekly FUFIRI regimen (25%) or a biweekly FOLFIRI (75%) regimen per institutional standard and those randomized to the 5-FU and leucovorin arm were treated with either a weekly continuous infusion 5-FU and leucovorin AIO regimen[116] or the biweekly LV5FU2 regimen.[47] Similar to the IFL study, this study found a statistically significant improvement in response rate, progression-free survival (PFS) and overall survival (OS) for the patients in the irinotecan combination arm compared to continuous infusion 5-FU and leucovorin.[110]

In addition to the two different 5-FU and leucovorin dosing strategies noted above, several randomized phase II and III studies provided evidence that irinotecan in combination with capecitabine in first-line management of patients with metastatic colorectal cancer is effective and tolerable on an every three-week schedule.[117–120] Given the demonstrated efficacy of both bolus and continuous infusion 5-FU and leucovorin and oral capecitabine in combination with irinotecan in the first-line treatment of metastatic colorectal cancer patients, the BICC-C study sought to determine the best method of fluoropyrimidine delivery to be used in combination with irinotecan. In the first phase of this study, 430 treatment naive patients were randomized to receive modified IFL, simplified FOLFIRI,[121] or CapeIRI. Patients treated with sFOLFIRI experienced a statistically significant improved progression free survival compared to mIFL (HR 1.51) and CapeIRI (HR 1.36), as well as a trend toward improved overall survival, although when bevacizumab was combined with either mIFL or sFOLFIRI in the second period of the study after bevacizumab approval, sFOLFIRI did achieve a statistically significant improved OS as noted below. In addition to being more effective, the sFOLFIRI was also associated with the lowest rates of diarrhea and febrile neutropenia. On the other hand, treatment with CapeIRI was associated with the highest rates of grade 3 or higher nausea, vomiting, diarrhea, dehydration, and hand–foot syndrome. For reasons of efficacy and tolerability, sFOLFIRI is thought to be superior to mIFL and CapeIRI, respectively.

The BICC-C study aided the understanding of the optimal delivery of fluoropyrimidines in combination with irinotecan in the first-line setting, including the increase in toxicity for combining irinotecan with capecitabine. For this reason, CapeIRI was not continued into the second period of the BICC-C study evaluating the addition of bevacizumab. In addition, the EORTC 40015 study, comparing FOLFIRI with CAPIRI, was stopped early because of increased non-disease-related deaths in the capecitabine/irinotecan arm. Similarly, given the results of the BICC-C study, decreased tolerability of IFL in other studies,[122] and overall better tolerance of continuous infusion 5-FU over bolus 5-FU, the combination of irinotecan with either bolus 5-FU or capecitabine is not commonly used in the management of patients with metastatic colorectal cancer.

2.2.2 *UGT1A1*

Uridine 5'-diphosphoglucoronosyltransferase 1A, or UGT1A, is an enzyme in the glucoronidation pathway responsible for the metabolism of a number of drugs, including the active metabolite of irinotecan, SN-38. The UGT1A1*28 polymorphism, located within the promoter region of the *UGT1A1* gene, is the most commonly characterized mutation, with studies indicating an association between UGT1A1*28 and incidence of neutropenia and diarrhea in patients treated with irinotecan.[123–126] In addition, patients homozygous for the UGT1A1*28 polymorphism appeared to have a higher response rate, though the exact mechanism by which this may be explained is unclear.[125,127] Presence of other UGT1A variants are associated with similar increased incidences of neutropenia, but are not clearly related to response rate.[127] Though the allele frequency of UGT1A1*28 is about 39% in Caucasians, and about 10% of Caucasians are homozygous for this allele, screening for UGT1A variants is not commonly done clinically.

2.3 *Alkylating agents*

2.3.1 *Oxaliplatin*

Although first and second generation platinum compounds have limited activity in the treatment of colorectal cancer,[128–131] oxaliplatin, a third generation diaminocyclohexane platinum complex, has become a commonly used agent in the management of colorectal cancer. Oxaliplatin differs from the diammine platinum agents cisplatin and carboplatin in that it has a bulky diaminocyclohexane moiety side chain that is retained after drug aquation. Although the mechanism of action is similar to that of cisplatin, the different side-chain moiety allows for the formation of bulkier DNA intrastrand adducts, causing blockage of DNA replication and transcription.[132,133] The molecular differences between oxaliplatin and the other platinum agents likely accounts for the fact that oxaliplatin is active in cisplatin-resistant tumors, including colorectal cancers, as well as the differences in side effects, including mild to moderate nausea, diarrhea, and mild myelosuppression and a unique dose-dependent, cold-related peripheral and pharyngolaryngeal paresthesia and dysesthesia. Table 3 lists all key studies using oxaliplatin in metastatic colorectal cancer.

Phase II studies in both the first-line setting, and in patients resistant to 5-FU-based therapies, report a 12–24% response rate in first-line phase II studies and a 10% response rate in phase II studies in the second-line of therapy.[134–137] However, a randomized phase III study comparing FOLFOX4 to LV5FU2 and single-agent oxaliplatin after progression on IFL demonstrated that single-agent oxaliplatin was no better than LV5FU2, and FOLFOX4 had superior overall response rates and time to progression.[138] Given this finding (and others reviewed below) few phase III studies have further evaluated single agent oxaliplatin, and as such single-agent oxaliplatin is not recommended to use in the treatment of patients with metastatic colorectal cancer.

Similar to irinotecan, *in vitro* studies show that oxaliplatin and 5-FU have synergistic anti-tumor activity in colorectal xenografts.[139,140] Clinical responses in the first line setting are also increased with the combination of 5-FU and oxaliplatin, exhibiting 37–62% response rates.[62,64,141–145] Historically, oxaliplatin was combined with chronomodulated 5-FU and leucovorin, with an improvement in response rate and PFS with no difference in OS when compared to chronomodulated 5-FU and leucovorin alone.[146] Although data suggests that chronomodulated delivery of chemotherapy is effective, it is difficult to deliver and, and such, is not widely used.

As a result most studies focused on combining 5-FU, leucovorin, and oxaliplatin with the 5-FU and leucovorin given either as a bolus, continuous infusion, and/or a combination of bolus and continuous infusion. Most commonly, a FOLFOX regimen is used, so-named because of the drugs used including **FOL**inic acid (leucovorin), **F**luorouracil given as a continuous infusion with or without a bolus, and **OX**aliplatin. Although FOLFOX4 and modified FOLFOX6 (mFOLFOX6) are currently the most commonly used FOLFOX regimens in clinical trials and practice, it is valuable to briefly review the development of these current dosing strategies through the early trials of the other FOLFOX regimens.

Initial phase II studies of pretreated patients with advanced colorectal cancer treated with FOLFOX1, a regimen consisting of continuously infused 5-FU and leucovorin on a 2-week cycle in combination with oxaliplatin 130 mg/m^2 every other cycle, resulted in a 30.7% response rate with tolerable side effects with grade 3 neuropathy.[147] Although FOLFOX1 was not evaluated further, this same study evaluated FOLFOX2 and FOLFOX3 regimens, both with the same 5-FU and leucovorin backbone but lower doses of oxaliplatin (100 mg/m^2 and 85 mg/m^2, respectively) given every cycle, and noted a 35% and 15.5% response rate, respectively, with only a 6% and 3% rate of neuropathy, respectively, when oxaliplatin was given every other week.[147] Independent phase II studies of pretreated patients with metastatic colorectal cancer treated with either FOLFOX2 or FOLFOX3 demonstrated a response rate of 46% and 20% and progression free survival rates of 7 and 6 months, respectively.[56,57] Furthermore, a multicenter phase II study of 100 pretreated patients treated with either FOLFOX3 or FOLFOX4 found response rates of 18.4% and 23.5% and progression free survival of 4.6 and 5.1 months. Grade 3/4 sensory neuropathy occurred in 27.5% of patients treated with FOLFOX3 and 15.8% with FOLFOX4, and neutropenia in 15% and 36.9% with FOLFOX3 and FOLFOX4, respectively.[58]

Although the response and adverse event rates in the phase II studies of FOLFOX2 and FOLFOX3 cannot be accurately compared, and this latter study was not randomized to compare the FOLFOX4 and FOLFOX3 regimens, no large randomized trials have compared these three regimens. Given the response rate and tolerability associated with FOLFOX4 and that FOLFOX4 comprised a standardly used bolus-continuous infusion 5-FU backbone in addition to oxaliplatin dosing more closely related to the single-agent oxaliplatin dosing of 130 mg/m^2 every three weeks, FOLFOX4 was evaluated in a phase III study in comparison to LV5FU2 in the first-line treatment for metastatic colorectal cancer. This study demonstrated improved response rate and progression-free survival, and a trend toward improved OS in patients treated with FOLFOX4. With the addition of oxaliplatin, patients had a higher rate of grades 3 and 4 neutropenia, diarrhea, and neurosensory toxicity, but this did not result in impairment in quality of life.[142] In addition, as noted above, a phase III study found that FOLFOX4 was also superior to both LV5FU2, and single-agent oxaliplatin after patients with metastatic disease progressed on IFL, with a statistically significant improvement in response rate and time to progression.[138] Similarly, a randomized phase II study of FOLFOX4 in the third line after progression on sequential 5-FU and leucovorin and irinotecan resulted in a statistically significant improvement in response rate, progression free survival, and symptomatic improvement, although no difference in overall survival, as compared to LV5FU2.[152] These studies established FOLFOX4 as a viable treatment option both in the first-line of therapy and after progression on an irinotecan-containing regimen in the treatment of patients with metastatic colorectal cancer.

Table 3 Oxaliplatin-containing regimens.

Study	Phase	Regimens	Pt #	RR (%)	OR (p)	SD (%)	PFS (m)	HR (p)	mOS (m)	HR (p)
First line										
Diaz-Rubio[134]	II	Oxaliplatin 130 mg/m² Q3W	25	12	—	32	4.0	—	14.5	—
Becouarn[148]	II	Oxaliplatin 130 mg/m² Q3W	37	24.3	—	40.5	4.2+	—	13.0	—
Cheeseman[60]	II	mFOLFOX6	25	72	—	12	10.6	—	16.7	—
DeGramont[142]	III	FOLFOX4	210	50.0	—	31.9	8.2	(0.0003)	16.2	(0.12)
		LV5FU2	210	21.9		51.0	6.0		14.7	
Zori Comba[149]	II	Oxaliplatin 85 mg/m² Q2W	35	9	—	8	2	—	NR	—
		Oxaliplatin 85 mg/m² Q2W + Mayo 5-FU/LV Q4W	38	41		6	3.9		NR	
OPTIMOX1[143]	III	FOLFOX4	311	58.5	—	28.3	9.0	1.06 (0.47)	19.3	0.93 (0.49)
		FOLFOX7 × 6 cycles then maintenance 5-FU × 12 cycles then FOLFOX7	309	59.2		27.2	8.7		21.2	
Scheithauer[150]	II	Capecitabine 2,000 mg/m² daily D1–14, oxaliplatin 130 mg/m² Q3W	45	42.2	—	44.4	6.0	2.15 (0.001)	NR	—
		Capecitabine 3,500 mg/m² daily D1–7, 14–21, oxaliplatin 85 mg/m² D1, 14 Q4W	44	54.5		27.3	10.5		NR	
Cassidy[63]	II	XELOX	96	45	—	31	7.7	—	19.5	—
Diaz-Rubio[145]	III	XELOX	174	37	0.539	29	8.9	1.18 (0.153)	18.1	1.22 (0.145)
		FUOX	174	46		25	9.5		20.8	

(Continued)

Table 3   (Continued)

Study	Phase	Regimens	Pt #	RR (%)	OR (p)	SD (%)	PFS (m)	HR (p)	mOS (m)	HR (p)
Cassidy[144]	III	XELOX +/- bevacizumab	1017	37	1.0	NR	8.0	1.04	19.8	0.99
		FOLFOX4 +/- bevacizumab	1017	37			8.5		19.6	
Second line and beyond										
Machover[136]	II	Oxaliplatin 130 mg/m² Q3W	106	10	—	37	NR	—	NR	—
DeGramont[147]	II	FOLFOX1	13	30.7		38.4	NR	—	11	—
		FOLFOX2	60	36.7		35.0			15	
		FOLFOX3	40	15.5		52.5			10	
DeGramont[56]	II	FOLFOX2	46	46	—	46	7	—	17	—
Andre[57]	II	FOLFOX3	30	20	—	50	6.0	—	13.2	—
Andre[58]	II	FOLFOX3	38	18.4	—	29	4.6	—	10.6	—
		FOLFOX4	51	23.5		31.4	5.1		11.1	
Maindrault-Goebel[59]	II	FOLFOX6	60	27	—	45	5.3	—	10.8	—
Cheeseman[60]	II	mFOLFOX6	37	12	—	35	4.8	—	10.7	—
Ryan[151]	II	mFOLFOX6	70	11	—	67	6.2	—	8.7	—
Maindrault-Goebel[61]	II	FOLFOX7	48	42	—	40	6.0	—	16.1	—
Rothenberg[138]	III	FOLFOX4	152	9.9	(<0.0001)	59.9	4.6	(<0.0001)	NR	—
		LV5FU2	151	0.0	(0.5)	45.7	2.7	(0.03)		
		Oxaliplatin 85 mg/m² Q2W	156	1.3		39.1	1.6			
Kemeny[152]	II	FOLFOX4	110	13	—	66	4.8	(<0.0001)	9.9	(0.20)
		LV5FU2	104	2.0		48	2.4		11.4	
Rothenberg[153]	III	XELOX	313	15	1.28	NR	4.7	0.97 (NR)	11.9	0.97
		FOLFOX4	314	12			4.8		12.6	

In order to attempt to improve on the response rates and tolerability, the 5-FU and oxaliplatin dosages have been further modified in other FOLFOX regimens. FOLFOX5 was designed to be identical to FOLFOX4 with the exception of a higher oxaliplatin dose at 100 mg/m^2, given findings of a higher phase II response rate with 100 mg/m^2 in the FOLFOX2 regimen.[56,147] FOLFOX5, however, was never evaluated in clinical trials. Instead, to make a more simplified regimen, the higher oxaliplatin dose was combined with a simplified LV5FU2 regimen (FOLFOX6). The phase II study of FOLFOX6 combined the higher dose of oxaliplatin with leucovorin, a single 5-FU bolus, and a 46-h continuous infusion of 2,400 mg/m^2 of 5-FU, which was increased to 3,000 mg/m^2 after two cycles if there were no grade 2 or higher toxicities. In the pretreated patients treated with FOLFOX6, there was a 27% response rate and 5.3-month progression-free survival. Of the 60 patients treated on this study, 16% had grade 3 peripheral neuropathy and 24% had grade 3 or 4 neutropenia. The authors noted that the response rate was lower than that seen with FOLFOX2, which they attributed to a combination of patient selection and a lower oxaliplatin dose intensity due to non-neurologic toxicity with FOLFOX6.[59]

To take advantage of the observed dose–response effect, the FOLFOX7 regimen was designed with a higher oxaliplatin dose (130 mg/m^2) but a lower total 5-FU dosage, using the simplified LV5FU2 regimen. A phase II study found a 42% response rate and six-month progression free survival in the second-line setting, with an 11% rate of grade 3 peripheral neuropathy.[61] In an attempt to mitigate the peripheral neuropathy associated with oxaliplatin, OPTIMOX1 a randomized phase III study compared six cycles of FOLFOX7 followed by 12 cycles without oxaliplatin followed by reintroduction of FOLFOX7, with FOLFOX4 administered continuously, until disease progression. Of note, a 5-FU bolus was included on day 1 in the phase II study of FOLFOX7, but was not used in the OPTIMOX1 study. Overall, this study demonstrated equivalent response rates and progression-free and overall survival, without any statistical difference in the rate of grade 3 peripheral neuropathy.[143]

Although evidence points to high response rates in the phase II studies using a high dose oxaliplatin in combination with a 5-FU and leucovorin, the goal of therapy for unresectable metastatic disease is centered on palliation and, as such, response rate is balanced with toxicity and ease of administration. Therefore, a modified FOLFOX6 regimen, using the simplified LV5FU2 backbone in combination with lower-dose oxaliplatin 85 mg/m^2, is the most commonly used FOLFOX regimen in the United States. Two phase II studies of this regimen found a 72% response rate in the first line and a 12–25% response rate in the second line, with 3% grade 3 neuropathy and 14–31% grade 3 or 4 neutropenia.[60,151]

In addition to the different schedules and dosing of 5-FU and oxaliplatin used in the numbered FOLFOX regimens, the combination of oxaliplatin with bolus 5-FU and leucovorin has also been evaluated. Phase II studies, in the both first-line use, and after progression on at least one prior regimen, found response rates comparable to those published for the FOLFOX regimens: ranging from 40–63% as first-line therapy, and about 20% in second-line use.[62,149,154–156] Although oxaliplatin in combination with bolus 5-FU and leucovorin has not been compared to the continuous infusion FOLFOX regimens, the bolus regimens are associated with high rates of grades 3 and 4 neutropenia, diarrhea, and stomatitis and, given comparable efficacy in phase II studies, oxaliplatin is most commonly given in combination with continuous infusion 5-FU.

Oxaliplatin has been evaluated in combination with capecitabine, and the combination is variably referred to as CapeOx, CAPOX, and XELOX. Unlike the numbered FOLFOX regimens, variations in schedule and dosing of both the capecitabine and oxaliplatin can occur in the published studies, and are not necessarily reflected in the regimens acronym. First-line studies with XELOX provided evidence that time to progression and median OS is comparable to continuous infusion 5-FU and oxaliplatin-containing regimens.[64,144,145] In the second-line setting, after progression on an irinotecan-containing regimen, XELOX is equivalent to FOLFOX4 in progression-free and overall survival.[153] While the occurrence of neuropathy and neutropenia are generally similar between XELOX and 5-FU-containing regimens, significantly more hand–foot syndrome occurs in patients undergoing treatment with XELOX.[64,144,145,153] Given clinical efficacy and general tolerability, oxaliplatin can be combined with either capecitabine or 5-FU and leucovorin in the management of patients with advanced colorectal cancer.

2.4 Oxaliplatin versus irinotecan

A comparison of FOLFOX4 with IFL found that patients treated with FOLFOX4 show a statistically significant improved response rate (45% vs. 31%), median time to tumor progression (8.7 vs. 6.9 months), and median OS (19.5 vs. 15.0 months).[122] In addition, there was increased toxicity with nausea, vomiting, diarrhea, and febrile neutropenia in the IFL arm compared to FOLFOX4, where only increased paresthesias were noted. Although the irinotecan-containing IFL regimen was shown to be inferior to the oxaliplatin-containing FOLFOX4 in this study, other studies have shown equivalent efficacy and suggest that toxicity related to dosing schedules may contribute to the differences in outcome. Notably, and in comparison, FOLFOX4 had similar response rate (31% vs. 34%), median time to progression (7.0 months), and median OS (14.0 months vs. 15.0 months) when compared to FOLFIRI.[157] Statistically significant differences in all grades of toxicity were noted for FOLFIRI, but not for grade 3/4 toxicity (except neurologic and thrombocytopenia for FOLFOX4).

Although direct comparisons between oxaliplatin- and irinotecan-comparing regimens are useful to aid in choosing a patient's first line of therapy, more prudent to the clinical decision-making is whether the order of therapy is of importance for a patient's long-term prognosis. One study found no statistically significant difference in median PFS or median OS when patients with metastatic colorectal cancer were treated with FOLFOX6 followed by FOLFIRI at progression or, conversely, FOLFIRI followed by FOLFOX6 at progression.[121] Recent data from CALGB/SWOG 80405 also suggests that FOLFIRI or mFOLFOX6 can be used in the first-line setting in combination with the biologics as outlined below.[158] Overall, either oxaliplatin or irinotecan in combination with continuous infusion 5-FU is a legitimate first-line treatment of metastatic colorectal cancer.

2.5 *Oxaliplatin and irinotecan combinations*

In vitro studies of SN38, the active metabolite of irinotecan, and oxaliplatin have demonstrated synergistic cytotoxicity in colorectal cell lines.[159] Several phase I and phase II studies also found that the combination of irinotecan and oxaliplatin was active and tolerable in patients with metastatic colorectal cancer who have failed treatment with 5-FU and leucovorin.[160–163] In N9741, a randomized phase III trial of first-line therapy, the combination of irinotecan and oxaliplatin (IROX) was compared to IFL and FOLFOX4. IROX was noted to have a higher response rate and longer median OS compared to IFL with no difference in time to progression. But, in comparison to FOLFOX4, the response rate and median time to progression were inferior for IROX.[122] Given a worse overall toxicity profile and lower efficacy, the combination of irinotecan and oxaliplatin has not been adopted as a treatment option for metastatic colorectal cancer.

With the clear benefit of doublet therapy with 5-FU/LV in combination with irinotecan or oxaliplatin as outlined above, the next logical hypothesis was that of further improvement in outcomes with triplet therapy. Two groups of investigators reported response rates of 58.1–72% in phase II studies combining two different dosing schedules of 5-FU and leucovorin, irinotecan, and oxaliplatin — both termed FOLFOXIRI — in the first-line management of metastatic colorectal cancer.[65,66] In phase III studies by the same two groups, however, the results are divergent. The Hellenic Oncology Research Group (HORG) performed a phase III study of FOLFOXIRI compared to FOLFIRI in untreated patients with metastatic colorectal cancer. In this study, the dosing and schedule of LV5FU2 as that same as that used in FOLFIRI group, and there was no statistically significant difference response rates (43% *vs.* 33.6%), median time to progression (8.4 *vs.* 6.9 months), or median OS (21.5 *vs.* 19.5months).[164] The Italian group, Gruppo Oncologico Nord Ovest

(GONO), similarly performed a phase III study of FOLFOXIRI with a simplified continuous infusion 5-FU backbone compared to the simplified FOLFIRI regimen. Their study, however, demonstrated a statistically significant improvement in response rate (60% *vs.* 34%), median PFS (9.8 *vs.* 6.9 months; HR 0.63), and median OS (22.6 *vs.* 16.7 months; HR 0.70).[165] Of note, the GONO study had a statistically significant improvement in patients undergoing secondary R0 resection of previously unresectable metastatic disease (15% *vs.* 6%), while the difference was not statistically significant in the HORG study (10% *vs.* 4%). There was also an increase in side effects with FOLFOXIRI compared to FOLFIRI, including neutropenia, neurotoxicity, diarrhea, and alopecia.

There were phase II/III studies tested the triplet cytotoxic regimens (with or without biological therapies) (Table 4). It seemed that the triplets increased the response rate and lead to benefits in PFS and OS in the phase III studies.[165,170]

3 Biologic Therapies

3.1 *VEGF inhibitors*

Angiogenesis is a complex and dynamic process regulated by a number of pro- and anti-angiogenic molecules, leading to neovascularization important for both tumor growth and metastatic dissemination. A key regulator of both physiologic and pathologic vascularization is the vascular endothelial growth factor (VEGF) family of proteins, six secreted glycoproteins that bind a number of different VEGF receptors on endothelial cells.[171] Stimulation of tumor angiogenesis by one of the secreted glycoproteins, VEGF-A, is thought to occur mainly through its interaction with one of the VEGF receptors, VEGFR-2.[172] Elevated levels of VEGF have been correlated with progression of colorectal cancer.[173,174] and preclinical studies have shown efficacy with anti-VEGF therapy both as single agents and in combination with cytotoxic chemotherapy. Several anti-VEGF therapies have shown activity in patients with metastatic colorectal cancer, including: bevacizumab, ziv-aflibercept, regorafenib, and ramucirumab (all clinic trials with anti-VEGF in combination were listed in Table 5).[184–194] Clinical studies of the multi-targeted tyrosine kinase inhibitors cedirinab and vatalanib, with activity against all of the VEGF receptors, however, failed to show significant efficacy in patients with metastatic colorectal cancer.[175–178]

3.1.1 *Bevacizumab*

Bevacizumab is a recombinant humanized monoclonal antibody directed against all isoforms of VEGF-A, a soluble growth factor that binds to both VEGFR-1 and

Table 4 Triplet cytotoxic regimens with and without biologic therapies.

Study	Phase	Regimens	Pt #	RR (%)	OR (p)	SD (%)	PFS (%)	HR (p)	mOS (m)	HR (p)
First line										
Falcone[166]	II	FOLFOXIRI	42	69	—	19	10.4	—	26.5	—
Souglakos[66]	II	FOLFOXIRI (HORG)	31	58.1	—	25.8	13	—	NR	—
Masi[65]	II	FOLFOXIRI (GONO)	32	72	—	22	10.8	—	28.4	—
HORG Souglakos[164]	III	FOLFOXIRI (HORG)	138	43.0	(0.168)	31.3	8.4	0.83 (0.17)	21.5	(0.337)
		FOLFIRI	147	33.6	—	26.7	6.9	—	19.5	—
GONO Falcone[165]	III	FOLFOXIRI (GONO)	122	60	(<0.0001)	21	9.8	0.63 (0.0006)	22.6	0.70 (0.032)
		sFOLFIRI	122	34	—	34	6.9	—	16.7	—
Masi[167]	II	FOLFOXIRI (GONO) + bevacizumab	57	77	—	23	13.1	—	30.9	—
Saridaki[168]	II	FOLFOXIRI (HORG) + cetuximab	30	70	—	26.7	10.2	—	30.3	—
Fornaro[169]	II	FOLFOXIRI (GONO) + panitumumab	37	89	—	8	11.3	—	NR	—
TRIBE[170]	III	FOLFOXIRI (GONO) + bevacizumab	252	65.1	1.64 (0.006)	24.6	12.1	0.75 (0.003)	25.8	0.79 (0.054)
		sFOLFIRI + bevacizumab	258	53.1	—	32.0	9.7	—	31.0	—

Table 5 Anti-VEGF therapy trials.

Study	Phase	Regimens	Pt #	RR (%)	OR (p)	SD (%)	PFS (%)	HR (p)	mOS (m)	HR (p)
First line										
AVF0780g[184]	II	5-FU/LV + LD bevacizumab	35	40	(0.029)	NR	9.0	0.46 (0.005)	21.5	0.63
		5-FU/LV	36	17	(0.434)	—	5.2	0.66 (0.217)	13.8	1.17
		5-FU/LV + HD bevacizumab	33	24	—	—	7.2	—	16.1	—
AVF2192g[185]	II	5-FU/LV (Roswell Park) + bevacizumab	104	26	(0.055)	NR	9.2	0.50 (.0002)	16.6	0.79 (0.16)
		5-FU/LV (Roswell Park)	105	15.2	—	—	5.5	—	12.9	—
AVF2107g[186]	III	IFL + bevacizumab	402	44.8	(0.004)	NR	10.6	0.54 (<.001)	20.3	0.66 (<0.001)
		IFL + placebo	411	34.8	—	—	6.2	—	15.6	—
BICC-C[53,111]	III	sFOLFIRI + bevacizumab	57	57.9	—	NR	11.2	(0.28)	28	1.79 (0.037)
		mIFL + bevacizumab	60	53.3	—	—	8.3	—	19.2	—
TREE-1, TREE-2[187]	II	mFOLFOX6	49	41	—	24	8.7	—	19.2	—
		mFOLFOX6 + bevacizumab	71	52	—	39	9.9	—	26.1	—
		bFOL	50	20	—	42	6.9	—	17.9	—
		bFOL + bevacizumab	70	39	—	37	8.3	—	20.4	—
		CapeOx	48	27	—	40	5.9	—	17.2	—
		CapeOx + bevacizumab	72	46	—	31	10.3	—	24.6	—
NO1696[188]	III	FOLFOX4 or XELOX + bevacizumab	700	38	1.00	NR	9.4	0.83 (.0023)	21.3	0.89 (.077)
		FOLFOX4 or XELOX + placebo	701	38	—	—	8.0	—	19.9	—
Garcia-Carbonero[189]	II	mFOLFOX6 + ramucirumab	48	58.3	—	35.5	11.5	—	20.4	—

(Continued)

Table 5   (*Continued*)

Study	Phase	Regimens	Pt #	RR (%)	OR (p)	SD (%)	PFS (%)	HR (p)	mOS (m)	HR (p)
Second line or beyond										
E3200[190]	III	FOLFOX4 + bevacizumab	286	22.7	—	NR	7.3	0.61	12.9	0.75
		FOLFOX4	291	8.6	—	—	4.7	—	10.8	—
		Bevacizumab	243	3.3	—	—	2.7	—	10.2	—
Tang[191]	II	Aflibercept 4 mg/kg Q2W (bevacizumab-naïve)	24	0	—	33.3	2.0	—	10.4	—
		Aflibercept 4 mg/kg Q2W (prior bevacizumab)	51	2		42	2.4	—	8.5	—
VELOUR[192]	III	sFOLFIRI + aflibercept	612	19.8	(<0.001)	65.9	6.9	0.76 (<0.0001)	13.5	0.82 (0.003)
		sFOLFIRI + placebo	614	11.1	—	64.9	4.7	—	12.1	—
CORRECT[193]	III	Regorafenib	505	1.0	(0.19)	40.0	1.9	0.49 (<0.0001)	6.4	0.77 (0.005)
		Placebo	255	0.4		14.6	1.7	—	5.0	—
RAISE[194]	III	sFOLFIRI + ramucirumab	536	13.4	(0.63)	60.6	5.7	0.793 (<0.0005)	13.3	0.84 (0.022)
		sFOLFIRI + placebo	536	12.5	—	56.3	4.5	—	11.7	—

VEGFR-2. In addition to the anti-angiogenic effects of bevacizumab, preclinical studies suggest that bevacizumab may decrease the elevated interstitial pressure within the tumor by normalizing the tumor vasculature structure and function and thus aid in the delivery of chemotherapy to the tumor.[179,180] Furthermore, colorectal cancer tumor cells express VEGFR-1, the activation of which leads to invasion and migration of tumor cells, including triggering of the epithelial to mesenchymal transition, and thus blocking activation of VEGFR-1 with bevacizumab is proposed to also have a potential direct effect on tumor cell function.[181,182] Furthermore, bevacizumab may play a role in immunomodulation by blocking the VEGF-A-mediated inhibition of dendritic cell maturation, inhibition of T cell development and cytotoxic activity, and infiltration of regulatory T cells into the tumor microenvironment.[183]

Phase II studies of bevacizumab (5 mg/m^2) in combination with bolus 5-FU and leucovorin (Roswell Park regimen) provided evidence for statistically significant superior response rates and median time to progression when compared to bolus 5-FU and leucovorin alone in previously untreated patients.[184,185] In both studies, while there was an improvement in OS with bevacizumab (HR 0.63 and 0.79, respectively), this difference was not statistically significant.

The first randomized, placebo controlled, phase III trial (AFV2017g) of bevacizumab evaluated it in combination with IFL and found a significant improvement in response rate, median PFS (HR 0.54), and median OS (HR 0.66) when compared to IFL alone.[186] In addition, the second phase of the BICC-C study (described above) also found the addition of bevacizumab to FOLFIRI resulted in an improvement in median OS compared to IFL (HR 1.79) with no statistically significant difference in response rate or median progression free survival.[111] With these findings, the continuous infusion schedule of 5-FU became the preferred irinotecan-containing regimen to be combined with bevacizumab.

Given that FOLFOX4 is to be superior to IFL in the first-line setting,[122] bevacizumab was evaluated in combination with several oxaliplatin-containing regimens. In the randomized phase II study, TREE-2, which evaluated mFOLFOX6, bFOL, and CapeOx in combination with bevacizumab, the reported response rates, median progression-free survival, and median OS were higher than those reported in TREE-1, a study that looked at mFOLFOX6, bFOL, and CapeOx alone. There were no statistical analyses comparing the bevacizumab cohort to the chemotherapy-alone cohort because the study was not designed initially to examine this difference.[187] In a separate phase III study, NO16966, the addition of bevacizumab to FOLFOX4 or CapeOx was evaluated in patients with previously untreated metastatic colorectal cancer. The addition of bevacizumab to FOLFOX4 or CapeOx resulted in a modest improvement in median progression free survival (HR 0.83), but no improvement in response rate or median overall survival. Subset analyses found an improvement in median PFS in patients treated with CapeOx and bevacizumab compared to CapeOx and placebo, but there was no difference in median OS in the group nor a difference in median progression-free and OS with the addition of bevacizumab to FOLFOX4.[188] The inconsistency in the addition of bevacizumab to the oxaliplatin-containing regimens in NO16966, where no OS benefit was noted, and irinotecan-containing regimens in AVF2107g and BICC-C remains a topic of debate. The authors suggest that a shortened duration of treatment may explain the difference in effect: patients in NO16966 received 27.1 weeks of oxaliplatin-containing regimen and bevacizumab,[188] whereas patients in the AVF2107g study received a median 40.4 weeks of IFL/bevacizumab therapy.[186] Furthermore, 71% of patients in NO16966 treated with bevacizumab discontinued bevacizumab prior to disease progression, as reflected in the differences in general (9.4 months) and on-treatment PFS (10.4 months), a difference that might be due to toxicity associated with the chemotherapy rather than the bevacizumab.[188,195]

Given improved efficacy with FOLFOXIRI as compared to FOLFIRI, the Italian GONO group performed the first-line phase III TRIBE study comparing 12 cycles of induction chemotherapy with FOLFOXIRI (GONO) and bevacizumab with simplified FOLFIRI and bevacizumab after a 77% response rate was seen with a five-drug regimen in a phase II study.[167] In the TRIBE study, treatment with the five-drug regimen led to a statistically significant improvement in response rate (65.1% *vs.* 53.1%) and median progression free survival (12.1 *vs.* 9.7 months; HR 0.75) but no difference in median OS compared to simplified FOLFIRI and bevacizumab. There was also no statistically significant difference in rates of R0 resection of metastatic lesions. Grade 3/4 neurotoxicity, stomatitis, diarrhea, and neutropenia were significantly higher in the FOLFOXIRI/bevacizumab arm.[170]

While there may have been debate on the role of bevacizumab in combination with oxaliplatin-containing regimens in chemotherapy-naïve metastatic colorectal cancer patients, the metastatic colorectal cancer patients who have progressed on an irinotecan-containing regimen who have not received prior bevacizumab benefited from the addition of high dose bevacizumab to FOLFOX4 in the ECOG study E3200. The combination of bevacizumab to FOLFOX4 improved response rates, median progression-free survival, and median OS compared to FOLFOX4 alone (PFS HR 0.61; OS HR 0.75) and to single-agent bevacizumab (which was determined to be inactive as a single agent).[190] Given that bevacizumab is commonly given in the first-line setting, this study does not answer the question as to whether continuing bevacizumab in the second-line setting despite progression on a bevacizumab-containing regimen is beneficial. This question, however, is addressed in other studies as discussed below.

Several meta-analyses have been completed on the trials outlined above. Overall, there is a significant improvement in median PFS and median OS when bevacizumab is combined with chemotherapy compared to chemotherapy alone or with a placebo in each of the three meta-analyses.[196–198] In addition, consistent with the findings in the individual studies discussed above, the incidence of grade 3 or 4 gastrointestinal perforation (OR 4.81), hypertension (OR 4.19), bleeding (OR 1.87), and thrombotic events (OR 1.75) were statistically increased in the bevacizumab-containing regimens.[197] Of note, however, the actual incidence of these side effects is relatively low. Given the tolerability and efficacy of bevacizumab in combination with both irinotecan- and oxaliplatin-containing regimens, bevacizumab is commonly used in the management of patients with metastatic colorectal cancer.

3.1.1.1 Bevacizumab after progression

Given the demonstrated benefit for combining bevacizumab with chemotherapy in both the treatment naïve and previously treated patients with metastatic colorectal cancer, the continuation of bevacizumab into the second-line setting at the time of first progression on a bevacizumab-containing regimens became of interest. Two prospective but observational cohort series found that the continuation of bevacizumab beyond first progression suggested a post-progression survival benefit compared to chemotherapy without bevacizumab: 19.2 months *vs.* 9.5 months (HR 0.48) in the BRiTE study[199] and 14.4 months *vs.* 10.6 months (HR 0.84) in the ARIES study.[200] A retrospective analysis also demonstrated similar results, with a 14.6-month post-progression median survival with continuing bevacizumab post-progression compared to 10.1 months in the chemotherapy alone post-progression cohort (HR 0.74).[201] Two RCTs confirmed a survival benefit for continuing bevacizumab beyond progression. The ML18147 study found an 11.2-month survival post-progression in the bevacizumab and chemotherapy group, whereas the chemotherapy alone group post-progression had a 9.8-month median survival (HR 0.81).[202] The BEBYP study, while closed early because of the results of the ML18147 study, found a 14.1-month survival post-progression compared to 15.5 months in the chemotherapy-alone arm. While the median post-progression survival is higher in the non-bevacizumab containing arm, the HR for post-progression survival favors the bevacizumab containing arm because of crossing survival curves.[203] Overall, the data support the continuation of bevacizumab post-progression on a bevacizumab-containing regimen.

3.1.2 *Aflibercept*

Aflibercept, also known as ziv-aflibercept or VEGF-trap, is a recombinant decoy fusion protein containing the second immunoglobulin domain of VEGFR-1 and the third immunoglobulin domain of VEGFR-2, fused to the constant region of a human IgG1 backbone. In contrast to the VEGF-A binding properties of bevacizumab, aflibercept binds to VEGF-A with higher affinity as well as to VEGF-B and placental growth factor, preventing the binding of these ligands to endogenous VEGF receptors.[204] Preclinical evidence suggests that aflibercept suppresses tumor growth a vascularization *in vivo* both alone[205] and in combination with chemotherapy such as 5-FU and irinotecan.[204]

A phase II study of single agent aflibercept in previously treated patients with metastatic colorectal cancer demonstrated modest activity. In patients with prior bevacizumab exposure, there was a 2% response rate, 2.4-month median PFS, and 8.5-month median OS. In those who had not received prior bevacizumab, none responded to aflibercept and there was a two-month median PFS and a 10.4-month median OS.[191] The pivotal, placebo-controlled, randomized phase III VELOUR trial compared patients with metastatic colorectal cancer who had progressed on a prior oxaliplatin-containing regimen, with or without bevacizumab, treated with simplified FOLFIRI with or without aflibercept. The addition of aflibercept led to a statistically significant improved response rate, median PFS (HR 0.76), and median OS (HR 0.82). In a planned subset analysis of the 30.4% of patients who had received prior bevacizumab, there was a statistically significant improvement in progression free survival (HR 0.66), but only a trend toward improvement in OS (HR 0.86) with the addition of aflibercept to simplified FOLFIRI. In the aflibercept treated group, there was an increase in grade 3 or 4 hypertension, hemorrhage, and arterial and venous thromboembolic events, although aside from the 19.3% incidence of grade 3 or 4 hypertension with aflibercept, the other side effects occurred in fewer than 10% of patients.[192] The results of this study led to the approval of aflibercept in combination with FOLFIRI for the treatment of patients with metastatic colorectal cancer following progression on an oxaliplatin-containing chemotherapy regimen.

3.1.3 *Ramucirumab*

In contrast to the ligand binding of both bevacizumab (VEGF-A) and aflibercept (VEGFA and VEGFB), ramucirumab is a human IgG-1 monoclonal antibody that targets the extracellular domain of VEGFR-2, preventing the binding of ligands such as VEGF-A.[206] In colorectal xenografts, ramucirumab inhibited angiogenesis and increased endothelial cell death.[207] Ramucirumab was approved by the FDA as second-line treatment for metastatic colorectal cancer in combination with FOLFIRI following the results of RAISE, a randomized, placebo-controlled, phase III study of sFOLFIRI with or without ramucirumab in patients who had progressed on a fluoropyrimidine, oxaliplatin, and bevacizumab regimen in the first line. There was prolonged PFS (5.7 months) and OS (13.3 months) for the ramucirumab-treated group compared to sFOLFIRI with placebo (4.5 months and 11.7 months, respectively). The adverse events associated with the addition of ramucirumab is consistent with other VEGF inhibitors, notably hypertension, proteinuria, and the incidence of thromboembolic events was low in both arms.[194] In addition to this phase III study, a phase II study of ramucirumab in combination with mFOLFOX6 has shown significant efficacy in first-line treatment of metastatic colorectal cancer, with response rates and PFS comparable with prior first-line studies of anti-VEGF therapies.[189] Without further evidence to support its use in combination with oxaliplatin-containing regimens and in the first-line setting, however, ramucirumab should be confined to use in the second line in combination with FOLFIRI.

3.1.4 *Regorefenib*

Regorafenib is a multikinase inhibitor that targets the angiogenic kinases found in VEGFR-1, VEGFR-2, VEGFR-3, PDGFR, FGFR-1, and TIE2 as well as the oncogenic kinases KIT, RET, RAF1, and BRAF. It has demonstrated potent anti-angiogenic activity in colorectal cancer xenografts.[208] After a 3.7% response rate and 70.4% stable disease rate was seen in an expanded cohort phase I study of regorafenib in patients with metastatic colorectal cancer, the phase III CORRECT study was designed comparing regorafenib to placebo in previously treated patients with metastatic colorectal cancer. Compared to placebo, the group treated with regorafenib experienced a statistically significant improvement in a median PFS (HR 0.49) and median OS (HR 0.77). The overall survival benefit was 1.4 months (6.4 months *vs*, 5.0 months). This benefit came at a cost of added side effects, including grade 3 or 4 hand–foot syndrome (17%), fatigue (7%), diarrhea (7%), hypertension (7%), and rash or desquamation (6%). Seventy-six percent of patients required a dose reduction of regorafenib, mostly due to side effects.[193] Given the improvement in median OS, regorafenib was approved by the FDA for use in patients with metastatic colorectal cancer who have progressed on other lines of therapy.

3.2 *EGFR inhibitors*

The epidermal growth factor receptor (EGFR) is a member of the ErbB tyrosine kinase receptor family whose gene expression is upregulated in colorectal cancer[209,210] and is associated with poorer prognosis.[211,212] Upon binding of ligands such as epidermal growth factor or TGF-α, the receptors homo- or hetero-dimerize, activating their intrinsic tyrosine kinase activity to autophosphorylate the receptor. This recruits and activates soluble factors within a cell to propagate downstream signaling pathways necessary for cellular proliferation, differentiation, migration, angiogenesis, and apoptosis, including but not limited to the RAS-RAF-MAPK, and PI3K-AKT-mTOR pathways.[213,214] Given the increased EGFR gene expression and association between poor prognosis and EGFR expression, targeting EGFR is an attractive treatment strategy. Currently, there are two FDA-approved anti-EGFR antibodies approved for the management of patients with metastatic colorectal cancer: cetuximab and panitumumab; the benefit of which is discussed in detail below. In the course of the development of these drugs, however, it was noted that patients with mutations in the EGFR-mediated MAPK pathway might respond differently to EGFR inhibitors, and so we will first discuss the *KRAS* and *BR AF* genes and their prognostic and potential therapeutic role in the management of patients with metastatic colorectal cancer. Table 6 lists all key studies with EGFR inhibitor.

3.2.1 *EGFR pathway mutations*

3.2.1.1 RAS mutations

The most important development in the use of anti-EGFR therapy is the recognition that these agents are active in colorectal cancers that do not harbor a mutation in the RAS proteins (referred to as "RAS wild type"). The RAS family of GTPase proteins, including KRAS, NRAS, and HRAS, are critical downstream effectors in the mitogen-activated protein kinase (MAPK) pathway that mediates transduction of activation signals from EGFR to intracellular signaling cascades. Point mutations within RAS proteins, most commonly KRAS, lead to constitutive activation of the MAPK pathway and thus oncogenesis in colorectal cancer development. Mutations in exon 2 of *KRAS* are the most common RAS mutations seen in advanced colorectal cancer, occurring in 37–45% of patients.[215–219] Other *KRAS* mutations in exon 3 are seen in 3.3–5.5% and exon 4 in 5.7-7.9% of patients. Mutations in *NRAS* are less common, with 3.0–4.8% with exon 2 mutations, 3.4–6.8% exon 3 mutations, and 0.1–1.2% exon 4 mutations. Overall, *RAS* mutations occur in about 53% of advanced colorectal cancer patients.[220]

Given that point mutations in the RAS proteins lead to constitutive activation of the MAPK pathway regardless of EGFR activation, it stands to reason that *RAS* mutant tumors would not be susceptible to EGFR inhibition. Although the first studies of anti-EGFR therapy did not select patients on RAS status, retrospective analyses of phase III studies of cetuximab and panitumumab compared to best supportive care observed a difference in response rate, PFS and OS were only in patients without a mutation in *KRAS* exon 2 codons 12 or 13.[218,219] While initial retrospective and *in vitro* studies suggested that, unlike *KRAS* codon 12 mutations, *KRAS* codon 13 (G13D) mutations responded to cetuximab therapy similar to *KRAS*

Table 6 Anti EGFR therapy trials.

Study	Phase	Regimens	Pt #	RR (%)	OR (p)	SD (%)	PFS (%)	HR (p)	mOS (m)	HR (p)
First line										
OPUS[215,225,242]	II	**All comers**								
		FOLFOX4 + cetuximab	169	46	1.52 (0.06)	45	7.2	0.93 (0.615)	18.3	1.02 (0.91)
		FOLFOX4	168	36	—	40	7.2	—	18.0	—
		KRAS WT								
		FOLFOX4 + cetuximab	82	57	—	29	8.3	0.57 (0.0064)	22.8	0.86 (0.39)
		FOLFOX4	97	34	—	43	7.2	—	18.5	—
		KRAS mutant								
		FOLFOX4 + cetuximab	77	34	—	47	5.5	1.72 (0.015)	13.4	1.29 (0.20)
		FOLFOX4	59	53	—	36	8.6	—	17.5	—
		KRAS/BRAF WT								
		FOLFOX4 + cetuximab	72	60	—	28	8.3	0.56 (0.0083)	22.8	0.89 (0.56)
		FOLFOX4	92	36	—	45	7.2	—	19.5	—
		Extended RAS mutation								
		FOLFOX4 + cetuximab	92	37.0	0.58 (0.087)	NR	5.6	1.54 (0.031)	13.5	1.29 (0.16)
		FOLFOX4	75	50.7	—	—	7.8	—	17.8	—
		Extended RAS WT								
		FOLFOX4 + cetuximab	38	57.9	3.33 (.008)	NR	12.0	0.53 (0.062)	19.8	0.94 (0.80)
		FOLFOX4	49	28.6	—	—	5.8	—	17.8	—

(Continued)

Table 6 (*Continued*)

Study	Phase	Regimens	Pt #	RR (%)	OR (p)	SD (%)	PFS (%)	HR (p)	mOS (m)	HR (p)
CRYSTAL[216,226,244]	III	**All comers**								
		FOLFIRI + cetuximab	599	46.9	1.40	37.4	8.9	0.851	19.9	0.878
		FOLFIRI	599	38.7	—	46.7	8.0	—	18.6	—
		KRAS WT								
		FOLFIRI + cetuximab	316	57.3	2.069	31.6	9.9	0.696	23.5	0.796
		FOLFIRI	350	39.7	—	46.3	8.4	—	20.0	—
		KRAS mutant								
		FOLFIRI + cetuximab	214	36.1	0.822	47.2	7.4	1.171	16.2	1.035
		FOLFIRI	183	31.3	—	45.9	7.7	—	16.7	—
		Extended *RAS WT*								
		FOLFIRI + cetuximab	178	66.3	3.11 (<0.001)	27.0	11.4	0.56 (<0.001)	28.4	0.69 (0.002)
		FOLFIRI	179	38.6	—	47.6	8.4	—	20.2	—
		Extended *RAS mutant*								
		FOLFIRI + cetuximab	246	31.7	0.85 (0.40)	47.2	7.4	1.10 (0.47)	16.4	1.05 (0.64)
		FOLFIRI	214	36.0	—	47.2	7.5	—	17.7	—
PRIME[217,245]	III	**All comers**								
		FOLFOX4 + panitumumab	593	NR	NR	NR	NR	NR	NR	NR
		FOLFOX4	590	—	—	—	—	—	—	—
		KRAS WT								
		FOLFOX4 + panitumumab	325	55	1.35	NR	9.6	0.80	23.9	0.83
		FOLFOX4	331	48	—	—	8.0	—	19.7	—

(*Continued*)

Table 6　(*Continued*)

Study	Phase	Regimens	Pt #	RR (%)	OR (p)	SD (%)	PFS (%)	HR (p)	mOS (m)	HR (p)
		KRAS mutant								
		FOLFOX4 + panitumumab	221	40	NR	NR	7.3	1.29	15.5	1.24
		FOLFOX4	219	40			8.8	—	19.3	—
		Extended RAS/BRAF WT								
		FOLFOX4 + panitumumab	228	NR	—	NR	10.8	0.68 (0.002)	28.3	0.74 (0.02)
		FOLFOX4	218	—	—		9.2	—	20.9	—
		Extended RAS/BRAF mutant								
		FOLFOX4 + panitumumab	296	NR	NR	NR	7.3	1.24 (0.03)	15.3	1.21 (0.06)
		FOLFOX4	305	—	—	—	8.0	—	18.0	—
			—	—	—	—	—	—	—	—
MRC COIN[229]	III	**All comers**								
		XELOX/mFOLFOX6 + cetuximab	815	NR	NR	NR	7.9	0.98	15.3	1.01
		XELOX/mFOLFOX6	815	—	—	—	8.1	—	15.8	—
			—	—	—	—	—	—	—	—
		KRAS WT								
		XELOX/mFOLFOX6 + cetuximab	367	64	1.35	NR	8.6	0.96	17.9	1.04
		XELOX/mFOLFOX6	362	57	—	—	8.6	—	17.0	—
			—	—	—	—	—	—	—	—
		KRAS mutant								
		XELOX/mFOLFOX6 + cetuximab	268	NR	—	NR	NR	—	14.8	0.98
		XELOX/mFOLFOX6	297	—	—	—	—	—	13.6	—
			—	—	—	—	—	—	—	—

(*Continued*)

Table 6 (*Continued*)

Study	Phase	Regimens	Pt #	RR (%)	OR (p)	SD (%)	PFS (%)	HR (p)	mOS (m)	HR (p)
		All WT (*NRAS, BRAF, KRAS*)								
		XELOX/mFOLFOX6 + cetuximab	NR	NR	NR	NR	NR	NR	20.1	1.02
		XELOX/mFOLFOX6	—	—	—	—	—	—	19.9	—
NORDIC-VII[243]	III	**All comers**							—	
		cNordic FLOX + cetuximab	194	49	1.35	NR	8.3	0.89	19.7	1.06
		Continuous NORDIC FLOX	185	41	—	—	7.9	—	20.4	—
		***KRAS* WT**								
		cNordic FLOX + cetuximab	97	46	0.96	—	7.9	1.07	20.1	1.14
		Continuous NORDIC FLOX	97	47	—	—	8.7	—	22.0	—
		***KRAS* mutant**								
		cNordic FLOX + cetuximab	72	49	1.44	—	9.2	0.71	21.1	1.03
		Continuous NORDIC FLOX	58	40	—	—	7.8	—	20.4	—
Second line or beyond										
Cunningham[240]	III	Cetuximab monotherapy	111	10.8	—	21.6	1.5	0.54	6.9	0.91
		Cetuximab + irinotecan	218	22.9	—	32.6	4.1	—	8.6	—
NCIC CTG CO.17237	III	Cetuximab + BSC	287	8	—	31.4	NR	0.68	6.1	0.77
		Best supportive care	285	0	—	10.9	NR	—	4.6	—
2002048[218,246]	III	**All comers**								
		Panitumumab + BSC	231	10	—	27	1.9	0.54	NR	1.00
		Best supportive care	232	0	—	10	1.7	—	NR	—

(*Continued*)

Table 6   (*Continued*)

Study	Phase	Regimens	Pt #	RR (%)	OR (p)	SD (%)	PFS (%)	HR (p)	mOS (m)	HR (p)
		KRAS WT								
		Panitumumab + BSC	124	17	—	34	2.8	0.45	NR	0.99
		Best Supportive Care	119	0	—	12	1.7	—	NR	—
		KRAS mutant								
		Panitumumab + BSC	84	0	NR	12	1.7	0.99	NR	1.02
		Best Supportive Care	100	0	—	8	1.7	—	NR	—
Karapetis[219]	III	*KRAS WT*								
		Cetuximab	117	12.8	NR	—	3.7	0.40	9.5	0.55
		Best supportive care	113	0	—	—	1.9	—	4.8	—
		KRAS mutant								
		Cetuximab	81	1.2	NR	NR	1.8	0.99	4.5	0.98
		Best supportive care	83	0	—	—	1.8	—	4.6	—
Sobrero[241]	III	*All comers*								
		Irinotecan + cetuximab	648	16.44.2	NR	45.1	4.0	0.692	10.7	0.975
		Irinotecan 350 mg/m^2 Q3W	650	—	—	41.7	2.6	—	10	—
20050181[247,248]	III	*KRAS mutant*								
		FOLFIRI + panitumumab	238	13.4	NR	55	5.3	0.94 (0.56)	11.8	0.93 (0.48)
		FOLFIRI	248	14.8	—	48	4.4	—	11.1	—
		KRAS WT								
		FOLFIRI + panitumumab	303	36	NR	38	6.7	0.82 (0.023)	14.5	0.92 (0.37)
		FOLFIRI	294	9.8	—	55	4.9	—	12.5	—

(*Continued*)

Table 6 (*Continued*)

Study	Phase	Regimens	Pt #	RR (%)	OR (p)	SD (%)	PFS (%)	HR (p)	mOS (m)	HR (p)
		Extended *RAS* mutant								
		FOLFIRI + panitumumab	299	NR	NR	NR	4.8	0.861 (0.144)	11.8	0.91 (.345)
		FOLFIRI	294	—	—	—	4.0	—	11.1	—
		Extended *RAS* WT								
		FOLFIRI + panitumumab	204	NR	NR	NR	6.4	0.695 (0.006)	16.2	0.803 (0.077)
		FOLFIRI	211	—	—	—	4.4	—	13.9	—
PICCOLO [230]	III	***KRAS* WT**								
		Irinotecan + panitumumab	230	34	4.12	24	NR	0.78	10.9	1.01
		Irinotecan	230	12	—	40	—	—	10.4	—
		Extended *RAS/BRAF/ PIK3CA* mutant								
		Irinotecan + panitumumab	70	12.9	NR	NR	NR	NR	NR	NR
		Irinotecan	67	10.4	—	—	—	—	—	—
		Extended *RAS/BRAF/ PIK3CA* WT								
		Irinotecan + panitumumab	160	43.8	NR	NR	NR	0.68	NR	0.92
		Irinotecan	163	12.3	—	—	—	—	—	—

wild-type tumors,[221,222] other studies showed that patients with *KRAS* G13D mutations do not respond to either cetuximab or panitumumab.[223,224] Furthermore, it was noted that not all *KRAS* exon 2 wild-type patients responded to anti-EGFR therapy. Retrospective analyses looking at other *RAS* mutations — termed new, extended, or expanded *RAS* mutations — found that patients who harbored other *KRAS* mutations codons 59 and 61 (exon 3) and codons 117 and 146 (exon 4) and *NRAS* codons 12 and 13 (exon 2), codons 59 and 61 (exon 3), or codons 117 and 146 (exon 4) mutations also did not respond to anti-EGFR therapy.[217,225,226] Although the sensitivity of both *KRAS* G13D mutations and extended *RAS* mutation analysis has not been evaluated in a prospective manner, it is recommended that all patients with metastatic colorectal cancer have their tumors, either a primary or metastatic lesion, be genomically tested for the presence of a *KRAS* or *NRAS* mutation prior to starting an anti-EGFR antibody.

3.2.1.2 BRAF mutations

BRAF is a serine-threonine kinase downstream of the RAS protein in the EGFR-mediated MAPK signaling pathway. Similar to RAS, constitutive activation of the MAPK pathway can occur with point mutations of the *BRAF* gene, notably within the activation segment at codon 600. *BRAF* V600E mutations are seen in 5–8% of colorectal cancers. Interestingly, *BRAF* mutant colorectal cancers appear to have a distinct phenotype, with a more aggressive appearing histology arising from serrated adenomas, occurring mostly on the right side of the colon and more often in women. *BRAF* V600E mutations are also associated with defective mismatch repair. Furthermore, patients with colorectal cancers harboring *BRAF* V600E mutations are associated with chemotherapy resistance and have a comparatively worse overall prognosis.[227,228]

While retrospective analysis from some trials of anti-EGFR inhibition suggest that EGFR therapy in *BRAF* mutant tumors is not efficacious,[229,230] debate continues as to whether *BRAF* mutation is in fact a negative predictive factor to EGFR-directed therapy.[216] In all studies with EGFR antibody therapy, however, no patients with a *BRAF* mutation had an objective response.[231] A meta-analysis of *BRAF* mutant patients in trials of either cetuximab or panitumumab suggested that, while patients with *BRAF* mutations had a worse OS compared to *BRAF* wild-type tumors, the observed difference in the effect of the anti-EGFR therapy on OS according to *BRAF* mutation was not statistically significant.[232]

Furthermore, drugs designed to target *BRAF* V600E mutations are ineffective when used as single agents against *BRAF* mutant colorectal cancers.[233] Given preclinical evidence suggesting that BRAF inhibitor resistance in *BRAF* mutant colorectal cancer cells is driven by upregulation of EGFR,[234,235] current clinical trials are examining combinations of EGFR and BRAF inhibitors. Until these data are mature, however, the role of anti-EGFR therapy in *BRAF* mutant colorectal cancers is unclear.

3.2.2 *Cetuximab*

Cetuximab is a mouse/human chimeric IgG1 monoclonal antibody that binds with high affinity to the extracellular domain of EGFR, causing decreased EGFR downstream signaling by competitive binding with endogenous ligands and downregulation of EGFR. It is dosed as 400 mg/m^2 on week 1, followed by 250 mg/m^2 weekly for subsequent doses.

An initial phase II study of single agent weekly cetuximab found a 9% response rate and 37% stable disease rate in pretreated patients with metastatic colorectal cancer.[236] When compared to best supportive care, the combination of weekly cetuximab with best supportive care in an unselected, pretreated population of patients with metastatic colorectal cancer improved response rate, time to progression, and median OS.[237] The benefit of cetuximab was even more pronounced in a retrospective analysis of *KRAS* exon 2 mutation analysis was completed on 69% of tumor tissues from patients in this study, with an even more pronounced improvement in response rate, median time to progression, and median OS in patients without *KRAS* exon 2 mutations treated with cetuximab compared to best supportive care. There was no difference between groups in patients whose tumors harbored a *KRAS* exon 2 mutation.[219]

Given the preclinical and clinical evidence of increased activity when cetuximab is combined with cytotoxic chemotherapy,[238,239] a combination of irinotecan and cetuximab was compared with cetuximab alone in unselected patients who had progressed on prior irinotecan. The combination resulted in a statistically significant improved response rate and time to progression but no significant difference in median OS.[240] An additional phase III study, EPIC, compared the combination of cetuximab and irinotecan to irinotecan alone in an unselected population of patients who had progressed through a first-line oxaliplatin-containing regimen. The addition of cetuximab to irinotecan significantly increased the response rate and median PFS, but there was no difference in the median OS, potentially confounded by the fact that 47% of patients who did not receive cetuximab on study received cetuximab after progression on study.[241] The effect of *RAS* mutation in the EPIC study is limited by the fact that *KRAS* was only assessable in 23% of the population treated.

In the first-line setting, the combination of cetuximab with both irinotecan- and oxaliplatin-containing regimens has been explored. Three major phase II or III studies examined cetuximab in combination with oxaliplatin-containing regimens:

OPUS evaluated FOLFOX4 with cetuximab versus FOLFOX4 alone,[242] MRC COIN evaluated mFOLFOX6 or XELOX with and without cetuximab,[229] and NORDIC-VII evaluated cetuximab in combination with continuous or intermittent NORDIC FLOX in comparison to continuous NORDIC FLOX.[243] In an unselected population, all three studies there was no difference in response rate, PFS, and median OS. On retrospective analysis for *KRAS* exon 2 mutation, however, mixed results were seen among the studies. In the phase II OPUS study, an initial subgroup analysis on 68% of the patients for *KRAS* exon 2 mutations found that patients with wild-type *KRAS* had an improved response rate and median PFS (HR 0.57).[242] When 93% of samples were analyzed for *KRAS* exon 2 mutation as well as *BRAF* mutations, those wild type for both continued to have an improved response rate and PFS (HR 0.56), but no difference in median OS (HR 0.89).[215] In the phase III studies MRC COIN and NORDIC-VII, however, 81% and 88% of patients had *KRAS* exon 2 mutation testing performed, respectively, and in those who were *KRAS* exon 2 wild type did not show a difference PFS (HR 0.96 and 1.07, respectively), or OS (HR 1.04 and 1.14, respectively), although there was an improved response rate in the MRC COIN study (OR 1.35).[229,243] Further genomic analysis for expanded *RAS* were done on 66% of patients from the OPUS study and a limited extended *RAS* (*KRAS* codon 12, 13, 61; *NRAS* codon 12, 61; and *BRAF* codon 600) on 81% of patients in the MRC COIN study. In OPUS, 74% of patients had an all-wild-type phenotype, and cetuximab therapy was associated with an improved response rate (OR 3.33) and PFS (HR 0.53) but no significant difference in OS (0.94).[225] In MRC COIN, there was no difference in OS when patients with all-wild-type genotype were treated with cetuximab (HR 1.02).[229]

In the CRYSTAL study, the addition of cetuximab to simplified FOLFIRI was compared to simplified FOLFIRI alone in a phase III, first-line setting. In an unselected population, there was a statistically significant improvement in response rate and PFS, but no difference in median OS.[244] When 89% of patient's tumor tissue was analyzed for presence of a *KRAS* exon 2 mutation, 37% of the samples contained a mutation. In patients who were *KRAS* exon 2 wild type, the addition of cetuximab to FOLFIRI improved the response rate (OR 2.1), PFS (HR 0.7), and median OS (HR 0.8).[216] The improvement in response rate, PFS, and median OS was even more pronounced when 65% of tumor tissues were assessed for extended *RAS* mutations, with an OR of 3.1, and HR of 0.56 and 0.69, respectively, in the all *RAS* wild-type population.[226]

Cetuximab has also been added to the FOLFOXIRI regimen. A phase II study of FOLFOXIRI (HORG) and cetuximab demonstrated a 70% response rate, 10.2-month PFS, and 30.3-month median OS. Toxicity included diarrhea, anemia, neutropenia, stomatitis, and fatigue.[168] Similar results were seen in a phase II study of FOLFOXIRI (GONO) with panitumumab, although the dose of irinotecan and continuous infusion 5-FU were decreased as a result of significant diarrhea with the combination.[169] Phase III studies of FOLFOXIRI and anti-EGFR therapy have not been completed.

3.2.3 *Panitumumab*

Panitumumab is a fully humanized IgG2 monoclonal antibody that binds with high affinity to the extracellular domain of EGFR, causing decreased EGFR downstream signaling by competitive binding with endogenous ligands and downregulation of EGFR. Compared to cetuximab, panitumumab has a longer half-life, allowing for dosing at 6 mg/kg every two weeks as opposed to weekly dosing with cetuximab. In addition, that it is a fully humanized antibody, the rate of infusion reactions is decreased, as is the development of neutralizing antibodies.

Similar to cetuximab, single-agent panitumumab resulting in an improvement in response rate and PFS in an unselected, chemotherapy-refractory population compared to best supportive care, but there was no difference in OS (study 2002048). This may have partially been related to 76% of the patients in the best supportive care arm receiving panitumumab at progression.[246] In the 92% of patients' tumor samples that could undergo *KRAS* exon 2 genomic analysis, a more dramatic improvement in response rate and PFS was noted in the *KRAS* wild-type population, but again the OS was no different.[218] Also in the chemotherapy-refractory setting, the combination of panitumumab and simplified FOLFIRI was compared to panitumumab alone (20050181)[247,248] and panitumumab in combination with irinotecan was compared irinotecan alone (PICCOLO).[230] In both studies, genomic testing for *KRAS* was done in a prospective manner, but while 20050181 selected for codons 12 and 13, PICCOLO selected codons 12, 13, and 61. Still, both studies found an improvement in response rate and PFS, but no difference in OS. The same trend was seen in both studies in tumors that were wild type for all *RAS* genes, although the PICCOLO study also included wild-type *PIK3CA* and *BRAF* in its analysis.[230,249]

In the PRIME study in the first-line setting, panitumumab was evaluated on combination with FOLFOX4 compared to FOLFOX4. Patients who were *KRAS* exon 2 wild type had a statistically significant improvement in PFS (HR 0.80), but only a trend toward improvement in response rate and median OS.[245] When accounting for the other *RAS* mutations as well as *BRAF* mutations, patients who were wild type for all mutations had an improvement in both PFS (0.68) and OS (0.02).[217]

In addition to individual studies showing the efficacy of cetuximab and pantiumumab in the treatment of *RAS* wild-type patients, the phase III ASPECCT trial compared cetuximab to panitumumab in chemotherapy-refractory *KRAS* exon 2 wild-type patients, and panitumumab was found to be non-inferior to cetuximab with respect to median overall survival with similar incidence of adverse events.[250] This suggests that either of these anti-EGFR therapies can be used in the treatment of metastatic colorectal cancer.

3.3 Biologic combinations

Preclinical studies suggest that a combination of EGFR and VEGF antibodies increases anti-tumor activity.[251–254] Despite phase II evidence showing safety and suggesting a benefit to combining cetuximab and bevacizumab in irinotecan-refractory patients,[255] two phase III studies suggest that the combination of anti-EGFR and anti-VEGF therapy leads to worse overall outcomes.[256,257] In PACCE, chemotherapy-naïve patients receiving panitumumab in combination with either an oxaliplatin- or irinotecan-containing regimen with bevacizumab had a worse PFS and median OS compared to either chemotherapy regimen in combination with bevacizumab alone. In addition, there was an increased incidence of rash, diarrhea, infections, and pulmonary emboli in the panitumumab arms, and the increased incidence of adverse events in combination with worse efficacy compared to controls led to premature closure of the trial after a planned interim analysis.[256] Similarly, chemotherapy-naïve patients treated with cetuximab added to XELOX and bevacizumab resulted a statistically significant decreased PFS but no significant difference in median OS compared to XELOX and bevacizumab.[257] The results seen in PACCE and CAIRO2 were irrespective of *KRAS* mutation, as *KRAS* exon 2 wild-type patients treated with anti-EGFR therapy in combination with chemotherapy and bevacizumab in both trials found decreased efficacy.[256,257] Despite encouraging preclinical evidence, it is clear that combinations of anti-EGFR with anti-VEGF therapies are not effective in the treatment of metastatic colorectal cancer.

3.4 Comparisons of biologic therapies

As outlined above, studies have shown that irinotecan- or oxaliplatin-containing regimens are effective as first-line therapies in patients with metastatic colorectal cancer. Moreover, the addition of both anti-VEGF and anti-EGFR therapies to these regimens is associated with improved efficacy. In order to try to discern which biologic and chemotherapy backbone is most effective, three RCTs have been completed. The randomized phase II PEAK trial evaluated mFOLFOX6 in combination with either bevacizumab or panitumumab in the first-line treatment of patients with *KRAS* exon 2 wild type metastatic colorectal cancer. Although there was no significant difference in response rate and PFS, patients treated with panitumumab had a statistically significant improved median OS (HR 0.62). A subset analysis evaluated the extended *RAS* wild-type population, patients treated with panitumumab had an improved PFS (HR 0.65) and a trend toward improved median OS.[258] The small sample size limits generalization of these results, however.

Similarly, in the phase III FIRE-3 study there was a statistically significant improvement in median OS in *KRAS* exon 2 wild type patients treated with simplified FOLFIRI and cetuximab compared to simplified FOLFIRI and bevacizumab (HR 0.77), but no difference in response rate or PFS. This was also true for patients who were wild type for all *RAS* mutations. The authors of this study caution that interpretation of the OS, a secondary endpoint of the trial, should be taken with caution, especially given the low number of events (343 of 592 patients) and wide confidence intervals.[259]

In contrast to both the PEAK and FIRE-3 studies, CALGB/SWOG 80405 found no significant difference in median OS when chemotherapy was combined with either cetuximab or bevacizumab. In the final design of this randomized phase III study, 1137 patients with *KRAS* wild-type (codons 12 and 13) metastatic colorectal cancer received either mFOLFOX6 or simplified FOLFIRI at the discretion of the treating physician and were randomized to receive either weekly cetuximab or biweekly bevacizumab. 73.4% of patients were treated with mFOLFOX6 and 26.6% were treated with simplified FOLFIRI, consistent with the prescribing practices in the United States and Canada. In total, there was no difference in PFS (HR 1.04) and median OS between patients treated with chemotherapy and bevacizumab (29.0 months) and patients treated with chemotherapy and cetuximab (29.9 months) (HR 0.925). For the patients treated with mFOLFOX6, there was also no difference in patients treated with cetuximab (30.1 months) versus bevacizumab (26.9 months). Similarly, there was no difference between the median OS in patients treated with cetuximab (28.9 months) and bevacizumab (33.4 months) in combination with simplified FOLFIRI.[158] In a subset of patients with expanded *RAS* testing (about 50%), 15% of the *KRAS* exon 2 wild-type patients harbored an additional *RAS* mutation. From the 526 patients wild type for expanded *RAS* mutations, there was no difference in PFS and median OS (HR 0.9) between patients treated with chemotherapy with bevacizumab compared to chemotherapy with cetuximab.[260] While further analyses still need to be completed, it appears that either mFOLFOX6 or FOLFIRI in combination with either bevacizumab or cetuximab are equivalent therapeutic options for the first-line treatment of patients with metastatic colorectal cancer without a *RAS* mutation.

4 Maintenance Therapy and Duration of Therapy

Controversy exists in regard to the optimal duration of therapy in patients with metastatic colorectal cancer. Traditionally, chemotherapy is continued until a patient experiences progressive disease, unacceptable toxicities, or clinical deterioration. Given that patients with metastatic colorectal cancer are now surviving for years and the cumulative toxicities of the regimens often lead to treatment discontinuation, intermittent chemotherapy with scheduled treatment breaks is attractive.

Several studies have compared the traditional use of continuous chemotherapy with intermittent chemotherapy with either a chemotherapy break or a maintenance regimen. In studies comparing continuous chemotherapy with induction chemotherapy, followed by a chemotherapy break and then re-introduction of the chemotherapy upon progression, there is no significant difference in OS.

4.1 *Chemotherapy breaks*

Few studies have compared continuous chemotherapy to intermittent chemotherapy with a treatment break. In a small randomized study of 58 patients there was no statistical difference in PFS or OS observed in patients treated with continuous FOLFIRI or a treatment break after achieving a response or stable disease after six cycles of FOLFORI and restarting FOLFIRI at progression.[261] Similarly, a study of 337 patients randomized to continuous FOLFIRI versus intermittent FOLFIRI on a two-month-on, two-month-off schedule demonstrated that intermittent FOLFIRI is not inferior to continuous FOLFIRI.[262] In MRC-COIN, comparison of either continuous therapy with either XELOX or mFOLFOX6 or induction XELOX or mFOLFOX6 for 12 weeks followed by observation round no difference in PFS (HR 1.052) or OS (HR 1.084), although the study did not show non-inferiority for a treatment break.[263] Overall, these studies suggest that there is no significant improvement for continuous therapy compared to a period of induction chemotherapy followed by a treatment break, although these studies both do not account for the use of biologic therapies as is commonplace in the treatment of metastatic colorectal cancer and do not compare a lower intensity maintenance regimen to either treatment breaks or intensive chemotherapy.

4.2 *Maintenance therapy*

On the other hand, there have been several studies that have evaluated maintenance therapy to either continuous chemotherapy with or without a biologic therapy or a treatment break. The OPTIMOX1 study compared maintenance therapy with sLV5FU2 to continuous chemotherapy in patients treated with oxaliplatin-containing regimens. In this study, 620 patients were randomized to continuous FOLFOX4 until progression or FOLFOX7 for six cycles followed by maintenance therapy with sLV5FU2 for 12 cycles followed by reintroduction of oxaliplatin. Although there was no difference in PFS (HR 1.06) or OS (HR 0.93) as well as no significant difference in sensory neuropathy, this study was limited by the fact that there was only a 40% reintroduction rate of FOLFOX7 in the intermittent therapy group and the two groups were not matched in the intensity of oxaliplatin given the differences in dosing in FOLFOX4 compared to FOLFOX7.[143] To circumvent this difference and evaluate the utility of maintenance therapy over a treatment break, OPTIMOX2 compared sLV5FU2 maintenance with observation after induction FOLFOX. In this study, 216 patients undergoing six cycles of upfront mFOLFOX7 therapy were randomized to maintenance sLV5FU2 or observation, with resumption of mFOL-FOX7 at progression. While this study demonstrated a significant improvement in PFS (HR 0.61) and duration of disease control (HR 0.71) in the maintenance arm, there was no difference in median OS (HR 0.88), suggesting that treatment breaks may safely be given without a decrease in OS.[264] OPTIMOX2, however, was underpowered as a result of early termination at the time of bevacizumab approval for use in metastatic colorectal cancer. In the absence of biologic therapy, studies indicate that either a maintenance strategy or scheduled treatment breaks in patients undergoing treatment with oxaliplatin-containing regimens for metastatic colorectal cancer.

Given the adoption of bevacizumab therapy in the treatment of patients with metastatic colorectal cancer, several studies evaluated bevacizumab maintenance or observation after induction chemotherapy and bevacizumab. Maintenance therapy with single-agent bevacizumab was assessed in the MACRO TTD study. In the MACRO TTD study, 480 patients treated initially treatment with six cycles of XELOX and bevacizumab were randomized to either XELOX/bevacizumab or bevacizumab maintenance, and there was no significant difference in PFS (HR 1.10) or OS (HR 1.05). Despite the lack of significant difference, the upper confidence interval for PFS crossed the predefined non-inferiority limit, so maintenance therapy with single-agent bevacizumab was not shown to be non-inferior to continuous chemotherapy.[265]

Two other studies evaluated a fluorouracil and bevacizumab combination maintenance compared to continuous chemotherapy: the CONcePT study and the TOGT study. In the CONcePT study, a small population was randomized to continuous therapy with mFOLFOX7 and bevacizumab or eight cycles of mFOLFOX7 and bevacizumab alternating with eight cycles of LV5FU2 and bevacizumab. Although the study was closed early by the data safety monitoring committee, the study reached its primary endpoint of improved time to treatment failure in those treated with intermittent oxaliplatin (HR 0.58).[266] Similarly, in the TOGT study maintenance therapy with capecitabine and bevacizumab after induction XELOX and bevacizumab for six cycles improved PFS (HR 0.60) but had no effect in OS compared to continuous XELOX and bevacizumab, suggesting that maintenance with capecitabine and bevacizumab is reasonable.[267]

The studies above suggest that maintenance therapy, or observation after a period of chemotherapy induction, are reasonable choices. To assess the optimal approach CAIRO3 randomized 558 patients who initially had stable disease or a response after six cycles of XELOX and bevacizumab to maintenance therapy with capecitabine and bevacizumab or observation, and XELOX and bevacizumab restarted at first progression. The maintenance group experienced a superior PFS after first progression (HR 0.67), although only a near statistically significant improvement in median OS was noted in the maintenance arm (HR 0.83; $p = 0.06$).[268,269]

While several maintenance strategies have been evaluated with bevacizumab, there have been few studies of evaluating maintenance therapy with anti-EGFR therapy. In the NORDIC VII study, 206 *KRAS* wild-type patients were randomized to continuous FLOX and cetuximab or induction FLOX and cetuximab for 16 weeks followed by maintenance cetuximab and reintroduction of FLOX at progression. There was no difference in both PFS and median OS in the maintenance versus continuous chemotherapy group.[243]

The studies outlined generally demonstrate that chemotherapy without treatment breaks, or induction chemotherapy with either maintenance therapy or treatment breaks are reasonable options for patients with metastatic colorectal cancer. In fact, a meta-analysis of 11 studies comparing continuous and intermittent chemotherapy strategies provides further evidence of no significant difference in patients treated with either continuous or intermittent chemotherapy (HR 1.03). In addition, a subgroup analysis of the three studies (MRC COIN, OPTIMOX2, CAIRO3) comparing induction chemotherapy followed by a treatment break to either continuous chemotherapy or maintenance chemotherapy found a statistically significant but not clinically relevant benefit to some form of continuous therapy compared to treatment breaks (HR 1.10).[270] In general, a maintenance strategy is generally preferred, but in select patients who have had a response to therapy and side effects may be significant, a treatment break may be reasonable.

5 Emerging Treatments: Immunotherapy

It is postulated that a higher tumor-specific mutational load leads to increased antigen presentation and activates the anti-tumor activity of cytotoxic T cells. Recognition of tumors with a high neoantigen presentation is theorized to be a driving force in recognizing patients who might respond to immunotherapies,[271] and may at least in part explain why treatment with anti-PD-1 or anti-CTLA-4 therapies are effective in melanoma and non-small cell lung cancer.[272–277] Despite having a high somatic mutation rate,[278] however, studies with CTLA-4 antagonists and anti-PD-1 or anti-PDL-1 antibodies are largely ineffective in the majority of colorectal cancer patients to date.[279–281] Still, isolated responses to immunotherapy in patients with colorectal cancer have been noted, particularly in patients with microsatellite unstable tumors.[282] This finding, in conjunction with studies showing microsatellite unstable (mismatch repair deficient) tumors harbor 10–100 times as many somatic mutations as microsatellite stable (mismatch repair proficient) tumors, prompted evaluation of the anti-PD-1 therapy pembrolizumab in patients with mismatch-repair-deficient metastatic colorectal cancer. This small phase II study demonstrated an improved PFS and OS benefit in patients treated with pembrolizumab with mismatch-repair-deficient metastatic colorectal cancer (both PFS and OS not reached), but not for mismatch-repair-proficient tumors (PFS 2.2 months; OS 5.5 months).[283] Although this is only a small study, the results are promising in the small subset of patients with mismatch repair deficient colorectal cancers.

6 Conclusions

Since the introduction of 5-FU in the 1950s, there have been many advances in the management of patients with metastatic colorectal cancer. While either oxaliplatin or irinotecan can be combined with 5-FU and bevacizumab or cetuximab (in *RAS* wild type patients) in the first-line setting, there is no definitive evidence that one regimen is superior to another. Although the anticipated side effect profile, individual patient preferences, and tumor characteristics must taken into account in choosing a patient's regimen, it is our practice to start with mFOLFOX6 in combination with bevacizumab for at least eight cycles, followed by maintenance 5-FU and bevacizumab; if a patient desires a treatment break, evidence does not refute the option to hold therapy if the patient has responding or stable disease. At progression, we would consider changing to sFOLFIRI with bevacizumab. If the patient is *RAS* wild type, we would then employ anti-EGFR therapy either alone or in combination with irinotecan in either the second- or third-line. At progression, given the modest benefits and adverse events of regorafenib, we would consider a patient for a clinical trial, perhaps with a targeted therapy or immunotherapy approach as described above, or regorafenib treatment. The availability of the many different options allows for individualized treatment plans for each patient, and is the likely reason for the improving overall survival in patients with metastatic colorectal cancer today.

References

1. Edwards BK, *et al.* Annual report to the nation on the status of cancer, 1975–2006, featuring colorectal cancer trends and impact of interventions (risk factors, screening, and treatment) to reduce future rates. *Cancer* 2010;**116**(3):544–573.
2. Yang DX, *et al.* Estimating the magnitude of colorectal cancers prevented during the era of screening: 1976 to 2009. *Cancer* 2014;**20**(18):2893–2901.
3. Brenner H, *et al.* Effect of screening sigmoidoscopy and screening colonoscopy on colorectal cancer incidence and mortality: Systematic review and meta-analysis of randomised controlled trials and observational studies. *BMJ* 2014;**348**:g2467.
4. Rahib L. *et al.* Projecting cancer incidence and deaths to 2030: The unexpected burden of thyroid, liver, and pancreas cancers in the United States. *Cancer Res* 2014;**74**(11): 2913–2921.
5. Siegel, R. *et al. Colorectal cancer statistics, 2014.* CA Cancer *J Clin*, 2014. **64**(2): p. 104–17.
6. Gill S, *et al.* Colorectal cancer. *Mayo Clin Proc* 2007;**82**(1):114–129.
7. Van Cutsem E, *et al.* Towards a pan-European consensus on the treatment of patients with colorectal liver metastases. *Eur J Cancer* 2006;**42**(14):2212–2221.
8. Kopetz S, *et al.* Improved survival in metastatic colorectal cancer is associated with adoption of hepatic resection and improved chemotherapy. *J Clin Oncol* 2009; **27**(22):3677–3683.
9. Slesser AA, *et al.* A meta-analysis comparing simultaneous versus delayed resections in patients with synchronous colorectal liver metastases. *Surg Oncol* 2013;**22**(1):36–47.
10. O'Dwyer PJ, Stevenson JP. Chemotherapy of advanced colorectal cancer. *Cancer Treat Res* 1998;**98**:111–152.
11. Leyland-Jones B, O'Dwyer PJ. Biochemical modulation: Application of laboratory models to the clinic. *Cancer Treat Rep* 1986;**70**(1):219–229.
12. Heidelberger C. Biochemical Mechanisms of action of fluorinated pyrimidines. *Exp Cell Res* 1963;**24**(Suppl. 9):462–471.
13. O'Dwyer PJ, *et al.* Fluorouracil modulation in colorectal cancer: Lack of improvement with N -phosphonoacetyl- l -aspartic acid or oral leucovorin or interferon, but enhanced therapeutic index with weekly 24-hour infusion schedule — an Eastern Cooperative Oncology Group/Cancer and Leukemia Group B Study. *J Clin Oncol* 2001;**19**(9): 2413–2421.
14. Chu E, *et al.* Thymidylate synthase inhibitors as anticancer agents: From bench to bedside. *Cancer Chemother Pharmacol* 2003;**52**(Suppl. 1):S80–S89.
15. Aschele C, *et al.* Novel mechanism(s) of resistance to 5-fluorouracil in human colon cancer (HCT-8) sublines following exposure to two different clinically relevant dose schedules. *Cancer Res* 1992;**52**(7):1855–1864.
16. Sobrero AF, *et al.* Fluorouracil in colorectal cancer — a tale of two drugs: Implications for biochemical modulation. *J Clin Oncol* 1997;**15**(1):368–381.
17. Evans RM, *et al.* Assessment of growth-limiting events caused by 5-fluorouracil in mouse cells and in human cells. *Cancer Res* 1980;**40**(11):4113–4122.

18. [No authors listed]. Comparison of antimetabolites in the treatment of breast and colon cancer. *JAMA* 1967;**200**(9):770–778.

19. Seifert P, *et al*. Comparison of continuously infused 5-fluorouracil with bolus injection in treatment of patients with colorectal adenocarcinoma. *Cancer* 1975;**36**(1):123–128.

20. Meta-analysis Group In Cancer, Piedbois P, *et al*. Efficacy of intravenous continuous infusion of fluorouracil compared with bolus administration in advanced colorectal cancer. *J Clin Oncol* 1998;**16**(1):301–308.

21. Hansen RM, *et al*. Phase III study of bolus versus infusion fluorouracil with or without cisplatin in advanced colorectal cancer. *J Natl Cancer Inst* 1996;**88**(10):668–674.

22. Weinerman B, *et al*. Systemic infusion versus bolus chemotherapy with 5-fluorouracil in measurable metastatic colorectal cancer. *Am J Clin Oncol* 1992;**15**(6):518–523.

23. Lokich JJ, *et al*. A prospective randomized comparison of continuous infusion fluorouracil with a conventional bolus schedule in metastatic colorectal carcinoma: A Mid-Atlantic Oncology Program Study. *J Clin Oncol* 1989;**7**(4):425–432.

24. [No authors listed]. Modulation of fluorouracil by leucovorin in patients with advanced colorectal cancer: Evidence in terms of response rate. Advanced Colorectal Cancer Meta-Analysis Project. *J Clin Oncol* 1992;**10**(6):896–903.

25. Thirion P, *et al*. Modulation of fluorouracil by leucovorin in patients with advanced colorectal cancer: An updated meta-analysis. *J Clin Oncol* 2004;**22**(18):3766–3775.

26. Moertel CG, *et al*. Therapy of advanced colorectal cancer with a combination of 5-fluorouracil, methyl-1,3-cis(2-chlorethyl)-1-nitrosourea, and vincristine. *J Natl Cancer Inst* 1975;**54**(1):69–71.

27. Moertel CG. Chemotherapy of gastrointestinal cancer. *N Engl J Med* 1978;**299**(19):1049–1052.

28. Boice JD, Jr., *et al*. Leukemia and preleukemia after adjuvant treatment of gastrointestinal cancer with semustine (methyl-CCNU). *N Engl J Med* 1983;**309**(18):1079–1084.

29. Poon MA, *et al*. Biochemical modulation of fluorouracil: Evidence of significant improvement of survival and quality of life in patients with advanced colorectal carcinoma. *J Clin Oncol* 1989;**7**(10):1407–1418.

30. Petrelli N, *et al*. A prospective randomized trial of 5-fluorouracil versus 5-fluorouracil and high-dose leucovorin versus 5-fluorouracil and methotrexate in previously untreated patients with advanced colorectal carcinoma. *J Clin Oncol* 1987;**5**(10):1559–1565.

31. Valone FH, *et al*. Treatment of patients with advanced colorectal carcinomas with fluorouracil alone, high-dose leucovorin plus fluorouracil, or sequential methotrexate, fluorouracil, and leucovorin: A randomized trial of the Northern California Oncology Group. *J Clin Oncol* 1989;**7**(10):1427–1436.

32. Herrmann R, *et al*. Sequential methotrexate and 5-fluorouracil (FU) *vs*. FU alone in metastatic colorectal cancer. Results of a randomized multicenter trial. The Association of Medical Oncology (AIO) of the German Cancer Society. *Ann Oncol* 1992;**3**(7):539–543.

33. Nordic Gastrointestinal Tumor Adjuvant Therapy Group. Superiority of sequential methotrexate, fluorouracil, and leucovorin to fluorouracil alone in advanced symptomatic colorectal carcinoma: A randomized trial. *J Clin Oncol* 1989;**7**(10):1437–1446.

34. Kemeny N, *et al*. Interferon alpha-2a and 5-fluorouracil for advanced colorectal carcinoma. Assessment of activity and toxicity. *Cancer* 1990;**66**(12):2470–2475.

35. Bedikian AY, *et al*. Chemotherapy for colorectal cancer with a combination of PALA and 5-FU. *Cancer Treat Rep* 1981;**65**(9–10):747–753.

36. Mayer RJ. Chemotherapy for metastatic colorectal cancer. *Cancer* 1992;**70**(5 Suppl.):1414–1424.

37. Evans RM, *et al*. Effect of excess folates and deoxyinosine on the activity and site of action of 5-fluorouracil. *Cancer Res* 1981;**41**(9 Pt. 1):3288–3295.

38. Santi DV, McHenry CS. 5-fluoro-2′-deoxyuridylate: Covalent complex with thymidylate synthetase. *Proc Natl Acad Sci U S A* 1972;**69**(7):1855–1857.

39. Berger SH, Hakala MT. Relationship of dUMP and free FdUMP pools to inhibition of thymidylate synthase by 5-fluorouracil. *Mol Pharmacol* 1984;**25**(2):303–309.

40. Waxman S, Bruckner H. The enhancement of 5-fluorouracil anti-metabolic activity by leucovorin, menadione and alpha-tocopherol. *Eur J Cancer Clin Oncol* 1982;**18**(7): 685–692.

41. Labianca R, *et al*. Folinic acid + 5-fluorouracil (5-FU) versus equidose 5-FU in advanced colorectal cancer. Phase III study of 'GISCAD' (Italian Group for the Study of Digestive Tract Cancer). *Ann Oncol* 1991;**2**(9):673–679.

42. Borner MM, *et al*. The impact of adding low-dose leucovorin to monthly 5-fluorouracil in advanced colorectal carcinoma: Results of a phase III trial. Swiss Group for Clinical Cancer Research (SAKK). *Ann Oncol* 1998;**9**(5):535–541.

43. Budd GT, *et al*. 5-fluorouracil and folinic acid in the treatment of metastatic colorectal cancer: A randomized comparison. A Southwest Oncology Group Study. *J Clin Oncol* 1987;**5**(2):272–277.

44. Leichman CG, *et al*. Phase II study of fluorouracil and its modulation in advanced colorectal cancer: A Southwest Oncology Group study. *J Clin Oncol* 1995;**13**(6): 1303–1311.

45. Sobrero AF, *et al*. Synergism and lack of cross-resistance between short-term and continuous exposure to fluorouracil in human colon adenocarcinoma cells. *J Natl Cancer Inst* 1993;**85**(23):1937–1944.

46. De Gramont A, *et al*. High-dose folinic acid and 5-fluorouracil bolus and continuous infusion in advanced colorectal cancer. *Eur J Cancer Clin Oncol* 1988;**24**(9):1499–1503.

47. De Gramont A, *et al*. Randomized trial comparing monthly low-dose leucovorin and fluorouracil bolus with bimonthly high-dose leucovorin and fluorouracil bolus plus continuous infusion for advanced colorectal cancer: A French intergroup study. *J Clin Oncol* 1997;**15**(2):808–815.

48. De Gramont A, *et al*. A review of GERCOD trials of bimonthly leucovorin plus 5-fluorouracil 48-h continuous infusion in advanced colorectal cancer: Evolution of a regimen. *Groupe d'Etude et de Recherche sur les Cancers de l'Ovaire et Digestifs* (GERCOD). *Eur J Cancer* 1998;**34**(5):619–626.

49. André T, *et al*. CPT-11 (irinotecan) addition to bimonthly, high-dose leucovorin and bolus and continuous-infusion 5-fluorouracil (FOLFIRI) for pretreated metastatic colorectal cancer. GERCOR. *Eur J Cancer* 1999;**35**(9):1343–1347.

50. Buroker TR, *et al*. Randomized comparison of two schedules of fluorouracil and leucovorin in the treatment of advanced colorectal cancer. *J Clin Oncol* 1994;**12**(1):14–20.

51. Petrelli N. *et al*. The modulation of fluorouracil with leucovorin in metastatic colorectal carcinoma: A prospective randomized phase III trial. Gastrointestinal Tumor Study Group. *J Clin Oncol* 1989;**7**(10):1419–1426.

52. Saltz LB, *et al*. Phase I clinical and pharmacokinetic study of irinotecan, fluorouracil, and leucovorin in patients with advanced solid tumors. *J Clin Oncol* 1996;**14**(11): 2959–2967.

53. Fuchs CS, *et al*. Randomized, controlled trial of irinotecan plus infusional, bolus, or oral fluoropyrimidines in first-line treatment of metastatic colorectal cancer: Updated results from the BICC-C study. *J Clin Oncol* 2008;**26**(4):689–690.

54. Ducreux M, *et al*. Irinotecan combined with bolus fluorouracil, continuous infusion fluorouracil, and high-dose leucovorin every two weeks (LV5FU2 regimen): A clinical dose-finding and pharmacokinetic study in patients with pretreated metastatic colorectal cancer. *J Clin Oncol* 1999;**17**(9):2901–2908.

55. De Gramont A, *et al*. Oxaliplatin with high-dose folinic acid and 5-fluorouracil 48 h infusion in pretreated metastatic colorectal cancer. *Proc Am Soc Clin Oncol* 1994;**13**:220 (Abstr.).

56. De Gramont A, *et al*. Oxaliplatin with high-dose leucovorin and 5-fluorouracil 48-hour continuous infusion in pretreated metastatic colorectal cancer. *Eur J Cancer* 1997;**33**(2):214–219.

57. André T, *et al*. Bimonthly high-dose leucovorin, 5-fluorouracil infusion and oxaliplatin (FOLFOX3) for metastatic colorectal cancer resistant to the same leucovorin and 5-fluorouracil regimen. *Ann Oncol* 1998;**9**(11):1251–1253.

58. André T, *et al*. Multicenter phase II study of bimonthly high-dose leucovorin, fluoroura-cil infusion, and oxaliplatin for metastatic colorectal cancer resistant to the same leucovorin and fluorouracil regimen. *J Clin Oncol* 1999;**17**(11):3560–3568.

59. Maindrault-Goebel F, *et al*. Oxaliplatin added to the simplified bimonthly leucovorin and 5-fluorouracil regimen as second-line therapy for metastatic colorectal cancer (FOLFOX6). GERCOR. *Eur J Cancer* 1999;**35**(9):1338–1342.

60. Cheeseman SL, *et al*. A 'modified de Gramont' regimen of fluorouracil, alone and with oxaliplatin, for advanced colorectal cancer. *Br J Cancer* 2002;**87**(4):393–399.

61. Maindrault-Goebel F, *et al*. High-dose intensity oxaliplatin added to the simplified bimonthly leucovorin and 5-fluorouracil regimen as second-line therapy for metastatic colorectal cancer (FOLFOX 7). *Eur J Cancer* 2001;**7**(8):1000–1005.

62. Sorbye H, *et al*. Multicenter phase II study of Nordic fluorouracil and folinic acid bolus schedule combined with oxaliplatin as first-line treatment of metastatic colorectal cancer. *J Clin Oncol* 2004;**22**(1):31–38.

63. Cassidy J, *et al*. XELOX (capecitabine plus oxaliplatin): Active first-line therapy for patients with metastatic colorectal cancer. *J Clin Oncol* 2004;**22**(11):2084–2091.

64. Porschen R, *et al*. Phase III study of capecitabine plus oxaliplatin compared with fluorouracil and leucovorin plus oxaliplatin in metastatic colorectal cancer: A final report of the AIO Colorectal Study Group. *J Clin Oncol* 2007;**25**(27):4217–4223.

65. Masi G, *et al.* First-line treatment of metastatic colorectal cancer with irinotecan, oxaliplatin and 5-fluorouracil/leucovorin (FOLFOXIRI): Results of a phase II study with a simplified biweekly schedule. *Ann Oncol* 2004;**15**(12):1766–1772.

66. Souglakos J, *et al.* Triplet combination with irinotecan plus oxaliplatin plus continuous-infusion fluorouracil and leucovorin as first-line treatment in metastatic colorectal cancer: A multicenter phase II trial. *J Clin Oncol* 2002;**20**(11):2651–2657.

67. Miwa M, *et al.* Design of a novel oral fluoropyrimidine carbamate, capecitabine, which generates 5-fluorouracil selectively in tumours by enzymes concentrated in human liver and cancer tissue. *Eur J Cancer* 1998;**34**(8):1274–1281.

68. Schuller J, *et al.* Preferential activation of capecitabine in tumor following oral administration to colorectal cancer patients. *Cancer Chemother Pharmacol* 2000;**45**(4): 291–297.

69. Cassidy J, *et al.* A Phase I study of capecitabine in combination with oral leucovorin in patients with intractable solid tumors. *Clin Cancer Res* 1998;**4**(11):2755–2761.

70. Van Cutsem E, *et al.* Capecitabine, an oral fluoropyrimidine carbamate with substantial activity in advanced colorectal cancer: Results of a randomized phase II study. *J Clin Oncol* 2000;**18**(6):1337–1345.

71. Hoff PM, *et al.* Comparison of oral capecitabine versus intravenous fluorouracil plus leucovorin as first-line treatment in 605 patients with metastatic colorectal cancer: Results of a randomized phase III study. *J Clin Oncol* 2001;**19**(8):2282–2292.

72. Van Cutsem E, *et al.* Oral capecitabine compared with intravenous fluorouracil plus leucovorin in patients with metastatic colorectal cancer: Results of a large phase III study. *J Clin Oncol* 2001;**19**(21):4097–4106.

73. Van Cutsem E, *et al.* Oral capecitabine vs intravenous 5-fluorouracil and leucovorin: Integrated efficacy data and novel analyses from two large, randomised, phase III trials. *Br J Cancer* 2004;**90**(6):1190–1197.

74. Cassidy J, *et al.* First-line oral capecitabine therapy in metastatic colorectal cancer: A favorable safety profile compared with intravenous 5-fluorouracil/leucovorin. *Ann Oncol* 2002;**13**(4):566–575.

75. Diasio RB, *et al.* Familial deficiency of dihydropyrimidine dehydrogenase. Biochemical basis for familial pyrimidinemia and severe 5-fluorouracil-induced toxicity. *J Clin Invest* 1988;**81**(1):47–51.

76. Harris BE, *et al.* Severe 5-fluorouracil toxicity secondary to dihydropyrimidine dehydrogenase deficiency. A potentially more common pharmacogenetic syndrome. *Cancer* 1991;**68**(3):499–501.

77. Lu Z, *et al.* Dihydropyrimidine dehydrogenase activity in human peripheral blood mononuclear cells and liver: Population characteristics, newly identified deficient patients, and clinical implication in 5-fluorouracil chemotherapy. *Cancer Res* 1993;**53**(22):5433–5438.

78. Meinsma R, *et al.* Human polymorphism in drug metabolism: Mutation in the dihydropyrimidine dehydrogenase gene results in exon skipping and thymine uracilurea. *DNA Cell Biol* 1995;**14**(1):1–6.

79. Mercier C, Ciccolini J. Severe or lethal toxicities upon capecitabine intake: Is *DPYD* genetic polymorphism the ideal culprit? *Trends Pharmacol Sci* 2007;**28**(12):597–598.

80. Van Kuilenburg AB, *et al.* Lethal outcome of a patient with a complete dihydropyrimidine dehydrogenase (DPD) deficiency after administration *of* 5-fluorouracil: Frequency of the common IVS14+1G>A mutation causing DPD deficiency. *Clin Cancer Res* 2001;**7**(5):1149–1153.

81. Ofverholm A, *et al.* Two cases of 5-fluorouracil toxicity linked with gene variants in the *DPYD* gene. *Clin Biochem* 2010;**43**(3):331–334.

82. Ciccolini J, *et al.* Routine dihydropyrimidine dehydrogenase testing for anticipating 5-fluorouracil-related severe toxicities: Hype or hope? *Clin Colorectal Cancer* 2010;**9**(4):224–228.

83. Collie-Duguid ES, *et al.* Known variant DPYD alleles do not explain DPD deficiency in cancer patients. *Pharmacogenetics* 2000;**10**(3):217–223.

84. Ezzeldin HH, *et al.* Methylation of the DPYD promoter: An alternative mechanism for dihydropyrimidine dehydrogenase deficiency in cancer patients. *Clin Cancer Res* 2005;**11**(24 Pt. 1):8699–8705.

85. Amstutz U, *et al.* Hypermethylation of the DPYD promoter region is not a major predictor of severe toxicity in 5-fluorouracil based chemotherapy. *J Exp Clin Cancer Res* 2008;**27**:54.

86. Savva-Bordalo J, *et al.* Promoter methylation and large intragenic rearrangements of *DPYD* are not implicated in severe toxicity to 5-fluorouracil-based chemotherapy in gastrointestinal cancer patients. *BMC Cancer* 2010;**10**:470.

87. Van Staveren MC, *et al.* Evaluation of predictive tests for screening for dihydropyrimidine dehydrogenase deficiency. *Pharmacogenomics J* 2013;**13**(5):389–395.

88. Johnson MR, Diasio RB. Importance of dihydropyrimidine dehydrogenase (DPD) deficiency in patients exhibiting toxicity following treatment with 5-fluorouracil. *Adv Enzyme Regul* 2001;**41**:151–157.

89. Van Kuilenburg AB, *et al.* High prevalence of the IVS14 + 1G>A mutation in the dihydropyrimidine dehydrogenase gene of patients with severe 5-fluorouracil-associated toxicity. *Pharmacogenetics* 2002;**12**(7):555–558.

90. Etienne MC, *et al.* Population study of dihydropyrimidine dehydrogenase in cancer patients. *J Clin Oncol* 1994;**12**(11):2248–2253.

91. Mattison LK, *et al.* Evidence for increased incidence of dihydropyrimidine dehydrogenase (DPD) deficiency in African Americans compared to Caucasians. *J Clin Oncol* 2005; **23**:16S(June 1 Suppl.). [in *ASCO Annu Meet Proc*]

92. Kawato Y, *et al.* Intracellular roles of SN-38, a metabolite of the camptothecin derivative CPT-11, in the antitumor effect of CPT-11. *Cancer Res* 1991;**51**(16):4187–4191.

93. Hsiang YH, *et al.* Camptothecin induces protein-linked DNA breaks via mammalian DNA topoisomerase I. *J Biol Chem* 1985;**260**(27):14873–14878.

94. Hsiang YH, *et al.* Arrest of replication forks by drug-stabilized topoisomerase I-DNA cleavable complexes as a mechanism of cell killing by camptothecin. *Cancer Res* 1989;**49**(18):5077–5082.

95. Schneider E, *et al.* DNA topoisomerases as anticancer drug targets. *Adv Pharmacol* 1990;**21**:149–183.

96. Hertzberg RP, *et al.* On the mechanism of topoisomerase I inhibition by camptothecin: Evidence for binding to an enzyme-DNA complex. *Biochemistry* 1989;**28**(11): 4629–4638.

97. Rougier P, *et al.* Phase II study of irinotecan in the treatment of advanced colorectal cancer in chemotherapy-naive patients and patients pretreated with fluorouracil-based chemotherapy. *J Clin Oncol* 1997;**15**(1):251–260.

98. Pitot HC, *et al.* Phase II trial of irinotecan in patients with metastatic colorectal carcinoma. *J Clin Oncol* 1997;**15**(8):2910–2919.

99. Firvida JL, *et al.* Phase II study of irinotecan as first-line chemotherapy for patients with advanced colorectal carcinoma. *Cancer* 2001;**91**(4):704–711.

100. Conti JA, *et al.* Irinotecan is an active agent in untreated patients with metastatic colorectal cancer. *J Clin Oncol* 1996;**14**(3):709–715.

101. Shimada Y, *et al.* Phase II study of CPT-11, a new camptothecin derivative, in metastatic colorectal cancer. CPT-11 Gastrointestinal Cancer Study Group. *J Clin Oncol* 1993; **11**(5):909–913.

102. Rothenberg ML, *et al.* Phase II trial of irinotecan in patients with progressive or rapidly recurrent colorectal cancer. *J Clin Oncol* 1996;**14**(4):1128–1135.

103. Van Cutsem E, *et al.* Clinical activity and benefit of irinotecan (CPT-11) in patients with colorectal cancer truly resistant to 5-fluorouracil (5-FU). *Eur J Cancer* 1999;**35**(1): 54–59.

104. Rothenberg ML, *et al.* A multicenter, phase II trial of weekly irinotecan (CPT-11) in patients with previously treated colorectal carcinoma. *Cancer* 1999;**85**(4):786–795.

105. Cunningham D, *et al.* Randomised trial of irinotecan plus supportive care versus supportive care alone after fluorouracil failure for patients with metastatic colorectal cancer. *Lancet* 1998;**352**(9138):1413–1418.

106. Rougier P, *et al.* Randomised trial of irinotecan versus fluorouracil by continuous infusion after fluorouracil failure in patients with metastatic colorectal cancer. *Lancet* 1998;**352**(9138):1407–1412.

107. Guichard S, *et al.* Sequence-dependent activity of the irinotecan-5FU combination in human colon-cancer model HT-29 *in vitro* and *in vivo*. *Int J Cancer* 1997;**73**(5): 729–734.

108. Pavillard V, *et al.* Combination of irinotecan (CPT11) and 5-fluorouracil with an analysis of cellular determinants of drug activity. *Biochem Pharmacol* 1998;**56**(10): 1315–1322.

109. Saltz LB, *et al.* Irinotecan plus fluorouracil and leucovorin for metastatic colorectal cancer. Irinotecan Study Group. *N Engl J Med* 2000;**343**(13):905–914.

110. Douillard JY, *et al.* Irinotecan combined with fluorouracil compared with fluorouracil alone as first-line treatment for metastatic colorectal cancer: A multicentre randomised trial. *Lancet* 2000;**355**(9209):1041–1047.

111. Fuchs CS, *et al.* Randomized, controlled trial of irinotecan plus infusional, bolus, or oral fluoropyrimidines in first-line treatment of metastatic colorectal cancer: Results from the BICC-C Study. *J Clin Oncol* 2007;**25**(30):4779–4786.

112. Van Cutsem E, *et al*. A phase II study of irinotecan alternated with five days bolus of 5-fluorouracil and leucovorin in first-line chemotherapy of metastatic colorectal cancer. *Ann Oncol* 1998;**9**(11):1199–1204.

113. Glimelius B, *et al*. Irinotecan combined with bolus 5-fluorouracil and folinic acid Nordic schedule as first-line therapy in advanced colorectal cancer. *Ann Oncol* 2002;**13**(12):1868–1873.

114. Glimelius B, *et al*. A randomized phase III multicenter trial comparing irinotecan in combination with the Nordic bolus 5-FU and folinic acid schedule or the bolus/infused de Gramont schedule (Lv5FU2) in patients with metastatic colorectal cancer. *Ann Oncol* 2008;**19**(5):909–914.

115. Fuchs CS, *et al*. Phase III comparison of two irinotecan dosing regimens in second-line therapy of metastatic colorectal cancer. *J Clin Oncol* 2003;**21**(5):807–814.

116. Kohne CH, *et al*. Effective biomodulation by leucovorin of high-dose infusion fluorouracil given as a weekly 24-hour infusion: Results of a randomized trial in patients with advanced colorectal cancer. *J Clin Oncol* 1998;**16**(2):418–426.

117. Rea DW, *et al*. A phase I/II and pharmacokinetic study of irinotecan in combination with capecitabine as first-line therapy for advanced colorectal cancer. *Ann Oncol* 2005**16**(7);1123–1132.

118. Bajetta E, *et al*. Randomized multicenter Phase II trial of two different schedules of irinotecan combined with capecitabine as first-line treatment in metastatic colorectal carcinoma. *Cancer* 2004;**100**(2):279–287.

119. Borner MM, *et al*. A randomized phase II trial of capecitabine and two different schedules of irinotecan in first-line treatment of metastatic colorectal cancer: Efficacy, quality-of-life and toxicity. *Ann Oncol* 2005;**16**(2):282–288.

120. Koopman M, *et al*. Sequential versus combination chemotherapy with capecitabine, irinotecan, and oxaliplatin in advanced colorectal cancer (CAIRO): A phase III randomised controlled trial. *Lancet* 2007;**370**(9582):135–142.

121. Tournigand C, *et al*. FOLFIRI followed by FOLFOX6 or the reverse sequence in advanced colorectal cancer: A randomized GERCOR study. *J Clin Oncol* 2004;**22**(2):229–237.

122. Goldberg RM, *et al*. A randomized controlled trial of fluorouracil plus leucovorin, irinotecan, and oxaliplatin combinations in patients with previously untreated metastatic colorectal cancer. *J Clin Oncol* 2004;**22**(1):23–30.

123. Ando Y, *et al*. Polymorphisms of UDP-glucuronosyltransferase gene and irinotecan toxicity: A pharmacogenetic analysis. *Cancer Res* 2000;**60**(24):6921–6926.

124. Innocenti F, *et al*. Genetic variants in the UDP-glucuronosyltransferase 1A1 gene predict the risk of severe neutropenia of irinotecan. *J Clin Oncol* 2004;**22**(8):1382–1388.

125. Toffoli G, *et al*. The role of UGT1A1*28 polymorphism in the pharmacodynamics and pharmacokinetics of irinotecan in patients with metastatic colorectal cancer. *J Clin Oncol* 2006;**24**(19):3061–3068.

126. Ruzzo A, *et al*. Pharmacogenetic profiling in patients with advanced colorectal cancer treated with first-line FOLFIRI chemotherapy. *Pharmacogenomics J* 2008;**8**(4):278–288.

127. Cecchin E, *et al*. Predictive role of the UGT1A1, UGT1A7, and UGT1A9 genetic variants and their haplotypes on the outcome of metastatic colorectal cancer patients treated with fluorouracil, leucovorin, and irinotecan. *J Clin Oncol* 2009;**27**(15):2457–2465.

128. Kemeny N, *et al*. Randomized study of continuous infusion fluorouracil versus fluorouracil plus cisplatin in patients with metastatic colorectal cancer. *J Clin Oncol* 1990;**8**(2):313–318.

129. Lokich J, *et al*. Protracted low-dose cisplatin infusion in advanced colorectal cancer. *Cancer Treat Rep* 1986;**70**(4):523–524.

130. DeSimone PA, *et al*. High-dose cisplatin in the treatment of advanced adenocarcinoma of the colon and rectum: A Southeastern Cancer Study Group trial. *Cancer Treat Rep* 1986;**70**(10):1229–1230.

131. Nole F, *et al*. Carboplatin in patients with advanced colorectal cancer pretreated with fluoropyrimidines. *Eur J Cancer* 1993;**29A**(9):1330–1331.

132. Raymond E, *et al*. Oxaliplatin: A review of preclinical and clinical studies. *Ann Oncol* 1998;**9**(10):1053–1071.

133. Saris CP, *et al*. *In vitro* formation of DNA adducts by cisplatin, lobaplatin and oxaliplatin in calf thymus DNA in solution and in cultured human cells. *Carcinogenesis* 1996;**17**(12):2763–2769.

134. Diaz-Rubio E, *et al*. Oxaliplatin as single agent in previously untreated colorectal carcinoma patients: A phase II multicentric study. *Ann Oncol* 1998;**9**(1):105–108.

135. Becouarn Y, *et al*. Phase II trial of oxaliplatin as first-line chemotherapy in metastatic colorectal cancer patients. Digestive Group of French Federation of Cancer Centers. *J Clin Oncol* 1998;**16**(8):2739–2744.

136. Machover D, *et al*. Two consecutive phase II studies of oxaliplatin (L-OHP) for treatment of patients with advanced colorectal carcinoma who were resistant to previous treatment with fluoropyrimidines. *Ann Oncol* 1996;**7**(1):95–98.

137. Levi F, *et al*. Oxaliplatin activity against metastatic colorectal cancer. A phase II study of 5-day continuous venous infusion at circadian rhythm modulated rate. *Eur J Cancer* 1993;**29A**(9):1280–1284.

138. Rothenberg ML, *et al*. Superiority of oxaliplatin and fluorouracil-leucovorin compared with either therapy alone in patients with progressive colorectal cancer after irinotecan and fluorouracil-leucovorin: Interim results of a phase III trial. *J Clin Oncol* 2003;**21**(11):2059–2069.

139. Raymond E, *et al*. Antitumor activity of oxaliplatin in combination with 5-fluorouracil and the thymidylate synthase inhibitor AG337 in human colon, breast and ovarian cancers. *Anticancer Drugs* 1997;**8**(9):876–885.

140. Fischel JL, *et al*. Search for the optimal schedule for the oxaliplatin/5-fluorouracil association modulated or not by folinic acid: Preclinical data. *Clin Cancer Res* 1998;**4**(10):2529–2535.

141. Levi FA, *et al*. Chronomodulated versus fixed-infusion-rate delivery of ambulatory chemotherapy with oxaliplatin, fluorouracil, and folinic acid (leucovorin) in patients with colorectal cancer metastases: A randomized multi-institutional trial. *J Natl Cancer Inst* 1994;**86**(21):1608–1617.

142. De Gramont A, *et al*. Leucovorin and fluorouracil with or without oxaliplatin as first-line treatment in advanced colorectal cancer. *J Clin Oncol* 2000;**18**(16):2938–2947.

143. Tournigand C, *et al*. OPTIMOX1: A randomized study of FOLFOX4 or FOLFOX7 with oxaliplatin in a stop-and-Go fashion in advanced colorectal cancer — a GERCOR study. *J Clin Oncol* 2006;**24**(3):394–400.

144. Cassidy J, *et al*. Randomized phase III study of capecitabine plus oxaliplatin compared with fluorouracil/folinic acid plus oxaliplatin as first-line therapy for metastatic colorectal cancer. *J Clin Oncol* 2008;**26**(12):2006–2012.

145. Diaz-Rubio E, *et al*. Phase III study of capecitabine plus oxaliplatin compared with continuous-infusion fluorouracil plus oxaliplatin as first-line therapy in metastatic colorectal cancer: Final report of the Spanish Cooperative Group for the Treatment of Digestive Tumors Trial. *J Clin Oncol* 2007;**25**(27):4224–4230.

146. Giacchetti S, *et al*. Phase III multicenter randomized trial of oxaliplatin added to chronomodulated fluorouracil-leucovorin as first-line treatment of metastatic colorectal cancer. *J Clin Oncol* 2000;**18**(1):136–147.

147. De Gramont A, *et al*. [Oxaliplatin, folinic acid and 5-fluorouracil (folfox) in pretreated patients with metastatic advanced cancer. The GERCOD]. *Rev Med Interne* 1997;**18**(10):769–775.

148. Becouarn Y, Rougier P. Clinical efficacy of oxaliplatin monotherapy: Phase II trials in advanced colorectal cancer. *Semin Oncol* 1998;**25**(2 Suppl. 5):23–31.

149. Zori Comba A, *et al*. A randomised phase II study of oxaliplatin alone versus oxaliplatin combined with 5-fluorouracil and folinic acid (Mayo Clinic regimen) in previously untreated metastatic colorectal cancer patients. *Eur J Cancer* 2001;**37**(8):1006–1013.

150. Scheithauer W, *et al*. Randomized multicenter phase II trial of two different schedules of capecitabine plus oxaliplatin as first-line treatment in advanced colorectal cancer. *J Clin Oncol* 2003;**21**(7):1307–1312.

151. Ryan DP, *et al*. A phase II study of modified deGramont 5-fluorouracil, leucovorin, and oxaliplatin in previously treated patients with metastatic colorectal cancer. *Cancer Invest* 2003;**21**(4):505–511.

152. Kemeny N, *et al*. Randomized multicenter phase II trial of bolus plus infusional fluorouracil/leucovorin compared with fluorouracil/leucovorin plus oxaliplatin as third-line treatment of patients with advanced colorectal cancer. *J Clin Oncol* 2004;**22**(23):4753–4761.

153. Rothenberg ML, *et al*. Capecitabine plus oxaliplatin (XELOX) versus 5-fluorouracil/folinic acid plus oxaliplatin (FOLFOX-4) as second-line therapy in metastatic colorectal cancer: A randomized phase III noninferiority study. *Ann Oncol* 2008;**19**(10):1720–1726.

154. Ravaioli A, *et al*. Bolus fluorouracil and leucovorin with oxaliplatin as first-line treatment in metastatic colorectal cancer. *J Clin Oncol* 2002;**20**(10):2545–2550.

155. Hochster H, *et al*. Oxaliplatin with weekly bolus fluorouracil and low-dose leucovorin as first-line therapy for patients with colorectal cancer. *J Clin Oncol* 2003;**21**(14):2703–2707.

156. Yang TS, *et al*. Oxaliplatin with weekly bolus 5-fluorouracil and leucovorin in pretreated advanced colorectal cancer patients: A phase II study. *Chemotherapy* 2003;**49**(4):194–199.

157. Colucci G, *et al.* Phase III randomized trial of FOLFIRI versus FOLFOX4 in the treatment of advanced colorectal cancer: A multicenter study of the Gruppo Oncologico Dell'Italia Meridionale. *J Clin Oncol* 2005;**23**(22):4866–4875.

158. Venook AP, *et al.* CALGB/SWOG 80405: Phase III trial of irinotecan/5-FU/leucovorin (FOLFIRI) or oxaliplatin/5-FU/leucovorin (mFOLFOX6) with bevacizumab (BV) or cetuximab (CET) for patients (pts) with KRAS wild-type (wt) untreated metastatic adenocarcinoma of the colon or rectum (MCRC). *ASCO Meet Abstr* 2014;**32** (18 Suppl.):LBA3.

159. Zeghari-Squalli N, *et al.* Cellular pharmacology of the combination of the DNA topoisomerase I inhibitor SN-38 and the diaminocyclohexane platinum derivative oxaliplatin. *Clin Cancer Res* 1999;**5**(5):1189–1196.

160. Scheithauer W, *et al.* Combined irinotecan and oxaliplatin plus granulocyte colony-stimulating factor in patients with advanced fluoropyrimidine/leucovorin-pretreated colorectal cancer. *J Clin Oncol* 1999;**17**(3):902–906.

161. Wasserman E, *et al.* Combination of oxaliplatin plus irinotecan in patients with gastrointestinal tumors: Results of two independent phase I studies with pharmacokinetics. *J Clin Oncol* 1999;**17**(6):1751–1759.

162. Goldwasser F, *et al.* Dose escalation of CPT-11 in combination with oxaliplatin using an every two weeks schedule: A phase I study in advanced gastrointestinal cancer patients. *Ann Onco,* 2000;**11**(11):1463–1470.

163. Kemeny N, *et al.* Phase I study of weekly oxaliplatin plus irinotecan in previously treated patients with metastatic colorectal cancer. *Ann Oncol* 2002;**13**(9):1490–1496.

164. Souglakos J, *et al.* FOLFOXIRI (folinic acid, 5-fluorouracil, oxaliplatin and irinotecan) vs FOLFIRI (folinic acid, 5-fluorouracil and irinotecan) as first-line treatment in metastatic colorectal cancer (MCC): A multicentre randomised phase III trial from the Hellenic Oncology Research Group (HORG). *Br J Cancer* 2006;**94**(6):798–805.

165. Falcone A, *et al.* Phase III trial of infusional fluorouracil, leucovorin, oxaliplatin, and irinotecan (FOLFOXIRI) compared with infusional fluorouracil, leucovorin, and irinotecan (FOLFIRI) as first-line treatment for metastatic colorectal cancer: The Gruppo Oncologico Nord Ovest. *J Clin Oncol* 2007;**25**(13):1670–1676.

166. Falcone A, *et al.* Biweekly chemotherapy with oxaliplatin, irinotecan, infusional Fluorouracil, and leucovorin: A pilot study in patients with metastatic colorectal cancer. *J Clin Oncol* 2002;**20**(19):4006–4014.

167. Masi G, *et al.* Bevacizumab with FOLFOXIRI (irinotecan, oxaliplatin, fluorouracil, and folinate) as first-line treatment for metastatic colorectal cancer: A phase 2 trial. *Lancet Oncol* 2010;**11**(9):845–852.

168. Saridaki Z, *et al.* A triplet combination with irinotecan (CPT-11), oxaliplatin (LOHP), continuous infusion 5-fluorouracil and leucovorin (FOLFOXIRI) plus cetuximab as first-line treatment in *KRAS* wt, metastatic colorectal cancer: A pilot phase II trial. *Br J Cancer* 2012;**107**(12):1932–1937.

169. Fornaro L, *et al.* FOLFOXIRI in combination with panitumumab as first-line treatment in quadruple wild-type (KRAS, NRAS, HRAS, BRAF) metastatic colorectal cancer patients: A phase II trial by the Gruppo Oncologico Nord Ovest (GONO). *Ann Oncol* 2013;**24**(8):2062–2067.

170. Loupakis F, *et al.* Initial therapy with FOLFOXIRI and bevacizumab for metastatic colorectal cancer. *N Engl J Med* 2014;**371**(17):1609–1618.

171. Hicklin DJ, Ellis LM. Role of the vascular endothelial growth factor pathway in tumor growth and angiogenesis. *J Clin Oncol* 2005;**23**(5):1011–1027.

172. Ferrara N. Vascular endothelial growth factor: Basic science and clinical progress. *Endocr Rev* 2004;**25**(4):581–611.

173. Takahashi Y, *et al.* Significance of vessel count and vascular endothelial growth factor and its receptor (KDR) in intestinal-type gastric cancer. *Clin Cancer Res* 1996;**2**(10):1679–1684.

174. Lee JC, *et al.* Prognostic value of vascular endothelial growth factor expression in colorectal cancer patients. *Eur J Cancer* 2000;**36**(6):748–753.

175. Hoff PM, *et al.* Cediranib plus FOLFOX/CAPOX versus placebo plus FOLFOX/CAPOX in patients with previously untreated metastatic colorectal cancer: A randomized, double-blind, phase III study (HORIZON II). *J Clin Oncol* 2012;**30**(29):3596–3603.

176. Schmoll HJ, *et al.* Cediranib with mFOLFOX6 versus bevacizumab with mFOLFOX6 as first-line treatment for patients with advanced colorectal cancer: A double-blind, randomized phase III study (HORIZON III). *J Clin Oncol* 2012;**30**(29):3588–3595.

177. Hecht JR, *et al.* Randomized, placebo-controlled, phase III study of first-line oxaliplatin-based chemotherapy plus PTK787/ZK 222584, an oral vascular endothelial growth factor receptor inhibitor, in patients with metastatic colorectal adenocarcinoma. *J Clin Oncol* 2011;**29**(15):1997–2003.

178. Van Cutsem E, *et al.* Randomized, placebo-controlled, phase III study of oxaliplatin, fluorouracil, and leucovorin with or without PTK787/ZK 222584 in patients with previously treated metastatic colorectal adenocarcinoma. *J Clin Oncol* 2011;**29**(15):2004–2010.

179. Willett CG, *et al.* Direct evidence that the VEGF-specific antibody bevacizumab has antivascular effects in human rectal cancer. *Nat Med* 2004;**10**(2):145–147.

180. Jain RK, Normalization of tumor vasculature: An emerging concept in antiangiogenic therapy. *Science* 2005;**307**(5706):58–62.

181. Ellis LM, Mechanisms of action of bevacizumab as a component of therapy for metastatic colorectal cancer. *Semin Oncol* 2006;**33**(5 Suppl. 10):S1–S7.

182. Shih T, Lindley C. Bevacizumab: An angiogenesis inhibitor for the treatment of solid malignancies. *Clin Ther* 2006;**28**(11):17791802.

183. Elamin YY, *et al.* Immune effects of bevacizumab: Killing two birds with one stone. *Cancer Microenviron* 2015;**8**(1):15–21.

184. Kabbinavar F, *et al.* Phase II, randomized trial comparing bevacizumab plus fluorouracil (FU)/leucovorin (LV) with FU/LV alone in patients with metastatic colorectal cancer. *J Clin Oncol* 2003;**21**(1):60–65.

185. Kabbinavar FF, *et al.* Addition of bevacizumab to bolus fluorouracil and leucovorin in first-line metastatic colorectal cancer: Results of a randomized phase II trial. *J Clin Oncol* 2005;**23**(16):3697–3705.

186. Hurwitz H, *et al.* Bevacizumab plus irinotecan, fluorouracil, and leucovorin for metastatic colorectal cancer. *N Engl J Med* 2004;**350**(23):2335–2342.

187. Hochster HS, *et al.* Safety and efficacy of oxaliplatin and fluoropyrimidine regimens with or without bevacizumab as first-line treatment of metastatic colorectal cancer: Results of the TREE Study. *J Clin Oncol* 2008;**26**(21):3523–3529.

188. Saltz LB, *et al.* Bevacizumab in combination with oxaliplatin-based chemotherapy as first-line therapy in metastatic colorectal cancer: A randomized phase III study. *J Clin Oncol* 2008;**26**(12):2013–2019.

189. Garcia-Carbonero R, *et al.* An open-label phase II study evaluating the safety and efficacy of ramucirumab combined with mFOLFOX-6 as first-line therapy for metastatic colorectal cancer. *Oncologist* 2014;**19**(4):350–351.

190. Giantonio BJ, *et al.* Bevacizumab in combination with oxaliplatin, fluorouracil, and leucovorin (FOLFOX4) for previously treated metastatic colorectal cancer: Results from the Eastern Cooperative Oncology Group Study E3200. *J Clin Oncol* 2007;**25**(12):1539–1544.

191. Tang PA, *et al.* Phase II clinical and pharmacokinetic study of aflibercept in patients with previously treated metastatic colorectal cancer. *Clin Cancer Res* 2012;**18**(21): 6023–6031.

192. Van Cutsem E, *et al.* Addition of aflibercept to fluorouracil, leucovorin, and irinotecan improves survival in a phase III randomized trial in patients with metastatic colorectal cancer previously treated with an oxaliplatin-based regimen. *J Clin Oncol* 2012; **30**(28):3499–3506.

193. Grothey A, *et al.* Regorafenib monotherapy for previously treated metastatic colorectal cancer (CORRECT): An international, multicentre, randomised, placebo-controlled, phase 3 trial. *Lancet* 2013;**381**(9863):303–312.

194. Tabernero J, *et al.* Ramucirumab versus placebo in combination with second-line FOLFIRI in patients with metastatic colorectal carcinoma that progressed during or after first-line therapy with bevacizumab, oxaliplatin, and a fluoropyrimidine (RAISE): A randomised, double-blind, multicentre, phase 3 study. *Lancet Oncol* 2015;**16**(5): 499–508.

195. Jenab-Wolcott J, Giantonio BJ. Antiangiogenic therapy in colorectal cancer: Where are we 5 years later? *Clin Colorectal Cancer* 2010;**9** Suppl. 1:S7–S15.

196. Wagner AD, *et al.* Anti-angiogenic therapies for metastatic colorectal cancer. *Cochrane Database Syst Rev* 2009;(3):CD005392.

197. Cao Y, *et al.* A meta-analysis of randomized controlled trials comparing chemotherapy plus bevacizumab with chemotherapy alone in metastatic colorectal cancer. *Int J Colorectal Dis* 2009;**24**(6):677–685.

198. Welch S, *et al.* Bevacizumab combined with chemotherapy for patients with advanced colorectal cancer: A systematic review. *Ann Oncol* 2010;**21**(6):1152–1162.

199. Grothey A, *et al.* Bevacizumab beyond first progression is associated with prolonged overall survival in metastatic colorectal cancer: Results from a large observational cohort study (BRiTE). *J Clin Oncol* 2008;**26**(33):5326–5334.

200. Grothey A, *et al.* Bevacizumab exposure beyond first disease progression in patients with metastatic colorectal cancer: Analyses of the ARIES observational cohort study. *Pharmacoepidemiol Drug Saf* 2014;**23**(7):726–734.

201. Cartwright TH, *et al.* Survival outcomes of bevacizumab beyond progression in metastatic colorectal cancer patients treated in US community oncology. *Clin Colorectal Cancer* 2012;**11**(4):238–246.

202. Bennouna J, *et al.* Continuation of bevacizumab after first progression in metastatic colorectal cancer (ML18147): A randomised phase 3 trial. *Lancet Oncol* 2013;**14**(1):29–37.

203. Masi G, *et al.* Continuation or reintroduction of bevacizumab beyond progression to first-line therapy in metastatic colorectal cancer: Final results of the randomized BEBYP trial. *Ann Oncol* 2015;**26**(4):724–730.

204. Gaya A, Tse V. A preclinical and clinical review of aflibercept for the management of cancer. *Cancer Treat Rev* 2012;**38**(5):484–493.

205. Holash J, *et al.* VEGF-Trap: A VEGF blocker with potent antitumor effects. *Proc Natl Acad Sci U S A* 2002;**99**(17):11393–11398.

206. Lu D, *et al.* Selection of high affinity human neutralizing antibodies to VEGFR2 from a large antibody phage display library for antiangiogenesis therapy. *Int J Cancer* 2002;**97**(3):393–399.

207. Bruns CJ, *et al.* Vascular endothelial growth factor is an *in vivo* survival factor for tumor endothelium in a murine model of colorectal carcinoma liver metastases. *Cancer* 2000;**89**(3):488–499.

208. Wilhelm SM, *et al.* Regorafenib (BAY 73–4506): A new oral multikinase inhibitor of angiogenic, stromal and oncogenic receptor tyrosine kinases with potent preclinical antitumor activity. *Int J Cancer* 2011;**129**(1):245–255.

209. Messa C, *et al.* EGF, TGF-alpha, and EGF-R in human colorectal adenocarcinoma. *Acta Oncol* 1998;**37**(3):285–289.

210. Porebska I, *et al.* Expression of the tyrosine kinase activity growth factor receptors (EGFR, ERB B2, ERB B3) in colorectal adenocarcinomas and adenomas. *Tumour Biol* 2000;**21**(2):105–115.

211. Mayer A, *et al.* The prognostic significance of proliferating cell nuclear antigen, epidermal growth factor receptor, and *mdr* gene expression in colorectal cancer. *Cancer* 1993;**71**(8):2454–2460.

212. Klapper LN, *et al.* Biochemical and clinical implications of the ErbB/HER signaling network of growth factor receptors. *Adv Cancer Res* 2000;**77**:25–79.

213. Mendelsohn J, Baselga J. The EGF receptor family as targets for cancer therapy. *Oncogene* 2000;**19**(56):6550–6565.

214. Ciardiello F, Tortora G. A novel approach in the treatment of cancer: Targeting the epidermal growth factor receptor. *Clin Cancer Res* 2001;**7**(10):2958–2970.

215. Bokemeyer C, *et al.* Efficacy according to biomarker status of cetuximab plus FOLFOX-4 as first-line treatment for metastatic colorectal cancer: The OPUS study. *Ann Oncol* 2011;**22**(7):1535–1546.

216. Van Cutsem E, *et al.* Cetuximab plus irinotecan, fluorouracil, and leucovorin as first-line treatment for metastatic colorectal cancer: Updated analysis of overall survival according to tumor *KRAS* and *BRAF* mutation status. *J Clin Oncol* 2011;**29**(15):2011–2019.

217. Douillard JY, *et al.* Panitumumab–FOLFOX4 treatment and *RAS* mutations in colorectal cancer. *N Engl J Med* 2013;**369**(11):1023–1034.

218. Amado RG, *et al.* Wild-type KRAS is required for panitumumab efficacy in patients with metastatic colorectal cancer. *J Clin Oncol* 2008;**26**(10):1626–1634.

219. Karapetis CS, *et al.* *K-ras* mutations and benefit from cetuximab in advanced colorectal cancer. *N Engl J Med* 2008;**359**(17):1757–1765.

220. Sorich MJ, *et al.* Extended *RAS* mutations and anti-EGFR monoclonal antibody survival benefit in metastatic colorectal cancer: A meta-analysis of randomized, controlled trials. *Ann Oncol* 2015;**26**(1):13–21.

221. De Roock W, *et al.* Association of KRAS p.G13D mutation with outcome in patients with chemotherapy-refractory metastatic colorectal cancer treated with cetuximab. *JAMA* 2010;**304**(16):1812–1820.

222. Tejpar S, *et al.* Association of KRAS G13D tumor mutations with outcome in patients with metastatic colorectal cancer treated with first-line chemotherapy with or without cetuximab. *J Clin Oncol* 2012;**30**(29):3570–3577.

223. Peeters M, *et al.* Mutant *KRAS* codon 12 and 13 alleles in patients with metastatic colorectal cancer: Assessment as prognostic and predictive biomarkers of response to panitumumab. *J Clin Oncol* 2013;**31**(6):759–765.

224. Gajate P, *et al.* Influence of *KRAS* p.G13D mutation in patients with metastatic colorectal cancer treated with cetuximab. *Clin Colorectal Cancer* 2012;**11**(4):291–296.

225. Bokemeyer C, *et al.* Treatment outcome according to tumor RAS mutation status in OPUS study patients with metastatic colorectal cancer (mCRC) randomized to FOLFOX4 with/without cetuximab. *ASCO Meet Abstr* 2014;**32**(15 Suppl.):3505.

226. Van Cutsem E, *et al.* Fluorouracil, leucovorin, and irinotecan plus cetuximab treatment and *RAS* mutations in colorectal cancer. *J Clin Oncol* 2015;**33**(7):692–700.

227. Lochhead P, *et al.* Microsatellite instability and BRAF mutation testing in colorectal cancer prognostication. *J Natl Cancer Inst* 2013;**105**(15):1151–1156.

228. Gonsalves WI, *et al.* Patient and tumor characteristics and *BRAF* and *KRAS* mutations in colon cancer, NCCTG/Alliance N0147. *J Natl Cancer Inst* 2014;**106**(7): pii: dju106.

229. Maughan TS, *et al.* Addition of cetuximab to oxaliplatin-based first-line combination chemotherapy for treatment of advanced colorectal cancer: Results of the randomised phase 3 MRC COIN trial. *Lancet* 2011;**377**(9783):2103–2114.

230. Seymour MT, *et al.* Panitumumab and irinotecan versus irinotecan alone for patients with *KRAS* wild-type, fluorouracil-resistant advanced colorectal cancer (PICCOLO): A prospectively stratified randomised trial. *Lancet Oncol* 2013;**14**(8):749–759.

231. Di Nicolantonio F, *et al.* Wild-type BRAF is required for response to panitumumab or cetuximab in metastatic colorectal cancer. *J Clin Oncol* 2008;**26**(35):5705–5712.

232. Rowland A, *et al.* Meta-analysis of *BRAF* mutation as a predictive biomarker of benefit from anti-EGFR monoclonal antibody therapy for RAS wild-type metastatic colorectal cancer. *Br J Cancer* 2015;**112**(12):1888–1894.

233. Falchook GS, *et al.* Dabrafenib in patients with melanoma, untreated brain metastases, and other solid tumours: A phase 1 dose-escalation trial. *Lancet* 2012;**379**(9829): 1893–1901.

234. Prahallad A, *et al.* Unresponsiveness of colon cancer to *BRAF*(V600E) inhibition through feedback activation of EGFR. *Nature* 2012;**483**(7387):100–103.

235. Corcoran RB, *et al.* EGFR-mediated re-activation of MAPK signaling contributes to insensitivity of BRAF mutant colorectal cancers to RAF inhibition with vemurafenib. *Cancer Discov* 2012;**2**(3):227–235.

236. Saltz LB, *et al.* Phase II trial of cetuximab in patients with refractory colorectal cancer that expresses the epidermal growth factor receptor. *J Clin Oncol* 2004;**22**(7): 1201–1208.

237. Jonker DJ, *et al.* Cetuximab for the treatment of colorectal cancer. *N Engl J Med* 2007;**357**(20):2040–2048.

238. Prewett MC, *et al.* Enhanced antitumor activity of anti-epidermal growth factor receptor monoclonal antibody IMC-C225 in combination with irinotecan (CPT-11) against human colorectal tumor xenografts. *Clin Cancer Res* 2002;**8**(5):994–1003.

239. Saltz L, *et al.* Cetuximab (IMC-C225) plus irinotecan (CPT-11) is active in CPT-11-refractory colorectal cancer (CRC) that expresses epidermal growth factor receptor (EGFR). *Proc Am Soc Clin Oncol* 2001;**20**(3a):Abstr. 7.

240. Cunningham D, *et al.* Cetuximab monotherapy and cetuximab plus irinotecan in irinotecan-refractory metastatic colorectal cancer. *N Engl J Med* 2004;**351**(4):337–345.

241. Sobrero AF, *et al.* EPIC: Phase III trial of cetuximab plus irinotecan after fluoropyrimidine and oxaliplatin failure in patients with metastatic colorectal cancer. *J Clin Oncol* 2008;**26**(14):2311–2319.

242. Bokemeyer C, *et al.* Fluorouracil, leucovorin, and oxaliplatin with and without cetuximab in the first-line treatment of metastatic colorectal cancer. *J Clin Oncol* 2009;**27**(5):663–671.

243. Tveit KM, *et al.* Phase III trial of cetuximab with continuous or intermittent fluorouracil, leucovorin, and oxaliplatin (Nordic FLOX) versus FLOX alone in first-line treatment of metastatic colorectal cancer: The NORDIC-VII study. *J Clin Oncol* 2012;**30**(15):1755–1762.

244. Van Cutsem E, *et al.* Cetuximab and chemotherapy as initial treatment for metastatic colorectal cancer. *N Engl J Med* 2009;**360**(14):1408–1417.

245. Douillard JY, *et al.* Randomized, phase III trial of panitumumab with infusional fluorouracil, leucovorin, and oxaliplatin (FOLFOX4) versus FOLFOX4 alone as first-line treatment in patients with previously untreated metastatic colorectal cancer: The PRIME study. *J Clin Oncol* 2010;**28**(31):4697–4705.

246. Van Cutsem E, *et al.* Open-label phase III trial of panitumumab plus best supportive care compared with best supportive care alone in patients with chemotherapy-refractory metastatic colorectal cancer. *J Clin Oncol* 2007;**25**(13):1658–1664.

247. Peeters M, *et al.* Randomized phase III study of panitumumab with fluorouracil, leucovorin, and irinotecan (FOLFIRI) compared with FOLFIRI alone as second-line treatment in patients with metastatic colorectal cancer. *J Clin Oncol* 2010;**28**(31): 4706–4713.

248. Peeters M, *et al.*, Final results from a randomized phase 3 study of FOLFIRI {+/-} panitumumab for second-line treatment of metastatic colorectal cancer. *Ann Oncol* 2014;**25**(1):107–116.

249. Peeters M, *et al.* Analysis of KRAS/NRAS mutations in phase 3 study 20050181 of panitumumab (pmab) plus FOLFIRI versus FOLFIRI for second-line treatment (tx) of metastatic colorectal cancer (mCRC). *ASCO Meet Abstr* 2014;**32**(3 Suppl.):LBA387.

250. Price TJ, *et al.* Panitumumab versus cetuximab in patients with chemotherapy-refractory wild-type KRAS exon 2 metastatic colorectal cancer (ASPECCT): A randomised,

multicentre, open-label, non-inferiority phase 3 study. *Lancet Oncol* 2014;**15**(6): 569–579.

251. Ciardiello F, *et al.* Antiangiogenic and antitumor activity of anti-epidermal growth factor receptor C225 monoclonal antibody in combination with vascular endothelial growth factor antisense oligonucleotide in human GEO colon cancer cells. *Clin Cancer Res* 2000;**6**(9):3739–3747.

252. Shaheen RM, *et al.* Inhibited growth of colon cancer carcinomatosis by antibodies to vascular endothelial and epidermal growth factor receptors. *Br J Cancer* 2001; **85**(4):584–589.

253. Jung YD, *et al.* Effects of combination anti-vascular endothelial growth factor receptor and anti-epidermal growth factor receptor therapies on the growth of gastric cancer in a nude mouse model. *Eur J Cancer* 2002;**38**(8):1133–1140.

254. Tonra JR, *et al.* Synergistic antitumor effects of combined epidermal growth factor receptor and vascular endothelial growth factor receptor-2 targeted therapy. *Clin Cancer Res* 2006;**12**(7 Pt. 1):2197–2207.

255. Saltz LB, *et al.* Randomized phase II trial of cetuximab, bevacizumab, and irinotecan compared with cetuximab and bevacizumab alone in irinotecan-refractory colorectal cancer: The BOND-2 study. *J Clin Oncol* 2007;**25**(29):4557–4561.

256. Hecht JR, *et al.* A randomized phase IIIB trial of chemotherapy, bevacizumab, and panitumumab compared with chemotherapy and bevacizumab alone for metastatic colorectal cancer. *J Clin Oncol* 2009;**27**(5):672–680.

257. Tol J, *et al.* Chemotherapy, bevacizumab, and cetuximab in metastatic colorectal cancer. *N Engl J Med* 2009;**360**(6):563–572.

258. Schwartzberg LS, *et al.* PEAK: A randomized, multicenter phase II study of panitumumab plus modified fluorouracil, leucovorin, and oxaliplatin (mFOLFOX6) or bevacizumab plus mFOLFOX6 in patients with previously untreated, unresectable, wild-type *KRAS* exon 2 metastatic colorectal cancer. *J Clin Oncol* 2014;**32**(21): 2240–2247.

259. Heinemann V, *et al.* FOLFIRI plus cetuximab versus FOLFIRI plus bevacizumab as first-line treatment for patients with metastatic colorectal cancer (FIRE-3): A randomised, open-label, phase 3 trial. *Lancet Oncol* 2014;**15**(10):1065–1075.

260. Lenz H, *et al.* 501OCALGB/SWOG 80405: Phase III trial of irinotecan/5-fu/leucovorin (FOLFIRI) or oxaliplatin/5-fu/leucovorin (mFOLFOX6) with bevacizumab (BV) or cetuximab (CET) for patients (Pts) with expanded ras analyses untreated metastatic adenocarcinoma of the colon or rectum (mCRC). *Ann Oncol* 2014;**25**(Suppl. 4), doi: 10.1093/annonc/mdu438.13.

261. Alexopoulos CG. Kotsori AA. Continuous versus intermittent chemotherapy in metastatic colorectal cancer. *ASCO Meet Abstr* 2006;**24**(18 Suppl.):3582.

262. Labianca R, *et al.* Intermittent versus continuous chemotherapy in advanced colorectal cancer: A randomised 'GISCAD' trial. *Ann Oncol* 2011;**22**(5):1236–1242.

263. Adams RA, *et al.*, Intermittent versus continuous oxaliplatin and fluoropyrimidine combination chemotherapy for first-line treatment of advanced colorectal cancer: Results of the randomised phase 3 MRC COIN trial. *Lancet Oncol* 2011;**12**(7):642–653.

264. Chibaudel B, *et al*. Can chemotherapy be discontinued in unresectable metastatic colorectal cancer? The GERCOR OPTIMOX2 Study. *J Clin Oncol* 2009;**27**(34): 5727–5733.

265. Diaz-Rubio E, *et al*. First-line XELOX plus bevacizumab followed by XELOX plus bevacizumab or single-agent bevacizumab as maintenance therapy in patients with metastatic colorectal cancer: Yhe phase III MACRO TTD study. *Oncologist* 2012;**17**(1):15–25.

266. Grothey A, *et al*. Intermittent oxaliplatin (oxali) administration and time-to-treatment-failure (TTF) in metastatic colorectal cancer (mCRC): Final results of the phase III CONcePT trial. *ASCO Meet Abstr* 2008;**26**(15 Suppl.):4010.

267. Yalcin S, *et al*. Bevacizumab + capecitabine as maintenance therapy after initial bevacizumab + XELOX treatment in previously untreated patients with metastatic colorectal cancer: Phase III 'Stop and Go' study results — a Turkish Oncology Group Trial. *Oncology* 2013;**85**(6):328–335.

268. Koopman M, *et al*. Final results and subgroup analyses of the phase 3 CAIRO3 study: Maintenance treatment with capecitabine + bevacizumab versus observation after induction treatment with chemotherapy + bevacizumab in metastatic colorectal cancer (mCRC). *ASCO Meet Abstr* 2014;**32**(15 Suppl.):3504.

269. Simkens LH, *et al*. Maintenance treatment with capecitabine and bevacizumab in metastatic colorectal cancer (CAIRO3): A phase 3 randomised controlled trial of the Dutch Colorectal Cancer Group. *Lancet* 2015;**385**(9980):1843–1852.

270. Berry SR, *et al*. Continuous versus intermittent chemotherapy strategies in metastatic colorectal cancer: A systematic review and meta-analysis. *Ann Oncol* 2015;**26**(3): 477–485.

271. Schumacher TN, Schreiber RD. Neoantigens in cancer immunotherapy. *Science* 2015;**348**(6230):69–74.

272. Hodi FS, *et al*. Improved survival with ipilimumab in patients with metastatic melanoma. *N Engl J Med* 2010;**363**(8):711–723.

273. Robert C, *et al*. Pembrolizumab versus ipilimumab in advanced melanoma. *N Engl J Med* 2015;**372**(26):2521–2532.

274. Postow MA, *et al*. Nivolumab and ipilimumab versus ipilimumab in untreated melanoma. *N Engl J Med* 2015;**372**(21):2006–2017.

275. Garon EB, *et al*. Pembrolizumab for the treatment of non-small-cell lung cancer. *N Engl J Med* 2015;**372**(21):2018–2028.

276. Brahmer J, *et al*. Nivolumab versus docetaxel in advanced squamous-cell non-small-cell lung cancer. *N Engl J Med* 2015;**373**(2):123–135.

277. Gettinger SN, *et al*. Overall Survival and long-term safety of nivolumab (anti-programmed death 1 antibody, BMS-936558, ONO-4538) in patients with previously treated advanced non-small-cell lung cancer. *J Clin Oncol* 2015;**33**(18):2004–2012.

278. Alexandrov LB, *et al*. Signatures of mutational processes in human cancer. *Nature* 2013;**500**(7463):415–421.

279. Topalian SL, *et al*. Safety, activity, and immune correlates of anti-PD-1 antibody in cancer. *N Engl J Med* 2012;**366**(26):2443–2454.

280. Chung KY, *et al.* Phase II study of the anti-cytotoxic T-lymphocyte-associated antigen 4 monoclonal antibody, tremelimumab, in patients with refractory metastatic colorectal cancer. *J Clin Oncol* 2010;**28**(21):3485–3490.

281. Brahmer JR, *et al.* Safety and activity of anti-PD-L1 antibody in patients with advanced cancer. *N Engl J Med* 2012;**366**(26):2455–2465.

282. Lipson EJ, *et al.* Durable cancer regression off-treatment and effective reinduction therapy with an anti-PD-1 antibody. *Clin Cancer Res* 2013;**19**(2):462–468.

283. Le DT, *et al.* PD-1 blockade in tumors with mismatch-repair deficiency. *N Engl J Med* 2015;**372**(26):2509–2520.

Chapter 14

Local and Locally Advanced Rectal Cancer

Bert H. O'Neil, Alyssa D. Fajardo, Andrew Wang and Safi Shahda

1 Introduction

Rectal cancer comprises approximately 30% of cases of cancers of the large intestine in the United States, with an expected incidence for 2014 of approximately 40,000 patients.[1] Prognosis for rectal cancer has improved over time, but is still slightly worse than cancer of the colon.[2] The rectum is defined as the portion of the large intestine that resides in the true pelvis (i.e. below the abdominal peritoneal reflection) (Figure 1). The typical endoscopic definition of a rectal vs. sigmoid colon tumor is 12–15 cm, but this number varies from person to person, and given the flexibility of the colonoscope, these measurements can be inaccurate compared with those obtained by rigid proctoscopy or even digital rectal examination. It should also be noted that there is no endoscopically definable landmark that defines the proximal boundary of the rectum. The dentate line defines the distal margin of the rectum endoscopically.

As is the case with colon cancer, the primary modality for cure of rectal cancer remains surgery. However, optimization of cure has come to involve chemotherapy and radiotherapy in more advanced cases due to the potential for this cancer to recur within the pelvis or to recur systemically. In this chapter, we outline the current options for therapy (of stages II, and III rectal cancer) with focus on areas of remaining controversy. We advocate for a risk-based approach to therapy that is based on adequate initial staging of the cancer and involves careful physical examination, endoscopic ultrasound or good quality pelvic magnetic resonance imaging (MRI), and imaging of the abdomen by computed tomography (CT) or MRI.

2 Local and Regional Staging

2.1 *Physical exam*

A physical exam should include a digital rectal exam (DRE) and proctoscopy to yield valuable information regarding tumor characteristics, including the location of the tumor and whether there is fixation to the sphincter muscles. The location, morphology, number of quadrants involved, degree or fixation and mobility, and direct continuity with other structures should all be noted. For a low rectal or anal canal tumor, inguinal lymph node evaluation should be included in the exam. Clinical staging systems exist, however the accuracy is not dependable and is related to examiner experience.[3] DRE use alone is inadequate and other adjuncts are needed to fully stage rectal cancer.

2.2 *Imaging*

The goals of imaging the primary tumor are as follows: (1) assess the T-stage (both from a standpoint of depth of penetration of the tumor through the bowel wall; this may be best accomplished by endoscopic ultrasound; (2) assess relationship of the tumor to adjacent structures such as the bladder, vagina, prostate or pelvic wall; this may best be accomplished by MRI; (3) assess local nodal status–the ability of MRI and ERUS for this goal are similar; (4) assess the relationship between the tumor and the mesorectum, likely best accomplished by MRI. Whether to choose endo-rectal ultrasound (ERUS), MRI or perform both remains somewhat controversial, but often depends on local imaging capabilities. Some groups have advocated that the imaging technologies are complementary and as such should both be performed routinely.[4] CT imaging is primarily useful for assessment of metastatic disease and less useful for distinguishing treatment-determining local characteristics of the tumor.[5]

2.2.1. *Endorectal ultrasound*

ERUS (Figure 1) can be performed after an enema to better evaluate the rectal mass after endoscopic assessment to evaluate both the T and N stages. A 360 degree rotating endorectal probe provides complete circular imaging, and either a 7 or 10 mHz transducer is used to provide a five layer model of the rectal wall. There are three hyperechoic concentric circles and two hypoechoic circles, corresponding to the interfaces between the different layers of the rectal wall.[6] ERUS is useful in establishing if a tumor breeches the muscularis propria which infers a uT3 lesion. It is also helpful in determining if the tumor extends into the

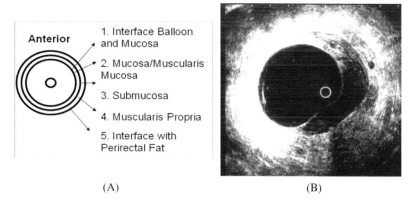

Figure 1   Illustration of ERUS in rectal carcinoma diagnosis.

submucosa (uT1) or involves the muscularis propria (uT2).[7,8] The perirectal tissues are also evaluated for evidence of lymph node involvement. Nodes that are visualized are considered metastatic.

The accuracy for evaluating rectal cancer stage is user dependent and variable. The accuracy ranges from 39–95%, and a significant percentage of patients are either under or overstaged.[9–13] There are lower accuracy rates for T1 and T2 lesions, and the accuracy for nodal involvement is about 75%.[10,14]

There are several limitations to the use of ERUS. These include a significant learning curve, user dependence, difficulty determining inflammatory verses neoplastic lymph nodes, difficulty to perform in high rectal cancers and near obstructing lesions, and patient discomfort. Furthermore, ERUS often cannot evaluate regional lymphatic involvement as it cannot detect nodes further away in the mesorectum or identify micrometastatic disease in a lymph node. The use of fine needle aspiration has not been shown to significantly improve nodal staging over ERUS alone, and therefore is not routinely used as it also has a potential risk of seeding tumor cells.[15]

2.2.2 *Magnetic resonance imaging*

Initial experience with using body-coil MRI was poor, however with advents in technology there are now high-resolution images without the need for an intra-rectal coil. This has improved accuracy rates when the acquired images obtained are directly parallel or perpendicular to the tumor and by distending the rectum with gel. Accuracy rates for T stage are ~80% and ~70–80% for nodal staging.[16,17] MRI T staging has been defined and can be seen in Table 1.[18]

Table 1   MRI Staging proposed by Brown *et al.*[18]

MRI T stage
T1:   Low signal in the submucosal layer or replacement of the submucosal layer by abnormal signal not extending into circular muscle layer.
T2:   Intermediate signal intensity within muscularis propria. Outer muscle coat replaced by tumor of intermediate signal intensity that does not extend beyond the outer rectal muscle into perirectal fat.
T3:   Broad-based bulge or nodular projection (not fine speculation) of intermediate signal intensity projecting beyond outer muscle coat.
T4:   Extension of abnormal signal into adjacent organ, extension of tumor signal through the peritoneal reflection.

The resolution of MRI limits the ability to distinguish between T1 and T2 lesions as it does not typically delineate the layers of the rectal wall. Another limitation of MRI is that lymph node involvement criteria by MRI have not been standardized. Size criteria are not adequate, and the criteria that is most predictable for determining lymph node metastasis are signal heterogeneity and an irregular border.[16] Newer technology using ultrasmall superparamagnetic iron oxide (UPSIO)-enhanced MRI has been shown to have a 93% sensitivity and 96% specificity for perirectal lymph node metastases, but these findings still need to be validated.[19] This modality is not clinically available at this point in time.

The circumferential resection margin (CRM) is now known to be an important predictor of locoregional recurrence in rectal cancer patients undergoing a radical proctectomy with total mesorectal excision.[20–23] A curative operation in patients with a positive CRM requires either an extended resection or tumor downstaging with neoadjuvant chemoradiation therapy as postoperative radiation does not reduce the risk of local recurrence.[24] A phased-array coil MRI can predict with high accuracy the distance of the tumor to the rectal fascia propria (Figure 2).[25,26]

2.2.3 *Distant metastases*

Widespread metastatic disease must be ruled out prior to consideration for resection. The most common sites of metastasis from rectal cancer are to the liver and lung. Computed tomography (CT) scan is universally available and the most common modality to evaluate for metastatic disease; however, it is not accurate in determining T and N stage of rectal cancer. Furthermore, CT can miss or underestimate the extent of disease in a significant proportion of patients.[27] Abdominal MRI, CT, and 18-fluorodeoxyglucose positron emission tomography (FDG-PET) have been compared to evaluate for metastatic disease, and FDG-PET has been more accurate to detect liver metastasis.[28]

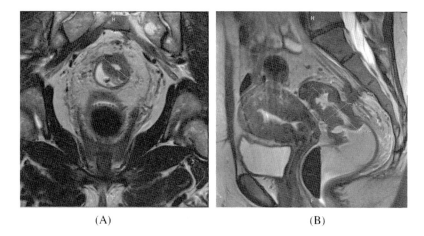

(A)   (B)

Figure 2 MRI of rectal carcinoma.

Once widespread metastatic disease has been ruled out, then the patient may be considered for resection. If a patient has metastatic disease to the lung or liver that is limited and felt to be able to be completely resected, he or she may still be a candidate for resection. The optimal therapy in these patients needs to be discussed via multidisciplinary setting between the oncologist, radiation oncologist, and surgeon and decided on a case-by-case basis, taking into account tumor biology and response to neoadjuvant treatment. Either staged or combined procedures may be recommended.[29,30] If there is concern for impending obstruction or the patient is obstructed, then the patient should be offered individualized therapy of fecal diversion verses stent placement.

3 Surgical Therapy

An ideal surgical treatment strategy for rectal cancer is one that is curative while preserving sphincter function with minimal morbidity. Local excision techniques can achieve this in well-selected patients. Local recurrence for local therapy of rectal cancer can be attributed to untreated involved lymph nodes, tumor implantation at the time of surgery, lymphatic spread or persistence at the time of surgery, or by a positive margin leaving residual cancer *in situ*. When deciding which operative approach is best for a patient, these must be taken into account.

3.1 *Local excision*

Patient selection for a local excision is paramount, and surgical candidates should have a low risk of lymph nodes metastasis, as lymph nodes are not addressed during local resection. Patients with an early T1 lesion without any high risk features are the most ideal candidates. High risk features include lymphovascular and perineural invasion, poorly differentiated tumors, tumor budding, and T2–T3 tumors.[31,32] T1 cancers can further be classified by sm levels (designated sm1, sm2, or sm3) in accordance with what third of the submucosa the lesion extends.[33] Submucosal level of penetration has been shown to significantly affect lymph node positivity. Incidences of lymph node metastases range from 0–4% for sm1 tumors, 8–21% for sm2, and 23–38.5% for sm3.[33–35] Patients with deeper tumors or high risk features that are poor surgical candidates for a radical resection may be offered a local resection in highly selected cases. These patients must be counseled that it is not the standard of care and could be suboptimal, which requires neoadjuvant or/and adjuvant chemoradiation treatment in conjuction with local treatment.

Operative approaches for transanal excision include a traditional local excision and minimally invasive options including transanal endoscopic microsurgery (TEM) and transanal minimally invasive surgery (TAMIS). The traditional transanal excision can be performed for distal rectal tumors. The patient is positioned depending on tumor location. Anal effacement can be achieved by either retractors or sutures. An operating protoscope is introduced to expose the mass. Stay sutures are placed at the lateral borders of the lesion. Electrocautery is then used to mark 1 cm margins around the lesion, and then a full thickness excision ensues. The specimen is removed *en bloc* and properly oriented for pathological review. The defect is then closed transversely and patency of the rectal lumen is ensured.

TEM and TAMIS involve using either an operating 4 cm proctoscope or TAMIS platform respectively, and each establish a pneumorectum by insufflating $CO2$. The operating microscope or laparoscope allows clear visualization of the lesion, and 1 cm margins are established by laparoscopic instrumentation using electrocautery. A full thickness excision (including as much of the mesorectum as desired) is then performed. It should be noted that for high lesions, especially anteriorly, that the abdominal cavity can be entered and requires repair and discussion with the patient regarding the potential need for an abdominal procedure to repair the defect and even a temporary ostomy. Complications include urinary retention, bleeding, development of rectovaginal or rectourethral fistulas in anterior lesions, perforation, infection, and temporary incontinence.

3.2 *Radical excision*

Patients who have T1 cancers with high risk features and any T2-T4 lesions along with any patients with nodal disease should be offered radical resection if no metastatic disease is identified. The decision as to what operation is best for the patient depends on the tumor stage, candidacy of the patient to tolerate an operation, preoperative incontinence, and tumor location. Tumor location will determine resectability and sphincter preservation or sacrifice. Tumors that are T3 or T4 or any nodal disease should be offered neoadjuvant chemoradiation prior to resection with adjuvant treatment after recovery from surgery. T1 or T2 tumors without nodal involvement may proceed directly to resection.

3.2.1 *Sphincter-sparing surgery*

Sphincter-sparing surgery includes performing a low anterior resection (LAR) with total mesorectal excision. A 2 cm distal margin is typically deemed sufficient in order to perform an anastomosis. An "ultralow" LAR implies that a coloanal anastomosis is created. Reconstruction of intestinal continuity can be achieve by a straight stapled anastomosis, a handsewn anastomosis, use of an end to side or side to end anastomosis, or by use of a colonic J pouch reservoir depending on patient factors and surgeon preference. Protection by a loop ileostomy is dependent on anastomosis level, presence of air leak during testing, prior radiation, use of pouch along with other patient factors, and again, surgeon preference. Anastomotic leak is the most feared complication and can occur in up to 17% of cases.[36]

3.2.2 *Abdominoperineal resection*

An abdominoperineal resection (APR) removes the mesorectum, rectum, levator muscles, and anus. This technique is used for low rectal tumors involving the sphincter complex, if adequate oncologic margins are unable to be obtained, and for rectal cancer radical excision candidates with fecal incontinence. An APR requires creation of a permanent colostomy. Like patients undergoing a LAR, infertility, impotence and ejaculatory complications can occur from the pelvic dissection and these sexual dysfunctions can occur in up to 67% of individuals.[37] Other common complications after APR include delayed wound healing or infection of the perineal wound, urinary dysfunction, and issues with the colostomy (pouching problems, retraction, stenosis, or peristomal hernia).

3.2.3 *Total mesorectal excision*

Total mesorectal excision (TME) in conjunction with an LAR or an APR involves precise sharp dissection and removal of the entire rectal mesentery, including that distal to the tumor, as an intact unit.[38] The rectal mesentery is removed sharply under direct visualization to preserve the autonomic nerves, minimize blood loss, and to avoid violation of the mesorectal envelope.[39] It is hypothesized that the field of rectal cancer spread is limited to this envelope and its total removal encompasses the tumor burden locally. Conventional surgery violates the circumference of the mesorectum during the blunt dissection along undefined planes. This leaves residual mesorectum in the pelvis and a higher rate of pelvic recurrence. The TME technique has a reported local failure rates from 5–7% for Stage II and Stage III cancers.[38,40,41] The "completeness" of the TME also correlates with prognosis.[42]

4 Adjuvant and Neuoadjuvant Therapy

4.1 *Adjuvant therapy*

The currently accepted standard of care for locally advanced rectal cancer in the United States involves preoperative chemoradiotherapy followed by surgical resection. This treatment paradigm was confirmed by the German Rectal Cancer Trial (CAO/ARO/AIO 94- described in more detail below),[43] but came as a culmination of many studies evaluating the benefits of radiotherapy and chemotherapy as described in this section. The need for and type of adjuvant therapy should be driven by the two major risks for these patients, the risk of local recurrence and the risk of distant metastasis after apparently adequate surgery. Due to its bony structure and presence of the major nerves and vessels of the lower extremities, local recurrence in the pelvis is a significant management issue that can lead to devastating morbidity for patients. A large combined analysis of several (postoperative therapy) randomized trials by Gunderson *et al.*[44] gives us an excellent picture of risk of local and distant recurrence for all potential T and N stage combinations. It should be noted that some of these recurrence rates are likely to be overestimated given that trials included in this analysis were performed in the pre-total mesorectal excision (TME) era. The major message of this analysis is that both T and N stage are independently important for risk of local recurrence (for example, a T1N1 tumor would have a similar chance of local recurrence as a tumor that is T3N0). Oncologists of all types should be familiar with these relative risks when assigning various treatment modalities to their patients.

4.1.1 *Postoperative chemoradiotherapy and continuous infusion fluorouracil*

The importance of postoperative chemoradiotherapy (versus surgery alone or surgery plus radiotherapy) was established over the two decades preceeding the publication of the German rectal cancer trial. The NSABP R02 trial randomized 694 patients with Dukes' B and C rectal cancer to either adjuvant chemotherapy or adjuvant chemoradiotherapy.[45] The addition of radiotherapy did not result in survival benefit but did reduce local recurrence risk (13% to 8% at 5-year, $p = 0.02$). The Mayo/NCCTG 79-47-51 trial studied the utility of concurrent chemotherapy with radiotherapy in the postoperative setting. It was a randomized phase III trial with 204 patients with T3-4 or N+ rectal cancer. The patients were randomized to postoperative chemoradiation or postoperative radiotherapy alone.[46] After a median follow-up of more than 7 years, the combined therapy reduced the recurrence of rectal cancer by 34 percent (63% to 41%, $p = 0.0016$) and distant metastasis by 37 percent ($p = 0.011$). It also demonstrated improvements in both cancer-related survival and OS (55% vs. 40%). The GITSG GI-7175 trial randomized 227 patients to surgery alone, adjuvant radiotherapy, adjuvant chemotherapy, and adjuvant chemoradiotherapy.[47] With a median follow up of 6.7 years, the chemoradiotherapy group had the lowest recurrence risk though there was no difference in survival between the groups. However, with longer follow up (7.8 years), the investigators reported a survival benefit for chemoradiotherapy arm compared to surgery alone arm.[48] Together, these trials established postoperative chemoradiotherapy for rectal cancer.

The importance of chemotherapy for local control was also demonstrated by the European Organization for Research and Treatment of Cancer (EORTC) trial 22921. It was a four-arm randomized trial of 1011 patients who received preoperative irradiation of 45 Gy with or without a concurrent bolus of 5-FU/LV followed by surgery with or without four cycles of adjuvant 5-FU/LV chemotherapy.[49] The EORTC trial revealed a significant decrease in the local failure rate (5 year) in those patients who receive chemoradiation compared with irradiation (8% to 10% vs. 17%; $p < 0.001$), however there was no difference in the 5-year OS (65%). At 10 years, cumulative incidence of local relapse was 22·4% with radiotherapy alone, 11·8% with neoadjuvant radiotherapy and chemotherapy, 14·5% with radiotherapy and adjuvant chemotherapy and 11·7% with both adjuvant and neoadjuvant chemotherapy ($p = 0·0017$).[50] It is notable in this study that approximately a quarter of patients assigned to post-radiation chemotherapy never received that chemotherapy.

A similar trial was conducted by the Fédération Francophone de la Cancérologie Digestive group that randomized 742 patients to preoperative radiotherapy of 45 Gy with or without bolus 5-FU/leucovorin.[51] It reported a similar decrease in local failure rates (8.1% vs. 16.5%; $p < 0.05$) with preoperative chemoradiation vs. irradiation alone, but no survival benefit (68% vs. 67%).

Continuous infusion of 5-FU during the entirety of radiotherapy was studied against a week 1 and 5 approach by the U.S. Intergroup. In that study, 660 patients were randomized to postoperative bolus fluorouracil (350 mg/m2 daily d1-5, 400 mg/m2 days 36–40) versus CIV FU at 225 mg/m2 daily. Both groups received the same chemotherapy before and after chemoradiation. This change in fluorouracil administration led to decreases in both recurrence-free (63% vs. 53% at 4 years), and overall (70% vs. 60% at 4 years) survival.[52]

4.2 Preoperative vs. postoperative chemoradiotherapy

There are numerous reasons to surmise that preoperative chemoradiation is of benefit compared to postoperative therapy. These include the ability to avoid positive circumferential margins, conversion of APR to LAR, and preservation of stool continence due to removal of irradiated bowel at time of surgery rather than radiating a newly formed colorectal or coloanal anastomosis.[53] The German Rectal Cancer Trial[45] confirmed preoperative therapy as the current standard practice for patients who are candidates for chemoradiation. This seminal study randomized 421 patients with T3/4 or N+ rectal cancer to preoperative chemoradiotherapy or postoperative chemoradiotherapy. The preoperative treatment consisted of 5040 cGy in 180 cGy per fraction and 5FU given in a 120-hour continuous infusion during the first and fifth weeks of radiotherapy. Postoperative regimen differs from the preoperative regimen by an additional boost of 540 cGy. While there was no survival difference (76% vs. 74%, $p = 0.8$), the 5-year LR was lower in preoperative group (6% vs. 13%, $p = 0.006$). Both the acute grade 3/4 and long-term toxicities were lower in the preoperative arm, 27% vs. 40%, $p = 0.001$ and 14% vs. 24%, $p = 0.01$. Preoperative chemoradiotherapy was also associated with more tumor downstaging (~18%). Moreover, patients who were deemed to require abdominoperineal excision, a statistically significant increase in sphincter preservation was achieved in the preoperative arm. The sole downside of the approach is the potential for overtreatment- if one compares the EUS results in the pre- vs. postoperative therapy groups, it is apparent that overstaging by EUS occurred in approximately 18% of patients, suggesting potential overtreatment for this group of patients. Generally speaking, it is felt that the benefits of the preoperative approach outweigh this potential negative.

The MRC CR07 and NCIC-CTG C016 trial is a large trial that randomized 1350 patients to preoperative short-course radiotherapy or to selective postoperative chemoradiotherapy (long course).[48] The primary endpoint was local recurrence. With a median follow up of 4 years, there was a significant decrease in local recurrence in favor of preoperative treatment (4.4% vs. 10.6%, $p < 0.0001$). There was improvement in DFS (77.5% vs. 71.5%, $p = 0.013$) but no OS benefit. NSABP R-03 also attempted to answer the question of preoperative versus postoperative treatment in rectal cancer.[54] The trial originally intended to enroll 900 patients and randomize them to either preoperative or postoperative chemoradiotherapy.

However, the trial was only able to enroll 267 patients. With a median follow up of 8.4 years, preoperative arm had a significantly higher 5-year DFS (64.7% vs. 53.4%, *p* = 0.011). However, there was no significant difference in OS (74.5% vs. 65.6%, *p* = 0.065).

4.3 Short-course radiotherapy vs. long-course chemoradiotherapy in the preoperative setting

There are two principle options for preoperative radiotherapy of rectal cancer. One is a short-course radiotherapy only regimen (without chemotherapy), and the other is a longer-course radiotherapy with concurrent chemotherapy regimen. The short-course radiation treatment is an intense, 25 Gy in 5 daily fractions, regimen that has an estimated biological dose of 42 to 50 Gy in 2 Gy fractions.[55] It was first studied in Northern Europe and is most commonly utilized in that region. The Swedish Rectal Cancer Trial was the first to report a significant benefit of short-term radiation and is the only trial demonstrating a survival benefit for radiotherapy as a single adjuvant modality. In the Swedish study, patients with cT1-3 rectal cancer were randomized to receive either preoperative 25 Gy in 1 week followed by surgery 1 week later or surgery alone. 1186 patients were enrolled between 1987 and 1990. At 5 year follow up, patients who received preoperative irradiation had a significant decrease in local recurrence rates (11% vs. 27%; *p* < 0.001) as well as a significant improvement in 5-year OS (58% vs. 48%; *p* = 0.004). After 13 years, the OS is still significantly improved (38% vs. 30%; *p* = 0.008).[56] However, it is worth noting that this trial was conducted in the pre-TME era and the local recurrence rate was 46% in node-positive patients who were treated with surgery alone, a number much higher than the typical local recurrence rates from TME surgery.

A second large randomized trial evaluating the short-course radiotherapy was conducted by the Dutch Colorectal Cancer Group.[57] It randomized 1861 patients with cT1 to T3 disease to TME or intensive short-course preoperative radiation therapy followed by TME between 1996 to 1999. They found that preoperative short-course radiotherapy decreased the local recurrence rate (8% vs. 2%; *p* < 0.0001), but there was no difference in the 2-year survival rate (82% vs. 81.8%). With longer follow-up, the 10-year local failure rate was higher with TME (11%) but was still significantly decreased (to 5%) with preoperative irradiation.[58]

Two randomized trials have attempted to compare the shorter-course radiotherapy with the longer chemoradiotherapy regimen. The Polish Rectal Trial randomized 312 patients with cT3-T4 resectable rectal cancer palpable to preoperative short-course followed by surgery within 7 days or longer course chemoradiotherapy (bolus 5-FU/LV) with surgery 4–6 weeks after completion.[59] The primary study end point was sphincter preservation, and at a median follow-up of 48 months there was no difference between the two arms (61% short-course RT and 58% after long-course ($p = 0.57$)). In addition, there were no differences in DFS or OS. Acute Grade 3/4 toxicity was higher in the CRT arm (3.2% vs. 18.2 %) with no difference in late toxicity. It is important to note that nearly 40% of the patients in the short-course arm had pathologic T1-T2 disease and should not have been included on study by eligibility criteria. Furthermore, the chemotherapy in the long-course treatment is given in bolus rather than continuous infusion. Lastly, the sphincter-preservation endpoint is controversial as it is highly dependent on surgeons' level of comfort with changing surgical approach based on tumor response.

A second randomized trial comparing long-course chemoradiotherapy (infusional 5FU) to short-course RT was conducted by the Trans-Tasman Radiation Oncology Group.[60] The trial randomized 326 patients with T3 N0-2 rectal adenocarcinoma. The primary study end point was 3-year LR. After median follow-up of 5.9 years, the 3-year LR was 7.5% for short-course and 4.4% for long-course ($p = 0.24$). There was no difference in distant metastases, DFS, or OS.

Both short-course and long-course treatments have their advantages and disadvantages. Short-course treatment tends to have less short-term toxicity and provides higher level of treatment compliance. Though not shown in trials, the concern with short-course treatment is long-term toxicity as larger dose per fraction have more damage to normal tissue than lower dose per fraction.[61] One of the benefits of long-course chemoradiotherapy is tumor down-staging. Even though the Polish and Austria trials did not show any difference between long and short-term treatment, the German Rectal Cancer trial demonstrated both tumor downstaging and higher rates of sphincter-sparing surgery in patients with low-lying rectal malignancies. Recent data also showed that longer duration between chemoradiotherapy and surgery can also increase the rate of pCR.[62] Since data have not shown a clear benefit for either approach, both regimens are utilized and the difference in practice pattern is geographic.

4.4 *Is chemotherapy after preoperative CRT and surgery necessary?*

This question has become controversial over the past few years. A meta-analysis of postoperative trials with chemotherapy versus no chemotherapy arms has suggested a survival advantage to fluorouracil-based chemotherapy. However, only one large trial, EORTC 22921, has examined the role of postoperative chemotherapy directly in the more currently relevant setting of treatment with preoperative CRT. This trial randomized over 1000 patients to preoperative RT vs. CRT, then to postoperative

CT (fluorouracil and leucovorin) versus no adjuvant therapy. Long-term follow-up from this study was recently reported,[52] and demonstrated no statistically significant improvement in overall survival in patients who received postoperative fluorouracil and leucovorin. It is notable, however, that the number of patients in the treatment arm who did not receive planned therapy was high, perhaps diluting the benefit of that therapy. One very interesting observation from the 22921 study was that patients with pyT0-1 tumors (presumably those with the greatest degree of downstaging from preoperative therapy) appeared to derive the most benefit from postoperative adjuvant therapy.[48] At present, the authors of this chapter do not feel there is definitive evidence that postoperative chemotherapy is beneficial when preoperative CRT has been utilized; however, there remains enough indirect evidence that chemotherapy benefits patients with node positive colorectal cancer in general that oncologists should not forgo postoperative FU/LV altogether. Our practice is to administer (at a minimum) 4 months of a fluoropyrimidine-based regimen after recovery from surgery. The National Cancer Center Network (NCCN)[2] continues to recommend postoperative therapy in patients with locally advanced rectal cancer, based more on extrapolation from studies of stage III colon cancer than on studies specific to patients with rectal cancer.

4.5 *Neoadjuvant chemoradiotherapy: Roles of capecitabine and oxaliplatin during radiotherapy*

A number studies in a variety gastrointestinal malignancies including colon cancer have demonstrated similar activity with capecitabine in comparison to infusional 5-FU.[63,64] The introduction of oxaliplatin in colorectal cancer has transformed the landscape of the adjuvant treatment of this disease. The addition of oxaliplatin to fluoropyrimidine-based therapy has improved disease free survival (DFS) and overall survival (OS) in patients with curatively resected colon cancer with lymph node involvement[65] in addition to improvement in progression free survival and OS in patients with metastatic disease over 5FU and leucovorin alone.[66]

The NSABP-04 study was conducted to address the question whether capecitabine has similar efficacy as 5-FU in combination with radiotherapy in the neoadjuvant setting, and to investigate whether adding oxaliplatin to both phases of treatment can improve outcomes. This study randomized patients in a 2×2 factorial design to receive infusional 5-FU (225 mg/m2/D $\times$ 5 days for weeks 1 and 5) versus capecitabine (825 md/m2 PO BID, 5 days per week) with or without oxaliplatin 50 mg/m2 weekly for 5 weeks.[67] The primary objective of this study was locoregional control with secondary outcomes of DFS and OS. After enrolling 1608 patients, there were no significant differences in 3 year locoregional tumor recurrence rate (11.2 vs. 11.8%), 5 year DFS (66.4 vs. 67.7%), and 5 year OS (79.9 vs. 80.8%) amongst regimens using 5-FU or capecitabine respectively. The addition of oxaliplatin to preoperative therapy was associated with significantly more overall toxicity and grade 3-4 diarrhea ($p < 0.0001$), without improvement in pathologic complete response rate, relapse rate, DFS or OS. The three-year rate of locoregional recurrence among all patients who underwent R0 resection ranged from 2.9–4.6%. An unplanned subset analysis did not show significant differences for the use of oxaliplatin regardless of T-stage or ypCR status. This study has led to widespread substitution of the more convenient oral capecitabine for infusional 5-fluorouracil during radiotherapy.

The ACCORD 12/0405-Prodige 2 study compared neoadjuvant capecitabine (800 mg/m2 BID 5 days/week) with radiation (45 Gy) to capecitabine and oxaliplatin with a higher dose of radiation (50 Gy) given in 25 fractions (CAPOX 50).[68] This study enrolled 598 patients that were randomized to these two treatment arms. The primary objective of the study was complete pathologic response to neoadjuvant therapy (ypCR). More preoperative grade 3–4 toxicity occurred in the CAPOX 50 group (25 vs. 11%; $p < 0.001$). Surgery was performed in 98% of patients in both groups. There were no differences between groups in the rate of sphincter-sparing surgery (75%) or postoperative deaths at 60 days (0.3%). The ypCR rate was 13.9% with Cap 45 and 19.2% with CAPOX 50 ($p = 0.09$). This study demonstrated lack of benefit of oxaliplatin (during radiotherapy) with increased toxicity, consistent with the findings of NSABP-04.[67]

4.6 *Role of oxaliplatin in postoperative chemotherapy*

The PETACC-6 study was designed to evaluate the addition of oxaliplatin to preoperative neoadjuvant capecitabine-based chemoradiotherapy in addition to postoperative adjuvant chemotherapy.[69] This trial randomized 1,094 patients with rectal cancer within 12 cm from the anal verge, T3-4 or N+ disease. The interim analysis of this study recently reported no difference in DFS between the two arms of treatment. This is in contrast to the CAO/ARO/AIO-94 trial,[70] which randomized 1,265 patients to receive (1) preoperative radiation plus infusional 5-FU (1 g/m2 days 1–5 and 29–33), followed by TME and 4 cycles of bolus 5-FU (500 mg/m2 for 5 days) or (2) preoperative radiation plus infusional 5-FU (250 mg/m2 days 1–14 and 22–35) and oxaliplatin (50 mg/m2 days 1, 8, 22, and 29), followed by TME and 8 cycles of adjuvant oxaliplatin (100 mg/m2), leucovorin (400 mg/m2) and infusional 5-FU (2,400 mg/m2 over 48 hours) every 2 weeks. The rate of DFS was 71.2% in Arm 1 and 75.9% in Arm 2 ($p = 0.03$). Delayed grade 3–4 toxicities were similar in both arms (23 vs. 26%; $p = 0.14$) and grade 3–4 sensory neuropathy in the oxaliplatin arm was 7% at the completion of therapy, which later improved to 3% at one year. This rate of neuropathy remains higher than what was previously reported in adjuvant oxaliplatin-based therapy in colon cancer.[65]

A third randomized trial, the ADORE study, randomized patients whose post-operative staging was ypStage II/III after completing neoadjuvant CRT and surgery,[71] *excluding* patients whose tumors were pyT0-2. An interesting feature of this trial was randomization after surgery, in contradistinction to the 3 trials mentioned above. This ensured that enrolled patients would receive assigned postoperative therapy. Patients were randomized to receive either 5-FU/LV bolus (380 mg/m2, LV 20 mg/m2 on days 1–5, every 4 weeks × 4 cycles), or FOLFOX (oxaliplatin 85 mg/m2, LV 200 mg/m2, 5-FU bolus 400 mg/m2 on day 1, 5-FU infusion 2400 mg/m2 for 46 hours, every 2 weeks × 16 weeks). The primary endpoint of 3 years DFS was superior in patients treated with FOLFOX compared to 5-FU/LV (71.6% vs. 62.9% respectively, with a hazard ratio (HR) of 0.657, $p = 0.047$) in the 321 treated patients. This design should be noted for future rectal adjuvant therapy trials, but results would be applicable only to patients who were not significantly downstaged by preoperative chemoradiation.

As summarized above, data suggest a potential benefit from adjuvant chemotherapy following a neoadjuvant chemoradiotherapy for patients with rectal cancer, but no conclusive evidence exists to date (particularly for overall survival).

Regarding the efficacy of oxaliplatin, the studies have come to somewhat different conclusions. None yet has confirmed an overall survival benefit; as such the role of oxaliplatin remains unclear. That said, in higher risk patients it certainly is reasonable to give oxaliplatin in addition to a fluoropyrimidine until data from some of the studies matures.

4.7 *Can some patients be spared radiotherapy?*

While neoadjuvant chemoradiotherapy is associated with improved local control compared to radiotherapy alone, the role of radiation has been debated in select patients with relatively low risk of local recurrence. A chemotherapy and surgery only approach is of potential value, as radiotherapy can result in a number of long-term issues including incontinence of stool or urine, sexual dysfunction, and late pelvic fractures. Pilot studies have evaluated the role of chemotherapy solely with intention to spare patients the late toxicity of radiation therapy, hopefully without detriment to outcome.

In a single-arm prospective trial, 53 patients with stage II/III rectal cancer were treated with mFOLFOX6 for 6 cycles (3 months) with a primary endpoint of preoperative response rate. The secondary endpoints were ypCR, R0 resection rate and sphincter preservation.[72] Surgery was performed in 78.8% of patients. The rates of R0 resection, ypCR, and sphincter preservation, were promising (91.0%, 10.3%, and 82.9%, respectively). Another pilot study evaluated the addition of bevacizumab to mFOLFOX in a neoadjuvant setting without the routine use of radiation. Thirty-two patients with locally advanced rectal cancer were enrolled.[73] Patients with clinically stage II and III rectal cancer received 6 cycles of mFOLFOX with bevacizumab during the first 4 cycles. Patients who achieved an objective response proceeded to TME; otherwise patients received chemoradiotherapy and then TME. The primary endpoint was R0 resection. Thirty patients completed chemotherapy; 2 patients experienced cardiac toxicity but were able to receive chemoradiotherapy. While this was a small study, it demonstrated very interesting results with a ypCR rate of 25%, and a 4 year DFS of 84%. Based on these results, the Alliance for Clinical Trials is conducting a very important randomized clinical trial (NCT01515787) in patients with locally advanced rectal cancer. The study compares standard neoadjuvant chemoradiotherapy to neoadjuvant chemotherapy (mFOLFOX6) alone, with chemoradiotherpy reserved in the chemo-alone arm for select patients who demonstrate inadequate response to therapy. The study will aim to show non-inferiority of the chemotherapy-alone approach and could potentially introduce a new standard of care.

4.8   *Induction chemotherapy followed by chemoradiation?*

The average patient with rectal cancer has a significantly higher chance of distant recurrence compared to local recurrence. This fact has led to consideration of moving systemic therapy to an earlier part of the treatment course to avoid potential growth of minimal metastatic disease to more significant disease while radiotherapy, surgery, and recovery from surgery occur. A single-arm prospective study has evaluated the potential role of induction chemotherapy followed by chemoradiotherapy, enrolling 77 patients with rectal cancer and high-risk features on MRI such as: tumors within 1 mm of mesorectal fascia, T3 tumors at or below levators, tumors extending 5 mm into perirectal fat, T4 tumors, and T1-4N2 tumors. Patients received 12 weeks of CAPOX followed by capecitabine-based chemoradiotherapy and TME.[74] This approach demonstrated symptomatic benefit in 86% of patients within 2 cycles of initiating therapy, and 88% had a radiographic response at completion of chemotherapy. Pathologic CR was reported in 24% of patients. This approach certainly represents a viable option for patients who meet the inclusion criteria and there is a concern of a more systemic disease or risk of obstruction from radiation-induced inflammatory response. Initiating systemic therapy earlier in the course may have improved the outcome, however this hypothesis has yet to be validated in randomized studies.

5 Role of Biologic Agents in Rectal Cancer

Cetuximab is a chimeric monoclonal antibody that has demonstrated activity in advanced KRAS wild type colorectal cancer.[75] Additionally, it has activity as a radiosensitizer in combination with external beam radiotherapy in patients with locally advanced head and neck cancer.[76] Cetuximab has been evaluated in several single arm phase II studies with various chemotherapy combinations.[77–80] These studies demonstrated low ypCR as compared to historic control. A randomized controlled trial evaluated 2 arms: CAPOX followed by capecitabine in combination with radiation and TME and adjuvant CAPOX, with the same treatment in addition to weekly cetuximab.[78] This study randomized 165 patients with KRAS and BRAF wild type tumors were to the two arms. The primary endpoint of this study was complete response (pathological and radiographic for nonsurgical patients). While cetuximab-treated patients had a higher response rate, however the primary end point was not different between the two arms (9 vs. 11%). The authors reported that patients who received cetuximab in addition to the chemotherapy and chemoradiotherapy experienced improved overall survival, however it is worth noting that the study was not powered to detect difference in overall survival.

Bevacizumab is a humanized monoclonal antibody targets VEGF-A and has a well-established role in the treatment of metastatic colorectal cancer. Phase II clinical trials evaluating the addition of bevacizumab to neoadjuvant chemotherapy and chemoradiotherapy have resulted in contradicting results. In one study, patients received mFOLFOX in combination with bevacizumab for 4 cycles and followed by the bevacizumab 5 mg/kg, oxaliplatin 50 mg/m2 weekly and infusional 5-FU 200 mg/m2/day with radiotherapy.[81] After enrolling 26 patients, this study was terminated early due to excessive toxicity. In contrast to this trial, two additional studies exploring the role of bevacizumab with fluoropyrimidine-based chemoradiotherapy resulted in manageable toxicity with preliminary activity.[82,83] There were no wound healing associated complications, which tend to be the major concern with anti-angiogenic agents. At present, while there was perhaps some hint of activity of bevacizumab as a radiosensitizer, there are no large studies are further evaluating either bevacizumab or cetuximab in rectal cancer.

6 Summary and Authors' Recommendations by Clinical Stage

In summary, much work has been done to refine and standardize the imaging, surgery, and adjuvant therapy that comprises current standards of care for the treatment of rectal cancer. Future goals will include further refining our understanding of risk of recurrence using molecular markers, such that therapy can be best tailored to individual patients. We also need to continue to explore the still unfulfilled promise of using targeted therapies to improve rates of cure in this deadly disease.

Recommended therapy by stage

uT3N0 low (≤ 8 cm)-: Preoperative CRT with CIV FU or capecitabine followed by surgery followed by 4 months of a fluoropyrimidine (regardless of pathologic findings) or participation in a trial of preoperative chemotherapy without radiation. **uT3N0 high (8-15 cm)-:** Either CRT as above, or consideration of surgery first, with CRT reserved for patients who are unexpectedly node positive or have closer than expected radial margins (at the mesorectum). This strategy is based on the fact that nearly 20% of patients are overstaged by EUS, and that functional outcomes are not worsened to the same degree for high rectal tumors with postoperative radiotherapy when compared to low-lying tumors. As above, 4 months of a fluoropyrimidine are recommended. As above, these patients could be considered for a trial of preoperative chemotherapy without radiation.

   uT4N0 or uT3N1-2: Preoperative CRT with CIV FU or capecitabine followed by surgery followed by 4 months FOLFOX (CapeOx) or a fluoropyrimidine. We recommend particular consideration of oxaliplatin for patients who are pathologically node positive.

References

1. Cancer Facts & Figures 2014. American Cancer Society 2015. Retrieved from http://www.cancer.org/acs/groups/content/@editorial/documents/document/acspc-044552.pdf access2015/11/01
2. Rectal Cancer. National Comprehensive Cancer Network 2015. Retrieved from http://www.nccn.org/professionals/physician_gls/PDF/rectal.pdf; access 2015/11/01
3. Nicholls RJ, *et al*. The clinical staging of rectal cancer. *The British Journal of Surgery* 1982;**69**:404–409.
4. Samdani T, Garcia-Aguilar J. Imaging in rectal cancer: magnetic resonance imaging versus endorectal ultrasonography. *Surgical Oncology Clinics of North America* 2014;**23**:59–77.
5. Krestin GP, *et al*. [Computed tomography and magnetic resonance tomography of rectal and sigmoid tumors]. *Rontgen-Blatter; Zeitschrift fur Rontgen-Technik und medizinisch-wissenschaftliche Photographie* 1990;**43**:426–429.
6. Nogueras J. Endorectal ultrasonography: technique, image interpretation, and expanding indications in 1995. *Semin Colon Rectal Surg* 1995;**6**:70–77.

7. Beynon J, *et al*. Endoluminal ultrasound in the assessment of local invasion in rectal cancer. *The British Journal of Surgery* 1986;**73**:474–477.

8. Hildebrandt U, Feifel G. Preoperative staging of rectal cancer by intrarectal ultrasound. *Diseases of the Colon and Rectum* 1985;**28**:42–46.

9. Mor I HT, *et al*. Rectal endosonography: just how good are we at its interpretation? *Int J Colorectal Dis* 2010;**25**:87–90.

10. Garcia-Aguila J PJ, *et al*. Accuracy of endorectal ultrasonography in preoperative staging of rectal tumors. *Diseases of the Colon and Rectum* 2002;**45**:10–5.

11. Puli S RJ, *et al*. Accuracy of endoscopic ultrasound to diagnose nodal invason by rectal cancer: meta-analysis and systematic review. *Ann Surg Oncol* 2009;**16**:1255–65.

12. Orrom WJ *et al*. Endorectal ultrasound in the preoperative staging of rectal tumors: A learning experience. *Diseases of the Colon and Rectum* 1990;**33**:654–9.

13. Rafaelsen S ST, *et al*. Transrectal ultrasonography and magnetic resonance imaging in the staging of rectal cancer. Effect of experience. *Scan J Gastroenterol* 2008;**43**: 440–6.

14. Puli SR, *et al*. Accuracy of endoscopic ultrasound to diagnose nodal invasion by rectal cancers: a meta-analysis and systematic review. *Ann Surg Oncol* 2009;**16**:1255–65.

15. Harewood GC, *et al*. A prospective, blinded assessment of the impact of preoperative staging on the management of rectal cancer. *Gastroenterology* 2002;**123**:24–32.

16. Brown G, *et al*. Morphologic predictors of lymph node status in rectal cancer with use of high-spatial-resolution MR imaging with histopathologic comparison. *Radiology* 2003;**227**:371–7.

17. Kim NK, *et al*. Preoperative staging of rectal cancer with MRI: accuracy and clinical usefulness. *Ann Surg Oncol* 2000;**7**:732–7.

18. Brown G, Daniels IR. Preoperative staging of rectal cancer: the MERCURY research project. Recent results in cancer research Fortschritte der Krebsforschung Progres dans les recherches sur le cancer 2005;**165**:58–74.

19. Lahaye MJ, *et al*. USPIO-enhanced MR imaging for nodal staging in patients with primary rectal cancer: predictive criteria. *Radiology* 2008;**246**:804–11.

20. Adam IJ, *et al*. Role of circumferential margin involvement in the local recurrence of rectal cancer. *Lancet* 1994;**344**:707–11.

21. Hall NR, *et al*. Circumferential margin involvement after mesorectal excision of rectal cancer with curative intent. Predictor of survival but not local recurrence? *Diseases of the Colon and Rectum* 1998;**41**:979–83.

22. Nagtegaal ID, *et al*. Circumferential margin involvement is still an important predictor of local recurrence in rectal carcinoma: not one millimeter but two millimeters is the limit. *The American Journal of Surgical Pathology* 2002;**26**:350–7.

23. Quirke P, *et al*. Local recurrence of rectal adenocarcinoma due to inadequate surgical resection. Histopathological study of lateral tumour spread and surgical excision. *Lancet* 1986;**2**:996–9.

24. Marijnen CA, *et al*. Radiotherapy does not compensate for positive resection margins in rectal cancer patients: report of a multicenter randomized trial. *International Journal of Radiation Oncology, Biology, Physics* 2003;**55**:1311–20.

25. Beets-Tan RG. MRI in rectal cancer: the T stage and circumferential resection margin. Colorectal disease: the official journal of the Association of Coloproctology of Great Britain and Ireland 2003;**5**:392–5.

26. Branagan G, *et al.* Can magnetic resonance imaging predict circumferential margins and TNM stage in rectal cancer? *Diseases of the Colon and Rectum* 2004;**47**:1317–22.

27. Stevenson G. Radiology in the detection and prevention of colorectal cancer. *European journal of cancer* 1995;31A:1121–6.

28. Bipat S, *et al.* Rectal cancer: local staging and assessment of lymph node involvement with endoluminal US, CT, and MR imaging — a meta-analysis. *Radiology* 2004;**232**: 773–83.

29. Cellini C, *et al.* Stage IV rectal cancer with liver metastases: is there a benefit to resection of the primary tumor? *World Journal of Surgery* 2010;**34**:1102–8.

30. Damjanov N, *et al.* Resection of the primary colorectal cancer is not necessary in nonobstructed patients with metastatic disease. *The Oncologist* 2009;**14**:963–9.

31. Chang HC, *et al.* Risk factors for lymph node metastasis in pT1 and pT2 rectal cancer: a single-institute experience in 943 patients and literature review. *Annals of Surgical Oncology* 2012;**19**:2477–84.

32. Glasgow SC, *et al.* Meta-analysis of histopathological features of primary colorectal cancers that predict lymph node metastases. *Journal of Gastrointestinal Surgery: Official Journal of the Society for Surgery of the Alimentary Tract* 2012;**16**:1019–28.

33. Kikuchi R, *et al.* Management of early invasive colorectal cancer. Risk of recurrence and clinical guidelines. *Diseases of the Colon and Rectum* 1995;**38**:1286–95.

34. Choi PW, *et al.* Risk factors for lymph node metastasis in submucosal invasive colorectal cancer. *World Journal of Surgery* 2008;**32**:2089–94.

35. Nascimbeni R, *et al.* Risk of lymph node metastasis in T1 carcinoma of the colon and rectum. *Diseases of the Colon and Rectum* 2002;**45**:200–6.

36. Jayne DG, *et al.* Randomized trial of laparoscopic-assisted resection of colorectal carcinoma: 3-year results of the UK MRC CLASICC Trial Group. *Journal of Clinical Oncology: Official Journal of the American Society of Clinical Oncology* 2007;**25**: 3061–8.

37. Williams NS, Johnston D. The quality of life after rectal excision for low rectal cancer. *The British Journal of Surgery* 1983;**70**:460–2.

38. RJ H. The 'Holy Plane' of rectal surgery. *J R Soc Med* 1988;**81**:503–8.

39. Havenga K DM, *et al.* Anatomical basis of autonomic nerve-preserving total mesorectal excision for rectal cancer. *Br J Surg* 1996;**83**:384–8.

40. Adam IJ MM, *et al.* Role of circumferential margin involvement in the local recurrence of rectal cancer. *Lancet* 1994;**344**:707–77.

41. Enker WE TH, *et al.* Total mesorectal excision in the operative treatment of carcinoma of the rectum. *J Am Coll Surg* 1995;**181**:335–46.

42. Nagtegaal ID vdVC, *et al.* Macroscopic evaluation of rectal cancer resection specimen: clinical significance of the pathologist in quality control. *J Clin Oncol* 2002;**20**:1729–34.

43. Sauer R, *et al.* Preoperative versus postoperative chemoradiotherapy for rectal cancer. *The New England Journal of Medicine* 2004;**351**:1731–40.

44. Gunderson LL, *et al*. Impact of T and N substage on survival and disease relapse in adjuvant rectal cancer: a pooled analysis. *International Journal of Radiation Oncology, Biology, Physics* 2002;**54**:386–96.

45. Wolmark N, *et al*. Randomized trial of postoperative adjuvant chemotherapy with or without radiotherapy for carcinoma of the rectum: National Surgical Adjuvant Breast and Bowel Project Protocol R-02. *Journal of the National Cancer Institute* 2000;**92**:388–96.

46. Krook JE, *et al*. Effective surgical adjuvant therapy for high-risk rectal carcinoma. *The New England Journal of Medicine* 1991;**324**:709–15.

47. Prolongation of the disease-free interval in surgically treated rectal carcinoma. Gastrointestinal Tumor Study Group. *The New England Journal of Medicine* 1985;**312**:1465–72.

48. Sebag-Montefiore D, *et al*. Preoperative radiotherapy versus selective postoperative chemoradiotherapy in patients with rectal cancer (MRC CR07 and NCIC-CTG C016): a multicentre, randomised trial. *Lancet* 2009;**373**:811–20.

49. Bosset JF, *et al*. Chemotherapy with preoperative radiotherapy in rectal cancer. *The New England Journal of Medicine* 2006;**355**:1114–23.

50. Bosset JF, *et al*. Fluorouracil-based adjuvant chemotherapy after preoperative chemoradiotherapy in rectal cancer: long-term results of the EORTC 22921 randomised study. *The Lancet Oncology* 2014;**15**:184–90.

51. Gerard JP, *et al*. Preoperative radiotherapy with or without concurrent fluorouracil and leucovorin in T3-4 rectal cancers: results of FFCD 9203. *Journal of Clinical Oncology: Official Journal of the American Society of Clinical Oncology* 2006;**24**:4620–5.

52. O'Connell MJ, *et al*. Improving adjuvant therapy for rectal cancer by combining protracted-infusion fluorouracil with radiation therapy after curative surgery. *The New England Journal of Medicine* 1994;**331**:502–7.

53. Glynne-Jones R, *et al*. Challenges in the neoadjuvant treatment of rectal cancer: balancing the risk of recurrence and quality of life. Cancer radiotherapie: *journal de la Societe francaise de radiotherapie oncologique* 2013;**17**:675–85.

54. Roh MS, *et al*. Preoperative multimodality therapy improves disease-free survival in patients with carcinoma of the rectum: NSABP R-03. *Journal of Clinical Oncology: Official Journal of the American Society of Clinical Oncology* 2009;**27**:5124–30.

55. Improved survival with preoperative radiotherapy in resectable rectal cancer. Swedish Rectal Cancer Trial. *The New England Journal of Medicine* 1997;**336**:980–7.

56. Folkesson J, *et al*. Swedish Rectal Cancer Trial: long lasting benefits from radiotherapy on survival and local recurrence rate. *Journal of Clinical Oncology: Official Journal of the American Society of Clinical Oncology* 2005;**23**:5644–50.

57. Kapiteijn E, *et al*. Preoperative radiotherapy combined with total mesorectal excision for resectable rectal cancer. *The New England Journal of Medicine* 2001;**345**:638–46.

58. van Gijn W, *et al*. Preoperative radiotherapy combined with total mesorectal excision for resectable rectal cancer: 12-year follow-up of the multicentre, randomised controlled TME trial. *The Lancet Oncology* 2011;**12**:575–82.

59. Bujko K, *et al*. Long-term results of a randomized trial comparing preoperative short-course radiotherapy with preoperative conventionally fractionated chemoradiation for rectal cancer. *The British Journal of Surgery* 2006;**93**:1215–23.

60. Ngan SY, *et al.* Randomized trial of short-course radiotherapy versus long-course chemoradiation comparing rates of local recurrence in patients with T3 rectal cancer: Trans-Tasman Radiation Oncology Group trial 01.04. *Journal of Clinical Oncology: Official Journal of the American Society of Clinical Oncology* 2012;**30**:3827–33.

61. Joye I, Haustermans K. Early and late toxicity of radiotherapy for rectal cancer. Recent results in cancer research Fortschritte der Krebsforschung Progres dans les recherches sur le cancer 2014;**203**:189–201.

62. Garcia-Aguilar J, *et al.* Optimal timing of surgery after chemoradiation for advanced rectal cancer: preliminary results of a multicenter, nonrandomized phase II prospective trial. *Annals of Surgery* 2011;**254**:97–102.

63. Cassidy J, *et al.* Randomized phase III study of capecitabine plus oxaliplatin compared with fluorouracil/folinic acid plus oxaliplatin as first-line therapy for metastatic colorectal cancer. *Journal of Clinical Oncology: Official Journal of the American Society of Clinical Oncology* 2008;**26**:2006–12.

64. Cunningham D, *et al.* Capecitabine and oxaliplatin for advanced esophagogastric cancer. *The New England Journal of Medicine* 2008;**358**:36–46.

65. Andre T, *et al.* Oxaliplatin, fluorouracil, and leucovorin as adjuvant treatment for colon cancer. *The New England Journal of Medicine* 2004;**350**:2343–51.

66. de Gramont A, *et al.* Leucovorin and fluorouracil with or without oxaliplatin as first-line treatment in advanced colorectal cancer. *Journal of Clinical Oncology: Official Journal of the American Society of Clinical Oncology* 2000;**18**:2938–47.

67. Allegra CJ, *et al.* Final results from NSABP protocol R-04: Neoadjuvant chemoradiation (RT) comparing continuous infusion (CIV) 5-FU with capecitabine (Cape) with or without oxaliplatin (Ox) in patients with stage II and III rectal cancer. *ASCO Meeting Abstracts* 2014;**32**:3603.

68. Gerard JP, *et al.* Comparison of two neoadjuvant chemoradiotherapy regimens for locally advanced rectal cancer: results of the phase III trial ACCORD 12/0405-Prodige 2. *Journal of Clinical Oncology: Official Journal of the American Society of Clinical Oncology* 2010;**28**:1638–44.

69. Schmoll H-J, *et al.* Preoperative chemoradiotherapy and postoperative chemotherapy with capecitabine and oxaliplatin versus capecitabine alone in locally advanced rectal cancer: Disease-free survival results at interim analysis. *ASCO Meeting Abstracts* 2014;**32**:3501.

70. Rodel C, *et al.* Preoperative chemoradiotherapy and postoperative chemotherapy with 5-fluorouracil and oxaliplatin versus 5-fluorouracil alone in locally advanced rectal cancer: Results of the German CAO/ARO/AIO-04 randomized phase III trial. *ASCO Meeting Abstracts* 2014;**32**:3500.

71. Hong YS, *et al.* Adjuvant chemotherapy with oxaliplatin/5-fluorouracil/leucovorin (FOLFOX) versus 5-fluorouracil/leucovorin (FL) for rectal cancer patients whose postoperative yp stage 2 or 3 after preoperative chemoradiotherapy: Updated results of 3-year disease-free survival from a randomized phase II study (The ADORE). *ASCO Meeting Abstracts* 2014;**32**:3502.

72. Koike J, *et al*. Neoadjuvant mFOLFOX6 for stage II/III rectal cancer patients with a T3/T4 tumor. *ASCO Meeting Abstracts* 2014;**32**:3554.

73. Schrag D, *et al*. Neoadjuvant chemotherapy without routine use of radiation therapy for patients with locally advanced rectal cancer: a pilot trial. *Journal of Clinical Oncology: Official Journal of the American Society of Clinical Oncology* 2014;**32**:513–8.

74. Chau I, *et al*. Neoadjuvant capecitabine and oxaliplatin followed by synchronous chemoradiation and total mesorectal excision in magnetic resonance imaging-defined poor-risk rectal cancer. *Journal of Clinical Oncology: Official Journal of the American Society of Clinical Oncology* 2006;**24**:668–74.

75. Bardelli A, Siena S. Molecular mechanisms of resistance to cetuximab and panitumumab in colorectal cancer. *Journal of Clinical Oncology: Official Journal of the American Society of Clinical Oncology* 2010;**28**:1254–61.

76. Specenier P, Vermorken JB. Cetuximab in the treatment of squamous cell carcinoma of the head and neck. *Expert review of anticancer therapy* 2011;**11**:511–24.

77. Velenik V, *et al*. A phase II study of cetuximab, capecitabine and radiotherapy in neoadjuvant treatment of patients with locally advanced resectable rectal cancer. *European Journal of Surgical Oncology: The Journal of the European Society of Surgical Oncology and the British Association of Surgical Oncology* 2010;**36**:244–50.

78. Horisberger K, *et al*. Cetuximab in combination with capecitabine, irinotecan, and radiotherapy for patients with locally advanced rectal cancer: results of a Phase II MARGIT trial. *International Journal of Radiation Oncology, Biology, Physics* 2009;**74**:1487–93.

79. Rodel C, *et al*. Phase I-II trial of cetuximab, capecitabine, oxaliplatin, and radiotherapy as preoperative treatment in rectal cancer. *International Journal of Radiation Oncology, Biology, Physics* 2008;**70**:1081–6.

80. Machiels JP, *et al*. Phase I/II study of preoperative cetuximab, capecitabine, and external beam radiotherapy in patients with rectal cancer. Annals of oncology: official journal of the European Society for Medical Oncology/ESMO 2007;**18**:738–44.

81. Dipetrillo T, *et al*. Neoadjuvant bevacizumab, oxaliplatin, 5-fluorouracil, and radiation for rectal cancer. *International Journal of Radiation Oncology, Biology, Physics* 2012;**82**:124–9.

82. Crane CH, *et al*. Phase II trial of neoadjuvant bevacizumab, capecitabine, and radiotherapy for locally advanced rectal cancer. *International Journal of Radiation Oncology, Biology, Physics* 2010;**76**:824–30.

83. Willett CG, *et al*. Efficacy, safety, and biomarkers of neoadjuvant bevacizumab, radiation therapy, and fluorouracil in rectal cancer: a multidisciplinary phase II study. *Journal of Clinical Oncology: Official Journal of the American Society of Clinical Oncology* 2009;**27**:3020–6.

Chapter 15

Adjuvant Chemotherapy of Colon Cancer: Histology *vs.* Biology

James J. Lee, Gaurav Goel and Edward Chu

1 Introduction

Colorectal cancer (CRC) is the third most common cancer and the second leading cause of cancer death in men and women in the United States.[1] Approximately 136,830 new cases of CRC will be diagnosed in 2014, and nearly 50,000 patients will die from this disease.[2] At the time of initial diagnosis, nearly 40% of colon cancer patients present with localized disease while another 37% of the patients present with tumor involvement of the regional lymph nodes.[1] Although surgical resection plays a critical role in the management of locoregional disease, it is usually not curative as a single modality. The long-term outcome with surgery alone is related to the extent of disease at presentation. Five-year survival rates vary with the stage at diagnosis (74% for stage I, 67% for stage IIA, and 28% for stage IIIC disease), which reflects the risk of tumor recurrence with surgery alone.[3]

A significant proportion of stage III colon cancer patients who undergo potentially curative surgical resection develop disease recurrence that is believed to be secondary to clinically occult micrometastatic disease present at the time of surgery. Administration of adjuvant chemotherapy after surgical resection of the tumor has the potential to eradicate these micrometastases, thereby increasing the chance of cure. The benefits of adjuvant chemotherapy have been most clearly demonstrated in stage III disease, but its potential benefit in unselected stage II colon cancer patients remains a subject of on-going debate.[4]

Herein, we review the role of adjuvant chemotherapy in the treatment of stages II and III colon cancer and the emerging clinical data regarding the potential role of molecular biomarkers as predictive factors that can identify the subset of patients who would most benefit from adjuvant therapy.

2 The Role of Fluoropyrimidines

Over the past 30 years, the combination of 5-fluorouracil (FU) and the reduced folate leucovorin (LV) has been the backbone of adjuvant chemotherapy for early-stage colon cancer (Figure 1).[5] The benefit of adjuvant 5-FU-based chemotherapy in stage III colon cancer was first demonstrated by the North Central Cancer Treatment Group (NCCTG) trial, which showed that 5-FU-containing regimen reduced the risk of cancer recurrence by 41% ($p < 0.0001$) and the overall death rate by 33% ($p = 0.006$) at a median follow-up of three years.[6] Several large randomized trials in the United States were conducted in follow-up to the landmark NSABP study, and these studies established the role of bolus 5-FU/LV as a standard treatment regimen for patients with stage III colon cancer following surgical resection.[7–9] GERCOR C96.1 trial was a randomized phase III randomized trial conducted in Europe, and this study compared infusional 5-FU/LV (LV5FU2 [de Gramont regimen]: LV 200 mg/m² by a 2-h IV infusion and 5-FU 400 mg/m² by IV bolus, followed by 5-FU 600 mg/m²/day via a 22-h continuous infusion for two consecutive days, repeated every two weeks) with bolus 5-FU/LV (Mayo Clinic regimen).[10,11] This trial showed that LV5FU2 was much better tolerated than bolus 5-FU/LV with similar clinical efficacy in terms of six-year disease-free survival

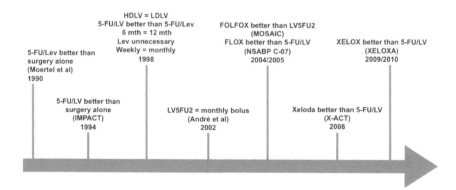

Figure 1   Evolution of adjuvant chemotherapy of early-stage colon cancer.

(DFS) and overall survival (OS).[10,11] Based on this study, the LV5FU2 regimen was adopted as a standard backbone regimen for many subsequent adjuvant combination trials, including MOSAIC trial.[10,11]

Capecitabine (XELODA®) is an oral fluoropyrimidine that offers increased convenience and potentially improved therapeutic benefit when compared to intravenous 5-FU-based chemotherapy.[12] Single-agent capecitabine was approved for the adjuvant therapy of stage III colon cancer in 2005, based on the results of the capecitabine in Adjuvant Colon Cancer Therapy (X-ACT) study.[13] This trial enrolled nearly 2,000 patients with stage III colon cancer and established the non-inferiority of capecitabine monotherapy when compared to bolus 5-FU/LV for the adjuvant treatment of stage III colon cancer patients. Of note, there were significant regional differences in the rates of treatment-related toxicities in patients receiving bolus 5-FU/LV and capecitabine in the adjuvant therapy of colon cancer.[14] Significantly more grade 3/4 adverse events (AEs), grade 4 AEs, and discontinuations of treatments were reported in U.S. patients compared with non-U.S. patients.[14]

3 Role of Oxaliplatin in Adjuvant Chemotherapy

Oxaliplatin is a third-generation diaminocyclohexane platinum compound that has been studied in the setting of adjuvant chemotherapy of surgically resected early-stage colon cancer. Three large randomized phase III clinical trials were conducted to demonstrate the benefit of adding oxaliplatin to fluoropyrimidine backbone in the adjuvant therapy of stage III colon cancer (Table 1).[15–19] The pivotal Multicenter International Study of Oxaliplatin/5-Fluorouracil/Leucovorin in the Adjuvant Treatment of Colon Cancer (MOSAIC) trial enrolled 2,246 patients with stage II (40%) and III (60%) colon cancer that were randomized to receive six months of adjuvant LV5FU2 versus oxaliplatin plus LV5FU2 (FOLFOX4: LV5FU2 and oxaliplatin 85 mg/m^2 administered via a 2-h IV infusion on day 1, repeated every two weeks)[15] The primary endpoint of this study was DFS, and the secondary endpoints were OS and safety. The three-year DFS rate was significantly improved in the oxaliplatin-containing arm (78.2% *vs.* 72.9%; hazard ratio [HR] 0.77; $p = 0.002$) when compared to LV5FU2. An updated analysis of MOSAIC clinical trial revealed that the addition of oxaliplatin to LV5FU2 also significantly improved five-year DFS (73.3% *vs.* 67.4%; HR 0.80; $p = 0.003$) and six-year OS (78.5% *vs.* 76.0%; HR 0.84; $p = 0.046$) in the adjuvant treatment of stages II and III colon cancer.[16] In a subgroup analysis, the addition of oxaliplatin was associated with statistically significant improvement in six-year OS among stage III patients (72.9% *vs.* 68.7%; HR 0.80; 95% CI 0.65–0.97; $p = 0.023$).

Table 1   Randomized clinical trials in the adjuvant treatment of early-stage colon cancer.

Study/Authors	Patients Enrolled (n)	Patient Population	Adjuvant Treatment Arms
NCCTG[6]	1,296	Dukes' B2 and C	5-FU/LEV vs. LEV alone vs. Observation
NSABP C-03[7]	1,081	Dukes' B and C	5-FU/lomustine/vincristine vs. 5-FU/LV
NSABP C-04[9]	2,151	Dukes' B and C	5-FU/LV vs. 5-FU/LEV vs. 5-FU/LV/LEV
IMPACT 1[22,23]	1,526	Dukes' B and C	5-FU/LV vs. Observation
O'Connell et al.[24]	317	Stages II and III	5-FU/LV vs. Observation
IMPACT 2[23]	1,016	Dukes' B2	5-FU/LV vs. Observation
Sargent et al.[25]	3,351	Stages II and III	5-FU/LV, or 5-FU/LEV vs. Observation alone
adjCCA-01[26]	702	Stage III	5-FU/LV vs. 5-FU/LEV
Dencausse et al.[27]	180	Stage III	5-FU/LEV vs. 5-FU/LV (12 months) vs. 5-FU/LV (6 months)
Intergroup 0089[28]	3,794	Stages II and III	5-FU/LV (Mayo Clinic) vs. 5-FU/LV (Roswell Park) vs. 5-FU/LV/LEV
MOSAIC[15,16]	2,246	Stages II and III	5-FU/LV (de Gramont) vs. FOLFOX4
NSABP C-07[17,18]	2,492	Stages II and III	5-FU/LV vs. FLOX
X-ACT[13]	1,987	Stage III	Capecitabine vs. 5-FU/LV
QUASAR[29]	3,283	Stage II (91%)	5-FU/LV (with our without LEV) vs. Observation
CALGB 89803[30]	1,264	Stage III	CPT-11/5-FU/LV (IFL) vs. 5-FU/LV
PETACC-3[31]	3,278	Stages II and III	CPT-11/5-FU/LV (FOLFIRI) vs. 5-FU/LV (de Gramont)

(Continued)

Table 1   (*Continued*)

Study/Authors	Patients Enrolled (*n*)	Patient Population	Adjuvant Treatment Arms
ACCORD02[32]	400	Stage III	CPT-11 plus 5-FU/LV *vs.* 5-FU/LV
NO16968 (XELOXA)[19]	1,886	Stage III	XELOX *vs.* 5-FU/LV (Mayo Clinic or Roswell Park)
NSABP C-08[20,33]	2,672	Stages II and III	mFOLFOX6/bevacizumab *vs.* mFOLFOX6 alone
BO17920 (AVANT)[34]	3,451	Stages II and III	FOLFOX4 *vs.* FOLFOX4/bevacizumab *vs.* XELOX/bevacizumab
NO147[21]	2,580	Stage III	mFOLFOX6/cetuximab *vs.* mFOLFOX6 alone

5-FU/LV (Mayo Clinic regimen)[28]: LV 20 mg/m^2 and 5-FU 425 mg/m^2 administered by IV bolus daily five times (days 1–5), repeated every four weeks for a total of six cycles (24 weeks);

5-FU/LV (Roswell Park regimen)[28]: LV 500 mg/m^2 administered by a 2-hour IV infusion and 5-FU 500 mg/m^2 by an IV bolus weekly six times (weeks 1–6), followed by a two-week rest period (weeks 7 and 8), for a total of four cycles (32 weeks);

LV5FU2 (de Gramont regimen)[15]: LV 200 mg/m^2 administered by a 2-h IV infusion followed by 5-FU 400 mg/m^2 by an IV bolus and then 5-FU 600 mg/m^2 by a 22-h continuous IV infusion on two consecutive days (days 1–2), repeated every two weeks, for a total of 12 cycles (24 weeks);

IFL regimen[30]: Irinotecan 125 mg/m^2 administered by a 90-min IV infusion, LV 20 mg/m^2 and 5-FU 500 mg/m^2 by an IV bolus, weekly four times (weeks 1–4) followed by a two-week rest period (weeks 5–6), for a total of five cycles (30 weeks);

FOLFIRI regimen[31]: LV5FU2 (de Gramont regimen) plus irinotecan 180 mg/m^2 administered by a 30- to 90-min IV infusion on day 1, repeated every two weeks, for a total of 12 cycles (24 weeks);

FLOX regimen[17]: 5-FU/LV (Roswell Park regimen) plus oxaliplatin 85 mg/m^2 administered by a 2-h IV infusions on days 1, 15, and 29, repeated every eight weeks, for a total of three cycles (24 weeks);

FOLFOX4 regimen[15]: LV5FU2 (de Gramont regimen) plus oxaliplatin 85 mg/m^2 by a 2-h IV infusion on day 1, repeated every two weeks, for a total of 12 cycles (24 weeks);

mFOLFOX6 regimen[20]: LV 400 mg/m^2 by an IV infusion on day 1, 5-FU 400 mg/m^2 by an IV bolus on day 1 followed by 5-FU 2,400 mg/m^2 by an IV continuous 46- to 48-h infusion, and oxaliplatin 85 mg/m^2 by a 2-h IV infusion on day 1, repeated every two weeks, for a total of 12 cycles (24 weeks);

XELOX regimen[19]: Oxaliplatin 130 mg/m^2 administered by a 2-h IV infusion on day 1 and capecitabine 1,000 mg/m^2 PO twice daily on days 1–14, repeated every three weeks, for a total of eight cycles (24 weeks).

Based on the three-year DFS improvement demonstrated by the MOSAIC study, FOLFOX4 was approved by the U.S. FDA in 2004 as a standard treatment regimen for adjuvant chemotherapy in patients with stage III colon cancer. However, most U.S. oncologists prefer to use modified FOLFOX6 regimen (mFOLFOX6 regimen: LV 400 mg/m^2 by a 2-h IV infusion, oxaliplatin 85 mg/m^2 by a 2-h IV infusion, and 5-FU 400 mg/m^2 by a IV bolus on day 1, followed by 5-FU 2,400 mg/m^2 by a 46- to 48-h continuous IV infusion, repeated every two weeks, for a total of 12 cycles) given its improved safety profile with reduced myelosuppression and gastrointestinal (GI) toxicity when compared with the original FOLFOX4 regimen.[20,21]

The National Surgical Adjuvant Breast and Bowel Project (NSABP) C-07 trial randomly assigned 2,492 patients with resected stage II (29%) or stage III (71%) colon cancer to receive weekly bolus 5-FU/LV (Mayo Clinic regimen) alone or the same 5-FU/LV regimen plus oxaliplatin (FLOX).[17] The FLOX regimen was associated with a statistically significant improvement in four-year DFS rates (73.2% *vs.* 67.0%; HR 0.80; 95% CI 0.69–0.93; $p < 0.004$) when compared to 5-FU monotherapy. An updated analysis of this trial done after eight years of median follow-up showed that FLOX remained superior in terms of five-year DFS rates (69.4% *vs.* 64.2 %; HR 0.82; 95% CI 0.72–0.93; $p = 0.002$).[18] However, 5-year OS rates were no significant statistic difference between the two treatment groups (80.2% *vs.* 78.4%; HR 0.88; 95% CI 0.75–1.02; $p = 0.08$). The toxicity profiles of the MOSAIC and NSABP-C07 trials were different with significantly more grade 3/4 diarrhea observed with FLOX than with FOLFOX while grade 3 sensory neuropathy was approximately the same with FOLFOX when compared to FLOX (12% *vs.* 8%). Of note, in patients treated with the bolus FLOX regimen, there were increased hospitalizations resulting from diarrhea. When comparing the two oxaliplatin-based regimens, the median dose of oxaliplatin administered per patient was higher in the MOSAIC trial than in the NSABP C-07 trial (810 mg/m^2 [9.5 cycles] versus 667 mg/m^2 [7.8 cycles]). As the overall clinical benefit appears to be similar between the two regimens, the findings from the FLOX study suggest that a lower cumulative dose of oxaliplatin can be given without compromising clinical outcome. FOLFOX is preferred over FLOX for the adjuvant chemotherapy of patients with colon cancer as a result of its improved safety profile and scheduling convenience.

NO16968 (XELOX in Adjuvant Colon Cancer Treatment [XELOXA]) trial randomized 1,886 patients with stage III colon cancer to the combination of capecitabine plus oxaliplatin (XELOX; $n = 944$) for 24 weeks or bolus 5-FU/LV (Mayo Clinic for 24 weeks or Roswell Park regimen for 32 weeks; $n = 942$) as adjuvant therapy.[19] The primary endpoint of this study was DFS. The three-year DFS rate was significantly higher in the XELOX arm than the bolus 5-FU/LV arm with a 20% reduction in the relative risk of disease recurrence (70.9% *vs.* 66.5%;

Table 2   Effect of adjuvant chemotherapy on three-year DFS.

Study	Treatment	Three-year DFS
NCCTG[6]	Observation	52%
IMPACT[22,23]	Observation	44%
IMPACT[22,23]	5-FU/LV	62%
Punt[35]	5-FU/LV	65%
Fields[36]	5-FU/LV	67%
André[10,11]	5-FU/LV	61%
MOSAIC[15,16]	5-FU/LV	65%
X-ACT[13]	Capecitabine	64%
MOSAIC[15,16]	FOLFOX4	72%
NSABP C-07[17,18]	FLOX	72%
NO16968[19]	XELOX	71%

HR 0.80; 95% CI 0.69–0.93; $p = 0.0045$). The difference in DFS was maintained in subsequent follow-up with the four-year DFS rate (68.4% *vs.* 62.3%) and five-year DFS rate (66.1% *vs.* 59.8%). The three-year recurrence-free survival (RFS) rate was also significantly higher in XELOX arm (72.1% *vs.* 67.5%; HR 0.78; 95% CI 0.67–0.92; $p = 0.0024$). After a median follow-up of 57 months, the XELOX arm was associated with a trend toward improved OS (79.1% *vs.* 76.1%; HR 0.87; 95% CI 0.72–1.05; $p = 0.1486$). To date, no direct randomized study has been conducted to compare the clinical efficacy of XELOX versus FOLFOX. As presented in Table 2, a cross-trial comparison suggests that XELOX confers similar DFS and OS benefit as is observed with FOLFOX4. As a result, XELOX is also considered a standard treatment option as adjuvant chemotherapy in patients with stage III colon cancer.

According to the ESMO clinical practice guidelines,[37] either FOLFOX or XELOX are preferred for the adjuvant therapy of patients with early-stage colon cancer. Although FLOX confers the same level of clinical benefit as FOLFOX or XELOX, its use in the United States has been limited by its significant GI toxicity. With the development of clinically relevant neurotoxicity resulting from FOLFOX/XELOX therapy, oxaliplatin should be stopped and fluoropyrimidine monotherapy (infusional 5-FU or capecitabine) continued to complete a full six-month course of treatment. In patients who are unable to tolerate oxaliplatin-based chemotherapy, such as older patients and those with impaired performance status resulting from comorbid illnesses, monotherapy with capecitabine or infusional 5-FU should be viewed as an appropriate treatment alternative to FOLFOX/XELOX.

The recent National Comprehensive Cancer Network (NCCN) guidelines recommend six months of adjuvant chemotherapy for patients with resected stage III disease.[38,39] The treatment options are FOLFOX or XELOX. While FLOX is also recommended, both FOLFOX and XELOX are the preferred regimens. In patients who are deemed to not be eligible for oxaliplatin-based chemotherapy, fluoropyrimidine monotherapy with capecitabine or 5-FU/LV is recommended.

4 The Role of Irinotecan in Adjuvant Chemotherapy

Irinotecan (CPT-11) containing regimens have been extensively evaluated in the adjuvant treatment of stage III colon cancer. Three large randomized clinical trials investigated the combination of CPT-11 with 5-FU/LV, and have failed to demonstrate improvement in three-year DFS or OS with such approach.[30–32] The first study was CALGB 89803, which was a randomized phase III study evaluating the role of irinotecan (CPT-11) plus bolus 5-FU/LV (IFL) in comparison to bolus 5-FU/LV (Roswell Park regimen) in the adjuvant chemotherapy of patients ($n = 1,264$) with resected stage III colon cancer.[30] The primary endpoints were OS and DFS. IFL did not improve DFS or OS in stage III disease, but significantly increased the incidence of grade 3/4 toxicities including severe neutropenia, febrile neutropenia, and treatment-related mortality (2.8% *vs.* 1.0%; $p = 0.008$).

ACCORD II was a multicenter phase III trial to evaluate the addition of irinotecan to LV5FU2 (FOLFIRI) in patients with resected colon cancer at high risk of relapse, which was defined as either N2 disease or N1 plus a perforated or obstructing primary lesion.[32] Patients ($n = 400$) were randomized to LV5FU2 (de Gramont regimen) or FOLFIRI, and the primary endpoint of this study was DFS. There was no significant improvement in three-year DFS (60% *vs.* 51%; HR 1.12; 95% CI 0.85–1.47; $p = 0.42$) and five-year OS (67% *vs.* 61%; HR 1.20; 95% CI 0.087–1.67; $p = 0.26$). Of note, the LV5FU2 plus irinotecan arm was associated with significantly more grade 3/4 neutropenia when compared to the LV5FU2 alone arm (28% *vs.* 4%; $p < 0.001$).

Pan-European Trial Adjuvant Colon Cancer (PETACC-3) was a randomized, multicenter, phase III trial to investigate whether the addition of irinotecan to infusional 5-FU/LV (FOLFIRI) would improve DFS in the adjuvant chemotherapy of patients with resected stage II or III colon cancer.[31] Van Cutsem *et al.* randomized 2,094 stage III patients to the combination of LV5FU2 plus irinotecan (FOLFIRI) or to LV5FU2 (de Gramont regimen) alone. The five-year DFS rate in patients ($n = 2,094$) with stage III colon cancer was 56.7% with FOLFIRI and 54.3% with LV5FU2 alone (HR 0.90; 95% CI 0.79–1.02; $p = 0.106$). There was no significant difference in five-year OS rate (73.6% *vs.* 71.3%; $p = 0.094$). Patients ($n = 880$) with stage II colon cancer also did not derive any significant survival benefit with the addition of irinotecan to LV5FU2 (FOLFIRI) compared with LV5FU2 in the five-year DFS (80.9% *vs.* 76.9%; HR 0.81; 95% CI 0.61–1.08; *p* = 0.158) and the five-year OS (90.0% *vs.* 88.8%; *p* = 0.344). However, FOLFIRI was associated with a substantial increase of severe GI toxicities (diarrhea, 11.9% *vs.* 5.6%) and neutropenia (28.2% *vs.* 6.0%).

Both the NCCN guidelines and the ESMO clinical practice guidelines do not recommend the use of irinotecan-containing regimens in the adjuvant setting for patients with stage II or III colon cancer.[37,39]

5 The Role of Biologics in Adjuvant Therapy

The monoclonal antibodies, bevacizumab and cetuximab, have been investigated in large clinical trials to determine their role in the adjuvant treatment for colon cancer based on their efficacy in the metastatic disease setting. NSABP C-08 was the first clinical trial to evaluate the potential benefit of bevacizumab to FOLFOX-based chemotherapy for the adjuvant treatment of early-stage colon cancer.[20,33] This study randomized 2,672 patients with stage II (25%) or stage III (75%) colon cancer to compare mFOLFOX6 regimen alone for six months versus mFOLFOX6 plus bevacizumab for six months followed by bevacizumab alone for additional six months. The addition of bevacizumab did not result in a significant increase in three-year DFS (77.9% *vs.* 75.1%; HR 0.93; 95% CI 0.81–1.08; *p* = 0.35) and five-year OS (82.5% *vs.* 80.7%; HR 0.95; 95% CI 0.79–1.13; *p* = 0.56). Interestingly, exploratory analyses revealed that the beneficial effect of bevacizumab on the DFS was significant during and immediately following its discontinuation up to 15 months (HR 0.61; 95% CI 0.48–0.78; *p* < 0.0001), while this benefit was entirely lost by 24 months (HR 1.19; 95% CI 0.99–1.42; *p* = 0.059).

The AVANT (BO17920) trial was a global, randomized phase 3 study to evaluate the role of bevacizumab in combination with FOLFOX4 or XELOX in the adjuvant treatment of patients (*n* = 3,451) with resected stage III or high-risk stage II colon cancer, with the primary endpoint being DFS.[34] Patients were randomly assigned to one of three treatment options: FOLFOX4 for six months followed by observation for six months (*n* = 1,151); FOLFOX4 plus bevacizumab for six months followed by bevacizumab alone for six months (*n* = 1,155); or XELOX plus bevacizumab for six months followed by bevacizumab alone for six months (*n* = 1,145). The addition of bevacizumab to FOLFOX4 or XELOX did not result in a significant increase in three-year DFS (76% *vs.* 73% *vs.* 75%; HR 1.17 for FOLFOX4/bevacizumab *vs.* FOLFOX4 [95% CI 0.98–1.39; *p* = 0.07]; HR 1.07 for

XELOX/bevacizumab *vs.* FOLFOX4 [95% CI 0.90–1.28; $p = 0.44$]) and five-year OS (85% *vs.* 81% *vs.* 82%; HR 1.27 for FOLFOX4/bevacizumab *vs.* FOLFOX4 [95% CI 1.03–1.57; $p = 0.02$]; HR 1.15 for XELOX/bevacizumab versus FOLFOX4 [95% CI 0.93–1.42; $p = 0.21$]). These data showed that the addition of bevacizumab to either FOLFOX or XELOX did not improve DFS or OS in resected stage III and high-risk stage II colon cancer. Despite the clear benefit of bevacizumab in the metastatic disease setting, the results of the NSABP C-08 and AVANT studies demonstrated that bevacizumab does not provide clinical benefit in the adjuvant setting when combined with oxaliplatin-containing chemotherapy.

The role of cetuximab in the adjuvant setting was evaluated in the NO147 clinical trial, which randomized stage III colon cancer patients (1,863 patients with wild-type *KRAS* exon 2 and 717 patients with mutant *KRAS* exon 2) to mFOLFOX6 plus cetuximab versus mFOLFOX6 alone.[21] The trial was terminated early as a pre-planned interim analysis failed to demonstrate a clinical benefit from the addition of cetuximab in any patient subgroup.

PETACC-8 was a randomized phase III study conducted in Europe to assess whether the addition of cetuximab to FOLFOX4 chemotherapy in patients with resected stage III colon cancer could improve DFS.[40] The protocol was amended to limit enrollment to patients with wild-type *KRAS* exon 2 tumors. Of 2,559 enrolled patients, 1,602 patients had wild-type *KRAS* exon 2 tumors ($n = 791$ in FOLFOX4 plus cetuximab arm; $n = 811$ in FOLFOX4 arm). The three-year DFS of the wild-type *KRAS* exon 2 intention-to-treat population was not significantly different between the FOLFOX4 plus cetuximab arm and FOLFOX4 arm (75.1% *vs.* 78.0%; HR 1.05; 95% CI 0.85–1.29; $p = 0.66$). There was no significant difference in the OS either (HR 1.09; 95% CI 0.81–1.47; $p = 0.56$). Of note, the three-year OS rates between the two treatment arms were not markedly different in the subgroup of patients ($n = 984$) with both wild-type *KRAS* exon 2 and wild-type *BRAF* tumors (89.7% *vs.* 91.2%; HR 0.98; 95% CI 0.67–1.44; $p = 0.92$) or in patients ($n = 742$) with mutant *KRAS* exon 2 tumors (87.2% *vs.* 88.1%; HR 1.06; 95% CI 0.73–1.53; $p = 0.76$). The addition of cetuximab to FOLFOX4 did not improve DFS in comparison to FOLFOX4 alone in patients with resected stage III colon cancer harboring wild-type *KRAS* exon 2. Taken together, the results of the NO147 and PETACC-8 studies demonstrated that cetuximab was unable to add clinical benefit to FOLFOX chemotherapy in the adjuvant treatment of resected stage III colon cancer.

Both the NCCN guidelines and the ESMO clinical practice guidelines do not recommend the use of the anti-VEGF antibody (bevacizumab) or the anti-EGFR antibodies (cetuximab or panitumumab) in the adjuvant setting for patients with stage II or III colon cancer.[37,39]

6 Stage II Colon Cancer

Despite years of on-going debate, the presently available data support the role of 5-FU-based adjuvant chemotherapy in patients with stage II colon cancer, although the absolute improvements are relatively small in stage II disease when compared with stage III disease.[22,29,41–43] The study that conclusively highlights the clinical benefit of adjuvant chemotherapy in stage II colon cancer is the Quick and Simple and Reliable (QUASAR) trial conducted in the United Kingdom. This study randomly assigned 3,238 resected early stage colon cancer patients (91% with stage II) to adjuvant chemotherapy with 5-FU plus LV (with or without LEV) or observation alone.[29] The relative risk of recurrence for stage II colon cancer with 5-FU/LV adjuvant chemotherapy compared to observation alone in the first two years after randomization was 0.71 (8% *vs.* 11.2%; 95% CI 0.49–1.01; $p = 0.01$). The relative risk of death from any cause with chemotherapy versus observation alone in patients with stage II colon cancer was 0.84 (95% CI 0.68–1.00; $p = 0.046$). These data show that adjuvant chemotherapy with 5-FU/LV improves the survival of patients with stage II colon cancer.

Several pooled studies and meta-analyses evaluated the role of adjuvant 5-FU-based chemotherapy in stage II colon cancer.[4,23,44–47] The Ontario Cancer Care Program systematically reviewed 37 randomized controlled trials and 11 meta-analyses that compared adjuvant chemotherapy versus observation in patients with stage II colon cancer.[44] Pooled data from 4,187 stage II patients showed that adjuvant chemotherapy reduced the risk of death by 13%, and this risk reduction in death approached statistical significance (HR 0.87; 95% CI 0.75–1.01; $p = 0.07$).

Sargent *et al.* analyzed the Adjuvant Colon Cancer Endpoints (ACCENT) database, a collection of individual patient data from 18 trials evaluating 5-FU-based adjuvant chemotherapy in more than 20,898 patients with stage II or III colon cancer in the initial eight-year follow-up period.[4] The real power of this analysis was the large number of patients, nearly 7,000, with stage II disease. Adjuvant chemotherapy in patients with stage II colon cancer resulted in a significant 5.4% improvement in eight-year OS rate in comparison to surgery alone (eight-year OS, 66.8% *vs.* 72.2%; $p = 0.026$).

The true benefit of oxaliplatin in patients with stage II colon cancer is presently uncertain given the small number of such patients in the MOSAIC and NSABP C-07 clinical trials.[16,17] An exploratory analysis of the MOSAIC trial data showed a trend toward improved five-year DFS in patients with high-risk stage II disease treated by FOLFOX4 compared with LV5FU2 (82.3% *vs.* 74.6%; HR 0.72; 95% CI 0.50–1.02).[16,17]

The ESMO clinical practice guidelines and the NCCN guidelines do not recommend the routine use of adjuvant chemotherapy for medically fit patients with stage II colon cancer. However, both guidelines recommend that adjuvant chemotherapy can be considered in patients with high-risk features: lymph node sampling <12; poorly differentiated tumor; vascular or lymphatic or perineural invasion; tumor presentation with obstruction or perforation, and pT4 stage.[37,39]

7 Treatment Considerations in the Elderly

The optimal regimen for adjuvant therapy of colon cancer in elderly patients has not been clearly established. Older patients derive a similar magnitude of benefit from adjuvant 5-FU-based chemotherapy as their younger counterparts.[25] This observation is based on the results from a pooled analysis of 3,351 patients with stages II and III colon cancer that were enrolled in seven different randomized phase III trials comparing 5-FU-based adjuvant chemotherapy versus surgery alone.[25] Adjuvant treatment had a significant positive effect on both OS and time to tumor recurrence, and was found to be of similar magnitude in four different age categories, ≤50, 51 to 60, 61 to 70, and >70 years. The X-ACT study showed that older patients, as defined by ≥70 years, with stage III colon cancer treated with capecitabine also had improved clinical outcome.[13]

The benefit from adjuvant oxaliplatin based chemotherapy in older patients has been somewhat conflicting. In a subgroup analysis of the MOSAIC study, the benefit of the addition of oxaliplatin to 5-FU/LV was seen only in patients under the age of 65 years.[16] Updated analyses of data from the NSABP C-07, MOSAIC, and the Adjuvant Colon Cancer Endpoints (ACCENT) database also suggest a reduced benefit from adjuvant oxaliplatin-based chemotherapy in patients older than 70 years of age.[18,48,49]

However, there are clinical data showing that older patients (≥70 years) can derive substantial benefit from oxaliplatin-containing adjuvant chemotherapy. Haller *et al.* analyzed DFS across age groups in the NO16968 study to determine the efficacy of XELOX in older patients as defined by ≥70 years.[50] Analysis of three-year DFS in patients of <70 and ≥70 years showed a similar advantage of XELOX over 5-FU/LV (HR 0.79 in <70 years [95% CI 0.66–0.94] versus 0.87 in ≥70 years [95% CI, 0.63–1.0]), a result that is at odds with the ACCENT database analysis and the MOSAIC study. The findings from Haller *et al.* are consistent with the results from a recent comparative effectiveness analysis of oxaliplatin versus non-oxaliplatin containing adjuvant chemotherapy that was conducted by Sanoff and colleagues in stage III colon cancer patients.[51] Sanoff *et al.* analyzed the survival data of stage III colon cancer patients ($n = 4,060$) who received adjuvant chemotherapy from five observational data sources (the Surveillance, Epidemiology, and End Results registry linked to Medicare claims [SEER-Medicare]; the New York State Cancer Registry [NYSCR] linked to Medicaid and Medicare claims; the NCCN Outcomes Database; and the Cancer Care Outcomes Research & Surveillance Consortium [CanCORS]), and compared them with pooled data from the ACCENT group ($n = 8,292$). This analysis found that older patients (70–74 years old) experienced clear survival benefit from oxaliplatin-containing adjuvant chemotherapy in SEER–Medicare (HR of death 0.66; 95% CI 0.52–0.84) and NYSCR–Medicare (HR of death 0.62; 95% CI 0.36–1.07).

The appropriate treatment of the elderly population in the adjuvant setting remains to be established. While there are conflicting data as to what the optimal therapy should be, there appears to be growing evidence to support considering the use of oxaliplatin-based adjuvant chemotherapy in elderly patients with stage III and high-risk stage II disease. It is clear that the decision to treat with more aggressive oxaliplatin-based chemotherapy should be based on the individual risk-benefit assessment, which should factor in performance status and presence of comorbid illnesses. The NCCN guidelines recommend that the addition of oxaliplatin to 5-FU/LV in older patients (>70 years old) should remain optional and needs to be individualized.[39]

8 Optimal Duration of Adjuvant Chemotherapy

The current standard of care for stage III colon cancer patients is FOLFOX, XELOX, or FLOX for six months based on the findings from three large trials: MOSAIC, NO16968, and NSABP C-07. However, these combination regimens are associated with significant toxicities, especially as it relates to oxaliplatin-induced, cumulative dose-dependent neurotoxicity. A reduced duration of adjuvant chemotherapy while maintaining the efficacy of adjuvant treatment would be advantageous to avoid these associated toxicities and maintain patient quality of life. At present, however, there is limited data supporting a shorter duration of adjuvant chemotherapy than the current standard of six months while keeping the same survival benefit.

To address this specific issue, Chau *et al.*[52] conducted an adjuvant treatment trial of 801 patients with stage II/III colon cancer to compare three months of protracted venous infusion (PVI) of 5-FU (300 mg/m^2/day for 12 weeks) and six months of standard bolus 5-FU/LV. The five-year RFS was 66.7% and 73.3% with bolus 5-FU/LV and PVI 5-FU, respectively (HR 0.8; 95% CI 0.62–1.04; $p = 0.10$), while the five-year OS was 71.5% and 75.7% with bolus 5-FU/LV and PVI 5-FU, respectively (HR 0.79; 95% CI 0.61–1.03; $p = 0.083$). Significantly less diarrhea, stomatitis, nausea and vomiting, alopecia, lethargy, and neutropenia ($p < 0.0001$) were observed with PVI 5-FU. Although the study did not meet its primary endpoint OS, which was superiority of the three-month treatment arm, it showed that the chance of the three-month regimen being inferior to the six-month treatment plan was extremely low ($p < 0.005$).

The data from the MOSAIC and NSABP C-07 trials showed that the benefit of six months of FOLFOX treatment in the MOSAIC study was identical with that of FLOX regimen in the NSABP C-07 study (five-year DFS, 73.3% *vs.* 69.4%), while the total cumulative dose of oxaliplatin in the FLOX regimen was 30% less than that of FOLFOX regimen, suggesting that lower cumulative doses of oxaliplatin can be used with similar clinical benefit. Of note, the planned dose of oxaliplatin in the study protocols was 1,020 mg/m^2 (12 cycles) in MOSAIC and 765 mg/m^2 (nine cycles) in NSABP C-07, but the median dose of oxaliplatin administered per patient was 810 mg/m^2 (9.5 cycles) and 667 mg/m^2 (7.8 cycles) in MOSAIC and NSABP C-07, respectively. These data raise an important question as to the optimal number of cycles of oxaliplatin that can be administered without compromising survival benefit of adjuvant chemotherapy and minimizing oxaliplatin-induced neurotoxicity.

The International Duration Evaluation of Adjuvant Chemotherapy (IDEA) collaboration was established to address whether a three-month course of oxaliplatin-based adjuvant therapy (FOLFOX4/mFOLFOX6 or XELOX) is non-inferior to the current standard six-month treatment for patients with stage III colon cancer. The primary endpoint of this study is three-year DFS, and the potential advantage of the study design is that it prospectively combined and analyzed data from several randomized trials conducted around the world with a target accrual goal of at least 10,500 patients by the end of 2013.[53] There are six clinical trials currently participating in the IDEA project:[53] the Italian Three or Six Colon Adjuvant (TOSCA) trial; the U.K. Short Course Oncology Treatment (SCOT) trial; the IDEA France trial; the Intergroup Cancer and Leukemia Group B/Southwest Oncology Group (CALGB/SWOG) trial 80702; the Greek Hellenic Oncology Research Group (HORG) trial; and the Japanese Adjuvant Chemotherapy for colon cancer with HIgh EVidencE (ACHIEVE) trial. It is expected that the data from the IDEA project will provide a definitive answer as to the optimal duration of adjuvant chemotherapy for patients with stage III colon cancer, and the results of this novel collaborative effort are eagerly awaited.

9 Risk Stratification Based on High-Risk Prognostic Features and Predictive Molecular Biomarkers

9.1 *High-risk prognostic features in stage II disease*

Significant efforts have been made towards identification of the clinical, pathological, and molecular features to help distinguish high-risk stage II patients with a greater risk of disease recurrence and who might derive a greater benefit from adjuvant chemotherapy. The clinical features that have been identified as being associated with poor prognosis in stage II disease are T4 stage, lymphovascular invasion (LVI), perineural invasion, bowel obstruction or perforation, inadequate LN sampling (<12 LN) in the surgical resection specimen, and poorly differentiated histologic features.[54–56] The recent ESMO and NCCN have endorsed these clinical risk factors for the identification of patients with high-risk stage II disease.[37,39]

At present, there is no clear evidence indicating that these high-risk features of poor prognosis in stage II disease are also predictive of the potential benefit of adjuvant therapy. In an exploratory analysis of the MOSAIC clinical trial data, there was a non-statistically significant trend towards improved DFS with FOLFOX4 compared with 5-FU/LV (82% *vs.* 75%; HR 0.72) in the subgroup of stage II patients with high-risk features (clinical T4, poorly differentiated histology, perforation, obstruction, or <10 LN in the surgical specimen).[48] OS was similar in both treatment groups (85% *vs.* 83%; *p* = 0.65).[48]

9.2 *Predictive molecular biomarkers for adjuvant therapy*

In addition to the high-risk clinical features of prognosis in stage II disease, several other factors have been evaluated for their potential role as predictive biomarkers of adjuvant chemotherapy. These markers include microsatellite instability (MSI), loss of heterozygosity (LOH) 18q, thymidylate synthase (TS) overexpression, gene expression signatures or recurrence score (RS) assays, circulating tumor cells, and genetic mutations such as *KRAS, BRAF* and *p53*.[57–59] Among all these biomarkers, only MSI status has been identified, to date, as playing a potential predictive role for adjuvant therapy.

MSI refers to a change in the length of DNA microsatellites due to the insertion or deletion of repeating short nucleotide sequences, that is caused by either a germline mutation in one of the four most common mismatch repair (MMR) genes (*MLH1, MSH2, MSH6, PMS2*) or epigenetic silencing of *MLH1* by the hypermethylation of the promoter regions.[60,61] MSI is thus considered to be the molecular fingerprint of a deficient MMR system. A reference panel of 5–10 microsatellite markers is used to determine MSI status, and MSI-High (MSI-H) is diagnosed when 40% or more of the microsatellite markers demonstrates instability.[60] Lack of expression of MMR proteins by immunohistochemistry (IHC) is diagnostic for defective MMR (dMMR) and is often used to determine MSI status as an alternative to PCR. MSI-H tumors are more prevalent in stage II as compared to stage III colon cancer (21% *vs.* 14 %).[62] They tend to be located more proximally, have a mucinous histology, show intense intratumoral lymphocytic infiltration, and are associated with a better prognosis than microsatellite stable (MSS) colon cancers.

Ribic *et al.* investigated the role of MSI status as a predictive biomarker of adjuvant chemotherapy in patients ($n = 570$) with stage II or III colon cancer enrolled in five randomized trials of 5-FU-based adjuvant chemotherapy.[63] Among 570 tissue specimens, 95 (16.7%) were MSI-H. Among patients who received adjuvant chemotherapy, MSI-H was not correlated with improvement of OS (HR for death 1.07; 95% CI 0.62–1.86; $p = 0.80$). Hutchins *et al.* evaluated the role of MMR status as prognostic and predictive biomarkers in patients from the QUASAR trial.[64] dMMR was associated with lower recurrence rate when compared with pMMR (11% *vs.* 26%; risk ratio 0.53; 95% CI 0.40–0.70; $p < 0.001$). MMR status was not significantly associated with the reduced risk of recurrence with chemotherapy. In addition, MMR status was not predictive of adjuvant chemotherapy benefit on OS. Popat *et al.* reported a systemic review of 32 adjuvant clinical trials, which enrolled 7,642 patients including 1,277 patients with MSI-H.[65] In patients treated with adjuvant 5-FU, patients with MSI-H tumor derived no benefit from adjuvant 5-FU (HR 1.24; 95% CI 0.72–2.14).

Sargent *et al.* investigated the role of MSI status as a predictive marker in 457 patients with stage II or III colon cancer who were previously enrolled in five randomized clinical trials of 5-FU-based adjuvant therapy.[66] Among 457 patients, 70 (15%) patients had dMMR tumor. Among patients with dMMR tumor, there was no improvement of DFS in the group receiving 5-FU adjuvant therapy in comparison to those assigned to surgery alone (HR 1.10; 95% CI 0.42–2.91; $p = 0.85$). Further analysis of the pooled data set of 1,027 patients ($n = 165$ with dMMR) from the previous report,[63] adjuvant chemotherapy was significantly associated with reduced OS in patients with dMMR stage II CRC (HR 2.95; 95% CI 1.02–8.54; $p = 0.04$).

Sinicrope *et al.* reported a clear difference in predictive value of MSI status for adjuvant 5-FU chemotherapy between tumors harboring germline mutations in MMR genes and sporadic dMMR tumors.[67] Survival data of stage II and III colon cancer patients ($n = 2,141$) were analyzed from randomized trials of 5-FU-based adjuvant therapy. dMMR was detected in 344 of 2,141 (16.1%) tumors. Tumors with dMMR were further categorized by presumed germline mutations in MMR genes versus sporadic origin by epigenetic silencing of *MLH1* expression. The frequency of suspected germline cancers was 4.6% (99 of 2,141 cancers). Adjuvant therapy with 5-FU-based treatment was associated with a statistically significant improvement in DFS in patients with colon cancer of suspected germline mutations in MMR genes, but not in sporadic cancers ($p = 0.006$). In stage III patients with suspected germline mutations of MMR genes in tumors, adjuvant 5-FU therapy was associated with a greater DFS (HR 0.26; 95% CI 0.09–0.77; $p = 0.009$), whereas no treatment benefit in DFS was observed in patients with sporadic dMMR stage III tumors (HR 0.79; 95% CI 0.35–1.80; $p = 0.577$).

The European Group on Tumor Markers (EGTM) recommends that MSI status may be analyzed in stage II patients who are being considered for adjuvant chemotherapy.[68] Given their improved overall prognosis, patients with MSI-H stage II CRC may not require adjuvant chemotherapy. However, MSI-H stage II patients with high-risk features such as pT4 or LVI should not be excluded from receiving chemotherapy.

The NCCN and ESMO clinical practice guidelines recommend that MSI testing should be considered for patients with stage II disease. The assessment of MSI status is particularly important as patients with stage II MSI-H colon cancer have a good overall prognosis and do not benefit from 5-FU-containing adjuvant therapy.[37,39]

9.3 Gene expression signatures

It is now well established that patients with stage II colon cancer not only differ in their cancer recurrence risk depending on the underlying tumor characteristics, but they also derive varying levels of benefit from adjuvant chemotherapy. The development of oxaliplatin-associated toxicity, especially as it relates to chronic peripheral neuropathy, has raised concerns as to the real benefit of adjuvant chemotherapy in unselected stage III colon cancer patients as well. As a consequence, significant efforts are being made to identify potential biomarkers that would help define the subset of stages II and III colon cancer patients expected to derive maximum clinical benefit from adjuvant treatment. Oncotype DX colon cancer assay and ColoPrint are the two most well-known of these biomarkers, out of the many gene expression profiling assays that have been developed over the past few years.

ColoPrint is an 18-gene signature that was validated in 206 stage I–III colon cancer tumor samples, and patients were stratified into low- and high-risk groups.[69] Patients with low-risk stage II disease were found to have significantly improved five-year RFS than patients with high-risk disease (87.6% *vs.* 67.2%; HR 2.5; $p = 0.005$). In a multivariate analysis, the gene signature was one of the most significant prognostic factors (HR 2.69; $p = 0.003$). The ColoPrint assay was subsequently revalidated by Salazar *et al.* as an independent prognostic marker in a pooled set of stage II colon cancer patients ($n = 320$) and also more exclusively in the T3 MSS subgroup ($n = 227$).[70]

The Oncotype DX assay was initially developed by measuring expression levels of 761 candidate genes using reverse transcription-polymerase chain reaction (RT-PCR) in stages II and III resected tumor specimens obtained from four independent clinical studies.[71] The recurrence score (RS) was initially determined based on the expression of 12 genes (seven recurrence genes and five reference genes) and then validated as an independent predictor of cancer recurrence in patients with stage II colon cancer, using 1,436 tumor blocks from the U.K. QUASAR trial.[72] Subsequently, using 690 patient samples from the Cancer and Leukemia Group B (CALGB) 9581 trial, the 12-gene RS was shown to be prognostic for clinical outcome and was revalidated as a significant predictor of recurrence risk in stage II CRC.[73]

Currently, the greatest utility of RS assay is to predict the recurrence risk in stage II colon cancer patients with T3 MSS tumors and in those without high-risk clinicopathologic features. A model estimate from the recent validation study of Oncotype DX assay based upon the data from NSABP C-07 clinical trial, has suggested a greater absolute oxaliplatin benefit with higher RS values, most notably in patients with stages II and IIIA/B disease.[74] However, in the absence of convincing data to support clinically meaningful impact on outcome, none of the currently available RS assays have been approved for use as a decision-making tool in the management of early-stage colon cancer patients at this time.[75] Because of insufficient supporting clinical data, the NCCN guidelines do not recommend the routine use of these multigene assays to determine adjuvant therapy in patients with stage II or III colon cancer.[39]

10 Pharmacoeconomic Considerations in Adjuvant Chemotherapy

Douillard *et al.* reported that capecitabine is more effective and less costly than two different intravenous regimens of 5-FU/LV (de Gramont and Mayo Clinic regimens) as adjuvant therapy in stage III colon cancer in France.[76] In the economic analysis including direct costs, such as drug acquisition and drug administration, capecitabine was significantly less costly (€3,654 per patient) than the Mayo Clinic regimen (€10,481 per patient) and de Gramont regimen (€7,204 per patient), respectively.

Aballea *et al.* analyzed the cost-effectiveness of FOLFOX4 in stage III patients from a U.S. Medicare perspective.[77] FOLFOX4 was found to be cost-effective when compared with 5-FU/LV in the adjuvant treatment of stage III colon cancer. Mean total lifetime disease-related costs were $56,300 with FOLFOX4 and $39,300 with 5-FU/LV. However, compared with 5-FU/LV, FOLFOX4 was estimated to cost $20,600 per life-year gained and $22,800 per quality-adjusted life-year (QALY) gained, discounting costs and outcomes at 3% per annum.

Chu *et al.* reported a retrospective, claim-based analysis of 1,396 colorectal cancer patients treated with capecitabine or 5-FU monotherapy for adjuvant therapy.[78] Adjuvant capecitabine monotherapy was associated with lower total medical and chemotherapy-related costs than 5-FU. Reduced complications and costs associated with capecitabine administration offset its higher acquisition cost. Capecitabine users incurred $740 less in total direct medical costs ($p = 0.003$) and $785 less in chemotherapy-related costs ($p < 0.0001$) than 5-FU users. Although drug acquisition cost was higher for capecitabine than for 5-FU ($958 *vs.* $71; $p < 0.0001$), chemotherapy administration cost was lower ($76 *vs.* $1,062; $p < 0.0001$). The unadjusted (610 *vs.* 1,960 events per 1,000 person-months) and adjusted risks (47%) were lower for capecitabine than 5-FU for any complication.

Eggington *et al.* evaluated the cost-effectiveness of adjuvant capecitabine and FOLFOX4 chemotherapy, using data from the MOSAIC and X-ACT trials.[79] The health economic analysis suggested that capecitabine is expected to produce cost-savings of approximately £3,320 per patient in comparison with intravenous 5-FU/LV (Mayo Clinic regimen). FOLFOX4 is estimated to cost £2,970 per additional QALY gained when compared to 5-FU/LV alone.

Cassidy *et al.* analyzed incremental direct and societal costs and gains in quality-adjusted life months (QALMs) in patients receiving adjuvant chemotherapy of capecitabine or intravenous 5-FU/LV.[12] Drug acquisition costs were higher for capecitabine than 5-FU/LV, but higher 5-FU/LV administration costs resulted in 57% lower chemotherapy costs for capecitabine. Chemotherapy-associated adverse events resulted in a cost savings of £3,653 with capecitabine. The reduction of societal costs, including patient travel/time costs, resulted in cost savings £1,318 with capecitabine with lifetime gain in QALMs of nine months.

There is now a growing body of evidence confirming that overall costs of treatment are reduced with XELOX when compared to FOLFOX. This cost difference driven by lower costs of capecitabine-based chemotherapy in administration of chemotherapy and management of chemotherapy-related complications provides support for the use of XELOX as adjuvant therapy of colon cancer.

11 On-Going Phase III Adjuvant Studies

11.1 *QUASAR-2 adjuvant trial*

QUASAR 2 is a multicenter international study comparing capecitabine with capecitabine plus bevacizumab as adjuvant treatment of patients ($n = 2,240$) with stage II or III colorectal cancer.[80] The primary endpoint of this study is three-year DFS. Patient enrollment was completed in October 2010, and the planned study completion is September 2014.

11.2 CALGB/SWOG colon trial C80702 (CLEAR Colon Trial); a phase III trial of 6 vs. 12 treatments of adjuvant FOLFOX plus celecoxib or placebo for patients with resected stage III colon cancer

This study is a randomized phase III trial to compare FOLFOX plus celecoxib with FOLOFX alone in patients with resected stage III colon cancer.[81] The target goal of accrual is 2,500 patients with stage III colon cancer, and the primary endpoint is DFS. One of the main goals of this U.S.-driven study is to determine whether a shorter course of adjuvant chemotherapy can confer the same level of clinical benefit as the standard six months of FOLFOX chemotherapy, which is similar to the IDEA study, outlined above. The rationale for this study comes from reports suggesting that aspirin and anti-inflammatory drugs (NSAIDs) use can lengthen survival in patients with colon cancer, especially in tumors with *PIK3CA* mutations.[82–84] This study evaluates whether the addition of celecoxib, a selective COX-2 inhibitor, to FOLFOX chemotherapy is able to extend the DFS and OS associated with FOLFOX chemotherapy. This study is actively accruing patients at multiple sites in the United States.

12 Future Directions

Recent advances in next-generation sequencing (NGS) technology are now providing unprecedented opportunities for the development of highly selective and personalized treatment options for patients with colon cancer. However, our understanding of cancer mutations and genetic changes in tumor tissues are still in its earliest stage of development, and it requires rigorous clinical research focusing on identification and validation of highly specific agents for each genetic mutations. Further efforts should focus on the identification of specific predictive molecular markers for adjuvant chemotherapy in colorectal cancer based on this genetic information.

There has been a steady increase of life expectancy during the last several decades, resulting in a substantial increase in the elderly population worldwide. In general, the incidence and prevalence of colorectal cancer increases rapidly after age 50. As discussed earlier, the elderly population has unique aging-related physical conditions and co-morbidities in comparison to younger population, which requires a more carefully tailored approach to the treatment of colorectal cancer patients in this population group.

Although the benefit of adjuvant chemotherapy in patients with stage II colon cancer has been demonstrated, the absolute benefit of adjuvant chemotherapy in this patient population is small relative to what is observed in stage III disease. As a result, a proper risk stratification of stage II disease including predictive markers is required to identify a subset of patients who may derive absolute benefit from adjuvant chemotherapy. The current risk stratification is mainly based on prognostic clinical factors and MSI status. Future research should focus on the identification and validation of biomarkers that can predict which adjuvant chemotherapy should be used in stage II disease.

Current adjuvant chemotherapy with either FOLFOX or XELOX chemotherapy provides significant survival benefit in patients with stage III or II colon cancer. However, a majority of stage III colon cancer patients will experience a recurrence of their disease even after adjuvant chemotherapy. Thus, there is a clear unmet need to develop biomarkers that can identify which patients are at increased risk for disease recurrence. Moreover, there is a real need to develop novel agents and combination therapies for the adjuvant treatment of early-stage colon cancer.

13 Conclusion

The benefit of adjuvant chemotherapy has been clearly established for patients with III colon cancer with risk reduction of death by absolute 5–10% in stage III with fluoropyrimidine monotherapy and additional 4–5% with oxaliplatin-containing regimen including FOLFOX and XELOX. Oxaliplatin-containing regimens (FOLFOX or XELOX administered for six months) are the current standard adjuvant chemotherapy options for stage III colon cancer patients. Clinical studies have also demonstrated 3–5% absolute risk reduction of death in stage II colon cancer. However, the risk stratification of patients with stage II colon cancer remains largely unproven at present, requiring further development and identification of reliable predictive biomarkers for adjuvant therapy in stage II disease. Current practice guidelines including the recent ESMO and NCCN guidelines suggest individualizing treatment decisions based on the presence or absence of high-risk clinicopathologic features, MSI status, and most importantly, a detailed discussion of benefit-risk ratio with these patients. FOLFOX/XELOX, 5-FU/LV, or single-agent capecitabine are considered to be reasonable options for high-risk stage II patients who decide in favor of adjuvant chemotherapy. Finally, despite all the encouraging data surrounding gene expression signatures, the role of recurrence score assays as a decision-making tool in the management of early-stage colon cancer is presently limited and therefore should not be used in routine clinical practice at this time.

References

1. Siegel R, *et al*. Colorectal cancer statistics, 2014. *CA Cancer J Clin* 2014;**64**:104–117.
2. Siegel R, *et al*. Cancer statistics, 2014. *CA Cancer J Clin* 2014;**64**:9–29.
3. Edge SB, *et al*. *AJCC (American Joint Committee on Cancer) Cancer Staging Manual*. 7th edition. New York: Springer, 2010.
4. Sargent D, *et al*. Evidence for cure by adjuvant therapy in colon cancer: Observations based on individual patient data from 20,898 patients on 18 randomized trials. *J Clin Oncol* 2009;**27**:872–877.
5. Pinedo HM, Peters GF. Fluorouracil: Biochemistry and pharmacology. *J Clin Oncol* 1998;**6**:1653–1664.
6. Moertel CG, *et al*. Levamisole and fluorouracil for adjuvant therapy of resected colon carcinoma. *N Engl J Med* 1990;**322**:352–358.
7. Wolmark N, *et al*. The benefit of leucovorin-modulated fluorouracil as postoperative adjuvant therapy for primary colon cancer: results from National Surgical Adjuvant Breast and Bowel Project protocol C-03. *J Clin Oncol* 1993;**11**:1879–1887.
8. Moertel CG, *et al*. Fluorouracil plus levamisole as effective adjuvant therapy after resection of stage III colon carcinoma: A final report. *Ann Intern Med* 1995;**122**:321–326.
9. Wolmark N, *et al*. Clinical trial to assess the relative efficacy of fluorouracil and leucovorin, fluorouracil and levamisole, and fluorouracil, leucovorin, and levamisole in patients with Dukes' B and C carcinoma of the colon: Results from National Surgical Adjuvant Breast and Bowel Project C-04. *J Clin Oncol* 1999;**17**:3553–3559.
10. André T, *et al*. Phase III study comparing a semimonthly with a monthly regimen of fluorouracil and leucovorin as adjuvant treatment for stage II and III colon cancer patients: Final results of GERCOR C96.1. *J Clin Oncol* 2007;**25**:3732–3738.
11. André T, *et al*. Semimonthly versus monthly regimen of fluorouracil and leucovorin administered for 24 or 36 weeks as adjuvant therapy in stage II and III colon cancer: Results of a randomized trial. *J Clin Oncol* 2003;**21**:2896–2903.
12. Cassidy J, *et al*. Pharmacoeconomic analysis of adjuvant oral capecitabine *vs*. intravenous 5-FU/LV in Dukes' C colon cancer: The X-ACT trial. *Br J Cancer* 2006;**94**: 1122–1129.
13. Twelves C, *et al*. Capecitabine as adjuvant treatment for stage III colon cancer. *N Engl J Med* 2005;**352**:2696–2704.
14. Haller DG, *et al*. Potential regional differences for the tolerability profiles of fluoropyrimidines. *J Clin Oncol* 2008;**26**(13):2118–2123.
15. André T, *et al*. Oxaliplatin, fluorouracil, and leucovorin as adjuvant treatment for colon cancer. *N Engl J Med* 2004;**350**:2343–2351.
16. André T, *et al*. Improved overall survival with oxaliplatin, fluorouracil, and leucovorin as adjuvant treatment in stage II or III colon cancer in the MOSAIC trial. *J Clin Oncol* 2009;**27**:3109–3116.
17. Kuebler JP, *et al*. Oxaliplatin combined with weekly bolus fluorouracil and leucovorin as surgical adjuvant chemotherapy for stage II and III colon cancer: Results from NSABP C-07. *J Clin Oncol* 2007;**25**:2198–2204.

18. Yothers G, *et al*. Oxaliplatin as adjuvant therapy for colon cancer: Updated results of NSABP C-07 trial, including survival and subset analyses. *J Clin Oncol* 2011;**29**: 3768–3774.

19. Haller DG, *et al*. Capecitabine plus oxaliplatin compared with fluorouracil and folinic acid as adjuvant therapy for stage III colon cancer. *J Clin Oncol* 2011;**29**:1465–1471.

20. Allegra CJ, *et al*. Phase III trial assessing bevacizumab in stages II and III carcinoma of the colon: Results of NSABP protocol C-08. *J Clin Oncol* 2011;**29**:11–16.

21. Alberts SR, *et al*. Effect of oxaliplatin, fluorouracil, and leucovorin with or without cetuximab on survival among patients with resected stage III colon cancer: A randomized trial. *JAMA*, 2012;**307**:1383–1393.

22. International Multicenter Pooled Analysis of Colon Cancer Trials (IMPACT) investigators. Efficacy of adjuvant fluorouracil and folinic acid in colon cancer. *Lancet* 1995;**345**: 939–944.

23. Marsoni S, International Multicenter Pooled Analysis of Colon Cancer Trials investigators. Efficacy of adjuvant fluorouracil and leucovorin in stage B2 and C colon cancer. *Semin Oncol* 2001;**28**:14–19.

24. O'Connell MJ, *et al*. Controlled trial of fluorouracil and low-dose leucovorin given for 6 months as postoperative adjuvant therapy for colon cancer. *J Clin Oncol* 1997;**15**: 246–250.

25. Sargent DJ, *et al*. A pooled analysis of adjuvant chemotherapy for resected colon cancer in elderly patients. *N Engl J Med* 2001;**345**:1091–1097.

26. Porschen R, *et al*. Arbeitsgemeinschaft Gastrointestinale Onkologie. Fluorouracil plus leucovorin as effective adjuvant chemotherapy in curatively resected stage III colon cancer: Results of the trial adjCCA-01. *J Clin Oncol* 2001;**19**:1787–1794.

27. Dencausse Y, *et al*. Adjuvant chemotherapy in stage III colon cancer with 5-fluorouracil and levamisole versus 5-fluorouracil and leucovorin. *Onkologie* 2002;**25**:426–430.

28. Haller DG, *et al*. Phase III study of fluorouracil, leucovorin, and levamisole in high-risk stage II and III colon cancer: Final report of Intergroup 0089. *J Clin Oncol* 2005;**23**: 8671–8678.

29. Quasar Collaborative Group, Gray R, *et al*. Adjuvant chemotherapy versus observation in patients with colorectal cancer: A randomised study. *Lancet* 2007;**370**:2020–2029.

30. Saltz LB, *et al*. Irinotecan fluorouracil plus leucovorin is not superior to fluorouracil plus leucovorin alone as adjuvant treatment for stage III colon cancer: Results of CALGB 89803. *J Clin Oncol* 2007;**25**:3456–3461.

31. Van Cutsem E, *et al*. Randomized phase III trial comparing biweekly infusional fluorouracil/leucovorin alone or with irinotecan in the adjuvant treatment of stage III colon cancer: PETACC-3. *J Clin Oncol* 2009;**27**:3117–3125.

32. Ychou M, *et al*. A phase III randomised trial of LV5FU2 + irinotecan versus LV5FU2 alone in adjuvant high-risk colon cancer (FNCLCC Accord02/FFCD9802). *Ann Oncol* 2009;**20**:674–680.

33. Allegra CJ, *et al*. Bevacizumab in stage II-III colon cancer: 5-year update of the National Surgical Adjuvant Breast and Bowel Project C-08 trial. *J Clin Oncol* 2012; **31**:359–364.

34. De Gramont A, *et al*. Bevacizumab plus oxaliplatin-based chemotherapy as adjuvant treatment for colon cancer (AVANT): A phase 3 randomised controlled trial. *Lancet Oncol* 2012;**13**:1225–1233.

35. Punt CJ, *et al*. Edrecolomab alone or in combination with fluorouracil and folinic acid in the adjuvant treatment of stage III colon cancer: A randomised study. *Lancet* 2002;**360**:671–677.

36. Fields AL, *et al*. Adjuvant therapy with the monoclonal antibody Edrecolomab plus fluorouracil-based therapy does not improve overall survival of patients with stage III colon cancer. *J Clin Oncol* 2009;**27**:1941–1947.

37. Labianca R, *et al*. Early colon cancer: ESMO Clinical Practice Guidelines for diagnosis, treatment and follow-up. *Ann Oncol* 2013;**24**(Suppl. 6):vi64–vi72.

38. Engstrom PF, *et al*. NCCN Clinical Practice Guidelines in Oncology: Colon cancer. *J Natl Compr Canc Netw* 2009;**7**:778–831.

39. Benson AB III, *et al*. Localized colon cancer, version 3.2013: Featured updates to the NCCN Guidelines. *J Natl Compr Canc Netw* 2013;**11**:519–528.

40. Taieb J, *et al*. Oxaliplatin, fluorouracil, and leucovorin with or without cetuximab in patients with resected stage III colon cancer (PETACC-8): An open-label, randomised phase 3 trial. *Lancet Oncol* 2014;**15**:862–873.

41. Moertel CG, *et al*. Intergroup study of fluorouracil plus levamisole as adjuvant therapy for stage II/Dukes' B2 colon cancer. *J Clin Oncol* 1995;**13**:2936–2943.

42. Moore HC, Haller DG. Adjuvant therapy of colon cancer. *Semin Oncol* 1999;**26**: 545–555.

43. Schippinger W, *et al*. A prospective randomised phase III trial of adjuvant chemotherapy with 5-fluorouracil and leucovorin in patients with stage II colon cancer. *Br J Cancer* 2007;**97**:1021–1027.

44. Figueredo A, *et al*. Adjuvant therapy for stage II colon cancer: a systematic review from the Cancer Care Ontario Program in evidence-based care's gastrointestinal cancer disease site group. *J Clin Oncol* 2004;**22**:3395–3407.

45. Figueredo A, *et al*. Adjuvant therapy for completely resected stage II colon cancer. *Cochrane Database Syst Rev* 2008;**3**:CD005390.

46. Gill S, *et al*. Pooled analysis of fluorouracil-based adjuvant therapy for stage II and III colon cancer: Who benefits and by how much? *J Clin Oncol* 2004;**22**:1797–1806.

47. Mamounas E, *et al*. Comparative efficacy of adjuvant chemotherapy in patients with Dukes' B versus Dukes' C colon cancer: results from four National Surgical Adjuvant Breast and Bowel Project adjuvant studies (C-01, C-02, C-03, and C-04). *J Clin Oncol* 1999;**17**:1349–1355.

48. Tournigand C, *et al*. Adjuvant therapy with fluorouracil and oxaliplatin in stage II and elderly patients (between ages 70 and 75 years) with colon cancer: Subgroup analyses of the Multicenter International Study of Oxaliplatin, Fluorouracil, and Leucovorin in the Adjuvant Treatment of Colon Cancer trial. *J Clin Oncol* 2012;**30**:3353–3360.

49. McCleary NJ, *et al*. Impact of age on the efficacy of newer adjuvant therapies in patients with stage II/III colon cancer: Findings from the ACCENT database. *J Clin Oncol* 2013;**31**:260–2606.

50. Haller DG, *et al*. Efficacy findings from a randomized phase III trial of capecitabine plus oxaliplatin versus bolus 5-FU/LV for stage III colon cancer (NO16968): Impact of age on disease-free survival (DFS). *J Clin Oncol* 2010;**28**(15 Suppl.):3521.

51. Sanoff HK, *et al*. Comparative effectiveness of oxaliplatin vs non-oxaliplatin-containing adjuvant chemotherapy for stage III colon cancer. *J Natl Cancer Inst* 2012;**104**: 211–227.

52. Chau I, *et al*. A randomised comparison between 6 months of bolus fluorouracil/ leucovorin and 12 weeks of protracted venous infusion fluorouracil as adjuvant treatment in colorectal cancer. *Ann Oncol* 2005;**16**:549–557.

53. André, T, *et al*. The IDEA (International Duration Evaluation of Adjuvant Chemotherapy) Collaboration: Prospective combined analysis of phase III trials investigating duration of adjuvant therapy with the FOLFOX (FOLFOX4 or Modified FOLFOX6) or XELOX (3 versus 6 months) Regimen for patients with stage iii colon cancer: Trial design and current status. *Curr Colorectal Cancer Rep* 2013;**9**:261–269.

54. Compton CC, *et al*. Prognostic factors in colorectal cancer. College of American Pathologists Consensus Statement 1999. *Arch Pathol Lab Med* 2000;**124**:979–994.

55. Benson AB III, *et al*. American Society of Clinical Oncology recommendations on adjuvant chemotherapy for stage II colon cancer. *J Clin Oncol* 2004;**22**:3408–3419.

56. Zlobec I, Lugli A. Prognostic and predictive factors in colorectal cancer. *J Clin Pathol* 2008;**61**:561–569.

57. Locker GY, *et al*., ASCO. ASCO 2006 update of recommendations for the use of tumor markers in gastrointestinal cancer. *J Clin Oncol* 25006;**24**:5313–5327.

58. Tejpar S, *et al*. Prognostic and predictive biomarkers in resected colon cancer: Current status and future perspectives for integrating genomics into biomarker discovery. *Oncologist* 2010;**15**:390–404.

59. Mettu NB, *et al*. Use of molecular biomarkers to inform adjuvant therapy for colon cancer. *Oncology (Williston Park)* 2013;**27**:746–754.

60. Umar A, *et al*. Revised Bethesda Guidelines for hereditary nonpolyposis colorectal cancer (Lynch syndrome) and microsatellite instability. *J Natl Cancer Inst* 2004;**96**: 261–268.

61. Wilson PM, *et al*. Predictive and prognostic markers in colorectal cancer. *Gastrointest Cancer Res* 2007;**1**:237–246.

62. Bertagnolli MM, *et al*. Microsatellite instability and loss of heterozygosity at chromo-somal location 18q: Prospective evaluation of biomarkers for stages II and III colon cancer — a study of CALGB 9581 and 89803. *J Clin Oncol* 2011;**29**:3153–3162.

63. Ribic CM, *et al*. Tumor microsatellite-instability status as a predictor of benefit from fluorouracil-based adjuvant chemotherapy for colon cancer. *N Engl J Med* 2003;**349**: 247–257.

64. Hutchins G, *et al*. Value of mismatch repair, *KRAS*, and *BRAF* mutations in predicting recurrence and benefits from chemotherapy in colorectal cancer. *J Clin Oncol* 2011;**29**:1261–1270.

65. Popat S, *et al*. Systematic review of microsatellite instability and colorectal cancer prognosis. *J Clin Oncol* 2005;**23**:609–618.

66. Sargent DJ, *et al*. Defective mismatch repair as a predictive marker for lack of efficacy of fluorouracil-based adjuvant therapy in colon cancer. *J Clin Oncol* 2010;**228**: 3219–3226.

67. Sinicrope FA, *et al*. DNA mismatch repair status and colon cancer recurrence and survival in clinical trials of 5-fluorouracil-based adjuvant therapy. *J Natl Cancer Inst* 2011;**103**:863–875.

68. Duffy MJ, *et al*. Tumor markers in colorectal cancer, gastric cancer and gastrointestinal stromal cancers: European group on tumor markers 2014 guidelines update. *Int J Cancer* 2014;**134**:2513–2522.

69. Salazar R, *et al*. Gene expression signature to improve prognosis prediction of stage II and III colorectal cancer. *J Clin Oncol* 2011;**29**:17–24.

70. Salazar R, *et al*. The PARSC trial, a prospective study for the assessment of recurrence risk in stage II colon cancer patients using ColoPrint. *J Clin Oncol* 2012;**30**(15 Suppl.):TPS10632.

71. O'Connell MJ, *et al*. Relationship between tumor gene expression and recurrence in four independent studies of patients with stage II/III colon cancer treated with surgery alone or surgery plus adjuvant fluorouracil plus leucovorin. *J Clin Oncol* 2010;**28**: 3937–3944.

72. Gray RG, *et al*. Validation study of a quantitative multigene reverse transcriptase-polymerase chain reaction assay for assessment of recurrence risk in patients with stage II colon cancer. *J Clin Oncol* 2011;**29**:4611–4619.

73. Venook AP, *et al*. Biologic determinants of tumor recurrence in stage II colon cancer: Validation study of the 12-gene recurrence score in cancer and leukemia group B (CALGB) 9581. *J Clin Oncol* 2013;**31**:1775–1781.

74. Yothers G, *et al*. Validation of the 12-gene colon cancer recurrence score in NSABP C-07 as a predictor of recurrence in patients with stage II and III colon cancer treated with fluorouracil and leucovorin (FU/LV) and FU/LV plus oxaliplatin. *J Clin Oncol* 2013;**31**:4512-4519.

75. Lee JJ, Chu E. Personalized medicine in the adjuvant chemotherapy of stage II colon cancer — are we there yet? *Oncology (Williston Park)* 2013;**27**:756–758.

76. Douillard JY, *et al*. Cost consequences of adjuvant capecitabine, Mayo Clinic and de Gramont regimens for stage III colon cancer in the French setting. *Oncology* 2007;**72**:248–254.

77. Aballea S, *et al*. Cost-effectiveness analysis of oxaliplatin compared with 5-fluorouracil/leucovorin in adjuvant treatment of stage III colon cancer in the US. *Cancer* 2007; **109**:1082–1089.

78. Chu E, *et al*. Costs associated with capecitabine or 5-fluorouracil monotherapy after surgical resection in patients with colorectal cancer. *Oncology* 2009;**77**:244–253.

79. Eggington S, *et al*. Cost-effectiveness of oxaliplatin and capecitabine in the adjuvant treatment of stage III colon cancer. *Br J Cancer* 2006;**95**:1195–1201.

80. http://www.octo-oxford.org.uk/alltrials/closed/q2.html.

81. ClinicalTrials.gov. Oxaliplatin, Leucovorin Calcium, and Fluorouracil With or Without Celecoxib in Treating Patients With Stage III Colon Cancer Previously Treated With Surgery. Retrived from http://clinicaltrials.gov/show/NCT01150045

82. Chia WK, *et al*. Aspirin as adjuvant therapy for colorectal cancer-reinterpreting paradigms. *Nat Rev Clin Oncol* 2012;**9**(10):561–570.
83. Bastiaannet E, *et al*. Use of aspirin postdiagnosis improves survival for colon cancer patients. *Br J Cancer* 2012;**106**(9):1564–1570.
84. Liao X, *et al*. Aspirin use, tumor PIK3CA mutation, and colorectal-cancer survival. *N Engl J Med* 2012;**367**(17):1596–1606.

Chapter 16

Hepatocellular Carcinoma: Liver Transplantation, Hepatic Resection, and Regional Treatment Options

Bhavin C. Shah and David A. Geller

1 Introduction

Hepatocellular carcinoma (HCC) occurs in 90% of patients with chronic liver disease and is the third leading cause of cancer-related mortality worldwide.[1–4] The incidence of HCC has been rising steadily in due to increasing incidence of hepatitis C and B, along with chronic alcoholism and fatty liver disease as additional contributing factors.[3–5] Nonalcoholic steatohepatitis (NASH) has also been recognized as a risk factor for HCC.[6] Furthermore, aflatoxin intake, diabetes, obesity, and hemochromatosis have been associated with a higher risk for developing HCC. Only approximately 30% of patients are resectable when diagnosed with HCC due to delayed diagnosis and coexisting cirrhosis.[5] Early detection of HCC in high risk patients using ultrasound as a screening modality has been successful in detecting many patients with early stage HCC who can potentially receive curative treatment.[7] The clinical course of HCC and the survival of patients depend not just on the stage of the tumor but also on the underlying liver disease at the time of diagnosis and the response to treatment.

Liver transplantation (LT) or liver resection (LR) are the only potential curative approaches to surgically treat HCC. LT is considered the treatment of choice and best option because it removes the cancer and the residual at risk diseased liver which can potentially have a recurrent tumor in future. LT provides a five year survival of more than 70%.[8] Mazzafero *et al.*[8] described excellent long term survival in patients with either single HCC nodule <5 cm, or 2–3 nodules with each being 3 cm or less which corresponds to stage II HCC by TNM classification. However, donor availability remains rate-limiting for LT in the setting of HCC. For example, in the USA, there are currently 15,654 patients waiting for a LT, but there were only 6,455 liver transplant performed in 2013 in the United States.[9] This disparity led to significant dropout, with 1,542 patients being removed from the wait list in 2013 because they died, and another 1,552 patients were removed because they became too sick to be transplanted.[9] Another way of looking at it is that eight patients on average per day were removed from the LT wait list because either the cirrhosis or the HCC tumor progressed, resulting in their demise. Liver resection has been a surgical option but has limited role in patients with underlying severe or end stage liver disease causing high morbidity, mortality and increased intrahepatic recurrences.[10,11] There has been a recent increase in incidence of liver resection for HCC with low morbidity and low mortality rates <5% compared to LT for patients with early tumors and relatively preserved liver function.[12–14]

Local ablative therapies such as microwave (MW) and radiofrequency ablation (RFA) have emerged to be safe and effective treatment modalities for providing good local control of the disease[15–18] as a bridge therapy to LT or when LR is not possible. RFA, MW, and Transarterial chemoembolization (TACE) have been used for patients who are unfit for surgical resections or those who have advanced unresectable tumors.[18,19] Systemic therapy with VEGF (vascular endothelial growth factor) and FGF (fibroblast growth factor) inhibitors has been used in advanced HCC recently with some success.[20] Only sorafenib has shown some beneficial effect in increasing survival in patients who are not operative or regional liver therapy candidates.[20] Patients with HCC according to a recent population based SEER (Surveillance, Epidemiology, and End Results) registry study had an overall one year survival of 47%; however, patients with localized HCC who received therapy was reported as 83% and those who received surgery was 91% at one year.[21] In this chapter we discuss the various approaches to treat hepatocellular carcinoma.

The algorithm for management of HCC is shown in Figure 1.

2 Surgical Resection or Liver Transplantation for Early HCC

2.1 *Liver transplantation*

Liver transplantation (LT) and liver resection (LR) are both potential curative approaches to treat HCC. In 1963, Starzl performed the first successful liver transplantation, and some of the earliest cases done were patients with hepatoblastoma

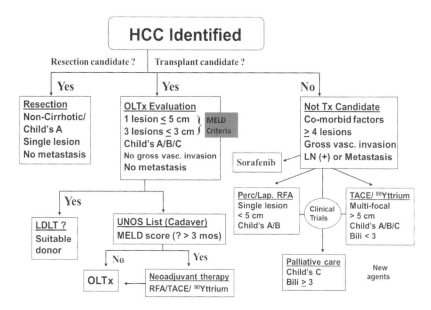

Figure 1 Algorithm for management of HCC.

or HCC.[22] Although LT was considered ideal approach for potential cure from primary hepatic malignancies, several initial reports[23,24] of LT for primary and metastatic liver cancer showed high recurrence rates and the strategy was soon dismissed. During the subsequent years, major breakthroughs such as the expansion of the organ donor pool by introduction of the brain death criteria, refined surgical techniques and introduction of immunosuppressive drugs like cyclosporine in 1979[25,26] led to significant increase in LT. In 1983, the NIH declared that LT was a valid therapy for end-stage liver disease.27 Initial results of LT in HCC were disappointing with high perioperative mortality, 80% tumor recurrence, and 5-year OS of 15%.[28,29] Other studies had similar results so LT for HCC was restricted to clinical trials until 1989. In 1991, Iwatsuki *et al.*[30] published better long-term survival after LT for HCC than after liver resection with similar recurrence rates (50% and 43%) after LR and LT respectively. In 1996, a landmark study by Mazzaferro *et al.*[8] established LT as standard indication for HCC within the "Milan criteria", which includes small HCC (1 lesion ≤5 cm, or 2 to 3 lesions each ≤3 cm), no macro-vascular invasion, and no regional nodal or distant metastasis. In this retrospective review of 48 patients, those who met these criteria showed a 4-year OS of 85% compared to those with HCC size that exceeded these criteria, had a 4-year OS of 50%.[8]

Initially, patients with HCC were at a distinct disadvantage in organ allocation. The time spent on the waitlist failed to correspond to risk of death till the model for end stage liver disease (MELD) score was adopted in 2002.[31,32] Patients diagnosed with HCC often show sufficient liver function and thus, their urgency for LT is not adequately represented in their MELD scores. Therefore, cirrhotic HCC patients within the United Network for Organ Sharing (UNOS) and Eurotransplant (ET) network receive exception MELD (eMELD) scoring when diagnosed as American Liver Tumor Study Group (ALTSG) stage II HCC (*i.e.* single HCC 2–5 cm or 2–3 lesions <3 cm) for UNOS patients and within Milan criteria for ET patients. The eMELD score given is equivalent to a 15% probability of death within 3 months, which is 22 points. Subsequently, this eMELD is increased every 3 months by the number of points equivalent to a 10% increase in mortality until transplantation or drop-out of Milan criteria. MELD is an accurate predictor of mortality in ESLD.[31,32]

Several studies using the Milan criteria have shown the survival benefit of LT in HCC.[33] A 20-year retrospective experience with orthotopic LT (OLT) showed overall survival (OS) at 1 year: 89%; 5 years: 69%; and 10 years: 41%, and disease free survival (DFS): 1 year: 86%; 5 years: 65%; 10 years: 40% and a disease-specific survival: 87% at 10 years.[34] A recent 20-year experience of LT in patients with HCC showed that HCV patients had lower survival post-LT. HCC alone had no impact on survival but patient survival decreased in the HCC+/HCV+ group and this was a consequence of HCV recurrence.[35] A major obstacle for LT as the gold standard treatment for HCC is tumor growth resulting in dropout from the waiting list for LT. In a study by Yao *et al.*,[36] predictors for dropout included two or three tumor nodules or a solitary lesion greater than 3 cm at initial presentation and previous hepatic resection. Expansion of the tumor size criteria has led to the University of California San Francisco (UCSF) criteria (single tumor nodule up to 6.5 cm; or 3 or fewer tumors, the largest ≤4.5 cm with the sum of the total tumor diameters (≤8 cm).[37] Yao *et al.*[37] showed that patients with HCC meeting the criteria: solitary tumor ≤6.5 cm, or ≤3 nodules with the largest lesion ≤4.5 cm and total tumor diameter ≤8 cm, had survival rates of 90% and 75.2%, at 1 and 5 years, respectively, after OLT versus a 50% 1-year survival for patients with tumors exceeding these limits (*p* = 0.0005). They concluded that the UNOS criteria for OLT based on tumor size may be modestly expanded while still preserving excellent survival after OLT. However, in another recent large (with 476 patients) French multicenter retrospective analysis,[38] the application of the UCSF criteria compared with the Milan criteria in the pre-transplantation setting (contemplating time on the waiting list close to zero) is associated with a low survival rate (≤50%) in those within UCFS criteria but outside the Milan criteria.

Due to many social reasons and non-availability of UNOS-like system, living donor liver transplantation (LDLT) in Asian countries[39–41] comprises the majority of liver transplantation procedures. LDLT has become an established treatment for HCC patients with end-stage liver disease and is increasingly being adopted for treatment of HCC patients in Western countries, which not only addresses the shortage of donor organs but also reduces the dropout rate on the waiting list.[41] It should be pointed out that the overall number of LDLT in the USA is relatively low, with only 252 reported LDLT of the 6,455 LT performed in 2013, thus LDLT represents less than 4% of total LT's in the USA.[9] This ratio is vastly different in Asia where LDLT represents the majority of LT cases due to lack of availability of cadaveric donors and cultural differences.

There have been some reports suggesting poorer outcome with LDLT versus DDLT (deceased donor liver transplantation) for patients with HCC. Park *et al.*[42] showed worse recurrence-free survival among 166 LDLT recipients (81% at 5 years) compared to 50 DDLT recipients (94% at 5 years; $p = 0.045$). They found that smaller the LDLT graft, the poorer the recurrence-free survival, suggesting that the physiology of the small graft may stimulate tumor recurrence. The initial results of the A2ALL cohort[43] in United States also found a higher recurrence rate within 3 years in LDLT than in DDLT group (29% *vs.* 0%, $p = 0.002$), but they had patients with aggressive tumor characteristics in the LDLT group. The same group recently published an updated report[44] in which HCC recurrence was significantly different between LDLT and DDLT after adjustment for tumor characteristics. They concluded that the higher recurrence observed after LDLT was likely due to differences in the tumor characteristics, pre-transplant HCC management, and waiting time. Vakili *et al.*[45] showed that although HCC recurrence rate of LDLT (29%) was significantly higher than that of DDLT (12%) ($p < 0.05$), the overall survival after LDLT was significantly better than that following DDLT for HCC during the same period ($p = 0.02$).

Hwang *et al.*s[46] performed a nationwide survey and found 1 and 3-year recurrence-free survival rates were 83% and 80%, and 88% and 82%, respectively, with no significant difference between them. Sotiropoulos *et al.*[47] (47) supported the comparable recurrence-free survival rates between LDLT and DDLT for HCC (75% *vs.* 81% at three years). A recent meta-analysis48 included 12 retrospective studies comparing the recurrence rates and recurrence-free survival between of 633 LDLTs and 1,232 DDLTs recipients. This study showed lower disease-free survival after LDLT compared with DDLT for HCC (HR = 1.59, 95% CI: 1.02–2.49; $p = 0.041$), but there was no difference in overall survival between LDLT and DDLT (HR = 0.97, 95% CI: 0.73–1.27; $p = 0.808$). The University of Tokyo experience[49] of LDLT in patients, where 30% patients had HCC found no association between graft regeneration/initial graft volume and tumor recurrence among 125 consecutive LDLTs for HCC cases. In the absence of a prospective study regarding the use of LDLT vs DDLT for HCC patients, they concluded that there is no evidence to support the higher HCC recurrence after LDLT than DDLT, and LDLT remains a reasonable treatment option for HCC patients with cirrhosis.

Thus benefits of LT are that it treats the underlying cause of disease by removing at risk organ and has lower risk of recurrence and much improved DFS than LR. Also, it can be used in Childs B and Childs C cirrhotics. The limitations of LT include risk of disease progression while awaiting transplant, need for lifelong immunosuppression, and it potentially reduces allografts for other ESLD patients. There is some evidence suggesting higher recurrence in patients with HCC receiving LDLT; however, it is unclear if tumor biology or small graft size is the cause of recurrence.

2.2 *Liver resection (LR)*

Although LT is the best theoretical curative treatment for HCC, shortage of donor availability makes liver resection a preferred first option in those patients eligible for resection. Liver resection (LR) has been limited by high morbidity and mortality and intrahepatic recurrence rates in past, all due to the underlying liver disease.[50–52] However, at present LR for HCC can be performed in high volume centers with a mortality rate of less than 5% and overall 5-year survival rates comparable to those of transplantation in early tumors.[52–55] Also, LR as first line approach preserves the possibility of second line treatment which may include salvage LT or a repeat resection.[52] When intention-to-treat survival is used as the outcome endpoint, LR potentially competes with LT as main curative first line treatment for HCC patients.[56]

Due to the scarcity of organ donors, most centers accept the goal of using LT in patient with HCC to achieve a 5-year survival rate greater than or equal to 50%.[56–58] Because of related cirrhosis and late diagnosis, less than 30% of patients are resectable when diagnosed with HCC.[5,59] The main limitation of LR is that survival results equivalent to LT are limited to patients with compensated cirrhosis.[52] Also, persistent underlying liver disease is associated with a risk of recurrence mainly due to *de novo* foci of HCC, accounting for lower disease-free survival than LT.[60]

An MSKCC study[61] of long-term outcomes of patients with early HCC within Milan criteria who would have been candidates for transplantation but were treated instead with LR showed the 1, 3, and 5-year overall survival was 85%, 74%, and 69%, respectively, with a median survival of 71 months. The 5-year disease-free survival was 48% with a median of 52 months. They concluded that partial hepatectomy in patients with early HCC who are otherwise eligible for transplantation can be performed with minimal morbidity and can achieve comparable 5-year survival to that reported for LT, so LR should be considered the standard therapy for patients with HCC who have adequate liver reserve.[61]

Yeh *et al.*[62] in a retrospective analysis of clinicopathological factors influencing long-term outcome of HCC patients with liver cirrhosis undergoing hepatectomy, showed an overall postoperative morbidity of 15.6% and mortality rate of 8.8%. The 1, 3, and 5-year disease-free survival rates were 51%, 34%, and 27%, respectively, and the overall cumulative survival rates at 1, 3, and 5 years were 63%, 42%, and 32%, respectively. They identified elevated alkaline phosphatase, tumor size >2 cm, presence of satellite lesions and vascular invasion as poor prognostic factors. Shimozawa *et al.*[63] in another retrospective review of 135 consecutive patients with one to three HCCs of diameter ≤3 cm who underwent curative hepatic resection between 1987 and 2001 showed a 3, 5, and 10-year disease-free survival after hepatic resection to be 49%, 30%, and 8%, respectively and the 3, 5, and 10-year overall survival percentages after hepatic resection were 73%, 55%, and 18%, respectively. Age more than 60 years was an independent unfavorable prognostic factor affecting disease-free survival, and the presence of liver cirrhosis was an independently significant factor of poor overall survival. The cumulative incidence of postoperative recurrence was 82%. The 5-year overall survival in patients with tumor recurrence undergoing repeat hepatectomy (85%) was significantly greater than in patients without second resection (41%). Six patients (4%) survived longer than 10 years after hepatic resection (four with recurrence and two without recurrence). All four of these patients with postoperative recurrence underwent repeat hepatectomy. They concluded that post resection survival of patients with small HCC will differ depending on the presence of liver cirrhosis and that repeat hepatectomy may contribute to the prolongation of survival in such patients with postoperative recurrence.[63] An 11-year European study of 93 patients who underwent LR for HCC with a median tumor size of 55 mm (5–250 mm) had a R0 resection rate of 95%. The postoperative morbidity was 61%. The study had high hospital mortality of 8.6% in the entire study period but decreased over time. Actuarial survival was 81% after 1 year, 58% after 3 years and 26% after 5 years. The T-stage was identified as a prognostic factor influencing survival.[64] Therefore the outcome of LR in HCC is highly based on the patient selection.

2.3 *Role of minimally invasive surgery*

Laparoscopic hepatectomy emerged in the early 1990s as a treatment option for patients with small peripheral tumors in the liver. It has now been established as safe and feasible for both benign and malignant liver lesions.[65–67] A recent review of 142 published papers on laparoscopic liver resection including 2,804 patients, where 50% of resections were for malignancy was performed with low postoperative mortality rate 0.3%.[65] HCC was the most common malignancy resected, followed by metastatic colorectal cancer. Another review of 31 studies that directly compared laparoscopic (LLR) with open liver resection (OLR) in 2,473 patients showed significant benefits for patients consisting of less blood loss, less narcotic requirements, and shorter length of hospital stay. There were no economic disadvantages to the laparoscopic approach, and case-cohort matched studies showed no difference in oncologic outcomes between the laparoscopic and open groups with similar 3-year and 5-year overall survival rates.[64] More than a dozen case-cohort retrospective studies matching LLR to OLR for HCC showed comparable 5-year DFS and 5-year OS rates.[67] A meta-analysis of 15 non-randomized, case-matched studies comparing 485 pts LLR vs. 753 OLR for HCC showed LLR had favorable outcomes for low blood loss, less blood transfused, decreased post-op morbidity, less postoperative hospital stay and there was no significant differences in surgical margins, 5-year overall survival, or recurrence-free survival between the two groups.[68] A study of salvage LT after 12 LR and 12 OLR for HCC showed that LLR facilitated the LT procedure as compared with OLR in terms of reduced operative time, blood loss and transfusion requirements. They concluded that LLR is preferred over OLR when feasible in potential transplant candidates since salvage LT was easier in the patients that underwent prior LLR compared to those that underwent prior OLR.[69]

2.4 *Liver resection versus liver transplantation decision making*

In a retrospective analysis using data from the 1998–2007 Surveillance, Epidemiology, and End Results-Medicare linked database, when patients 66 years of age and older with early HCC were selected, 47% of all patients with early HCC received no surgical therapy. About 33% patients with solitary, unilobar tumors and microscopic confirmation of HCC and 51% patients with no liver-related comorbidities did not receive surgical therapy.[70] In reality, only a small subset of patients would be candidates for both LR and OLT. Although there is a certain degree of surgeon preference, both LT and LR have equivalent results for stage II HCC in terms of survival, but LR has higher recurrences.

In early HCC, an European study[71] involving 132 patients from two centers reported a <1% 90-day mortality, and a median survival of 74.5 months with a 5-year survival rate of 70% (63% in patients with cirrhosis). The median time to recurrence was 31.6 months and the 5-year recurrence rate was 68%. Presence of satellite nodules and platelet count <150,000/µL were independently associated with survival whereas presence of satellite nodules, cirrhosis, and non-anatomic resection were independently associated with recurrence. Patients with a single HCC ≤2 cm and platelet count ≥150,000/µL achieved a median survival of 138 months and a 5-year survival rate of 81%, respectively. They concluded that LR of HCC ≤2 cm is safe and achieves excellent results and should continue to be considered a primary treatment modality in patients with small HCC and well-preserved liver function.[71]

The Liver Cancer Study Group of Japan have reported the largest series of patients undergoing resections for HCC with curative intent (*n* = 6,785). They reported a DFS at 1 year, 3 years, 5 years and 10 years of 85%, 64%, 45%, and 21% respectively (72). Multivariable analysis revealed tumor differentiation as the strongest predictor of death from recurrent HCC within 5 years. They concluded that long-term recurrence-free survival is possible after liver resection for HCC, particularly in patients with a single lesion measuring less than 5 cm with a simple nodular appearance and low tumor marker levels.[72] Margarit *et al.*[73] have compared the outcome of 37 liver resection (LR) patients with well-matched 36 patients who underwent liver transplantation (LT) for single, early HCC in Child–Turcotte–Pugh class A patients with cirrhosis younger than 70 years of age. The mortality was higher and hospital stay longer in the LT group. Tumor recurrence was higher in the LR group (59% vs. 11%), extrahepatic recurrences predominated after LT and hepatic recurrences after LR. The overall survival was similar in both groups but the disease-free survival was significantly better after LT. Only 27.6% of resected patients were eligible for LT.[73] Salvage LT was performed in 16.2% of resected patients, with older age being the main contraindication. Outcome of salvage LT was similar to that of primary LT.

Primary LR followed by LT for recurrence or deterioration of liver function has been recently suggested as a rational strategy for patients with HCC under Milan criteria and preserved liver function. Poon *et al.*[53] performed a study evaluating survival and pattern of recurrence after resection of potentially transplantable small HCC in patients with preserved liver function, with special reference to determine feasibility of salvage transplantation. They reported overall survival rates at 1, 3, 5, and 10 years of 90%, 76%, 70%, and 35%, respectively, and the corresponding disease-free survival rates were 74%, 50%, 36%, and 22%. Patients with concomitant oligonodular tumors and cirrhosis had worse 5-year overall survival rate of 48% and a disease-free survival rate of 0%, compared with other subgroups. At a median follow-up of 48 months, 67 patients had recurrence and 79% of them were considered eligible for salvage transplantation. Decompensation from Child–Pugh class A to B or C without recurrence occurred in only six patients. So they concluded that for Child–Pugh class A patients with small HCC, LR is a reasonable first-line treatment associated with a favorable 5-year overall survival rate.

There is no clear consensus regarding the best treatment strategy for patients with advanced HCC. Facciuto *et al.*[74] studied patients with HCC and cirrhosis beyond Milan criteria who underwent LR or LT at a single institution. 23 HCC patients were primarily treated by LR, 5 of whom eventually underwent salvage LT. 32 patients underwent primary LT. The overall actuarial survival rates at 3 and 5 years were 35% after LR, and 69% and 60%, respectively, after primary LT. Recurrence-free survival at 5 years was significantly higher after LT (65%) than after LR (26%). Of the patients who underwent LR, 11 (48%) experienced recurrence only in the liver; 6 of these 11 presented with advanced recurrence, poor medical status, or short disease-free intervals and were not considered for transplantation. Salvage LT was performed in 5 patients with early stage recurrence (45% of patients with hepatic recurrence after LR and 22% of all patients who underwent LR). At a median of 18 months after salvage LT, all 5 patients were alive, 4 were free of disease, and 1 developed HCC recurrence 16 months after salvage LT. They suggested for patients with HCC beyond Milan criteria, multimodality treatment approach including LR, salvage LT, and primary LT results in long-term survival in half of the patients.[74] When indicated, LR can optimize the use of scarce donor organs by leaving LT as a reserve option for early stage HCC recurrence.

Several studies support a strategy based on LR as first line therapy and salvage LT in case of transplantable tumor recurrence or severe liver decompensation. There are several limitations in these studies. First, they generally compare therapies from a transplantation perspective only, since the main inclusion criterion is the fulfillment of Milan criteria.[57] These studies present a selection bias in terms of liver function or tumor characteristics and aggressiveness.[75] Conversely, none of the studies in this comparison were done from a LR perspective: i.e. analyzing LT performance in resectable HCC patients with compensated cirrhosis independently from fulfillment of the Milan criteria. In this subgroup of patients, instead of expansion of current selection criteria for LT it would be better substantiate biologically (i.e. increasing prevalence of microvascular invasion [MVI]) why LT is contraindicated in this population.[75] Second, comparison between LT and LR is usually limited to a 5-year survival perspective, while it is well known that the survival advantage of LT is probably higher after this time-point. Third, intention-to-treat survival is the ideal outcome endpoint to be used in well-designed prospective studies, but it cannot be used as a good treatment decision tool since it is strictly dependent on local waiting list characteristics.[76,77] Patients with same tumor characteristics but with longer waiting times have intrinsically lower intention-to-treat survival perspectives than patients with a lower number of competitors or lower priority points. An innovative priority-allocation endpoint has been recently introduced in LT, the transplant survival benefit.[78] This endpoint is based on the ratio and/or difference between post-LT outcome and outcome before/without LT.[75]

Vitale *et al.*[75] used number of patients/organs needed to transplant (NTT) as an indicator of the benefit of LT over LR, and generated a decision model derived from large multi-center cohorts and evaluating both a 5-year and a 10-year post-surgical scenario. 5-year post-LR and post-LT survival predictions were used to calculate the benefit of LT over LR in resectable HCC using NTT as benefit endpoint. LT became an effective therapy (NTT <5) for all patients without MVI whenever tumor extension and for oligonodular HCC with MVI within conventional LT criteria. In their study,[75] an attempt is made to measure the transplant benefit in resectable HCC for patients either within or beyond the Milan criteria and using NTT as benefit measure. The strong impact of MVI on LT benefit and the high prevalence of this aggressive feature also in small tumors undergoing LR,[76] suggest that resectable HCC is a contraindication to LT when a 5-year time horizon is adopted. The 10-year scenario, conversely, increased the transplant benefit in all subgroups of resectable patients, and LT became an effective therapy (NTT <5) for all patients without MVI whenever tumor extension and for oligonodular HCC with MVI within conventional LT criteria.

Mazzaferro *et al.*[79] conducted a multi institutional web based survey of specialists to evaluate outcomes of patients who underwent transplantation for HCC despite exceeding Milan criteria. The survival of these patients was correlated retrospectively with the size of the largest tumor nodule, number of nodules, and presence or absence of microvascular invasion detected at pathology to have generate a Metroticket prognostic model with 3-year and 5-year survival endpoints and they also tried to identify subgroup of patients who have outcomes similar to those undergoing LT for Milan criteria tumors. Their results show a median size of the largest nodule was 40 mm (range 4–200) and the median number of nodules was 4.[1–20] Four hundred and fifty-four of 1,112 patients (41%) had MVI and, for those transplanted outside the Milan criteria, 5-year overall survival was 54%, compared with 73% for those that met the criteria. A total of 283 patients without microvascular invasion, but who fell within the Up-to-seven criteria (HCC with 7 as the sum of the size of the largest tumor in cm and the number of tumors) achieved a 5-year overall survival of 71%. They concluded that more patients can undergo transplant if the current approach to candidacy based on strict Milan criteria were replaced with a more precise estimation of survival contouring individual tumor characteristics and use of the up-to-seven criteria.[79]

Nathan *et al.*[80] conducted a physician survey to quantify the impact of clinical factors on choice of therapy for early HCC by gastroenterologists and hepatologists. Physicians who treat HCC were invited to complete a web-based survey including ten case scenarios that systematically varied across seven clinical factors. Choice of therapy-LT, LR, RFA or regional intra-arterial therapy-was analyzed using multinomial logistic regression models. Tumor number and size, type of resection required, biological MELD score, and platelet count had the largest effects on choice of therapy. For example, LR was more likely to be recommended over LT for patients with small solitary tumors versus multiple tumors, those who would require a minor versus major LR , those with lower biological MELD score (6 vs. 10; relative risk ratio [RRR] 1.95), and those with a higher platelet count (150,000 vs. 70,000/μL). In contrast, serum α-fetoprotein level and etiology of cirrhosis were not associated with choice of therapy. To compare LT with LR, a randomized controlled trial would be ideal but is not likely feasible as a large number of patients would be required, and there is a great deal of regional variability in wait times as well as treating physician preference.

Non randomized comparisons have been made by pooling patients from retrospective studies. Dhir et al.[81] performed a meta-analysis of 1,763 patients undergoing LR vs. LT for early HCC within the Milan criteria. The 5-year OS for all patients was 58% (transplantation: 63%; resection: 53%). Meta-analysis of all 10 studies revealed a survival advantage for LT. Analysis of only those reports that utilized an "intention-to-treat" strategy failed to demonstrate a survival advantage for either treatment approach.[81] In the current guidelines of the German Cancer Society and the updated European Association for the Study of the Liver and European Organization for Research and Treatment of Cancer guidelines for treatment of HCC, patients with solitary tumors should undergo anatomic LR as first-line therapy in case platelets are at least at 100,000 and the venous pressure gradient is less than or equal to 10 mm Hg.[82,83] Proneth et al.[84] conducted a systematic review and meta-analysis of studies investigating LR and/or LT on patients who are candidates for both and showed that LR and LT are both treatment options that lead to similar 5-year OS. This conclusion was drawn from seven retrospective studies, which investigated LR and LT in a case-controlled manner, including ITT data from LT. Comparing data from 70 selected studies in which data of either LT or LR were reported alone or in comparing fashion, without respecting ITT, results favor LT, reflected by a significantly better 5-year OS and 3- and 5-year DFS after LT. They proposed that survival rates for LT in publications without ITT are estimated as too high since time on waitlist is not included in them and drop out of waitlist or mortality can affect outcome. This waitlist time can thus serve as a selection period for patients with the best prognosis, because only patients with stable disease undergo transplantation. This probably leads to lower recurrence than in resected patients who did not undergo this selection process and might be one reason for the higher recurrence-free survival after LT. Another reason for better OS in unselected studies might be that LT represents a cure for the underlying cirrhosis, which is the main risk factor for development of HCC.[84]

3 Tumor Biology

To refine our current staging systems, many morphological or chemical factors have been studied, including microscopic vascular invasion, encapsulation, plasma albumin mRNA, and serum alphafetoprotein.[85,86] Current radiologic techniques are not yet sufficient to perfectly define tumor number and size and are unlikely to be able to determine MVI. Some new staging systems require pretreatment biopsy, which poses a small but real risk of tumor seeding. To understand the biological behavior and identify genes associated with survival after LT, Marsh *et al.*[87,88] at the University of Pittsburgh performed microdissection on explanted tissue and studied DNA mutations near 9 tumor-associated gene loci to create an index of cumulative mutational damage, termed the fractional allelic imbalance (FAI). They found that FAI and vascular invasion were the strongest independent predictors of tumor-free survival. Thus, incorporation of gene mutational data allows desegregation of HCC patients from imprecise, morphology-based staging systems and allows improved prognostication.[86–88]

4 Local Therapy

Local ablative therapies are used when liver transplantation cannot be offered or in patients who are not candidates for surgical resection or transplantation, or as a bridge to transplantation.[89] A single tumor <3 cm in a cirrhotic would be ablated in a patient not eligible for transplantation or as bridge therapy to transplant. The various techniques are RFA, microwave ablation (MW), and percutaneous ethanol injection therapy (PEI). PEI is a popular treatment with good results and has been adopted throughout the world.[90–92] The mechanism is that ethanol causes dehydration and subsequent necrosis. Pure alcohol also blocks blood flow to the tumor bed resulting in small blood vessels thrombosis and tumor necrosis.[93] The technique is ideal in patients with a cirrhotic liver with a highly vascular and soft HCC. However, PEI has limitations when treating patients with multiple tumors because of the need for repeated puncture. It is contraindicated in patients with gross ascites, coagulopathy that cannot be corrected, obstructive jaundice due to the potential risk of bleeding and biliary peritonitis and main portal vein thrombosis. Increased risks of bleeding and peritoneal tumor seeding must be considered when the tumors are situated on the liver surface. Tumors which are immediately sub diaphragmatic or too close to vital structures (bile ducts, hepatic veins, portal vein branches, stomach) would also pose a problem for PEI. Many studies have shown that patients treated with surgical resection have significantly better long-term outcome or tumor-free survival than those treated with PEI.[91] A prospective study in Taiwan[94] comparing PEI with surgical resection showed no statistical difference in recurrence and survival between the two treatment groups; however, tumor size greater than 2 cm and alpha-fetoprotein over 200 ng/mL correlated with higher recurrence rate, and Child class B liver cirrhosis correlated with shorter overall survival. PEI had nearly the same effectiveness with 5-year survival of 60% as compared to resection of small HCCs after an average follow-up of 37.7 months.[94]

RFA is performed by a needle that is inserted into the liver percutaneously under ultrasonography or CT guidance, or inserted intraoperatively by open or laparoscopic techniques. The RF generator supplies RF power to the tissue through the electrode.[95] It produces RF voltage between the electrode and the grounding pad, which establishes lines of electric field. Resistive energy loss results in frictional heat. This thermal energy generated through frictional heat produced by rapid agitation of adjacent cells and produces liquefactive necrosis of the tumor cells. The volume of tissue destroyed by RFA depends on the temperature distribution of the RFA treated lesion with highest temperature, and therefore the highest degree of necrosis, occurs in the center of the RFA lesion. Untreated tumor cells can remain at the periphery where temperatures are not high enough.[95] The endpoint of local ablative therapy is complete tumor necrosis with a margin of normal tissue and this is based on either temperature or impedance, depending on the needle manufacturer. Of the methods of ablation, PEI and RFA have been compared. For tumors less than 5 cm, the percentages of complete necrosis for treated lesions are approach 90% with RFA;[89,96] however, the percentage of complete necrosis is lower for PEI.[96] A prospective randomized study has shown that RFA is superior to PEI in terms of local recurrence rate[97] and some show that the number of sessions required for RFA is also less than that of PEI.[98] Previous randomized studies failed to show a statistically significant difference in overall survival between patients who received RF ablation and those treated with PEI; however, RFA has shown lower local recurrence rate (2–18% at 2 years) when compared with PEI (11–45%).[97,99–100] Therefore, current European guidelines recommend the use of PEI in cases where RFA is not feasible for technical reasons[101] like subcapsular location or adjacent to the hepatic hilum.[101,102] A randomized controlled trial of 139 cirrhotic patients in Child–Pugh classes A or B[103] showed significantly better 1-year complete response rate of 65.7% and 36.2% of patients treated by RFA and PEI, respectively ($p = 0.0005$). However, the overall survival rate was not significantly different and there was an incremental health-care cost of €8,286 for each additional patient successfully treated by RFA.[103]

MWA on the other hand, uses dielectric hysteresis to produce heat. Tissue destruction occurs when tissues are heated to lethal temperatures from an applied electromagnetic field, typically at 900–2500 MHz. Polar molecules in tissue (primarily H_2O) are forced to continuously realign with the oscillating electric field, increasing their kinetic energy and, hence, the temperature of the tissue so tissues with a high percentage of water (as in solid organs and tumors) are most conducive to this type of heating.[104] RFA and microwave are comparable and no single therapy is superior.

Dong *et al.*[105] reported 93% complete response with no residual tumor and overall survival of 56% in patients with HCC who underwent percutaneous microwave ablation without severe complications. Lu *et al.* retrospectively compared patients who underwent microwave or radiofrequency ablation with no significant difference in survival or complication rates between the two groups.[106] Most authors[106,107] report shorter ablation times in the liver with microwave than with RFA, which translates to more efficient use of equipment and personnel and decreased operative time under general anesthesia. In addition, the speed of treatment gives microwaves an advantage for treating multiple lesions during one ablation session.[107] Ianitti *et al.*[108] reported outcomes from the first multi-institutional clinical trial in the United States using MWA for patients with unresectable HCC or metastatic liver cancer. They showed an overall survival of 47% (all tumor types) at 19-month follow up with no procedure related mortality. Ablative techniques are sometimes combined with chemotherapy or regional therapy. A retrospective comparative study by the Kagoshima Liver Cancer Study Group[109] who evaluated patients with MELD <13 undergoing curative hepatic resection or initial RFA percutaneously or surgically (thoracoscopic, laparoscopic, and open) for HCC within Milan criteria. They reported similar one year mortality after therapy for both LR and RFA groups. The group that underwent LR showed a trend towards better survival and significantly better disease-free survival compared to the RFA group. The advantage of LR was more evident for patients with single tumors and patients with Child's A cirrhosis whereas, patients with multinodular tumors survived longer when treated with RFA, regardless of the Child's grade of liver damage. Surgical RFA had survival benefits similar to those of hepatic resection for single tumors, and that it had the best efficacy for treating multinodular tumors or unresectable compared to percutaneous RFA. A meta-analysis[110] of non randomized studies comparing RFA with LR for small HCC published from 1997 to 2009 showed the overall survival was significantly higher in patients treated with LR than in those treated with RFA at 3 years and at 5 year and RFA had higher rates of local intrahepatic recurrence compared to LR. LR also had significantly higher 1, 3, and 5 years disease-free survival rates than RFA. The postoperative morbidity was higher with LR, but no significant differences were found in mortality. For tumors ≤3 cm, LR and RFA had similar results. They concluded that LR was superior to RFA in the treatment of patients with small HCC eligible for surgical treatments, particularly for tumors >3 cm.[110] The only prospective randomized controlled trial comparing LR with RFA shows nearly equivalent survival, however, in this study 21% who were randomized for RFA arm were converted to LR.[111] Laparoscopic and open approaches for RFA increase the chance of detection of unknown intrahepatic and extrahepatic tumors because they allow complete abdominal exploration and intraoperative ultrasound assessment. The additional advantages of open and laparoscopic approaches are the accurate placement of electrodes and the possible treatment of tumors in percutaneously inaccessible areas of the liver and tumors in close proximity to or invading the adjacent organs.[112]

Cryoablation and interstitial laser coagulation (ILC) are other modalities for local ablative approach. In cryoablation, a cylindrical probe is inserted into the lesion like RFA after confirming position with ultrasound guidance intraoperative or percutaneous. Liquid nitrogen is then circulated at temperatures no greater than $-195°C$ to create a tumor freeze. Tumor freezing is monitored by ultrasonography until an ice ball enveloped the tumor with a 1 cm margin of normal tissue. A multicenter randomized controlled trial-[113] comparing percutaneous cryoablation with RFA for the treatment of patients with HCC in Child class A or B cirrhosis and one or two HCC lesions ≤4 cm, showed that cryoablation resulted in a significantly lower local tumor progression, although both cryoablation and RFA were equally safe and effective with similar 5-year survival rate.[113] A recent non randomized comparison of patients with primary HCCs <5 cm treated by cryoablation or RFA/ MWA showed that patients with tumors >2 cm had lower local recurrence rates in the cryoablation group compared with the RFA/MW group (21% vs. 56 % at 2 years; $p = 0.006$).[114] A review of[115] ablative therapies when compared with TACE showed that complete tumor necrosis can be achieved in 60–100% of patients treated with ablative therapies versus only 17–62% response after TACE while complete tumor response is rare (0–4.8%) as viable tumor cells remain after TACE. Five-year survival rates were lower with TACE (1–8%), compared to PEI (0–70%) and cryoablation (40%). RFA was associated with fewer treatment sessions and a higher complete necrosis rate. Cryoablation was associated with a higher morbidity rate. They concluded that TACE is a valuable therapy with survival benefits in strictly selected patients with unresectable HCC. RFA and PEI should be considered as the local ablative techniques of choice for the treatment of, preferably small, HCC.[115] When tumors are located close to bile ducts or large vessels, PEI is preferred. Completeness of ablation can be more easily monitored during cryoablation and another advantage of cryoablation is the possibility of edge freezing. The results of ILC are comparable to RFA with only few side effects and high tumor response rates.

Irreversible electroporation (IRE) is a non-thermal ablation technique that uses electrical gradient that across cell membranes to create cellular damage. The application of high voltage direct electrical current across the cell has the ability to alter the transmembrane potential and disrupt the lipid bilayer. This leads to the creation of small nanopores that allow for exchange of intra and extra-cellular components via a mechanism that is not yet fully understood. When the voltage applied is sufficiently high these pores become permanent and contribute to cell death.[116] This is a new technology being studied for safety and efficacy. In an early study, patients with unresectable tumors and tumors not amenable for radiofrequency ablation because of their vicinity to organs that are vulnerable to thermal damage such as the bowel, stomach or because they were close to large blood vessels that would limit efficacy of ablation due to the heat sink effect were treated with irreversible electroporation using percutaneous ultrasound and/or computed tomography guided electrode placement. After IRE therapy, 72% of lesions were completely ablated with 93% success for lesions ≤3 cm. The local recurrence-free period was 18 ± 4 months. These preliminary results suggested that IRE is a safe and feasible technique for local ablation of HCC, particularly for lesions less than 3 cm. No major complications were encountered during this study even for tumors close to essential structures or organs.[117] A similar study where IRE was performed in patients not eligible for surgery and lesions abutting large vessels or bile ducts showed a 71% success rate with no local recurrence at more than a year of follow up. In one case, intervention was terminated and abdominal bleeding required laparotomy while in two cases, a post-interventional hemothorax required intervention. No complications related to the bile ducts occurred. They had higher complication rate in HCC associated with perivascular lesions in using IRE.[118]

5 Regional Therapy

TACE and Yttrium-90 (Y-90) glass microspheres are used for those patients who are not eligible for local control or for those who are not surgical candidates.[119] TACE with cisplatin versus adriamycin can be used in multiple sessions to control or downstage an HCC. A prospective study[120] evaluated pre-OLT TACE on preventing tumor progression while on the waiting list in patients within Milan criteria and also analyzed a separate group of patients with advanced-stage HCC outside the Milan criteria but with at least 50% tumor reduction after TACE (downstaging) to expand current criteria. They reported 1, 2, and 5-year intention-to-treat survival of 98%, 98%, and 94% respectively and the 1, 2, and 5-year survival rates after OLT of 98%, 98%, and 93% in patients within Milan criteria. No patient dropped out of list and tumor recurrence was seen in one patient (2.5%). They concluded that TACE followed by OLT is associated with an excellent outcome in selected patients and is highly efficacious in preventing tumor progression while waiting for OLT. Although TACE reduced tumor burden preoperatively, it failed to show a beneficial effect on patient survival in advanced-stage HCCs with a high tumor recurrence of 30% of patients after OLT.[120] Chapman *et al.*[121] evaluated outcomes of downstaging patients with advanced (American liver tumor study group stage III/IV) HCC with TACE to allow eligibility for OLT. There were 23.7% of patients who had adequate downstaging to qualify for OLT under the Milan criteria. By Response Evaluation Criteria in Solid Tumors (RECIST) criteria, 35.5% patients had a partial response, 29% had stable disease, and 35.5% had progressive disease. Responses to TACE (with ≥90% tumor necrosis) was shown in 75% of patients who had OLT. A good

94% intermediate survival at a median of 19.6 months was observed. The authors suggested that selected patients with stage III/IV HCC can be downstaged to Milan criteria with TACE but more importantly, patients who are successfully downstaged and transplanted have excellent midterm disease-free and overall survival, similar to stage II HCC. TACE is combined with local ablation to achieve better local control and survival benefit. A prospective, randomized, controlled trial[122] comparing RFA/MWA ablation alone with combined ablation and TACE in patients with HCC ≤7 cm showed that the patients in the TACE-RFA or TACE-MWA group had better overall survival than the RFA or MWA group and showed better recurrence-free survival than the RFA or MWA group.[122] Another randomized controlled trial[123] on patients with HCC less than 7 cm showed that 1, 3, and 4-year overall survivals for the TACE-RFA group and the RFA group were 92.6%, 66.6%, and 61.8% and 85.3%, 59%, and 45.0%, respectively. The corresponding recurrence-free survivals were 79.4%, 60.6%, and 54.8% for TACE-RFA and 66.7%, 44.2%, and 38.9% for RFA group. Thus, patients in the TACE-RFA group had better overall survival and recurrence-free survival than patients in the RFA group suggesting that combined treatment has more benefit.[123]

Selective internal radiation therapy (SIRT) is performed by intra-arterial injection of Y-90glass microspheres for treatment of unresectable hepatocellular carcinoma (HCC) in the presence of an acceptable liver function.[124] Initial studies showed that Y-90 treatment is well tolerated and is safe in patients with compromised portal venous flow in one or both first order and related segmental portal venous branches and no evidence of cavernous transformation without causing significant liver dysfunction.[124] Long term studies[125] have shown that in patients with unresectable HCC Y-90 treatment can be performed with a 30-day mortality rate of 3% with reasonable response rates and acceptable morbidity. Child's A patients, with or without portal vein thrombosis (PVT), benefited the most from Y-90, while Child's B patients with PVT had poor overall survival and poor TTP survival. A multicenter European study[126] in patients with Child–Pugh A cirrhosis with good performance status who received unilobar or whole liver Y-90 treatments for predominantly multinodular disease (75.9%) invading both lobes (53.1%) and/or portal vein occlusion and advanced Barcelona Clinic Liver Cancer (BCLC) staging (BCLC C, 56.3%) or intermediate staging (BCLC B, 26.8%) showed a median overall survival of 12.8 months, with acceptable morbidity. This analysis showed that Y-90 radioembolization provides survival benefit for patients with advanced HCC with low mortality rates. A study comparing effectiveness and toxicity of TACE and Y-90 microspheres in patients with unresectable HCC[127] showed that disease progression and median overall survival was similar for both groups after 6 months and Grade 3 or higher toxicity was observed in 34% patients. This preliminary study suggested that chemoembolization and radioembolization provided similar effectiveness and toxicity in patients with unresectable HCC.[127] Another retrospective study[128] comparing safety and efficacy of Y-90 radioembolization with that of chemoembolization in patients with unresectable HCC has no significant difference in survival between the two groups but in patients who underwent chemoembolization, there was a significantly higher rates of hospitalization for postembolization syndrome after treatment. The rates of other complications and rehospitalization were similar between groups.[128]

6 Systemic Therapy

6.1 *Systemic therapy for advanced/metastatic disease*

HCC is a well-vascularized tumor so one approach designed to treat it involves targeted therapy with anti-angiogenic factors, such as vascular endothelial growth factor (VEGF) and the platelet-derived growth factor receptor (PDGFR). Sorafenib, with activity on tumor cell proliferation and angiogenesis via interactions with receptor RAF kinase, Raf-1, B-Raf, VEGF, PDGFR and c-Kit receptors, causing a marked antitumoral effect[129,130] is the only oral systemic agent to demonstrate overall survival (OS) benefit as first-line therapy in advanced HCC.[20,131,132] An uncontrolled phase II study involving Child's class A or B patients with advanced HCC showed a median overall survival of 9.2 months and a median time to progression (TTP) of 5.5 months when using Sorafenib.[132] Sorafenib was approved for the treatment of patients with advanced HCC on the basis of the efficacy and the safety results reported by two international RCTs, the SHARP (Sorafenib HCC Assessment Randomized Protocol) and the Asia-Pacific trials.[20,133] In the SHARP multicenter, phase III, double-blind, placebo-controlled trial,[20] they randomly assigned 602 patients with advanced HCC who had not received previous systemic treatment to receive either sorafenib (at a dose of 400 mg twice daily) or placebo. They showed that in patients with advanced HCC, the median survival and the time to radiologic progression were nearly 3 months longer for patients treated with sorafenib than for those given placebo.[20] Although, there was no difference in the median time to symptomatic progression, a significant advantage for sorafenib over placebo was reported for time to radiologic progression (TTP).[20] In both SHARP and Asia-Pacific trials, more than 95% of patients were Child's A cirrhosis[20,133] and so the potential benefits of sorafenib in Child's B patients could not be investigated in those trials. There have been some observational studies to validate this. Kim *et al.*[134] in an Asian cohort of 225 patients with HCC evaluated according to Child–Pugh score (68 with Child–Pugh B). The disease control rate was higher in patients with Child's A than Child's B cirrhosis, but did not differ among patients with Child–Pugh score B7 and those with Child–Pugh score B8 or B9. No differences in the rate of grade 3/4 AEs were reported among patients with different Child–Pugh classes. About 25% patients with Child's B 8 and B-9 had to stop sorafenib due to cirrhosis-related complications. They concluded that HCC patients with Child's score B7 can be included in future clinical trials, in order to collect further evidence on the treatment with sorafenib in this group of patients. Hollebecque et al.135 reported the results of a prospective experience on sorafenib efficacy in 120 patients with advanced HCC that showed decreased OS in Child's B patients compared to Child's A. This was attributed to poorer liver function in Child's B patients. Many efforts have been tried in the investigation of more effective biologic/target oriented agents for HCC. However, there has no approval at phase III level.

Like VEGF, fibroblast growth factor (FGF) is also a key factor in angiogenesis in HCC[136] and FGF may have direct and indirect effects on tumors.[137,138] The upregulation of alternate angiogenic signals, such as FGF, may play a role in avoiding resistance to VEGF-targeted therapy.[139,140] Combined administration of anti-FGF and anti-VEGF antibodies in a mouse HCC model has shown additive antitumor activity.[141] Thus, targeting to block both VEGF and FGF may offer therapeutic advantages over a blockade of VEGF alone. Brivanib, a tyrosine kinase inhibitor with dual inhibitor of FGF and VEGF signaling, has antiangiogenic and antiproliferative effects on tumor cells from multiple tumor types, including liver.[142,143] It demonstrated antitumor activity in xenograft HCC models expressing FGF receptors and in those resistant to sorafenib.[144] In a phase II studies, brivanib showed evidence of antitumor activity in patients with previously untreated advanced HCC as well as in those who had experienced prior antiangiogenic therapy failure.[145,146] In a phase III BRISK-PS study of HCC patients who experienced sorafenib treatment failure, brivanib did not significantly improve OS as compared with placebo but it improved time to progression (TTP), objective response rate (ORR), and disease control rate (DCR) according to modified Response Evaluation Criteria in Solid Tumors (mRECIST).[147] A phase III trial compared brivanib with sorafenib as first-line treatment for advanced HCC. The median OS was 9.9 months for sorafenib and 9.5 months for brivanib. TTP, ORR, and DCR were similar between the study arms. The study did not meet the OS non inferiority goal of primary end point brivanib versus sorafenib.[148] Brivainib is not FDA approved, however, it is being used in Europe and Asia (based on the phase II data). Similarly, sunitinib, another multikinase inhibitor with broad activity inhibiting all VEGFRs and PDGFRs, c-KIT, Flt-3, RET, and CSF-1R, was evaluated against sorafenib in a large phase III trial.[149] This trial was stopped prematurely, after inferior outcomes were noted with sunitinib. Linifanib, an inhibitor mainly with the VEGFRs and PDGFRs, was compared with sorafenib as first-line therapy in a noninferiority phase III trial.[150] The median OS was 9.1 months with linifanib and 9.8 months with sorafenib, which failed the prespecified boundaries for noninferiority even with improved TTP (5.4 months with linifanib vs. 4.0 with sorafenib, $p = 0.001$) and response rate (RR) (13.0% with linifanib vs. 6.9 % with sorafenib).

6.2 *Adjuvant therapy*

Numerous studies have investigated the use of adjuvant chemotherapy for primary HCC patients. There has been no randomized study indicate the benefit of systemic therapy after LR or LT. A recent meta-analysis of 13 RCTs and 35 observational studies to evaluate the efficacy of adjuvant chemotherapy in HCC patients after hepatectomy suggests that hepatectomy plus adjuvant chemotherapy being superior to hepatectomy alone in DFS and OS at 1, 3, and 5 years. However, subgroup and sensitivity analysis revealed that only adjuvant TACE had significant survival benefits. The meta-analysis of studies involving patients with portal vein tumor thrombus (PVTT) had more likely benefit from adjuvant chemotherapy.[129]

With sorafenib bringing systemic therapy benefits, efforts are attempted for increasing the overall outcome for HCC patients who have locally advanced disease but not surgical candidates. A prospective phase II, open label, trial investigating the safety and efficacy of the combination of sorafenib and conventional TACE in patients from the Asia-Pacific region with intermediate HCC. The combination achieved a disease control rate of 91.2% while the overall response rate was 52.4%. Thus showing safety and efficacy of concurrent sorafenib and TACE therapy in intermediate HCC.[151] A large randomized phase III to assess the benefits of systemic sorafenib and TACE combination in locally advanced HCC has been conducted in the United States (E1208, NCT01004978); unfortunately, the study was stopped recently because of poor recruiting. At the same time, a similar phase III randomized study in UK (TACE2, NCT01324076) is still on going, and the results will be available in 2016.

7 Conclusions

LT is the gold-standard treatment for HCC. Patients with small HCC (<3 cm) and preserved liver function have comparable survival between LR and LT. Considering donor shortages and wait times, LR is preferable in Child's A patients with HCC as first line curative approach. Some other factors to consider are: Patient factors — would they ever be OLT candidates? Do they need to be bridged to transplant? Tumor factors — microvascular invasion, satellite lesions, tumor >3 cm, poorly differentiated. Liver factors — presence of cirrhosis, portal hypertension, hepatitis C. Geographic factors — availability of donors, differences in the allocation system, differences in the potential waiting time, and differences in regional and national organ transplant law. In addition to taking into account these factors, LT candidates with HCC should be informed of risks and benefits of the waiting time for DDLT may lead to the dropout due to HCC progression. This could potentially be avoided by LDLT or bridging therapies like local ablation or liver resection. Local therapy like RFA or microwave are comparable and can be used in solitary tumor <3cm with good long term results or as a second choice for patients who are not candidates for surgical resection or transplantation. It can also be used as a bridging therapy while awaiting transplant. Regional therapy with TACE or Y-90 gives reasonable response and disease stabilization rates in unresectable patients and also used for patients who are not surgical candidates and not eligible for local ablative therapy. It can sometimes be combined with local or systemic therapies. Management of HCC is complex and should be performed in a multidisciplinary manner.

References

1. Jemal A, *et al*. Global cancer statistics. *CA Cancer J Clin* 2011;**61**:69–90.
2. Edwards BK, *et al*. Annual report to the nation on the status of cancer, 1975–2006, featuring colorectal cancer trends and impact of interventions (risk factors, screening, and treatment) to reduce future rates. *Cancer* 2010;**116**:544–573.
3. Bosch FX, *et al*. Primary liver cancer: worldwide incidence and trends. *Gastroenterology* 2004; **127**(5 Suppl. 1):S5–S16.
4. World Health Organization. Cancer. Retrieved from http://www.who.int/mediacentre/factsheets/fs297/en/index.html. Accessed Sept. 1, 2014.
5. Llovet JM, *et al*. Hepatocellular carcinoma. *Lancet*. 2003;**362**:1907–1917.
6. Caldwell SH, *et al*. Obesity and hepatocellular carcinoma. Gastroenterology. 2004;**127**:S97–S103.
7. Sangiovanni A, *et al*. Increased survival of cirrhotic patients with hepatocellular carcinoma detected during surveillance. Gastroenterology. 2004;**126**:1005–1014.
8. Mazzaferro V, *et al*. Liver transplantation for the treatment of small hepatocellular carcinomas in patients with cirrhosis. *N Engl J Med* 1996;**334**:693–699.
9. Organ Procurement and Transplantation Network. Homepage. Retrieved from http://optn.transplant.hrsa.gov Accessed Sept. 3, 2014.
10. Bismuth H, *et al*. Liver resection versus transplantation for hepatocellular carcinoma in cirrhotic patients. *Ann Surg* 1993;**218**:145–151.
11. Belghiti J, *et al*. Intrahepatic recurrence after resection of hepatocellular carcinoma complicating cirrhosis. *Ann Surg* 1991;**214**:114–117.
12. Poon RT, *et al*. Improving survival results after resection of hepatocellular carcinoma: a prospective study of 377 patients over 10 years. *Ann Surg* 2001;**234**:63–70.
13. Grazi GL, *et al*. Improved results of liver resection for hepatocellular carcinoma on cirrhosis give the procedure added value. *Ann Surg* 2001;**234**:71–78.

14. Cherqui D, *et al*. Liver resection for transplantable hepatocellular carcinoma: long-term survival and role of secondary liver transplantation. *Ann Surg* 2009;**250**(5):738–746.

15. Shiina S, *et al*. A randomized controlled trial of radiofrequency ablation with ethanol injection for small hepatocellular carcinoma. *Gastroenterology* 2005;**129**:122–130.

16. Saitsu H, Nakayama T. Microwave coagulo-necrotic therapy for hepatocellular carcinoma. *Nippon Rinsho* 1993;**51**:1102–1107.

17. Shibata T, *et al*. Small hepatocellular carcinoma: comparison of radiofrequency ablation and percutaneous microwave coagulation therapy. *Radiology* 2002;**223**: 331–337.

18. Heckman JT, *et al*. Bridging locoregional therapy for hepatocellular carcinoma prior to liver transplantation. *Ann Surg Oncol* 2008;**15**:3169–3177.

19. Poon RT, *et al*. Transarterial chemoembolization for inoperable hepatocellular carcinoma and postresection intrahepatic recurrence. *J Surg Oncol* 2000;**73**:109–114.

20. Llovet JM, *et al*. Sorafenib in advanced hepatocellular carcinoma. *N Engl J Med* 2008; Jul 24;**359**(4):378–90. doi: 10.1056/NEJMoa0708857.

21. Altekruse SF, *et al*. Hepatocellular Carcinoma incidence, Mortality and Survival Trends in United States from 1975 to 2005. *J Clin Oncol* 2009;**27**(9):1485–1491.

22. Starzl TE, *et al*. Orthotopic homotransplantation of the human liver. *Ann Surg* 1968;**168**:392–415.

23. van der Putten AB, *et al*. Selection criteria and decisions in 375 patients with liver disease, considered for liver transplantation during 1977–1985. *Liver* 1987;**7**(2):84–90.

24. Houben KW, McCall JL. Liver transplantation for hepatocellular carcinoma in patients without underlying liver disease: a systematic review. *Liver Transpl Surg* 1999 Mar; **5**(2):91–95.

25. Starzl TE, *et al*. Liver transplantation, 1980, with particular reference to cyclosporin-A. *Transplant Proc* 1981;**13**:281–285.

26. Starzl TE, *et al*. Liver transplantation with use of cyclosporin A and prednisone. *N Engl J Med* 1981;**305**:266–269.

27. National Institutes of Health Consensus Development Conference Statement: liver transplantation — June 20–23, 1983. *Hepatology* 1984;**4**:107S–110S.

28. Ringe B, *et al*. Surgical treatment of hepatocellular carcinoma: experience with liver resection and transplantation in 198 patients. *World J Surg* 1991;**15**:270–285.

29. Iwatsuki S, *et al*. Role of liver transplantation in cancer therapy. *Ann Surg* 1985 Oct; **202**(4):401–407.

30. Iwatsuki S, *et al*. Hepatic resection versus transplantation for hepatocellular carcinoma. *Ann Surg* 1991;**214**:221–228; discussion 228–229.

31. Kamath PS, *et al*. "A model to predict survival in patients with end-stage liver disease". *Hepatology* 2001;**33**(2):464–70.

32. Kamath PS, Kim WR (March 2007). "The model for end-stage liver disease (MELD)". *Hepatology* **45**(3):797–805.

33. Mazzaferro V, *et al*. Milan criteria in liver transplantation for hepatocellular carcinoma: an evidence-based analysis of 15 years of experience. *Liver Transpl* 2011;17 Suppl 2:S44–S57.

34. Doyle MB, *et al*. Liver transplantation for hepatocellular carcinoma: long-term results suggest excellent outcomes. *J Am Coll Surg*. 2012 Jul; 215(1):19–28; discussion 28–30. doi: 10.1016/j.jamcollsurg.2012.02.022. Epub 2012 May 18.

35. Dumitra S, *et al*. Hepatitis C infection and hepatocellular carcinoma in liver transplantation: a 20-year experience. HPB (Oxford). 2013 Sep; 15(9):724–31. doi: 10.1111/hpb.12041. Epub 2013 Mar 14.

36. Yao FY, *et al*. Liver transplantation for hepatocellular carcinoma: analysis of survival according to the intention-to-treat principle and dropout from the waiting list. *Liver Transpl* 2002 Oct; **8**(10):873–883.

37. Yao FY, *et al*. Liver transplantation for hepatocellular carcinoma: expansion of the tumor size limits does not adversely impact survival. *Hepatology* 2001;**33**:1394–1403.

38. Decaens T, *et al*. Impact of UCSF criteria according to pre- and post-OLT tumor features: analysis of 479 patients listed for HCC with a short waiting time. *Liver Transpl* 2006;**12**:1761–1769.

39. de Villa V, Lo CM. Liver transplantation for hepatocellular carcinoma in Asia. *Oncologist* 2007;**12**:1321–1331.

40. Lee Cheah Y, K H Chow P. Liver transplantation for hepatocellular carcinoma: an appraisal of current controversies. *Liver Cancer* 2012;**1**:183–189.

41. Hwang S, *et al*. Liver transplantation for HCC: its role: Eastern and Western perspectives. *J Hepatobiliary Pancreat Sci* 2010;**17**:443–448.

42. Park MS, *et al*. Living-donor liver transplantation associated with higher incidence of hepatocellular carcinoma recurrence than deceased-donor liver transplantation. Transplantation.

43. Fisher RA, *et al*. Hepatocellular carcinoma recurrence and death following living and deceased donor liver transplantation. *Am J Transplant* 2007;**7**:1601–1608.

44. Kulik LM, *et al*. Outcomes of living and deceased donor liver transplant recipients with hepatocellular carcinoma: results of the A2ALL cohort. *Am J Transplant* 2012;**12**: 2997–3007.

45. Vakili K, *et al*. Living donor liver transplantation for hepatocellular carcinoma: Increased recurrence but improved survival. *Liver Transpl* 2009;**15**:1861–1866.

46. Hwang S, *et al*. Liver transplantation for adult patients with hepatocellular carcinoma in Korea: comparison between cadaveric donor and living donor liver transplantations. *Liver Transpl* 2005;**11**:1265–1272

47. Sotiropoulos GC, *et al*. Liver transplantation for hepatocellular carcinoma: University Hospital Essen experience and metaanalysis of prognostic factors. *J Am Coll Surg* 2007;**205**:661–675.

48. Grant RC, *et al*. Living vs. deceased donor liver transplantation for hepatocellular carcinoma: a systematic review and meta-analysis. *Clin Transplant* 2013;**27**:140–147.

49. Akamatsu N, *et al*. Living-donor vs. deceased-donor liver transplantation for patients with hepatocellular carcinoma. *World J Hepatol* 2014 Sep 27; 6(9):626–31. doi: 10.4254/wjh.v6.i9.626.

50. Bismuth H, *et al*. Liver resection versus transplantation for hepatocellular carcinoma in cirrhotic patients. *Ann Surg* 1993;**218**:145–151.

51. Belghiti J, *et al*. Intrahepatic recurrence after resection of hepatocellular carcinoma complicating cirrhosis. *Ann Surg* 1991;**214**:114–117.

52. Cherqui D, *et al*. Liver resection for transplantable hepatocellular carcinoma: long-term survival and role of secondary liver transplantation. *Ann Surg* 2009 Nov; 250(5):738–46. doi: 10.1097/SLA.0b013e3181bd582b.

53. Poon RT, *et al*. Improving survival results after resection of hepatocellular carcinoma: a prospective study of 377 patients over 10 years. *Ann Surg* 2001;**234**:63–70.

54. Grazi GL, *et al*. Improved results of liver resection for hepatocellular carcinoma on cirrhosis give the procedure added value. *Ann Surg* 2001;**234**:71–78.

55. Bryant R, *et al*. Liver resection for hepatocellular carcinoma. *Surg Oncol Clin N Am* 2008;**17**:607– 633.

56. Fuks D, *et al*. Benefit of initial resection of hepatocellular carcinoma followed by transplantation in case of recurrence: an intention-to-treat analysis. *Hepatolology* 2012;**55**:132–140.

57. Clavien PA, *et al*. Recommendations for liver transplantation for hepatocellular carcinoma: an international consensus conference report. *Lancet Oncol* 2012;**13**:11–22.

58. Rahbari NN, *et al*. Hepatocellular carcinoma: current management and perspectives for the future. *Ann Surg* 2011;**253**:453–469.

59. Forner A, *et al*. Current strategy for staging and treatment: the BCLC update and future prospects. *Semin Liver Dis* 2010;**30**:61–74.

60. Figueras J, *et al*. Resection or transplantation for hepatocellular carcinoma in cirrhotic patients: outcomes based on indicated treatment strategy. *J Am Coll Surg* 2000;**190**: 580–587.

61. Cha CH, *et al*. Resection of hepatocellular carcinoma in patients otherwise eligible for transplantation. *Ann Surg* 2003 Sep; 238(3):315–21; discussion 321–3.

62. Yeh CN, *et al*. Prognostic factors of hepatic resection for hepatocellular carcinoma with cirrhosis: univariate and multivariate analysis. *J Surg Oncol* 2002 Dec; **81**(4): 195–202.

63. Shimozawa N, Hanazaki K. Longterm prognosis after hepatic resection for small hepatocellular carcinoma. *J Am Coll Surg* 2004 Mar; **198**(3):356–65.

64. Neeff H, *et al*. Hepatic resection for hepatocellular carcinoma — results and analysis of the current literature Zentralbl Chir. 2009 Apr; **134**(2):127–135. doi: 10.1055/s-0028–1098881. Epub 2009 Apr 20.

65. Nguyen KT, *et al*. World review of laparoscopic liver resection — 2,804 patients. *Ann Surg* 2009;**250**:831–41.

66. Buell JF, *et al*. The international position on laparoscopic liver surgery: the Louisville statement, 2008. *Ann Surg* 2009;**250**:825–30.

67. Nguyen KT, *et al*. Comparative benefits of laparoscopic vs open hepatic resection: a critical appraisal. *Arch Surg* 2011;**146**:348–56.

68. Yin Z, *et al*. Short- and long-term outcomes after laparoscopic and open hepatectomy for hepatocellular carcinoma: a global systematic review and meta-analysis. *Ann Surg Oncol* 2013 Apr; 20(4):1203–15. doi: 10.1245/s10434-012-2705-8. Epub 2012 Oct 26.

69. Laurent A, *et al*. Laparoscopic liver resection facilitates salvage liver transplantation for hepatocellular carcinoma. *J Hepatobiliary Pancreat Surg*. 2009; 16(3):310-4. doi: 10.1007/s00534-009-0063-0. Epub 2009 Mar 12.

70. Nathan H, *et al*. Surgical therapy for early hepatocellular carcinoma in the modern era: a 10-year SEER-medicare analysis. *Ann Surg*. 2013 Dec;**258**(6):1022–1027. doi: 10.1097/SLA.0b013e31827da749.

71. Roayaie S, *et al*. Resection of hepatocellular cancer ≤2 cm: results from two Western centers. *Hepatology* 2013 Apr; **57**(4):1426–35. doi: 10.1002/hep.25832. Epub 2013 Jan 25.

72. Eguchi S, *et al*. Recurrence-free survival more than 10 years after liver resection for hepatocellular carcinoma. *Br J Surg* 2011 Apr; **98**(4):552–557. doi: 10.1002/bjs.7393. Epub 2011 Jan 25.

73. Margarit C, *et al*. Resection for hepatocellular carcinoma is a good option in Child-Turcotte-Pugh class A patients with cirrhosis who are eligible for liver transplantation. *Liver Transpl* 2005 Oct;**11**(10):1242–51.

74. Facciuto ME, *et al*. Surgical treatment of hepatocellular carcinoma beyond Milan criteria. Results of liver resection salvage transplantation, and primary liver transplantation. *Ann Surg Oncol* 2008 May;**15**(5):1383–91. doi: 10.1245/s10434-008-9851-z. Epub 2008 Mar 5.

75. Vitale A, *et al*. Is resectable hepatocellular carcinoma a contraindication to liver transplantation? A novel decision model based on "number of patients needed to transplant" as measure of transplant benefit. *J Hepatol* 2014 Jun;**60**(6):1165–71. doi: 10.1016/j.jhep.2014.01.022. Epub 2014 Feb 6.

76. Adam R, *et al*. Resection or transplantation for early hepatocellular carcinoma in a cirrhotic liver: does size define the best oncological strategy? *Ann Surg* 2012;**256**: 883–891.

77. Koniaris LG, *et al*. Is surgical resection superior to transplantation in in the treatment of hepatocellular carcinoma? *Ann Surg* 2011;**254**:527–537.

78. Schaubel DE, *et al*. Survival benefit-based deceased-donor liver allocation. *Am J Transplant* 2009;**9**:970–981.

79. Mazzaferro V, *et al*. Predicting survival after liver transplantation in patients with hepatocellular carcinoma beyond the Milan criteria: a retrospective, exploratory analysis. *Lancet Oncol* 2009;**10**:35–43.

80. Nathan H, *et al*. Clinical decision-making by gastroenterologists and hepatologists for patients with early hepatocellular carcinoma. *Ann Surg Oncol* 2014 Jun; 21(6): 1844–51. doi: 10.1245/s10434-014-3536-6. Epub 2014 Feb 13.

81. Dhir M, *et al*. Comparison of outcomes of transplantation and resection in patients with early hepatocellular carcinoma: a meta-analysis. HPB (Oxford) 2012;**14**:635–645.

82. Clavien PA, *et al*. Recommendations for liver transplantation for hepatocellular carcinoma: an international consensus conference report. *Lancet Oncol* 2012;**13**: e11–22.

83. Llovet JM, *et al*. Prognosis of hepatocellular carcinoma: the BCLC staging classification. *Semin Liver Dis* 1999;**19**:329–38.

84. Proneth A, *et al.* Is resection or transplantation the ideal treatment in patients with hepatocellular carcinoma in cirrhosis if both are possible? A systematic review and metaanalysis. *Ann Surg Oncol* 2014 Sep; 21(9):3096–107. doi: 10.1245/s10434-014-3808-1. Epub 2014 May 28.

85. Mazzaferro V, *et al.* Liver transplantation for hepatocellular carcinoma. *Ann Surg Oncol* 2008 Apr; 15(4):1001–7. doi: 10.1245/s10434-007-9559-5. Epub 2008 Jan 31.

86. Bruix J, *et al.* Liver transplantation for hepatocellular carcinoma: Foucault pendulum versus evidence based decision. *Liver Transpl* 2003;**7**:700–2.

87. Marsh JW, *et al.* Genotyping of hepatocellular carcinoma in liver transplant recipients adds predictive power for determining recurrence-free survival. *Liver Transpl* 2003;**7**:664–71.

88. Finkelstein SD, *et al.* Microdissection-based allelotyping discriminates de novo tumor from intrahepatic spread in hepatocellular carcinoma. *Hepatology* 2003;**4**:871–9.

89. Livraghi T, *et al.* Sustained complete response and complications rates after radiofrequency ablation of very early hepatocellular carcinoma in cirrhosis: Is resection still the treatment of choice? *Hepatology* 2008;**47**:82–89.

90. Livraghi T, *et al.* Hepatocellular carcinoma and cirrhosis in 746 patients: long-term results of percutaneous ethanol injection. *Radiology* 1995;**197**:101–108.

91. Shiina S, Tagawa K, Unuma T, *et al.* Percutaneous ethanol injection therapy for hepatocellular carcinoma: results in 146 patients. *Am J Radiol* 1993;**160**:1023–1028.

92. Yamamoto J, *et al.* Treatment strategy for small hepatocellular carcinoma: comparison of long-term results after percutaneous ethanol injection therapy and surgical resection. *Hepatology* 2001;**34**:707–713.

93. Mathurin P, *et al.* Review article: Overview of medical treatments in unresectable hepatocellular carcinoma; an impossible meta-analysis? *Aliment Pharmacol Ther* 1998;**12**:111–126.

94. Huang GT, *et al.* Percutaneous ethanol injection versus surgical resection for the treatment of small hepatocellular carcinoma: a prospective study. *Ann Surg* 2005 Jul; **242**(1):36–42.

95. Rhim H, *et al.* Essential Techniques for Successful Radio-frequency Thermal Ablation of Malignant Hepatic Tumors. *RadioGraphics* 2001;**21**:S17–S39.

96. Livraghi T, *et al.* Small hepatocellular carcinoma: treatment with radio-frequency ablation versus ethanol injection. Radiology 1999;**210**:655–661.

97. Lencioni RA, *et al.* Small hepatocellular carcinoma in cirrhosis: randomized comparison of radio-frequency thermal ablation versus percutaneous ethanol injection. Radiology. 2003 Jul;**228**(1):235–40

98. Lencioni RA, *et al.* Percutaneous treatment of small hepatocellular carcinoma in cirrhosis: radio-frequency thermal ablation vs ethanol injection; a prospective, randomized trial (final report). Radiology 1999; 213 (suppl): 123.

99. Lin SM, *et al.* Radiofrequency ablation improves prognosis compared with ethanol injection for hepatocellular carcinoma ≤4 cm. Gastroenterology 2004;**127**:1714–1723.

100. Shiina S, *et al.* A randomized controlled trial of radiofrequency ablation with ethanol injection for small hepatocellular carcinoma. Gastroenterology. 2005;**129**:122–130.

101. European Association for the Study of the Liver, European Organisation for Research and Treatment of Cancer. EASL-EORTC clinical practice guidelines: management of hepatocellular carcinoma. *J Hepatol.* 2012;**56**:908–943

102. Ebara M, *et al.* Percutaneous ethanol injection for small hepatocellular carcinoma: Therapeutic efficacy based on 20-year observation. *J Hepatol* 2005;**43**:458–464.

103. Brunello F, *et al.* Radiofrequency ablation versus ethanol injection for early hepatocellular carcinoma: A randomized controlled trial. *Scand J Gastroenterol.* 2008;**43**(6):727–735. doi: 10.1080/00365520701885481.

104. Lubner MG, *et al.* Microwave Tumor Ablation: Mechanism of Action, Clinical Results and Devices. J Vasc Interv Radiol. Aug 2010; 21(8 Suppl): S192–S203. doi:10.1016/j.jvir.2010.04.007.

105. Dong B, *et al.* Percutaneous sonographically guided microwave coagulation therapy for hepatocellular carcinoma: results in 234 patients. AJR *Am J Roentgenol* 2003;**180**(6):1547–1555.

106. Lu MD, Xu HX, Xie XY, *et al.* Percutaneous microwave and radiofrequency ablation for hepatocellular carcinoma: a retrospective comparative study. *J Gastroenterol* 2005;**40**(11):1054–1060.

107. Boutros C, *et al.* Microwave coagulation therapy for hepatic tumors: Review of the literature and critical analysis. *Surg Oncol* 2009.

108. Iannitti DA, *et al.* Hepatic tumor ablation with clustered microwave antennae: the US Phase II Trial. HPB (Oxford) 2007;**9**(2):120–124.

109. Ueno S, *et al.* Surgical resection versus radiofrequency ablation for small hepatocellular carcinomas within the Milan criteria. *J Hepatobiliary Pancreat Surg.* 2009; 16(3):359–66. doi: 10.1007/s00534-009-0069-7. Epub 2009 Mar 20.

110. Zhou Y, *et al.* Meta-analysis of radiofrequency ablation versus hepatic resection for small hepatocellular carcinoma. *BMC Gastroenterol* 2010 Jul 9;**10**:78. doi: 10.1186/1471–230X-10-78.

111. Chen MS, *et al.* A prospective randomized trial comparing percutaneous local ablative therapy and partial hepatectomy for small hepatocellular carcinoma. *Ann Surg* 2006; **243**:321–328

112. Lau WY, *et al.* The current role of radiofrequency ablation in the management of hepatocellular carcinoma: a systematic review. *Ann Surg* 2009;**249**:20–25.

113. Wang C, *et al.* A multicenter randomized controlled trial of percutaneous cryoablation versus radiofrequency ablation in hepatocellular carcinoma. *Hepatology* 2014 Oct 6. doi: 10.1002/hep.27548. [Epub ahead of print]

114. Ei S, *et al.* Cryoablation Provides Superior Local Control of Primary Hepatocellular Carcinomas of >2 cm Compared with Radiofrequency Ablation and Microwave Coagulation Therapy: An Underestimated Tool in the Toolbox. *Ann Surg Oncol* 2014 Oct 7. [Epub ahead of print]

115. Jansen MC, *et al.* Outcome of regional and local ablative therapies for hepatocellular carcinoma: a collective review. *Eur J Surg Oncol* 2005 May;**31**(4):331–347.

116. Rubinsky, B. Irreversible electroporation in medicine. Technol Cancer Res Treat 6, 255–260 (2007).

117. Cheung W, *et al.* Irreversible electroporation for unresectable hepatocellular carcinoma: initial experience and review of safety and outcomes. *Technol Cancer Res Treat* 2013 Jun; 12(3):233-41. doi: 10.7785/tcrt.2012.500317. Epub 2013 Jan 25.

118. Eller A, *et al.* Local Control of Perivascular Malignant Liver Lesions Using Percutaneous Irreversible Electroporation: Initial Experiences. *Cardiovasc Intervent Radiol* 2014 May 6. [Epub ahead of print]

119. Dong W, *et al.* Clinical outcome of small hepatocellular carcinoma after different treatments: a meta-analysis. *World J Gastroenterol* 2014 Aug 7; **20**(29):10174–82. doi: 10.3748/wjg.v20.i29.10174.

120. Graziadei IW, *et al.* Chemoembolization followed by liver transplantation for hepatocellular carcinoma impedes tumor progression while on the waiting list and leads to excellent outcome. *Liver Transpl* 2003 Jun;**9**(6):557–563.

121. Chapman WC, *et al.* Outcomes of neoadjuvant transarterial chemoembolization to downstage hepatocellular carcinoma before liver transplantation. *Ann Surg* 2008 Oct;**248**(4):617–25. doi: 10.1097/SLA.0b013e31818a07d4.

122. Yi Y, *et al.* Radiofrequency ablation or microwave ablation combined with transcatheter arterial chemoembolization in treatment of hepatocellular carcinoma by comparing with radiofrequency ablation alone. *Chin J Cancer Res* 2014 Feb;**26**(1):112–118. doi: 10.3978/j.issn.1000-9604.2014.02.09.

123. Peng ZW, *et al.* Radiofrequency ablation with or without transcatheter arterial chemoembolization in the treatment of hepatocellular carcinoma: a prospective randomized trial. *J Clin Oncol* 2013 Feb 1;**31**(4):426–32. doi: 10.1200/JCO.2012.42.9936. Epub 2012 Dec 26.

124. Salem R, *et al.* Use of Yttrium-90 glass microspheres (TheraSphere) for the treatment of unresectable hepatocellular carcinoma in patients with portal vein thrombosis. *J Vasc Interv Radiol* 2004 Apr;**15**(4):335–45.

125. Salem R, *et al.* Radioembolization for hepatocellular carcinoma using Yttrium-90 microspheres: a comprehensive report of long-term outcomes. *Gastroenterology* 2010 Jan; 138(1):52–64. doi: 10.1053/j.gastro.2009.09.006. Epub 2009 Sep 18.

126. Sangro B, *et al.* European Network on Radioembolization with Yttrium-90 Resin Microspheres (ENRY). Survival after yttrium-90 resin microsphere radioembolization of hepatocellular carcinoma across Barcelona clinic liver cancer stages: a European evaluation. *Hepatology* 2011 Sep 2;**54**(3):868–78. doi: 10.1002/hep.24451. Epub 2011 Jun 30.

127. Kooby DA, *et al.* Comparison of yttrium-90 radioembolization and transcatheter arterial chemoembolization for the treatment of unresectable hepatocellular carcinoma. *J Vasc Interv Radiol* 2010 Feb; 21(2):224–30. doi: 10.1016/j.jvir.2009.10.013. Epub 2009 Dec 21.

128. Lance C, *et al.* Comparative analysis of the safety and efficacy of transcatheter arterial chemoembolization and yttrium-90 radioembolization in patients with unresectable hepatocellular carcinoma. *J Vasc Interv Radiol* 2011 Dec; 22(12):1697–705. doi: 10.1016/j.jvir.2011.08.013. Epub 2011 Oct 8.

129. Zheng Z, *et al*. Adjuvant chemotherapy for patients with primary hepatocellular carcinoma: A meta-analysis. *Int J Cancer* 2014 Sep 10. doi: 10.1002/ijc.29203. [Epub ahead of print]

130. Liu L, *et al*. Sorafenib blocks the RAF/MEK/ERK pathway, inhibits tumor angiogenesis, and induces tumor cell apoptosis in hepatocellular carcinoma model PLC/PRF/5. *Cancer Res* 2006;**66**:11851–11858.

131. Forner A, *et al*. Hepatocellular carcinoma. *Lancet* 2012; 379(9822):1245–1255.

132. Abou-Alfa GK, *et al*. Phase II study of sorafenib in patients with advanced hepatocellular carcinoma. *J Clin Oncol* 2006;**24**:4293–4300.

133. Cheng AL, *et al*. Efficacy and safety of sorafenib in patients in the Asia-Pacific region with advanced hepatocellular carcinoma: a phase III randomised, double-blind, placebo-controlled trial. *Lancet Oncol* 2009;**10**(1):25–34.

134. Kim JE, *et al*. Sorafenib for hepatocellular carcinoma according to Child-Pugh class of liver function. *Cancer Chemother Pharmacol* 2011 Nov; 68(5):1285–90. doi: 10.1007/s00280-011-1616-x. Epub 2011 Mar 29.

135. Hollebecque A, *et al*. Safety and efficacy of sorafenib in hepatocellular carcinoma: the impact of the Child-Pugh score. Aliment. *Pharmacol Ther* 2011;**34**(10):1193–1201.

136. Presta M, *et al*. (2005) Fibroblast growth factor/fibroblast growth factor receptor system in angiogenesis. *Cytokine Growth Factor Rev* 16:159–178.

137. Grose R, Dickson C (2005) Fibroblast growth factor signaling in tumorigenesis. *Cytokine Growth Factor Rev* 16:179–186.

138. Mise M, *et al*. (1996) Clinical significance of vascular endothelial growth factor and basic fibroblast growth factor gene expression in liver tumor. *Hepatology* 23:455–464.

139. Bergers G, Hanahan D (2008) Modes of resistance to anti-angiogenic therapy. *Nat Rev Cancer* 8:592–603.

140. Pàez-Ribes M, *et al*. (2009) Antiangiogenic therapy elicits malignant progression of tumors to increased local invasion and distant metastasis. *Cancer Cell* 15:220–231.

141. Wang L, *et al*. (2012) A novel monoclonal antibody to fibroblast growth factor 2 effectively inhibits growth of hepatocellular carcinoma xenografts. *Mol Cancer Ther* 11:864–872.

142. Cai ZW, *et al*. (2008) Discovery of brivanib alaninate ((S)-((R)-1-(4-(4-fluoro-2-methyl-1H-indol-5-yloxy)-5-methylpyrrolo[2,1-f][1,2,4]   triazin-6-yloxy) propan-2-yl)2-aminopropanoate), a novel prodrug of dual vascular endothelial growth factor receptor-2 and fibroblast growth factor receptor-1 kinase inhibitor (BMS-540215) *J Med Chem* **51**:1976–1980.

143. Huynh H, *et al*. (2008) Brivanib alaninate, a dual inhibitor of vascular endothelial growth factor receptor and fibroblast growth factor receptor tyrosine kinases, induces growth inhibition in mouse models of human hepatocellular carcinoma. *Clin Cancer Res* **14**:6146–6153.

144. Bhide RS, *et al*. (2010) The antiangiogenic activity in xenograft models of brivanib, a dual inhibitor of vascular endothelial growth factor receptor-2 and fibroblast growth factor receptor-1 kinases. *Mol Cancer Ther* **9**:369–378.

145. Park JW, *et al.* (2011) Phase II, open-label study of brivanib as first-line therapy in patients with advanced hepatocellular carcinoma. *Clin Cancer Res* **17**:1973–1983.

146. Finn RS, *et al.* (2012) Phase II, open-label study of brivanib as second-line therapy in patients with advanced hepatocellular carcinoma. *Clin Cancer Res* **18**:2090–2098.

147. Llovet JM, *et al.* (2013) Brivanib in patients with advanced hepatocellular carcinoma who were intolerant to sorafenib or for whom sorafenib failed: Results from the randomized phase III BRISK-PS study. *J Clin Oncol* **31**:3509–3516.

148. Johnson PJ, *et al.* Brivanib versus sorafenib as first-line therapy in patients with unresectable, advanced hepatocellular carcinoma: results from the randomized phase III BRISK-FL study. *J Clin Oncol* 2013 Oct 1;**31**(28):3517–3524. doi: 10.1200/ JCO.2012.48.4410. Epub 2013 Aug 26.

149. Cheng A-L, *et al.* Sunitinib versus sorafenib in advanced hepatocellular cancer: results of a randomized phase III trial. *J Clin Oncol* 2013;**31**:4067–75.

150. Cainap C, *et al.* Phase III trial of linifanib versus sorafenib in patients with advanced hepatocellular carcinoma (HCC). *J Clin Oncol* 2013;**31**(Suppl 4, abstr 249).

151. Chung YH, *et al.* Interim analysis of START: Study in Asia of the combination of TACE (transcatheter arterial chemoembolization) with sorafenib in patients with hepatocellular carcinoma trial. *Int J Cancer* 2013 May 15;**132**(10):2448–2458. doi: 10.1002/ijc.27925. Epub 2012 Nov 28.

Chapter 17

Cholangiocarcinoma and Gallbladder Cancer

Anuj Patel and Weijing Sun

1 Introduction

Biliary tract cancers are rare cancers resulting from malignant transformation of epithelial cells within the bile system. These cancers arise from the gallbladder and the bile duct system. Historically, the name *cholangiocarcinoma* was applied only to tumors arising from the intrahepatic bile ducts.[1] In recent use, however, the term refers to cancers of the entire biliary tree. Cholangiocarcinoma is divided into intrahepatic and extrahepatic, with extrahepatic further divided into hilar (or perihilar) and distal tumors. There is increasing recognition that these separate anatomic origins of biliary tract cancers have distinct biological and clinical characteristics.

2 Anatomy and Classification

Beginning with the individual bile ductules within each liver lobule, the biliary tree drains bile from the liver in an anastomosing system of ducts of increasing diameter. Segmental bile ducts drain each of the eight liver segments and join to form the left and right hepatic ducts. The left hepatic duct drains segments 2, 3, and 4 and the right hepatic duct drains segments 5, 6, 7, and 8; these exit the liver and join with receive bile ducts from segment 1 before joining in the liver hilum to form the common hepatic duct. The gallbladder lies underneath the right liver, in a fossa between the right and quadrate lobes. Bile flows to and from the gallbladder via the cystic duct. The common hepatic duct receives the cystic duct to form the common

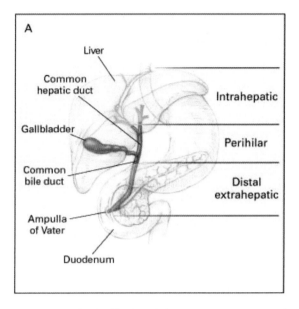

Figure 1   Anatomy and anatomic classification of biliary tract cancers. Adapted with permission from *N Engl J Med*. 1999;341(18):1368–1378.[1]

bile duct, which eventually joins with the pancreatic duct at the ampulla of Vater. There can be significant variations in this biliary anatomy.[2,3]

The second-order bile ducts act as the division point between intrahepatic and extrahepatic cholangiocarcinomas (Figure 1). The division between hilar and distal extrahepatic cholangiocarcinoma is generally made at the level of the cystic duct, though this is complicated by significant variability in this anastomotic site.

2.1 *Hilar classification*

Hilar cholangiocarcinoma can be further classified by tumor location and extent, according to the Bismuth–Corlette schema (Figure 2):

- Type I: Limited to the common hepatic duct, below the confluence of right and left hepatic ducts
- Type II: Involving the confluence of the right and left hepatic ducts.
- Type III: Involving the confluence and either the right (IIIA) or left (IIIB) hepatic duct, to their respective intrahepatic bifurcations
- Type IV: Involving confluence and both right and left hepatic ducts to their respective intrahepatic bifurcations OR multicentric disease

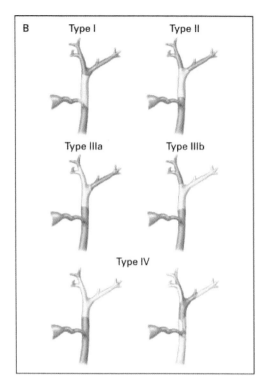

Figure 2 Bismuth–Corlette classification of perihilar cholangiocarcinomas. Yellow areas represent tumor, and green areas normal bile duct. Adapted with permission from *N Engl J Med.* 1999;341(18):1368–1378.[1]

This classification has traditionally been used to guide the choice of procedure when pursuing curative resection is possible (see Section 5.3 for details).[4]

2.2 Epidemiology

Biliary tract cancers represent 3–5% of all gastrointestinal malignancies.[5] Approximately 7,500 cases of biliary tract cancer are diagnosed in the United States every year; about 5,000 of these are gallbladder cancer, the remaining 2,000–3,000 are cholangiocarcinomas.[6] The distribution of new cases is heterogeneous across the world.[7]

Cholangiocarcinoma is the second most common primary hepatic malignancy, after hepatocellular carcinoma (HCC).[8] Incidence increases with age; the peak incidence is in the seventh decade of life and nearly 75% of cases occur at age 65 or later.[9,10] Age-adjusted incidence and mortality are both slightly higher in men.[10]

New cases in the United States are found most frequently in Hispanics and Asians, and least frequently in non-Hispanic whites and blacks.[10]

Extrahepatic tumors comprise the majority of cholangiocarcinoma diagnoses. Sixty to seventy percent are hilar tumors and 20–30% are distal extrahepatic tumors. Intrahepatic tumors are the least prevalent, representing only 5–10% of cases; intrahepatic cholangiocarcinoma does make up 10–20% of primary liver cancers[11]. Epidemiologic studies have shown that incidence of and mortality associated with intrahepatic cholangiocarcinoma are rising worldwide.[12–16] Conversely, rates of incidence and mortality from extrahepatic cholangiocarcinoma appear to be falling.[13,15] The reason for the increasing rate of intrahepatic cholangiocarcinoma is unclear, though studies show that this rise appears to be independent of misclassification or improved diagnostic techniques.[16]

Gallbladder cancer follows a prevalence pattern correlating with gallstone disease.[17] Unlike most cancers, gallbladder cancer is a female-predominant disease. Incidence is up to three times higher in women than in men.[18] Incidence and mortality also increase with age.[19] While rare in developed countries, very high rates of gallbladder cancer are seen in certain parts of South America and Asia, particularly regions of Chile, Bolivia, India, Ecuador, and Peru.[20,21] In the United States, gallbladder cancer rates are highest among Native Americans and Hispanics.[22]

2.2.1 *Risk factors for cholangiocarcinoma*

In the majority of patients with cholangiocarcinoma, no clear etiology or predisposing risk factor is found. While several risk factors for cholangiocarcinoma have been established, these are identified in less than 30% of all cases.[23]

In the United States, primary sclerosing cholangitis (PSC) is the most common and best-defined risk factor for cholangiocarcinoma. PSC is an autoimmune hepatobiliary disease characterized by chronic inflammation of the biliary tree. This inflammation can lead to biliary fibrosis and strictures, with resultant cholestasis. As the disease advances, progressive bile duct destruction and fibrosis leads to cirrhosis and end-stage liver disease. Unlike most autoimmune disorders, PSC is found more commonly in men, with a 2:1 predominance.[24] Greater than two-thirds of PSC is associated with an inflammatory bowel disease, particularly ulcerative colitis.[24,25]

Cholangiocarcinoma is the most fatal complication of PSC, occurring in approximately 8–13% of PSC patients.[26–29] Given this close relationship, many regard PSC as a premalignant condition. Even with this awareness, diagnosis of cholangiocarcinoma at early stages remains difficult. Many PSC patients are found to have cholangiocarcinoma following transplantation, despite extended pre-transplant evaluation.[27,30] Screening algorithms have been proposed and utilized for PSC patients, often incorporating imaging and tumor markers;[31–33] however, these approaches have not been validated and have been refuted by other studies.[34] Cholangiocarcinoma tends to present earlier in the setting of PSC, often between the ages of 30–50.[35,36] One-third to one-half of patients with PSC who develop cholangiocarcinoma are diagnosed within two years of their PSC diagnosis;[26,27] however, there does not appear to be an association between underlying cirrhosis or the duration of PSC and the incidence of cholangiocarcinoma.[27,35,37]

The most common cause of cholangiocarcinoma throughout Asia is liver fluke infection. Infection occurs primarily through ingestion of raw and uncooked fish.[38] Adult flukes enter the biliary system and lay eggs, also leading to chronic biliary inflammation. Two liver fluke species, *Opisthorchis viverrini* and *Clonorchis sinensis*, have been classified as Group 1 carcinogens by the International Agency for Research on Cancer.[39] In Northeast Thailand, where opisthorchitis is extremely common, cholangiocarcinoma is the most common malignancy. Data suggests that *O. viverrini* infection might be responsible for over two-thirds of the cholangiocarcinoma cases in that region.[40,41] *C. sinensis* is endemic in a number of other Asian countries, namely the Republic of Korea, China, Taiwan, and Vietnam, and has also been tied to the prevalence of cholangiocarcinoma.[42–45]

Certain other exposures have been clearly linked with cholangiocarcinoma. Chronic hepatolithiasis, or intrahepatic biliary stones, is another risk factor identified primary in Asia;[45–48] it is seen uncommonly in Western cholangiocarcinoma patients.[49] These calculi lead to intrahepatic cholestasis and are though to result in chronic inflammation and infection. Choledochal cysts have also been identified as a risk factor for cholangiocarcinoma. They are also seen more frequently in certain Asian populations.[50] These cysts are congenital cystic dilations of the bile ducts. Some forms of the cysts may predispose patients to the reflux of pancreatic enzymes which, when combined with stagnant bile and increased intraductal bile acid concentrations, lead to chronic inflammation and carcinogenesis.[50,51]

Thorotrast, a radioactive compound previously used as a radiocontrast agent, was found to be strongly associated with the development of cholangiocarcinoma. Thorotrast is no longer licensed for use; however, with a biological half-life of approximately 400 years, the risk for cholangiocarcinoma in exposed patients is delayed, with a latency period that may last over 50 years.[9]

Other potential carcinogens, including cigarette smoke and alcohol have been examined; however, these associations have not been clearly established and the findings are frequently inconsistent.[45,48,52–56] While hepatitis B virus (HBV) and hepatitis C virus (HCV) infections have been clearly associated with HCC, their relationship with cholangiocarcinoma has been less clear. More recent studies appear to show evidence for a relationship between HBV and HCV infection and cholangiocarcinoma in endemic regions of the world.[57,58]

2.2.2 *Risk factors for gallbladder cancer*

The most prominent risk factor for gallbladder cancer is a prior history of gall-stones, particularly chronic symptomatic gallstones. The large majority of patients with gallbladder cancer, 60–90%, have a history of cholelithiasis.[59] In studies of gallstone-associated gallbladder cancer, larger stone size, volume, and number appear to be associated with increased risk.[60] Some groups have proposed prophylactic cholecystectomy in patients following cholelithiasis in certain settings; however, most argue against it, given the overall rarity of malignancy.[61–64] Despite the high relative increase in risk associated with gallstone disease, gallbladder cancer only occurs in less than 3% of patients with cholelithiasis.[65]

Chronic infections of the gallbladder are also associated with gallbladder cancer. Chronic *Salmonella typhi* carrier state is the best reported of these infections and a key risk factor in endemic regions, conveying a 3–8 fold risk of gallbladder cancer.[66,67] Increased levels of of DNA and RNA from *Helicobacter* species have been found in the bile of patients with gallbladder cancer, though it is unclear whether this relationship is causative or simply representative of increased colonization in endemic regions with high rates of gallbladder cancer.[68–71]

Calcification of the gallbladder wall, or porcelain gallbladder, occurs as an uncommon result of chronic gallbladder inflammation. Traditionally, it has been seen as an indication for cholecystectomy due to an increased risk of gallbladder cancer. More recent studies, however, have argued that this risk — if present — is much lower than previously believed.[72–75]

Anomalous junction of the pancreaticobiliary duct has also been held as an indication for prophylactic cholecystectomy.[76] This variation in the pancreatic outflow can lead to chronic reflux of pancreatic secretions into the biliary tree. Pancreatobiliary maljunction can be seen in 10–20% of Asian patients with gall-bladder cancer.[77–79]

Obesity has also been clearly linked with increased incidence and mortality from gallbladder cancer;[80,81] this risk appears to persist independent of the increased rate of gallstones in obese patients.[82] Diabetes mellitus may also be a risk factor for gallbladder cancer, though this association is confounded by the relationships between diabetes, obesity, and gallstones.[56,83] Cigarette smoking has also been linked with gallbladder cancer mortality.[56,84]

2.3 *Pathology*

Classically, biliary tract cancers appear microscopically as mucin-producing adeno-carcinomas within a prominent desmoplastic and hypovascularized stroma.[85] Histologically, over 90% of biliary tract cancers are adenocarcinomas. Squamous cell and adenosquamous carcinomas are the second most common, with small cell carcinomas, sarcomas, and lymphomas found rarely. Adenocarcinomas are divided by histologic grade, as well-, moderately-, or poorly-differentiated, based on the remaining glandular structure seen in the tumor.

Intrahepatic cholangiocarcinoma can be subdivided by macroscopic growth patterns into four subtypes: mass-forming, periductal-infiltrating, intraductal, and undefined.[86] The mass-forming subtype is the most common form and presents as a defined mass located within the liver parenchyma. At earlier stages, mass-forming intrahepatic cholangiocarcinoma metastasizes through the liver through the portal venous system, in a manner similar to HCC.[87] Only at later stages does it tend to involve the lymphatic vessels and spread along Glisson's sheath. The periductal-infiltrating subtype generally grows via infiltration along the axis of the bile duct, occasionally extending into surrounding blood vessels or liver parenchyma.[88] This bile duct involvement can often result in dilatation of more peripheral intrahepatic bile ducts. Periductal-infiltrating tumors frequently spread within Glisson's sheath, again via the lymphatic vessels. Intraductal tumors grow toward and within the lumen of the bile duct and can often form papillary or tubular polypoid lesions.[89] Outcomes for intrahepatic cholangiocarcinoma following resection appears to vary by subtype and different surgical approaches for each subtype have been suggested.[90–93] The intraductal subtype is associated with the best prognosis;[51] mass-forming and periductal-infiltrating tumors appear to have generally poorer outcomes, though it is unclear whether one is significantly worse than the other.[88,92,94,95] Mixed forms of these macroscopic substypes are also seen. The mass-forming plus periductal-infiltrating subtype is commonly encountered and appears to have significantly higher rates of recurrence following resection and overall poorer survival.[96,97]

Extrahepatic cholangiocarcinoma can also be classified by macroscopic appearance. It is most commonly subdivided into nodular, sclerosing (or periductal-infiltrating), and papillary forms;[98] these correspond approximately to their intrahepatic analogues. Approximately 70% of hilar cholangiocarcinoma is of the sclerosing subtype. It is characterized by longitudinal bile duct involvement and extensive fibrosis of the surrounding tissue. Nodular extrahepatic cholangiocarcinoma presents with a defined mass protruding from the ductal mucosa. Papillary tumors protrude into the lumen with characteristic cauliflower-like masses. The papillary subtype is both the least common form and the form associated with the best overall prognosis.[99]

In both intrahepatic and extrahepatic cholangiocarcinoma, the intraductal or papillary subtypes appear have to have significantly better prognosis. There has been increasing evidence that papillary cholangiocarcinoma represents a biliary intraductal papillary mucinous neoplasm (IPMN), with features in common with pancreatic IPMN.[100,101,102] Both mucin-producing and non-mucin producing papillary lesions were adopted together as a distinct entity in the 2010 World Health Organization (WHO) classification as intraductal papillary neoplasm of the bile duct.

2.3.1 Molecular pathogenesis

Recent studies have begun to uncover the genetic and molecular processes underlying carcinogenesis in the bile ducts and gallbladder. These paint the picture of the repetitive accumulation of mutations in rapidly proliferating cells in the setting of chronic inflammation or infection.

Genomic profiling has demonstrated characteristic profiles for intrahepatic and extrahepatic cholangiocarcinoma. Next generation sequencing of a series of biliary tract cancers showed key variations in certain mutations based on tumor location.[103] Highlighted in this series were the specificity for IDH1/2 and FGFR mutations for intrahepatic cholangiocarcinoma. Similar findings had been noted in earlier studies. Mutations in the IDH1 and IDH2 genes have consistently been shown to be more frequent in intrahepatic versus extrahepatic cholangiocarcinoma or gallbladder carcinoma.[104–106]. In a genetically-engineered mouse model, IDH mutations caused inhibition of HNF-4α, leading to impaired hepatocyte differentiation and increased cell proliferation.[107] In human cholangiocarcinoma, these mutations have been associated with clear cell change, poorly differentiated histology[104] and, in one series, longer time-to-recurrence and overall survival.[108]

Intrahepatic specificity of FGFR mutations, specifically in FGFR2, has also been noted previously.[109,110] In one series, FGFR2 mutations were associated with the production of two fusion kinase genes, FGFR2-AHCYL1 and FGFR2-BICC1, and were mutually exclusive with KRAS/BRAF mutations. Following xenografts of these mutated cells into immunocompromised mice, treatment with the FGFR kinase inhibitors suppressed tumor transformation.[109] In one series, median cancer-specific survival was significantly longer for patients whose tumors contained FGFR2 translocations.[110]

Mutational profiles also appear to be influenced by etiology. In one example, Chan-on et al. revealed the results of exome sequencing of 209 cholangiocarcinoma samples from Asia and Europe.[106] One hundred eight of the cases had been caused by infection with the O. viverrini; the other 101 cases had been caused by non-O. viverrini-related etiologies. Whole-exome sequencing was performed on a discover set of 15 samples; fifteen genes were then selected for prevalence screening on the remaining 194 samples. This process had been validated on 54 samples, previously reported and included in this analysis.[111] TP53 was mutated in 40% of cholangiocarcinoma samples caused by O. viverrini, significantly higher when compared to 9% in the non-O. viverrini samples (p < 0.001). SMAD4 was mutated more frequently in non-*O. viverrini* cholangiocarcinomas (6% vs 19%, p = 0.006). IDH1 and IDH2 mutations were seen in 22.2% of non-*O. viverrini* intrahepatic cholangiocarcinoma samples and only 3.2% of *O. viverrini*-related intrahepatic cholangiocarcinom.

Activating mutations in cell proliferation oncogenes lead to uncontrolled cell growth and survival. The Ras/MAPK signaling pathway plays a key role in cell growth, differentiation, survival, and migration. Gain-of-function mutations in KRAS are present in approximately 45–55% of intrahepatic cholangiocarcinomas and 10–15% of extrahepatic cholangiocarcinomas.[112–116] BRAF, an important downstream effector of KRAS, was found to be mutated in 22% of intrahepatic cholangiocarcinomas post-hepatectomy.[114] In the same study, no tumors with KRAS mutations had BRAF mutations; however, KRAS mutations were seen in 20% of tumors with BRAF mutations. The ErbB family consists of 4 receptor kinases, including ErbB1 (or EGFR) and ErbB2 (or HER2). In one study, mutations in the EGFR gene were seen in 15% of cholangiocarcinoma cases.[117] MET is an oncogene that encodes for the hepatocyte growth factor (HGF) receptor. Preclinical and clinical data have suggested a role for the MET/HGF pathway in the development and progression of cholangiocarcinoma.[118] Studies have demonstrated MET overexpression by immunohistochemistry in over 80% of intrahepatic cholangiocarcinomas.[119,120]

Loss-of-function mutations in tumor suppressor genes also play a role in cholangiocarcinogenesis. CDKN2A negatively regulates proliferation in normal cells and is capable of cell cycle arrest. This tumor suppressor gene was highly mutated in reports from two studies, with 55% loss-of-function in intrahepatic cholangiocarcinoma and 83% in extrahepatic cholangiocarcinoma.[113] TP53 is one of the principal regulators of cell division. It appears to be inactivated in approximately one-third of cholangiocarcinoma, both intra- and extrahepatic. SMAD4, in conjunction with the other SMAD proteins, is an end effector in the TGFβ pathway, directly regulating the activity of genes controlling cell proliferation. In cholangiocarcinoma, TGFβ promotes epithelial-mesenchymal transition, a key process in multiple malignancies.[121] Mutations in SMAD4 were described in 4–20% of cholangiocarcinomas.[111,122]

3 Diagnosis

3.1 *Clinical presentation*

The majority of patients with cholangiocarcinoma or gallbladder cancer are diagnosed with late-stage disease, as they are generally asymptomatic at early stages. Late-stage presentation varies by tumor location.[123] With hilar and distal extrahepatic tumors, symptoms of hyperbilirubinemia due to biliary obstruction are the most common causes for initial presentation; these include painless jaundice, pruritus, dark urine, and pale stools. Intrahepatic tumors, conversely, generally do not develop significant hyperbilirubinemia, as the liver is able to compensate for unilateral intrahepatic bile duct obstruction. Rather, these patients generally present with nonspecific symptoms of malignancy, such as fatigue, weight loss, abdominal pain, fever, and night sweats.

3.2 *Laboratory studies*

Laboratory tests are usually most notable for findings of cholestatic liver injury, particularly elevated serum bilirubin, alkaline phosphatase and gamma-glutamyl transpeptidase; transaminase levels may also be moderately elevated.

Serum tumor markers are often ordered and may help guide diagnosis; however, none of these markers are specific for cholangiocarcinoma. The most commonly elevated serum markers are carbohydrate antigen (CA) 19–9, carcinoembryonic antigen (CEA), and CA-125. Changes in serum CA19-9 are commonly monitored with treatment and used as a surrogate for response. However, both the sensitivity and specificity of CA19-9 and CEA are limited for biliary tract cancers.[124,125] Both markers can be elevated in nonmalignant conditions, including PSC, pancreatitis, and cirrhosis. Also, CA 19-9 is related to the Lewis blood group antigens. Those 7–10% of the population negative for the Lewis blood group antigen are generally unable to produce CA 19-9 at all.[126]

Serum and biliary immunoglobulin G4 (IgG4) levels may also be tested to help rule out IgG4-associated cholangiopathy, an inflammatory disorder which can involve the pancreatic and bile ducts. IgG4-associated cholangiopathy can mimic cholangiocarcinoma and should be excluded in suspected cases.[127] Studies have proposed cutoffs of serum IgG4 to distinguish between the two diseases;[128,129] these approaches require validation.

3.3 *Radiographic studies*

The most common study ordered on presentation with jaundice, right-upper quadrant abdominal pain, or cholestatic lab studies is an abdominal ultrasound. Ultrasound can be useful in ruling out other causes of biliary obstruction, such as calculi;[130] however, it has limited sensitivity or specificity for diagnosing cholangiocarcinoma, particularly intrahepatic disease.[131,132] Doppler ultrasound can help assess for tumor-related vascular compression, invasion, or thrombosis.[133,134] Ultrasonography does have an increased role in the diagnosis of gallbladder cancer,

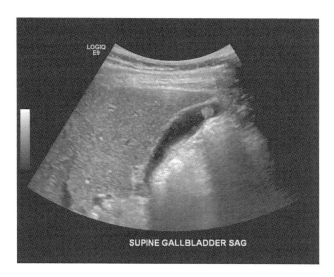

Figure 3   Ultrasound demonstrating a gallbladder polyp.

as certain findings on ultrasound may specifically distinguish between benign and malignant gallbladder disease (Figure 3).[135,136]

Computed tomography (CT) with intravenous contrast appears to have higher sensitivity for cholangiocarcinoma diagnosis than ultrasound, but still remains limited in assessing the extent and structure of tumor involvement. CT does, however, provide critical information regarding disease staging of both cholangiocarcinoma and gallbladder cancer, through the identification of lymphadenopathy and distal metastases (Figure 4). It can also provide evaluation of vascular and adjacent organ involvement.[137] Triphasic CT, including arterial phase, venous phase, and equilibrium phase imaging can also be helpful in distinguishing intrahepatic cholangiocarcinoma masses from HCC.[89]

Evaluation of the bile ducts through cholangiography is critical in diagnosing and assessing cholangiocarcinoma. Magnetic resonance imaging (MRI) with magnetic resonance cholangiography (MRCP) is useful, noninvasive study which provides an initial alternative to invasive cholangiographic procedures. These procedure, endoscopic retrograde cholangiography (ERCP) and percutaneous transhepatic cholangiography (PTC), are required if a therapeutic intervention is required and ERCP is often necessary for brush cytology and biopsy. All forms of cholangiography provide crucial three-dimensional images that can detect subtle ductal involvement not seen in other forms of imaging (Figure 5). Conversely, the gallbladder is not routinely visualized on cholangiography. The MRI component of the procedure, however, can provide critical information regarding hepatic and bile duct invasion and lymph node involvement.[138]

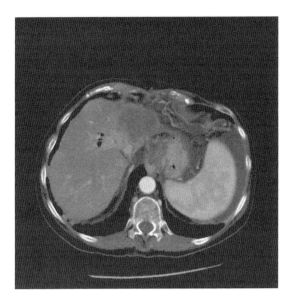

Figure 4 Contrast-enhanced computed tomography (CT) showing left hepatic mass from cholangiocarcinoma.

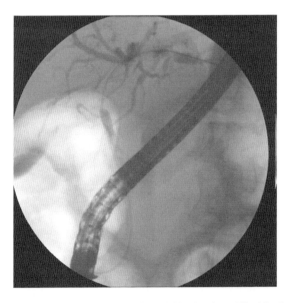

Figure 5 Endoscopic retrograde cholangiography (ERCP) showing a hilar bile duct stricture concerning for cholangiocarcinoma.

Endoscopic ultrasound (EUS) is increasingly becoming a standard component of diagnosis and staging. EUS has increased sensitivity and specificity for cholangiocarcinoma, when compared to extracorporeal ultrasound, and is the most sensitive method for diagnosing hilar cholangiocarcinoma.[139] It also provides key information for T staging of gallbladder cancer.[140,141] It also allows for evaluation and aspiration of regional lymphadenopathy and gallbladder masses; aspiration does increase sensitivity.[142,143] There is some limited concern, however, that routine aspiration might lead to tumor displacement and seeding of needle track.[144]

Positron emission tomography (PET) has an unclear role in the diagnosis of biliary tract cancers. PET appears to be sensitive and specific for the diagnosis of the primary tumor and of distant metastases in cholangiocarcinoma. In gallbladder cancer, it can help distinguish benign and malignant findings from other imaging modalities.[145,146] In both settings, however, it has shown poor sensitivity for evaluating regional lymph node involvement.[147–150] PET appears to be more sensitive to intrahepatic tumors than extrahepatic tumors. False-positive studies have been reported in the setting of chronic inflammation, such as in patients with PSC or active infection.[149,150] Mucinous tumors with extensive mucin deposition may have also false negative PET scans, due to poor FDG uptake.[150]

4 Staging

Three major staging systems exist for cholangiocarcinoma: the American Joint Cancer Committee (AJCC)/Union for International Cancer Control (UICC), the Liver Cancer Study Group of Japan (LCSGJ), and the National Cancer Center of Japan (NCCJ). The most recent 7th edition of the AJCC/ UICC staging system now has separate staging for intrahepatic, hilar, and distal extrahepatic cholangiocarcinomas, distinct from each other and from primary HCC (Tables 1a-c). This system is the only one which has a separate staging schema for distal extrahepatic tumors.

Significant efforts have focused on improving assessment of prognosis and resectability in hilar cholangiocarcinoma. As noted previously, the Bismuth–Corlette classification schema provides a description of tumor location and extent in hilar cholangiocarcinoma. It is not a staging system, however, and does not predict outcomes associated with resection or survival. The most recent AJCC/UICC TNM staging system addressed this to some degree by separating hilar and distal extrahepatic disease and by expanding on the definitions for tumor extension and lymph node involvement. This new edition does better predict survival, but still lacks discrimination with early and intermediate T stage tumors.[151,152] Staging systems have been proposed which incorporate location and extent of bile duct involvement, tumor size, portal vein and hepatic artery involvement, hepatic lobar

Table 1a.   AJCC/UICC TNM staging for intrahepatic bile duct tumors.

	Stage	T	N	M
T: Primary Tumor	Stage 0	Tis	N0	M0
TX: Primary tumor cannot be assessed	Stage I	T1	N0	M0
T0: No evidence of primary tumor				
Tis: Carcinoma *in situ* (intraductal tumor)	Stage II	T2	N0	M0
T1: Solitary tumor without vascular invasion	Stage III	T3	N0	M0
T2a: Solitary tumor with vascular invasion				
T2b: Multiple tumors, with or without vascular invasion	Stage IVA	T4	N0	M0
T3: Tumor perforating the visceral peritoneum or		Any T	N1	M0
involving the local extra hepatic structures by direct	Stage IVB	Any T	Any N	M1
invasion				
T4: Tumor with periductal invasion				

N: Regional Lymph Nodes
NX: Regional lymph nodes cannot be assessed
N0:   No regional lymph node metastasis
N1:   Regional lymph node metastasis present

M: Distant Metastasis
M0:   No distant metastasis
M1:   Distant metastasis present

Table 1b   AJCC/UICC TNM staging for perihilar bile duct tumors.

	Stage	T	N	M
T: Primary Tumor	Stage 0	Tis	N0	M0
TX: Primary tumor cannot be assessed	Stage I	T1	N0	M0
T0: No evidence of primary tumor				
Tis: Carcinoma *in situ*	Stage II	T2	N0	M0
T1: Tumor confined to the bile duct, with extension up	Stage IIIA	T3	N0	M0
to the muscle layer or fibrous tissue	Stage IIIB	T1-3	N1	M0
T2a: Tumor invades beyond the wall of the bile duct to				
surrounding adipose tissue	Stage IVA	T4	N0-1	M0
T2b: Tumor invades adjacent hepatic parenchyma	Stage IVB	Any T	N2	M0
T3: Tumor invades unilateral branches of the PV or HA				
T4: Tumor invades main portal vein or its branches		Any T	Any N	M1
bilaterally; or the common HA; or the 2nd-order				
biliary radicals bilaterally; or unilateral 2nd-order				
biliary radicals with contralateral PV or HA				
involvement				

(Continued)

Table 1b (*Continued*)

	Stage	T	N	M

N: Regional Lymph Nodes

NX: Regional lymph nodes cannot be assessed

N0: No regional lymph node metastasis

N1: Regional lymph node metastasis (including nodes along the cystic duct, common bile duct, HA, and PV)

N2: Metastasis to periaortic, pericaval, superior mesenteric artery, and/or celiac artery lymph nodes

M: Distant Metastasis

M0: No distant metastasis

M1: Distant metastasis present

Abbreviations: PV, portal vein; HA, hepatic artery.

Table 1c AJCC/UICC TNM staging for distal bile duct tumors.

	Stage	T	N	M
T: Primary Tumor	Stage 0	Tis	N0	M0
TX: Primary tumor cannot be assessed	Stage IA	T1	N0	M0
T0: No evidence of primary tumor				
Tis: Carcinoma *in situ*	Stage IB	T2	N0	M0
T1: Tumor confined to the bile duct histologically	Stage IIA	T3	N0	M0
T2: Tumor invades beyond the wall of the bile duct				
T3: Tumor invades the gallbladder, pancreas, duodenum,	Stage IIB	T1	N1	M0
or other adjacent organs without involvement of the		T2	N1	M0
celiac axis, or the superior mesenteric artery		T3	N1	M0
T4: Tumor involves the celiac axis, or the superior	Stage III	T4	Any N	M0
mesenteric artery	Stage IV	Any T	Any N	M1

N: Regional Lymph Nodes

N0: No regional lymph node metastasis

N1: Regional lymph node metastasis present

M: Distant Metastasis

M0: No distant metastasis

M1: Distant metastasis present

Table 1d   AJCC/UICC TNM staging for gallbladder cancer.

	Stage	T	N	M
T: Primary Tumor	Stage 0	Tis	N0	M0
TX: Primary tumor cannot be assessed	Stage I	T1	N0	M0
T0: No evidence of primary tumor				
Tis: Carcinoma *in situ*	Stage II	T2	N0	M0
T1a: Tumor invades lamina propria	Stage IIIA	T3	N0	M0
T1b: Tumor invades muscle layer				
T2: Tumor invades perimuscular connective tissue; no	Stage IIIB	T1-3	N1	M0
extension beyond serosa or into liver	Stage IVA	T4	N0-1	M0
T3: Tumor perforates the serosa and/or directly invades	Stage IVB	Any T	N2	M0
the liver and/or one other adjacent organ or structures				
T4: Tumor invades main portal vein or hepatic artery or		Any T	Any N	M1
invades two or more extrahepatic organs or structures				

N: Regional Lymph Nodes
N0:   No regional lymph node metastasis
N1:   Regional lymph node metastasis present

M: Distant Metastasis
M0:   No distant metastasis
M1:   Distant metastasis present

atrophy, macroscopic subtype, liver remnant volume post-resection, and underlying liver disease.[153,154]

The AJCC system is currently the primary staging system utilized in the literature for gallbladder cancer (Table 1d). Two older staging systems for gallbladder cancer include the modified Nevin system and the Japanese Biliary Surgical Society (JBSS) system have also been used. The modified Nevin system places more emphasis on lymph node metastases, compared with the AJCC and JBSS systems, rating all patients with nodal involvement as stage IV (out of five stages). Conversely, the JBSS schema has patients with early nodal involvement classified as only stage II. The most recent 7th edition added major vascular or nearby organ invasion as criteria for stage IV disease.

5 Surgical Resection

As in the majority of solid tumors, surgical resection remains the only potentially curative treatment option for cancers of the biliary tract. Due to the complicated anatomy of the biliary tree and adjacent structures, and the propensity for patients to remain asymptomatic until later-stage disease, less than 35% of biliary tract tumors are resectable at presentation. The nature of the surgery required depends both on the site of the tumor and its degree of spread.

5.1 *Intrahepatic cholangiocarcinoma*

Surgical resection in intrahepatic cholangiocarcinoma follows similar paradigms to liver surgery for HCC and hepatic metastases from other malignancies. As in those diseases, a primary goal of preoperative planning is to identify the amount and nature of resection required to achieve negative surgical margins, or an R0 resection. Compared with HCC, intrahepatic cholangiocarcinoma more often arises in normal underlying liver parenchyma,[155] allowing for larger portions of the liver to be safely resected. The majority of patients require hemihepatectomy.[156] When more extensive resection is required, portal vein embolization may be considered prior to surgery to increase residual liver volume.

Five-year overall survival following resection in intrahepatic cholangiocarcinoma varies widely, generally between 15% and 50% in more recent series.[94,95,157–166] The two factors dominating overall survival are positive surgical margins and lymph node involvement; other described prognostic factors include age, tumor size, intrahepatic metastases, macroscopic growth pattern, tumor differentiation, and preoperative CA19-9 levels.[94,95,158–160,164–167] Despite the clear prognostic implications of regional lymph node involvement, the role of routine lymphadenectomy with hepatic resection is not clearly understood, with conflicting data regarding its benefit.[168–170]

5.2 *Distal cholangiocarcinoma*

The resectability rate for distal extrahepatic cholangiocarcinoma is generally higher than with intrahepatic or hilar disease.[171] The standard surgery for distal resection is the Whipple procedure, or pancreatoduodenectomy. In certain settings, when the tumor is limited to the biliary tree without extension to the duodenum, a pylorus-sparing surgery may also be considered. In either case, regional lymphadenectomy is a standard component of surgery in this setting.

Five-year survival following resection in distal cholangiocarcinoma ranges between 20% and 40% are generally better than intrahepatic disease.[172–176] As with intrahepatic disease surgical margins and lymph node involvement are key determinants of survival; tumor differentiation and perineural invasion may also be prognostic factors.[173,176]

5.3 *Hilar cholangiocarcinoma*

Recently reported 5-year survival after surgery in hilar cholangiocarcinoma has ranged from 13% and 40% in larger series.[177] Klatskin tumors present specific obstacles for surgical planning and resection.[171] Their location often makes staging and determination of resectability difficult. Moreover, the surgery itself is often complicated, involving components of liver resection, biliary resection with anastomosis, and vascular reconstructions. Preoperative biliary drainage or portal vein embolization often have to be considered prior to surgery as well.

The Bismuth–Corlette classification, described above, was designed to help guide surgical planning and is often used to help determine the type of resection needed.[4] Type I and II tumors require *en bloc* resection of the extrahepatic bile duct, gallbladder with regional lymphadenectomy, and Roux-en-Y hepaticojejunostomy. Type III tumors require the addition of a right or left hepatectomy, in addition to aforementioned procedures. For type IV disease, an extended right or left hepatectomy is required, in addition to aforementioned procedures for types I and II tumors.

Hilar cholangiocarcinoma often involves some degree of vascular involvement. Previously, portal vein or hepatic artery invasion was generally considered a contraindication to resection; however, vascular resection and reconstruction are increasingly being performed as a part of surgery with curative intent in select patients, though the associated benefit remains controversial.[178–181]

5.4 *Gallbladder cancer*

The surgical approach for gallbladder cancer depends on the extent of local progression. In-situ carcinoma, involving only the gallbladder mucosa, and T1a disease, invading into the lamina propria, may be appropriate for simple cholecystectomy.[182] With T2 or greater disease, invading into or beyond the perimuscular layer of the gallbladder, or with any evidence of regional lymph node involvement, optimal resection includes cholecystectomy, regional lymphadenectomy, and resection of hepatic segments IVB and V. Management of T1b tumors remain unclear.[182–186] Gallbladder cancer is often found incidentally, either intraoperatively during cholecystectomy or on pathology evaluation following cholecystectomy. For cancer discovered during cholecystectomy, guidelines recommend conversion to an extended cholecystectomy if the tumor appears appropriate for curative resection; this may be dependent on the surgical expertise available. Patients with T1a disease found incidentally after the procedure can be safely observed.[187] More advanced tumors, which are considered resectable, generally benefit from a second operation for completion lymphadenectomy and limited hepatic resection[184,186–188]. Staging laparoscopy may play an important role in determining resectability, given a high prevalence of distant lymph node involvement and peritoneal metastases.[189,190]

5.5 *Adjunct operative procedures*

Preoperative biliary drainage can be performed in selected cases to relieve biliary obstruction prior to surgery. Its role as a routine component of surgical resection, however, is controversial. Preoperative obstructive jaundice has been associated with increased postoperative mortality.[191] Studies, however, have failed to demonstrate a benefit in morbidity or mortality from preoperative biliary drainage.[192] Moreover, drainage is associated with complications including acute cholangitis, acute pancreatitis, and bleeding.[193–195] There is also concern that percutaneous transhepatic biliary drainage may be associated with peritoneal tumor seeding;[196,197] endoscopic biliary drainage may serve as an alternative to a percutaneous approach.

Selective embolization of a portal vein prior to resection can induce a compensatory hypertrophy of the remaining liver. This is sometimes performed to increase residual volume of the liver remnant in patients requiring extensive liver resection, with the goal of preventing postoperative liver failure. Residual volume less than 40% is often used as an indication for portal vein embolization (PVE).[198,199] Studies have shown that preoperative PVE can be performed safely, without increases in perioperative mortality.[200,201] And while PVE does effectively increase residual liver volume, its effect on survival remains unclear.[200–203]

5.6 *Adjuvant therapy*

Disease recurrence patterns following surgery differ between cholangiocarcinoma and gallbladder cancer. In cholangiocarcinoma, recurrence is primarily local, while gallbladder cancer tends to recur distally.[204,205] Both radiotherapy and systemic chemotherapy have been evaluated in an adjuvant role; however, the data supporting these therapies is primarily retrospective (Table 2). Both the National Comprehensive Cancer Network (NCCN) and European Society for Medical Oncology (ESMO) guidelines recommend consideration of adjuvant treatment following surgical resection in certain settings, such as the presence of either positive resection margins or positive lymph nodes.[206,207] A majority of practitioners incorporate adjuvant chemotherapy and/or radiation in their management of resected hilar cholangiocarcinoma and gallbladder cancer, particularly in the Americas.[208,209]

Table 2   Selected comparative studies of adjuvant therapy in cholangiocarcinoma and gallbladder cancer.

Study	Pt Dx	n	Adjuvant Therapy	Results
Schoenthaler et al. 1994[210]	CC	45	RT [EBRT]	mOS: 11mo vs 14mo vs 6.5mo
		22	RT [CP]	
		45	none	
Pitt et al. 1995[211]	HiCC	14	RT	mOS: 20mo vs 20mo [NS]
		17	none	
Todoroki et al. 2000[212]	HiCC [R1]	28	RT	mOS: 32mo vs 10mo
		19	none	5yOS: 33.9% vs 13.5%
Serafini et al. 2001[213]	CC	34	CRT	mOS: 42mo vs 29mo [NS]
		50	none	DCC: mOS: 41mo vs 25mo
Gerhards et al. 2003[214]	HiCC	71	RT	mOS: 24mo vs 8mo
		20	none	
Takada et al. 2002[215]	CC	58	CT	5yDFS 20.7% vs 15.0% [NS]
		60	none	5yOS: 26.7% vs 24.1% [NS]
	GBC	69	CT	5yDFS: 20.3% vs 11.6%
		43	none	5yOS 26.0% vs 14.4%
Sagawa et al. 2005[216]	HiCC	39	RT	mOS: 23mo vs 20mo [NS]
		30	none	5yOS: 24% vs 30% [NS]
Balachandran et al. 2006[217]	GBC	73	CRT	mOS: 24mo vs 11mo
		44	none	5yOS: 35% vs 16%
Mojica et al. 2007[218]	GBC	1930	RT/CRT	mOS: 14mo vs 8mo
		395	none	
Wang et al. 2008[219]	GBC	3420	RT/CRT	mOS: 15mo vs 8mo
		760	none	
Borghero et al. 2008[220]	EHCC	42	CRT	mOS: 32mo vs 31mo;
		23	none	5yOS: 36% vs 42% [NS]
Gold et al. 2009[221]	GBC [stage I or II]	25	CRT	mOS: 4.8yrs vs 4.2yrs [NS]
		48	none	
Shinohara et al. 2009[222]	EHCC	701	RT	mOS: 16.0mo vs 9.0mo
		1372	none	HR 0.91 [NS]
Murakami et al. 2009[223]	CC, GBC	50	CT	5yOS: 57% vs 24%
		53	none	
Wirasorn et al. 2013[224]	CC	138	CT	mOS: 21.6 vs 13.4;
		125	none	3yOS: 40.1% vs 29.4%

Abbreviations: Pt Dx, patient diagnosis; CC, cholangiocarcinoma; RT, radiation therapy; EBRT, external beam radiation therapy; CP, charged-particle; mOS, median overall survival; HiCC, hilar cholangiocarcinoma; NS, not significant; R1, R1 resection; 5yOS, 5-year overall survival; CRT, chemoradiation; DCC, distal cholangiocarcinoma; CT, chemotherapy; 5yDFS, 5-year disease-free survival; GBC, gallbladder cancer; EHCC, extrahepatic cholangiocarcinoma; HR, hazard ratio; 3yOS, 3-year overall survival.

Despite this widespread use of adjuvant therapy, however, no survival benefit for this approach has been proven in a randomized trial.

Only one phase III trial has been completed in this setting.[215] 508 patients with resected pancreatobiliary cancers were randomized to surgery followed by adjuvant chemotherapy with 5-fluorouracil (5-FU) and mitomycin C versus surgery alone; 279 of these patients had cholangiocarcinoma or gallbladder cancer. Subgroup analyses were performed based on tumor type. Only in those patients with gallbladder cancer did treatment with adjuvant chemotherapy demonstrate a significant improvement in 5-year disease-free survival (20.3% vs 11.6%; p = 0.021). In patients with cholangiocarcinoma, a nonsignificant trend towards improved disease-free survival was seen.

In a meta-analysis of studies between 1960 and 2010, Horgan *et al.* studied the benefit of adjuvant therapy in biliary tract cancers.[225] They reviewed 20 studies involving 6,712 patients, which compared either adjuvant chemotherapy, radiotherapy, or combination chemoradiation following curative resection with resection alone. In the overall pooled data, there was trend towards improved survival in patients who received adjuvant therapy following resection, compared with those who underwent surgery alone (OR 0.74; p = 0.06). Survival benefit was significantly higher in patients who received chemotherapy (OR 0.39; p < 0.01) or chemoradiation (OR 0.61; p = 0.049), when compared to those who received radiotherapy alone (OR 0.98; p = 0.90). There was no difference between patients with cholangiocarcinomas or with gallbladder cancers. Patients with node-positive disease (OR 0.49; p = 0.004) and positive surgical margins (OR 0.36; p = 0.002) derived the greatest benefit from adjuvant therapy. Seventy-seven percent of those patients with lymph node involvement received chemotherapy alone; the remainder received chemoradiation. Sixty-three percent of those patients with positive surgical margins received radiotherapy alone.

5.7 *Liver transplantation*

Early outcomes for orthotopic liver transplantation as a treatment option for cholangiocarcinoma were poor, with high rates of disease recurrence and low rates of survival. Unfavorable results were described in a number of retrospective series[30,226–231]. Because of this, cholangiocarcinoma has been frequently listed as a contraindication to transplantation at most centers. More recently, research has focused on the combination of neoadjuvant radiotherapy and chemotherapy prior to liver transplantation, particularly in hilar cholangiocarcinoma. In a study from the University of Nebraska, 17 patients with localized hilar cholangiocarcinoma were treated with a neoadjuvant chemoradiation protocol consisting of intraluminal bile duct brachytherapy and continuous intravenous 5-flourouracil (5-FU) daily until transplantation.[232] Forty-five percent of patients were alive without evidence of disease recurrence at the time of publication. This concept for neoadjuvant therapy was adopted and modified by the Mayo Clinic for liver transplantation in a select population of hilar cholangiocarcinoma patients.[233] Patients with either unresectable locally-advanced hilar cholangiocarcinoma or resectable cholangiocarcinoma arising in the setting of PSC were treated with concurrent chemoradiation with external beam radiation therapy (EBRT) followed by intraluminal bile duct brachytherapy; daily continuous intravenous 5-FU was given through the radiation phase, capecitabine was then given daily until the peri-transplantation period. In a description of the outcomes of patients treated under this protocol, 5-year survival for all patients entering the protocol was 54%; five-year survival following transplantation was 73%. These results, while promising, were obtained under tightly controlled research protocols in very select patient populations and require validation.

5.8 Locoregional therapy

As noted, the majority of biliary tract cancers are unresectable at presentation. Major causes of death for locally-advanced disease, in cholangiocarcinoma particularly, are liver failure or refractory biliary obstruction with associated cholangitis. An increasing numbers of techniques are being developed for locoregional control of disease.

5.8.1 Radiation therapy

There is limited data regarding the role of radiation therapy, with or without chemotherapy, in unresectable cholangiocarcinoma (Table 3). Radiotherapy generally takes three forms in cholangiocarcinoma: EBRT, sterotactic beam radiotherapy (SBRT), and brachytherapy with iridium-192; intraoperative radiotherapy (IORT) can also be administered. Palliative radiotherapy has frequently been combined with chemotherapy, primarily fluoropyrimidine-based regimens.

5.8.2 Transarterial chemoembolization

Transarterial chemoembolization (TACE) is a mainstay of locoregional treatment in primary HCC and metastases to the liver, particularly from colorectal cancer. Studies have also demonstrated a role for TACE in unresectable cholangiocarcinoma (Table 4). TACE acts on hepatic tumors through two primary mechanisms. Embolization of the hepatic arteries supplying the tumor disrupts oxygen and nutrient delivery to malignant tissue. The local concentration of chemotherapy delivered

Table 3 Selected studies of radiation therapy in biliary tract cancer.

Study	Pt Dx	n	Therapies	mPFS (mo)	mOS (mo)
Alden and Mohiuddin 1994[234]	EHCC	24	EBRT (46Gy) + ILBT + CT	NR	12
		24	CT	NR	5.5
Foo *et al.* 1997[235]	EHCC	14	EBRT (23–68Gy) + ILBT ± CT	NR	12.8
Urego *et al.* 1999[236]	CC	34	EBRT (5–85Gy) ± ILBT ± CT	NR	14.0
Crane *et al.* 2002[237]	EHCC	27	EBRT (30Gy) ± ILBT ± CT	9	11
		14	EBRT (36–50Gy) ± ILBT ± CT	11	8
		11	EBRT (54–85Gy) ± ILBT ± CT	15	11
Shin *et al.* 2003[238]	EHCC	17	EBRT (36–55Gy)	NR	5
		14	EBRT (45–55Gy) + ILBT	NR	9
Park *et al.* 2006[239]	EHCC	19	EBRT (45Gy) + CT	13	14.0
Ben-David *et al.* 2006[240]	EHCC, GBC	52	EBRT (23–86Gy) ± CT	11	13.1
Deodato *et al.* 2006[241]	EHCC	22	EBRT (40–50Gy) ± ILBT + CT	16.3	23.0
Chen *et al.* 2010[242]	IHC	35	EBRT (30–60 Gy) ± TACE	NR	9.5
		84	no EBRT ± TACE	NR	5.1
Kopek *et al.* 2010[243]	HiCC, IHCC	27	SBRT (45)	6.7	10.6

Abbreviations: Pt Dx, patient diagnosis; mPFS, median progression-free survival; mOS, median overall survival; EHCC, extrahepatic cholangiocarcinoma; EBRT, external beam radiation therapy; ILBT, intraluminal brachytherapy; CT, chemotherapy; NR, not reported; CC, cholangiocarcinoma; GBC, gallbladder cancer; HiCC, hilar cholangiocarcinoma; IHC, intrahepatic cholangiocarcinoma; TACE, transarterial chemoembolization; SBRT, stereotactic beam radiotherapy.

to the tumor is much higher, and remains present for longer durations due to interference with drug washout out due to embolization. Similarity in survival and benefit following TACE, in patients with and without extrahepatic metastases suggested that liver disease is the primary determinant of survival in intrahepatic cholangiocarcinoma patients.[244,245] TACE has also been evaluated in an adjuvant role, following curative resection of intrahepatic cholangiocarcinoma.

Table 4   Selected studies of TACE in cholangiocarcinoma.

Study	Pt Dx/ Setting	n	Agents	Results
Kiefer *et al.* 2011[246]	IHCC	62	TACE (Cis, Dox, MMC)	mTTP: 8mo; 1yPFS 28% mOS: 15mo; 3yOS: 8%
Park *et al.* 2011[244]	IHCC, tx-naïve	72	TACE (Cis)	mOS: 12.2mo vs 3.3mo
		115	BSC	
Shen *et al.* 2011[247]	IHCC, adjuvant	53	TACE	1yRFS: 24.5% vs 33.3% [NS] 1yOS: 69.8% vs 54.2%
		72	obs	5yOS: 28.3% vs 20.8%
Wu *et al.* 2012[248]	IHCC, adjuvant	57	TACE	1yOS: 72% vs 54% 5yOS: 19% vs 10%
		57	obs	

Abbreviations: Pt Dx, patient diagnosis; IHC, intrahepatic cholangiocarcinoma; TACE, transarterial chemoembolization; Cis, cisplatin; Dox, doxorubicin; MMC, mitomycin-C; mTTP, median time-to-progression; 1yPFS, 1-year progression-free survival; mOS, median overall survival; 3yOS, 3-year overall survival; tx-naïve, treatment-naïve; BSC, best supportive care; obs, observation; NS, not significant; 5yOS, 5-year overall survival.

5.8.3 *Radiofrequency ablation*

Percutaneous radiofrequency ablation (RFA) involves the delivery of high-frequency alternating current to heat tissue and destroy tumor. RFA has been demonstrated to be effective and safe for local control of primary and secondary hepatic tumors. Unlike chemoembolization, it is not dependent on tumor vascularity. Studies have suggested a relationship between failure of ablation and the size of the lesions being treated.[249,250]

5.8.4 *Photodynamic therapy*

Photodynamic therapy (PDT) is a newer method for locoregional ablation, involving administration of a photosensitizing agent in combination with application of irradiation from laser light in either the visible or infrared wavelength. It has been studied in cholangiocarcinoma, often in combination with bile duct stenting. Retrospective analyses and earlier randomized trials demonstrated significant overall survival benefits following PDT.[251,252] However, a multicenter phase III trial of porfimer sodium PDT plus stenting, compared to stenting alone, was stopped early after overall survival was found to be significantly higher in the control arm.[253]

6 Systemic Chemotherapy

Cytotoxic chemotherapy remains the mainstay of treatment for patients with unresectable or metastatic biliary tract cancer. Given the rarity of this disease, clinical trials evaluating chemotherapy regimens in this setting have been small and have almost always been combined with various biliary tract cancers. Very few randomized trials have been conducted.The majority of trials have been performed with either fluoropyrimidine- or gemcitabine-based chemotherapy regimens. 5-fluorouracil (5-FU) had been tested in small trials, both as monotherapy and in combinations (Table 5). Overall response rates in these studies varied from 0 to 41%; median survival also varied notably, from 5 to 16 months.

Table 5 Selected studies of fluoropyrimidine-based regimens in advanced biliary tract cancers.

Study	n	Treatment Regimen	RR (%)	mPFS (mo)	mOS (mo)
Ellis *et al.* 1995[254]	20	5-FU + Epi + Cis	40	NR	11
Patt *et al.* 1996[255]	35	5-FU + IFN	34	9.5	12.0
Chen *et al.* 1998[256]	18	5-FU + LV	33	NR	7.0
Ducreux *et al.* 1998[257]	25	5-FU + Cis	24	NR	10
Raderer *et al.* 1999[258]	20	5-FU + LV + MMC	25	4	9.5
Choi *et al.* 2000[259]	28	5-FU + LV	32	NR	6.0
Patt *et al.* 2001[260]	41	5-FU + IFN + Dox + Cis	21	6.0	14.0
Chen *et al.* 2001[261]	25	5-FU + LV + MMC	26	3	6
Kim *et al.* 2003[262]	42	Cape + Cis	21	3.7	9.1
Kornek *et al.* 2004[263]	26	Cape + MMC	31	5.3	9.2
Ueno *et al.* 2004[264]	19	S-1	21	3.7	8.3
Rao *et al.* 2005[265]	27	5-FU + Epi + Cis	19	5.2	9.0
	27	5-FU + LV + etoposide	15	7.3	12.0
Cho *et al.* 2005[266]	44	Cape + Gem	32	6.0	14.0
Cho *et al.* 2005[267]	24[b-]	Cape + Gem	33	6.0	16.0
Ducreux *et al.* 2005[268]	28	5-FU	7	3.3	5.0
	28	5-FU + LV + Cis	19	3.3	8.0
Park *et al.* 2006[269]	43	Cape + Epi + Cis	40	5.2	8.0
Hong *et al.* 2007[270]	32	Cape + Cis	41	3.5	12.4
Feisthammel *et al.* 2007[271]	30	5-FU + irinotecan	10	3.8	6.3
Furuse *et al.* 2009[272]	61	UFT + Dox	7	1.6	6.5

Abbreviations: RR, response rate; mPFS, median progression-free survival; mOS, median overall survival; 5-FU, 5-fluorouracil; Epi, epirubicin; Cis, cisplatin; NR, not reported; IFN, interferon alfa-2b; LV, leucovorin; UFT, uracil-tegafur; MMC, mitomycin-C; Dox, doxorubicin; Cape, capecitabine; Gem, gemcitabine.

In the only randomized phase III trial involving 5-FU, Rao *et al.* randomized patients between ECF (epirubicin, cisplatin, 5-FU) and FELV (5-FU/LV, etoposide).[265] 54 patients with previously untreated advanced biliary cancer were randomized to either epirubicin, cisplatin, 5-FU (ECF) or 5-FU, etoposide, and leucovorin (FELV). The median OS was not significantly different between the two arms, ECF with 9.02 months compared to FELV with 12.03 months (p = 0.2059). Objective response rates were also similar, ECF 19.2% vs FELV 15% (p = 0.72). Patients were also evaluated for symptom resolution; greater than 60% of patients in each arm demonstrated resolution of pain, anorexia, weight loss, and nausea. Toxicities were generally similar in both groups, though grade 3 and 4 neutropenia was significantly with FELV compared to ECF. Given these findings, the authors of the study suggested that the study provided evidence that combination chemotherapy regimens could improve survival and symptomatic relief in advanced biliary cancer patients.

A mainstay of treatment in pancreatic cancer, gemcitabine has also been studied frequently in advanced biliary cancers (Table 6). Studies of gemcitabine monotherapy with varied dosing schemes demonstrated response rates ranging from 0% to 30%. Gemcitabine has also been tried in combination with multiple other agents, including 5-FU, capecitabine, cisplatin, oxaliplatin, and irinotecan. In these studies, response rates and survival varied significantly.

Several retrospective studies have attempted to compare varied combination regimens of chemotherapy. Yonemoto *et al.* performed a retrospective review of 304 consecutive patients with unresectable biliary tract cancers from nine central hospitals in Japan.[293] Of the 179 patients who received chemotherapy, 58 (19.1%) received gemcitabine, 45 (14.5%) received a cisplatin-based regimen, 30 (9.9%) received a 5-FU-based regimen, 27 (8.9%) took 5-FU, doxorubicin, and mitomycin (FAM), and 20 (6.6%) took S-1 — another fluoropyrimidine. No patients received gemcitabine in combination with other agents. The adjusted hazard ratio for gemcitabine monotherapy was 0.53 (95% CI 0.34–0.82) and 0.49 (95% CI 0.36–0.99) for the cisplatin regimens. The cisplatin-based treatments were associated with a higher frequencies of toxicities.

Eckel and Schmid performed a systematic review of chemotherapy trials published between 1985 and 2006.[294] One hundred and four trials, consisting of 112 trial arms, were pooled in the analysis. Pooled response rate was 22.6%; tumor control rate was 57.3%. Subgroup analyses, defined by treatment type, showed that regimens containing both gemcitabine and a platinum agent had significantly higher pooled response and tumor control rates when compared to either fluoropyrimidine or gemcitabine monotherapy or fluoropyrimidine-plus-platinum regimens.

This support for the combination of gemcitabine and platinum-based therapy was validated in the United Kingdom-based Advanced Biliary Care (ABC)-02 trial,

Table 6   Selected studies of gemcitabine-based regimens in advanced biliary tract cancers.

Study	n	Treatment Regimen	RR (%)	mPFS (mo)	mOS (mo)
Raderer *et al.* 1999[258]	19	Gem	16	2.5	6.5
Penz *et al.* 2001[273]	32	Gem	22	5.6	11.5
Gebbia *et al.* 2001[274]	18	Gem	22	3.4	8
	22	Gem + 5-FU + LV	36	4.1	11
Kuhn *et al.* 2002[275]	43	Gem + docetaxel	9	NR	11.0
Bhargava *et al.* 2003[276]	14	Gem + irinotecan	14	1.5	NR
Kornek *et al.* 2004[263]	25	Gem + MMC	20	4.2	6.7
Andre *et al.* 2004[277]	23	Gem + Ox	22	3.9	7.6
Knox *et al.* 2004[278]	27	Gem + 5-FU	33	3.7	5.3
Alberts *et al.* 2005[279]	42	Gem + 5-FU + LV	10	4.6	9.7
Thongprasert *et al.* 2005[280]	40	Gem + Cis	28	4.8	8.4
Knox *et al.* 2005[281]	45	Gem + Cape	31	7	14
Cho *et al.* 2005[266]	44	Gem + Cape	32	6.0	14
Cho *et al.* 2005[267]	24[b]	Gem + Cape	33	6.0	16
Lee *et al.* 2006[282]	24[a]	Gem + Cis	21	5.0	9.3
Kim *et al.* 2006[283]	29	Gem + Cis	34	3.0	11.0
Harder *et al.* 2006[284]	31	Gem + Ox	26	6.5	11
Manzione *et al.* 2007[285]	34	Gem + Ox	41	NR	10
Alberts *et al.* 2007[286]	58	Gem + Pem	NR	3.8	6.6
Riechelmann *et al.* 2007[287]	75	Gem + Cape	29	6.2	12.7
Lee *et al.* 2008[288]	39	Gem + Cis	17	3.2	8.6
Andre *et al.* 2008[289]	67	Gem + Ox	15	349	8.8
Meyerhardt *et al.* 2008[290]	33	Gem + Cis	21	6.3	9.7
Kim *et al.* 2009[291]	40	Gem + Ox	15	4.2	8.5
Jang *et al.* 2010[292]	53	Gem + Ox	19	4.8	8.3

Abbreviations: RR, response rate; mPFS, median progression-free survival; mOS, median overall survival; Gem, gemcitabine; NR, not reported; 5-FU, 5-fluorouracil; LV, leucovorin; MMC, mitomycin-C; Cis, cisplatin; Cape, capecitabine; Ox, oxaliplatin; Pem, pemetrexed.

whose results were published in 2010 and established the current standard-of-care for first-line systemic therapy.[295] In this study, 410 patients with nonresectable, recurrent, or metastatic biliary tract cancer were randomized to receive either gemcitabine alone or cisplatin followed by gemcitabine. The trial included patients with cholangiocarcinoma, gallbladder cancer, or ampullary cancer. Patients in the combination arm received cisplatin 25 mg/m^2 and gemcitabine 1000 mg/m^2 on days 1 and 8 of a 3-week cycle, for 8 cycles; patients in the gemcitabine monotherapy arm received gemcitabine 1000 mg/m^2 on days 1, 8, and 15 of a 4-week cycle, for 6 cycles. After a median follow-up of 8.2 months, the median OS was 11.7 months in the cisplatin–gemcitabine arm, compared to 8.1 months in the gemcitabine arm (HR = 0.64; p < 0.001). The median PFS was similarly improved, with 8.0 months and 5.0 months in the cisplatin–gemcitabine and gemcitabine arms respectively (HR = 0.64; p < 0.001). Disease control rate was also significantly increased in the cisplatin–gemcitabine arm (81.4% vs. 71.8%; p = 0.049). Severe hematologic toxicities were seen more frequently in the cisplatin-gemcitabine arm. Severe liver toxicities were significantly increased in the gemcitabine-alone arm.

Since the publication of ABC-02, the combination of gemcitabine and cisplatin has been accepted as the standard-of-care for unresectable and metastatic biliary tract cancers by most societies. Current trials have attempted different approaches to further improving overall survival. One such approach has been utilizing therapies targeting potential key mutations in biliary tract carcinogenesis. The heterogeneity in biliary tract cancers and their underlying molecular changes complicates this process. Recent trials have incorporated agents, primarily against EGFR and VEGF, in the form of both monoclonal antibodies and tyrosine kinase inhibitors (Table 7).[296]

Table 7   Selected studies of molecular targeted agents in advanced biliary tract cancers.

Agent/Study	n	Treatment Regimen	RR (%)	mPFS (mo)	mOS (mo)
Erlotinib [EGFR]					
Philip et al. 2006[297]	43	Erlot	8	2.6	7.5
Chiorean et al. 2012[298]	11	Erlot + docetaxel	0	NR	5.7
Lee et al. 2012[299]	135	Erlot + Gem + Ox	30	5.8[NS]	9.5[NS]
	133	Gem + Ox	16	4.2[NS]	9.5[NS]
Cetuximab [EGFR]					
Paule et al. 2007[300]	9[a]	Cet + Gem + Ox	11	4	7
Malka et al. 2014[301]	76	Cet + Gem + Ox	24[NC]	6.1[NC]	11.0[NC]
	74	Gem + Ox	23[NC]	5.5[NC]	12.4[NC]
Panitumumab [EGFR]					
Jensen et al. 2011[302]	46	Pan + Gem + Ox	33	8.3	10.0
Sohal et al. 2013[303]	35	Pan + Gem + irinotecan	31	9.7	12.9

(Continued)

Table 7 (*Continued*)

Agent/Study	n	Treatment Regimen	RR (%)	mPFS (mo)	mOS (mo)
Bevacizumab [VEGF-A]					
Zhu *et al.* 2010[304]	35	Bev + Gem + Ox	40	7.0	12.7
Sorafenib [VEGFR-2/3, PDGFR, RAF]					
Bengala *et al.* 2010[305]	46	Soraf	2	2.3	4.4
El-Khoueiry *et al.* 2012[306]	31	Soraf	0	3	9
Sunitinib [VEGFR, PDGFR, cKit]					
Yi *et al.* 2012[307]	56	sunitinib	9	1.7	4.8
Cediranib [VEGFR-1/2/3]					
Valle *et al.* 2014[308]	62	Ced + Gem + Cis	43	7.7	14.1
	62	placebo + Gem + Cis	19	7.4	11.9
Lapatinib [HER2]					
Ramanathan *et al.* 2009[309]	17	Lapatinib	0	1.8	5.2
Selumetinib [MEK1/2]					
Bekaii-Saab *et al.* 2011[310]	28	Selumetinib	12	3.7	9.8
Combinations					
Lubner *et al.* 2010[311]	49	Erlot + Bev	12	4.4	9.9
El-Khoueiry *et al.* 2014[312]	34	Erlot + Soraf	6	2	6

Abbreviations: RR, response rate; mPFS, median progression-free survival; mOS, median overall survival; EGFR, epidermal growth factor receptor; Erlot, erlotinib; NR, not reported; Gem, gemcitabine; Ox, oxaliplatin; Cet, cetuximab; Pan, panitumimab; VEGF, vascular endothelial growth factor; Bev, bevacizumab; VEGFR, vascular endothelial growth factor receptor; PDGFR, platelet-derived growth factor receptor; RAF, rapidly accelerated fibrosarcoma; Soraf, sorafenib; Ced, cediranib; HER2, human epidermal growth factor receptor 2; MEK, mitogen-activated protein kinase/extracellular-signal regulated kinase.

One phase III trial utilizing a targeted agent in biliary tract cancer has been completed. Lee *et al.*[299] reported the results of an open-label, randomized phase III trial of erlotininb plus chemotherapy with gemcitabine and oxaliplatin compared to chemotherapy alone. 268 patients with metastatic biliary tract adenocarcinoma were randomized. Both median progression-free survival and median overall survival were not significantly different between the two arms. Objective response rate was significantly higher in the erlotinib-containing arm.

7 Future Directions

Despite advances in treatment, biliary tract cancers remain associated with poor survival. Treatment options are limited and overall survival rates are low. Further research is needed to better understand the heterogeneity of these diseases. In addition to clear differences by anatomic classification, there are significant variations related geographic and etiological background. As we begin to better understand these differences, we may be able to tailor screening, prognostication, localized and systemic therapies. With a better understanding of the underlying risk factors, we may also develop greater strategies for primary prevention.

Genetic and molecular profiling is steadily uncovering the processes underlying carcinogenesis in the biliary tract. Numerous agents are being developed and studied in these cancers. Early results in some studies have been promising; however, these regimens need to be compared against the current standard-of-care, gemcitabine and cisplatin, for clear survival benefits. Greater efforts also need to be made to incorporate these findings with locoregional therapies as adjuvant, neoadjuvant, or palliative treatments.

References

1. de Groen PC, *et al.* Biliary tract cancers. *N Engl J Med* 1999;**341**(18):1368–1378. doi:10.1056/NEJM199910283411807.
2. Castaing D. Surgical anatomy of the biliary tract. *MHPB* 2008;**10**(2):72–76. doi:10.1080/13651820801992518.
3. Jurkovikj D. Important biliary drainage variations of left liver lobe. *Prilozi* 2009; **30**(2):81–92.
4. Bismuth H, Nakache R, Diamond T. Management strategies in resection for hilar cholangiocarcinoma. *Ann Surg* 1992;**215**(1):31–38.
5. Augustine MM, Fong Y. Epidemiology and risk factors of biliary tract and primary liver tumors. *Surg Oncol Clin N Am* 2014;**23**(2):171–188. doi:10.1016/j.soc.2013.10.001.
6. Lazaridis KN, Gores GJ. Cholangiocarcinoma. *Gastroenterology* 2005;**128**(6): 1655–1667.
7. Shaib Y, El-Serag HB. The epidemiology of cholangiocarcinoma. *Semin Liver Dis* 2004;**24**(2):115–125. doi:10.1055/s-2004-828889.
8. Gatto M, Bragazzi MC, Semeraro R, *et al.* Cholangiocarcinoma: update and future perspectives. *Dig Liver Dis* 2010;**42**(4):253–260. doi:10.1016/j.dld.2009.12.008.
9. Tyson GL, El-Serag HB. Risk factors for cholangiocarcinoma. *Hepatology* 2011;**54**(1):173–184. doi:10.1002/hep.24351.
10. Everhart JE, Ruhl CE. Burden of digestive diseases in the United States Part III: Liver, biliary tract, and pancreas. *Gastroenterology* 2009;**136**(4):1134–1144. doi:10.1053/j. gastro.2009.02.038.

11. Altaee MY, *et al*. Etiologic and clinical characteristics of peripheral and hilar cholangiocarcinoma. *Cancer* 1991;**68**(9):2051–2055.

12. Patel T. Increasing incidence and mortality of primary intrahepatic cholangiocarcinoma in the United States. *Hepatology* 2001;**33**(6):1353–1357. doi:10.1053/jhep.2001.25087.

13. Taylor-Robinson SD, *et al*. Increase in mortality rates from intrahepatic cholangiocarcinoma in England and Wales 1968–1998. *Gut* 2001;**48**(6):816–820.

14. Patel T. Worldwide trends in mortality from biliary tract malignancies. *BMC Cancer* 2002;**2**(1):10. doi:10.1186/1471–2407-2-10.

15. Khan SA, *et al*. Changing international trends in mortality rates for liver, biliary and pancreatic tumours. *J Hepatol* 2002;**37**(6):806–813.

16. Shaib YH, *et al*. Rising incidence of intrahepatic cholangiocarcinoma in the United States: a true increase? *J Hepatol* 2004;**40**(3):472–477. doi:10.1016/j.jhep.2003.11.030.

17. Reid KM, *et al*. Diagnosis and surgical management of gallbladder cancer: a review. *J Gastrointest Surg* 2007;**11**(5):671–681. doi:10.1007/s11605-006-0075-x.

18. Lazcano-Ponce EC, *et al*. Epidemiology and molecular pathology of gallbladder cancer. *CA Cancer J Clin* 2001;**51**(6):349–364.

19. Hundal R, Shaffer EA. Gallbladder cancer: epidemiology and outcome. *Clin Epidemiol* 2014;**6**:99–109. doi:10.2147/CLEP.S37357.

20. Randi G, *et al*. Gallbladder cancer worldwide: geographical distribution and risk factors. *Int J Cancer* 2006;**118**(7):1591–1602. doi:10.1002/ijc.21683.

21. Randi G, *et al*. Epidemiology of biliary tract cancers: an update. *Ann Oncol* 2009;**20**(1):146–159. doi:10.1093/annonc/mdn533.

22. Castro FA, *et al*. Biliary tract cancer incidence in the United States-Demographic and temporal variations by anatomic site. *Int J Cancer* 2013;**133**(7):1664–1671. doi:10.1002/ijc.28161.

23. Khan SA, *et al*. Guidelines for the diagnosis and treatment of cholangiocarcinoma: an update. *Gut* 2012;**61**(12):1657–1669. doi:10.1136/gutjnl-2011-301748.

24. Worthington J, Chapman R. Primary sclerosing cholangitis. *Orphanet J Rare Dis* 2006;**1**(1):41. doi:10.1186/1750-1172-1-41.

25. Aadland E, *et al*. Primary sclerosing cholangitis: a long-term follow-up study. *Scand J Gastroenterol*. 1987;**22**(6):655–664.

26. Rosen CB, Nagorney DM. Cholangiocarcinoma complicating primary sclerosing cholangitis. *Semin Liver Dis*. 1991;**11**(1):26–30. doi:10.1055/s-2008-1040419.

27. Broomé U, *et al*. Natural history and prognostic factors in 305 Swedish patients with primary sclerosing cholangitis. *Gut*. 1996;**38**(4):610–615. doi:10.1016/j.jhep.2003.11.030.

28. Kornfeld D, *et al*. Survival and risk of cholangiocarcinoma in patients with primary sclerosing cholangitis. A population-based study. *Scand J Gastroenterol*. 1997;**32**(10):1042–1045.

29. Morris-Stiff G, *et al*. Cholangiocarcinoma complicating primary sclerosing cholangitis: a 24-year experience. *Dig Surg* 2008;**25**(2):126–132. doi:10.1159/000128169.

30. Ghali P, *et al*. Liver transplantation for incidental cholangiocarcinoma: analysis of the Canadian experience. *Liver Transpl* 2005;**11**(11):1412–1416. doi:10.1002/lt.20512.

31. Nichols JC, *et al.* Diagnostic role of serum CA 19-9 for cholangiocarcinoma in patients with primary sclerosing cholangitis. *Mayo Clin Proc.* 1993;**68**(9):874–879.

32. Ramage JK, *et al.* Serum tumor markers for the diagnosis of cholangiocarcinoma in primary sclerosing cholangitis. *Gastroenterology.* 1995;**108**(3):865–869.

33. Tangkijvanich P, *et al.* Diagnostic role of serum interleukin 6 and CA 19–9 in patients with cholangiocarcinoma. *Hepatogastroenterology* 2004;**51**(55):15–19.

34. Fisher A, *et al.* CA19-9 does not predict cholangiocarcinoma in patients with primary sclerosing cholangitis undergoing liver transplantation. *Liver Transpl Surg.* 1995; **1**(2):94–98.

35. Bergquist A, *et al.* Risk factors and clinical presentation of hepatobiliary carcinoma in patients with primary sclerosing cholangitis: a case-control study. *Hepatology.* 1998;**27**(2):311–316. doi:10.1002/hep.510270201.

36. Chalasani N, *et al.* Cholangiocarcinoma in patients with primary sclerosing cholangitis: a multicenter case-control study. *Hepatology* 2000;**31**(1):7–11. doi:10.1002/hep.510310103.

37. Burak K, *et al.* Incidence and risk factors for cholangiocarcinoma in primary sclerosing cholangitis. *The American Journal of Gastroenterology* 2004;**99**(3):523–526. doi:10.1111/j.1572-0241.2004.04067.x.

38. Sithithaworn P, *et al.* Roles of liver fluke infection as risk factor for cholangiocarcinoma 2014;**21**(5):301–308. doi:10.1002/jhbp.62.

39. Bouvard V, *et al.* A review of human carcinogens--Part B: biological agents. *The lancet oncology.* April 2009:321–322.

40. Parkin DM, *et al.* Liver cancer in Thailand. I. A case-control study of cholangiocarcinoma. *Int J Cancer.* 1991;**48**(3):323–328.

41. Honjo S, *et al.* Genetic and environmental determinants of risk for cholangiocarcinoma via Opisthorchis viverrini in a densely infested area in Nakhon Phanom, northeast Thailand. *Int J Cancer* 2005;**117**(5):854–860. doi:10.1002/ijc.21146.

42. Shin HR, *et al.* Hepatitis B and C virus, Clonorchis sinensis for the risk of liver cancer: a case-control study in Pusan, Korea. *Int J Epidemiol.* 1996;**25**(5):933–940.

43. Choi D, *et al.* Cholangiocarcinoma and Clonorchis sinensis infection: a case-control study in Korea. *J Hepatol* 2006;**44**(6):1066–1073. doi:10.1016/j.jhep.2005.11.040.

44. Lim MK, *et al.* Clonorchis sinensis infection and increasing risk of cholangiocarcinoma in the Republic of Korea. *Am J Trop Med Hyg* 2006;**75**(1):93–96.

45. Lee TY, *et al.* Hepatitis B virus infection and intrahepatic cholangiocarcinoma in Korea: a case-control study. *The American Journal of Gastroenterology* 2008;**103**(7):1716–1720. doi:10.1111/j.1572-0241.2008.01796.x.

46. Huang MJ, *et al.* Comparison of intravenous radionuclide cholescintigraphy and endoscopic retrograde cholangiography in the diagnosis of intrahepatic gall-stones. *Br J Radiol.* 1981;**54**(640):302–306.

47. Chen MF. Peripheral cholangiocarcinoma (cholangiocellular carcinoma): clinical features, diagnosis and treatment. *J Gastroenterol Hepatol.* 1999;**14**(12):1144–1149.

48. Zhou Y-M, *et al.* Risk factors for intrahepatic cholangiocarcinoma: a case-control study in China. *World J Gastroenterol* 2008;**14**(4):632–635. doi:10.3748/wjg. 14.632.

49. Guglielmi A, *et al*. Hepatolithiasis-associated cholangiocarcinoma: results from a multi-institutional national database on a case series of 23 patients. *Eur J Surg Oncol* 2014;**40**(5):567–575. doi:10.1016/j.ejso.2013.12.006.

50. Söreide K, *et al*. Bile duct cysts in adults. *Br J Surg* 2004;**91**(12):1538–1548. doi:10.1002/bjs.4815.

51. Ohtsuka T, *et al*. Carcinoma arising in choledochocele. *Endoscopy* 2001;**33**(7): 614–619. doi:10.1055/s-2001-15324.

52. Yamamoto S, *et al*. Hepatitis C virus infection as a likely etiology of intrahepatic cholangiocarcinoma. *Cancer Sci* 2004;**95**(7):592–595.

53. Shaib YH, *et al*. Risk factors of intrahepatic cholangiocarcinoma in the United States: a case-control study. *Gastroenterology* 2005;**128**(3):620–626.

54. Shaib YH, *et al*. Risk factors for intrahepatic and extrahepatic cholangiocarcinoma: a hospital-based case-control study. *The American Journal of Gastroenterology* 2007;**102**(5):1016–1021. doi:10.1111/j.1572-0241.2007.01104.x.

55. Welzel TM, *et al*. Risk factors for intrahepatic and extrahepatic cholangiocarcinoma in the United States: a population-based case-control study. *Clin Gastroenterol Hepatol* 2007;**5**(10):1221–1228. doi:10.1016/j.cgh.2007.05.020.

56. Grainge MJ, *et al*. The antecedents of biliary cancer: a primary care case-control study in the United Kingdom. *Br J Cancer* 2009;**100**(1):178–180. doi:10.1038/sj.bjc.6604765.

57. Shin H-R, *et al*. Epidemiology of cholangiocarcinoma: an update focusing on risk factors. *Cancer Sci* 2010;**101**(3):579–585. doi:10.1111/j.1349-7006.2009.01458.x.

58. Ralphs S, Khan SA. The role of the hepatitis viruses in cholangiocarcinoma. *J Viral Hepat* 2013;**20**(5):297–305. doi:10.1111/jvh.12093.

59. Stinton LM, Shaffer EA. Epidemiology of gallbladder disease: cholelithiasis and cancer. *Gut Liver* 2012;**6**(2):172–187. doi:10.5009/gnl.2012.6.2.172.

60. Shrikhande SV, *et al*. Cholelithiasis in gallbladder cancer: coincidence, cofactor, or cause! *Eur J Surg Oncol* 2010;**36**(6):514–519. doi:10.1016/j.ejso.2010.05.002.

61. Archibald JD, *et al*. The role of prophylactic cholecystectomy versus deferral in the care of patients after endoscopic sphincterotomy. *Can J Surg* 2007;**50**(1):19–23.

62. Choi SY, *et al*. Is it necessary to perform prophylactic cholecystectomy for asymptomatic subjects with gallbladder polyps and gallstones? *J Gastroenterol Hepatol* 2010; **25**(6):1099–1104. doi:10.1111/j.1440-1746.2010.06288.x.

63. Kapoor VK. Cholecystectomy in patients with asymptomatic gallstones to prevent gall bladder cancer--the case against. *Indian J Gastroenterol* 2006;**25**(3):152–154.

64. McAlister VC, *et al*. Cholecystectomy deferral in patients with endoscopic sphincterotomy. *Cochrane Database Syst Rev* 2007;(4):CD006233. doi:10.1002/14651858. CD006233.pub2.

65. Carriaga MT, Henson DE. Liver, gallbladder, extrahepatic bile ducts, and pancreas. *Cancer*. 1995;**75**(1 Suppl):171–190.

66. Shukla VK, *et al*. Carcinoma of the gallbladder--is it a sequel of typhoid? *Dig Dis Sci* 2000;**45**(5):900–903.

67. Nagaraja V, Eslick GD. Systematic review with meta-analysis: The relationship between chronic Salmonella typhi carrier status and gall-bladder cancer. *Alimentary Pharmacology & Therapeutics* 2014;**39**(8):745–750. doi:10.1111/apt.12655.

68. Matsukura N, *et al*. Association between Helicobacter bilis in bile and biliary tract malignancies: H. bilis in bile from Japanese and Thai patients with benign and malignant diseases in the biliary tract. *Jpn J Cancer Res* 2002;**93**(7):842–847.

69. Murata H, *et al*. Helicobacter bilis infection in biliary tract cancer. *Alimentary Pharmacology & Therapeutics* 2004;**20** Suppl 1:90-94. doi:10.1111/j.1365-2036. 2004.01972.x.

70. Kobayashi T, *et al*. Helicobacter genus DNA fragments are commonly detectable in bile from patients with extrahepatic biliary diseases and associated with their pathogenesis. *Dig Dis Sci* 2005;**50**(5):862–867.

71. Metz DC. Helicobacter colonization of the biliary tree: Commensal, pathogen, or spurious finding? *The American Journal of Gastroenterology*. 1998;**93**(10):1996–1998. doi:10.1111/j.1572–0241.1998.01996.x.

72. Stephen AE, Berger DL. Carcinoma in the porcelain gallbladder: A relationship revisited. *Surgery* 2001;**129**(6):699–703. doi:10.1067/msy.2001.113888.

73. Towfigh S, *et al*. Porcelain gallbladder is not associated with gallbladder carcinoma. *Am Surg* 2001;**67**(1):7–10.

74. Puia IC, Puia A. Porcelain gallbladder and cancer — an association to be revised. *J Gastrointestin Liver Dis* 2013;**22**(3):358–359.

75. Schnelldorfer T. Porcelain gallbladder: A benign process or concern for malignancy? *J Gastrointest Surg* 2013;**17**(6):1161–1168. doi:10.1007/s11605-013-2170-0.

76. Funabiki T, *et al*. Surgical strategy for patients with pancreaticobiliary maljunction without choledocal dilatation. *Keio J Med*. 1997;**46**(4):169–172.

77. Elnemr A, *et al*. Anomalous pancreaticobiliary ductal junction without bile duct dilatation in gallbladder cancer. *Hepatogastroenterology* 2001;**48**(38):382–386.

78. Hu B, Gong B, Zhou D-Y. Association of anomalous pancreaticobiliary ductal junction with gallbladder carcinoma in Chinese patients: an ERCP study. *Gastrointest Endosc* 2003;**57**(4):541–545. doi:10.1067/mge.2003.136.

79. Deng Y-L, *et al*. Relationship between pancreaticobiliary maljunction and gallbladder carcinoma: meta-analysis. *HBPD INT* 2011;**10**(6):570–580. doi:10.1016/S1499-3872(11)60098-2.

80. Calle EE, *et al*. Overweight, obesity, and mortality from cancer in a prospectively studied cohort of U.S. adults. *N Engl J Med* 2003;**348**(17):1625–1638. doi:10.1056/NEJMoa021423.

81. Larsson SC, Wolk A. Obesity and the risk of gallbladder cancer: a meta-analysis. *Br J Cancer* 2007;**96**(9):1457–1461. doi:10.1038/sj.bjc.6603703.

82. Hsing AW, *et al*. Body size and the risk of biliary tract cancer: a population-based study in China. *Br J Cancer* 2008;**99**(5):811–815. doi:10.1038/sj.bjc.6604616.

83. Shebl FM, *et al*. Diabetes in relation to biliary tract cancer and stones: a population-based study in Shanghai, China. *Br J Cancer* 2010;**103**(1):115–119. doi:10.1038/sj. bjc.6605706.

84. Yagyu K, *et al*. Cigarette smoking, alcohol drinking and the risk of gallbladder cancer death: a prospective cohort study in Japan. *Int J Cancer* 2008;**122**(4):924–929. doi:10.1002/ijc.23159.

85. Sirica AE, Gores GJ. Desmoplastic stroma and cholangiocarcinoma: Clinical implications and therapeutic targeting. *Hepatology* 2014;**59**(6):2397–2402. doi:10.1002/hep.26762.

86. Yamasaki S. Intrahepatic cholangiocarcinoma: macroscopic type and stage classification. *J Hepatobiliary Pancreat Surg* 2003;**10**(4):288–291. doi:10.1007/s00534-002-0732-8.

87. Sasaki A, *et al.* Intrahepatic peripheral cholangiocarcinoma: mode of spread and choice of surgical treatment. *Br J Surg.* 1998;**85**(9):1206–1209.doi:10.1046/j.1365-2168. 1998.00815.x.

88. Uno M, *et al.* Periductal infiltrating type of intrahepatic cholangiocarcinoma: a rare macroscopic type without any apparent mass. *Surg Today* 2012;**42**(12):1189–1194. doi:10.1007/s00595-012-0145-5.

89. Chung YE, *et al.* Varying appearances of cholangiocarcinoma: radiologic-pathologic correlation. *Radiographics* 2009;**29**(3):683–700. doi:10.1148/rg.293085729.

90. Yamamoto J, *et al.* Surgical treatment of intrahepatic cholangiocarcinoma: four patients surviving more than five years. *Surgery.* 1992;**111**(6):617–622.

91. Ohashi K, *et al.* Clinical characteristics and proliferating activity of intrahepatic cholangiocarcinoma. *J Gastroenterol Hepatol.* 1994;**9**(5):442–446.

92. Hirohashi K, *et al.* Macroscopic types of intrahepatic cholangiocarcinoma: clinicopathologic features and surgical outcomes.*Hepatogastroenterology* 2002;**49**(44):326–329.

93. Ariizumi S-I, Yamamoto M. [Surgical treatment of intrahepatic cholangiocarcinoma based on the macroscopic subtype]. *Nihon Shokakibyo Gakkai Zasshi* 2012;**109**(11):1885–1894.

94. Morimoto Y, *et al.* Long-term survival and prognostic factors in the surgical treatment for intrahepatic cholangiocarcinoma. *J Hepatobiliary Pancreat Surg* 2003;**10**(6):432–440. doi:10.1007/s00534-002-0842-3.

95. Guglielmi A, *et al.* Intrahepatic cholangiocarcinoma: prognostic factors after surgical resection. *World J Surg* 2009;**33**(6):1247–1254. doi:10.1007/s00268-009-9970-0.

96. Yamamoto M, *et al.* Does gross appearance indicate prognosis in intrahepatic cholangiocarcinoma? *J Surg Oncol.* 1998;**69**(3):162–167.

97. Shimada K, *et al.* Surgical outcomes of the mass-forming plus periductal infiltrating types of intrahepatic cholangiocarcinoma: a comparative study with the typical mass-forming type of intrahepatic cholangiocarcinoma. *World J Surg* 2007;**31**(10):2016–2022. doi:10.1007/s00268-007-9194-0.

98. Esposito I, Schirmacher P. Pathological aspects of cholangiocarcinoma. *MHPB* 2008;**10**(2):83–86. doi:10.1080/13651820801992609.

99. Castellano-Megías VM, *et al.* Pathological aspects of so called "hilar cholangiocarcinoma". *World J Gastrointest Oncol* 2013;**5**(7):159–170. doi:10.4251/wjgo.v5.i7.159.

100. Zen Y, *et al.* Biliary papillary tumors share pathological features with intraductal papillary mucinous neoplasm of the pancreas. *Hepatology* 2006;**44**(5):1333–1343. doi:10.1002/hep.21387.

101. Rocha FG, *et al.* Intraductal papillary neoplasm of the bile duct: a biliary equivalent to intraductal papillary mucinous neoplasm of the pancreas? *Hepatology* 2012;**56**(4):1352–1360. doi:10.1002/hep.25786.

102. Barton JG, *et al.* Intraductal papillary mucinous neoplasm of the biliary tract: a real disease? *HPB (Oxford)* 2009;**11**(8):684–691. doi:10.1111/j.1477-2574.2009.00122.x.

103. Ross JS, *et al.* Comprehensive genomic profiling of biliary tract cancers to reveal tumor-specific differences and genomic alterations. *J Clin Oncol* 2015;**33**(No 3_ suppl):231.

104. Kipp BR, *et al.* Isocitrate dehydrogenase 1 and 2 mutations in cholangiocarcinoma. *Hum Pathol* 2012;**43**(10):1552–1558. doi:10.1016/j.humpath.2011.12.007.

105. Borger DR, *et al.* Frequent mutation of isocitrate dehydrogenase (IDH)1 and IDH2 in cholangiocarcinoma identified through broad-based tumor genotyping. *The Oncologist* 2012;**17**(1):72–79. doi:10.1634/theoncologist.2011-0386.

106. Chan-on W, *et al.* Exome sequencing identifies distinct mutational patterns in liver fluke-related and non-infection-related bile duct cancers. *Nat Genet* 2013;**45**(12): 1474–1478. doi:10.1038/ng.2806.

107. Saha SK, *et al.* Mutant IDH inhibits HNF-4α to block hepatocyte differentiation and promote biliary cancer. *Nature* 2014;**513**(7516):110-114. doi:10.1038/nature13441.

108. Wang P, *et al.* Mutations in isocitrate dehydrogenase 1 and 2 occur frequently in intrahepatic cholangiocarcinomas and share hypermethylation targets with glioblastomas. *Oncogene* 2013;**32**(25):3091–3100. doi:10.1038/onc.2012.315.

109. Arai Y, *et al.* Fibroblast growth factor receptor 2 tyrosine kinase fusions define a unique molecular subtype of cholangiocarcinoma. *Hepatology* 2014;**59**(4):1427–1434. doi:10. 1002/hep.26890.

110. Graham RP, *et al.* Fibroblast growth factor receptor 2 translocations in intrahepatic cholangiocarcinoma. *Hum Pathol* 2014;**45**(8):1630–1638. doi:10.1016/j.humpath.2014.03.014.

111. Ong CK, *et al.* Exome sequencing of liver fluke-associated cholangiocarcinoma. *Nat Genet* 2012;**44**(6):690–693. doi:10.1038/ng.2273.

112. Ohashi K, *et al.* Ki-ras mutations and p53 protein expressions in intrahepatic cholangiocarcinomas: relation to gross tumor morphology. *Gastroenterology.* 1995;**109**(5): 1612–1617.

113. Tannapfel A, *et al.* Frequency of p16(INK4A) alterations and K-ras mutations in intrahepatic cholangiocarcinoma of the liver. *Gut* 2000;**47**(5):721–727.

114. Tannapfel A, *et al.* Mutations of the BRAF gene in cholangiocarcinoma but not in hepatocellular carcinoma. *Gut* 2003;**52**(5):706–712.

115. Isa T, *et al.* Analysis of microsatellite instability, K-ras gene mutation and p53 protein overexpression in intrahepatic cholangiocarcinoma. *Hepatogastroenterology* 2002;**49**(45):604–608.

116. Rashid A, *et al.* K-ras mutation, p53 overexpression, and microsatellite instability in biliary tract cancers: a population-based study in China. *Clin Cancer Res* 2002;**8**(10):3156–3163.

117. Leone F, *et al.* Somatic mutations of epidermal growth factor receptor in bile duct and gallbladder carcinoma. *Clin Cancer Res* 2006;**12**(6):1680–1685. doi:10.1158/1078-0432.CCR-05-1692.

118. Miyamoto M, *et al.* Prognostic significance of overexpression of c-Met oncoprotein in cholangiocarcinoma. *Br J Cancer* 2011;**105**(1):131–138. doi:10.1038/bjc.2011.199.

119. Terada T, *et al.* Immunohistochemical demonstration of MET overexpression in human intrahepatic cholangiocarcinoma and in hepatolithiasis. *Hum Pathol.* 1998;**29**(2): 175–180.

120. Farazi PA, *et al.* Chronic bile duct injury associated with fibrotic matrix microenvironment provokes cholangiocarcinoma in p53-deficient mice. *Cancer Res* 2006; **66**(13):6622–6627. doi:10.1158/0008-5472.CAN-05-4609.

121. Sato Y, *et al.* Epithelial-mesenchymal transition induced by transforming growth factor-{beta}1/Snail activation aggravates invasive growth of cholangiocarcinoma. *The American Journal of Pathology* 2010;**177**(1):141–152. doi:10.2353/ajpath.2010.090747.

122. Hahn SA, *et al.* Mutations of the DPC4/Smad4 gene in biliary tract carcinoma. *Cancer Res.* 1998;**58**(6):1124–1126.

123. Nakeeb A, *et al.* Cholangiocarcinoma. A spectrum of intrahepatic, perihilar, and distal tumors. *Ann Surg.* 1996;**224**(4):463–73–discussion473–5.

124. Björnsson E, *et al.* CA 19-9 and CEA are unreliable markers for cholangiocarcinoma in patients with primary sclerosing cholangitis. *Liver.* 1999;**19**(6):501–508.

125. Patel AH, *et al.* The utility of CA 19-9 in the diagnoses of cholangiocarcinoma in patients without primary sclerosing cholangitis. *The American Journal of Gastroenterology* 2000;**95**(1):204–207. doi:10.1111/j.1572-0241.2000.01685.x.

126. Steinberg W. The clinical utility of the CA 19-9 tumor-associated antigen. *The American Journal of Gastroenterology.* 1990;**85**(4):350–355.

127. Delemos AS, Pratt DS. Immunoglobulin g4-associated cholangitis: the next great masquerader. *Gastroenterol Hepatol (N Y)* 2013;**9**(4):255–256.

128. Oseini AM, *et al.* Utility of serum immunoglobulin G4 in distinguishing immunoglobulin G4-associated cholangitis from cholangiocarcinoma. *Hepatology* 2011; **54**(3):940–948. doi:10.1002/hep.24487.

129. Boonstra K, *et al.* Serum immunoglobulin G4 and immunoglobulin G1 for distinguishing immunoglobulin G4-associated cholangitis from primary sclerosing cholangitis. *Hepatology* 2014;**59**(5):1954–1963. doi:10.1002/hep.26977.

130. Foley WD, Quiroz FA. The role of sonography in imaging of the biliary tract. *Ultrasound Q* 2007;**23**(2):123–135. doi:10.1097/01.ruq.0000263851.53549.a5.

131. Robledo R, *et al.* Extrahepatic bile duct carcinoma: US characteristics and accuracy in demonstration of tumors. *Radiology.* 1996;**198**(3):869–873. doi:10.1148/radiology. 198.3.8628885.

132. Hann LE, *et al.* Cholangiocarcinoma at the hepatic hilus: sonographic findings. *AJR Am J Roentgenol.* 1997;**168**(4):985–989. doi:10.2214/ajr.168.4.9124155.

133. Neumaier CE, *et al.* Staging of hilar cholangiocarcinoma with ultrasound. *J Clin Ultrasound.* 1995;**23**(3):173–178.

134. Bach AM, *et al.* Portal vein evaluation with US: comparison to angiography combined with CT arterial portography. *Radiology.* 1996;**201**(1):149–154. doi:10.1148/radiology.201.1.8816536.

135. Wibbenmeyer LA, *et al*. Sonographic diagnosis of unsuspected gallbladder cancer: imaging findings in comparison with benign gallbladder conditions. *AJR Am J Roentgenol*. 1995;**165**(5):1169–1174. doi:10.2214/ajr.165.5.7572497.

136. Pandey M, *et al*. Carcinoma of the gallbladder: role of sonography in diagnosis and staging. *J Clin Ultrasound* 2000;**28**(5):227–232. doi:10.1002/(SICI)1097-0096(200006)28:5<227::AID-JCU4>3.0.CO;2-4.

137. Ohtani T, *et al*. Spread of gallbladder carcinoma: CT evaluation with pathologic correlation. *Abdom Imaging*. 1996;**21**(3):195–201.

138. Schwartz LH, *et al*. Gallbladder carcinoma: findings at MR imaging with MR cholangiopancreatography. *J Comput Assist Tomogr* 2002;**26**(3):405–410.

139. Garrow D, *et al*. Endoscopic ultrasound: a meta-analysis of test performance in suspected biliary obstruction. *Clin Gastroenterol Hepatol* 2007;**5**(5):616–623. doi:10.1016/j.cgh.2007.02.027.

140. Fujita N, *et al*. Diagnosis of the depth of invasion of gallbladder carcinoma by EUS. *Gastrointest Endosc*. 1999;**50**(5):659–663.

141. Sadamoto Y, *et al*. Preoperative diagnosis and staging of gallbladder carcinoma by EUS. *Gastrointest Endosc* 2003;**58**(4):536–541.

142. Navaneethan U, *et al*. Endoscopic ultrasound in the diagnosis of cholangiocarcinoma as the etiology of biliary strictures: a systematic review and meta-analysis. *Gastroenterol Rep*. August 2014:gou057. doi:10.1093/gastro/gou057.

143. Wu L-M, *et al*. Endoscopic ultrasound-guided fine-needle aspiration biopsy in the evaluation of bile duct strictures and gallbladder masses: a systematic review and meta-analysis. *Eur J Gastroenterol Hepatol* 2011;**23**(2):113–120. doi:10.1097/MEG.0b013e3283426313.

144. Levy MJ, *et al*. Endoscopic ultrasound staging of cholangiocarcinoma. *Curr Opin Gastroenterol* 2012;**28**(3):244–252. doi:10.1097/MOG.0b013e32835005bc.

145. Rodríguez-Fernández A, *et al*. Positron-emission tomography with fluorine-18-fluoro-2-deoxy-D-glucose for gallbladder cancer diagnosis. *Am J Surg* 2004;**188**(2):171–175. doi:10.1016/j.amjsurg.2003.12.070.

146. Oe A, *et al*. Distinguishing benign from malignant gallbladder wall thickening using FDG-PET. *Ann Nucl Med* 2006;**20**(10):699–703.

147. Kluge R, *et al*. Positron emission tomography with [(18)F]fluoro-2-deoxy-D-glucose for diagnosis and staging of bile duct cancer. *Hepatology* 2001;**33**(5):1029–1035. doi:10.1053/jhep.2001.23912.

148. Wakabayashi H, *et al*. Significance of fluorodeoxyglucose PET imaging in the diagnosis of malignancies in patients with biliary stricture. *Eur J Surg Oncol* 2005;**31**(10):1175–1179. doi:10.1016/j.ejso.2005.05.012.

149. Petrowsky H, *et al*. Impact of integrated positron emission tomography and computed tomography on staging and management of gallbladder cancer and cholangiocarcinoma. *J Hepatol* 2006;**45**(1):43–50. doi:10.1016/j.jhep.2006.03.009.

150. Fritscher-Ravens A, *et al*. FDG PET in the diagnosis of hilar cholangiocarcinoma. *Nucl Med Commun* 2001;**22**(12):1277–1285.

151. de Jong MC, *et al.* Hilar Cholangiocarcinoma: Tumor Depth as a Predictor of Outcome. *Arch Surg* 2011;**146**(6):697–703. doi:10.1001/archsurg.2011.122.

152. Juntermanns B, *et al.* Comparison of the sixth and the seventh editions of the UICC classification for perihilar cholangiocarcinoma. *Ann Surg Oncol* 2013;**20**(1):277–284. doi:10.1245/s10434-012-2486-0.

153. Jarnagin WR, *et al.* Staging, Resectability, and Outcome in 225 Patients With Hilar Cholangiocarcinoma. *Ann Surg* 2001;**234**(4):507-2195. doi:10.1007/s00330-008-1006-x.

154. Deoliveira ML, *et al.* New staging system and a registry for perihilar cholangiocarcinoma. *Hepatology* 2011;**53**(4):1363–1371. doi:10.1002/hep.24227.

155. Jang S, *et al.* High throughput molecular profiling reveals differential mutation patterns in intrahepatic cholangiocarcinomas arising in chronic advanced liver diseases. *Mod Pathol* 2014;**27**(5):731–739. doi:10.1038/modpathol.2013.194.

156. Lee SY, Cherqui D. Operative management of cholangiocarcinoma. *Semin Liver Dis* 2013;**33**(3):248–261. doi:10.1055/s-0033-1351784.

157. Uenishi T, *et al.* Serosal invasion in TNM staging of mass-forming intrahepatic cholangiocarcinoma. *J Hepatobiliary Pancreat Surg* 2005;**12**(6):479–483. doi:10.1007/s00534-005-1026-8.

158. Yamashita Y-I, *et al.* The impact of surgical treatment and poor prognostic factors for patients with intrahepatic cholangiocarcinoma: retrospective analysis of 60 patients. *Anticancer Res* 2008;**28**(4C):2353–2359.

159. Nakagohri T, *et al.* Surgical outcome and prognostic factors in intrahepatic cholangiocarcinoma. *World J Surg* 2008;**32**(12):2675–2680. doi:10.1007/s00268-008-9778-3.

160. Jiang B-G, *et al.* Retrospective analysis of histopathologic prognostic factors after hepatectomy for intrahepatic cholangiocarcinoma. *Cancer J* 2009;**15**(3):257–261. doi:10.1097/PPO.0b013e31819e3312.

161. Jonas S, *et al.* Extended liver resection for intrahepatic cholangiocarcinoma: A comparison of the prognostic accuracy of the fifth and sixth editions of the TNM classification. *Ann Surg* 2009;**249**(2):303–309. doi:10.1097/SLA.0b013e318195e164.

162. Ercolani G, *et al.* Intrahepatic cholangiocarcinoma: primary liver resection and aggressive multimodal treatment of recurrence significantly prolong survival. *Ann Surg* 2010;**252**(1):107–114. doi:10.1097/SLA.0b013e3181e462e6.

163. Lanthaler M, *et al.* Surgical treatment of intrahepatic cholangiocarcinoma--a single center experience. *Am Surg* 2010;**76**(4):411–417.

164. Cho SY, *et al.* Survival analysis of intrahepatic cholangiocarcinoma after resection. *Ann Surg Oncol* 2010;**17**(7):1823–1830. doi:10.1245/s10434-010-0938-y.

165. de Jong MC, *et al.* Intrahepatic cholangiocarcinoma: an international multi-institutional analysis of prognostic factors and lymph node assessment. *J Clin Oncol* 2011;**29**(23):3140-3145. doi:10.1200/JCO.2011.35.6519.

166. Ribero D, *et al.* Surgical Approach for Long-term Survival of Patients With Intrahepatic Cholangiocarcinoma: A Multi-institutional Analysis of 434 Patients. *Arch Surg* 2012;**147**(12):1107–1113. doi:10.1001/archsurg.2012.1962.

167. Liu Z-H, *et al.* Factors influencing the prognosis of patients with intrahepatic cholangiocarcinoma. *Acta Gastroenterol Belg* 2012;**75**(2):215–218.

168. Shimada M, *et al.* Value of lymph node dissection during resection of intrahepatic cholangiocarcinoma. *Br J Surg* 2001;**88**(11):1463–1466. doi:10.1046/j.0007-1323.2001.01879.x.

169. Clark CJ, *et al.* Lymphadenectomy in the staging and treatment of intrahepatic cholangiocarcinoma: a population-based study using the National Cancer Institute SEER database. *HPB (Oxford)* 2011;**13**(9):612-620. doi:10.1111/j.1477-2574.2011.00340.x.

170. Li D-Y, *et al.* Routine lymph node dissection may be not suitable for all intrahepatic cholangiocarcinoma patients: results of a monocentric series. *World J Gastroenterol* 2013;**19**(47):9084–9091. doi:10.3748/wjg.v19.i47.9084.

171. Schulick RD. Criteria of unresectability and the decision-making process. *MHPB* 2008;**10**(2):122–125. doi:10.1080/13651820801993540.

172. Sakamoto Y, *et al.* Prognostic factors of surgical resection in middle and distal bile duct cancer: an analysis of 55 patients concerning the significance of ductal and radial margins. *Surgery* 2005;**137**(4):396–402. doi:10.1016/j.surg.2004.10.008.

173. Allen PJ, *et al.* Extrahepatic cholangiocarcinoma: a comparison of patients with resected proximal and distal lesions. *MHPB* 2008;**10**(5):341–346. doi:10.1080/13651820802276630.

174. van der Gaag NA, *et al.* Survival analysis and prognostic nomogram for patients undergoing resection of extrahepatic cholangiocarcinoma. *Ann Oncol* 2012;**23**(10):2642–2649. doi:10.1093/annonc/mds077.

175. Tan X, *et al.* Prognostic factors of distal cholangiocarcinoma after curative surgery: a series of 84 cases. *Hepatogastroenterology* 2013;**60**(128):1892–1895.

176. Kim HJ, *et al.* The prognostic factors for survival after curative resection of distal cholangiocarcinoma: perineural invasion and lymphovascular invasion. *Surg Today* 2014;**44**(10):1879–1886. doi:10.1007/s00595-014-0846-z.

177. Popescu I, Dumitrascu T. Curative-intent surgery for hilar cholangiocarcinoma: prognostic factors for clinical decision making. *Langenbecks Arch Surg* 2014;**399**(6):693–705. doi:10.1007/s00423-014-1210-x.

178. Ebata T, *et al.* Hepatectomy with portal vein resection for hilar cholangiocarcinoma: audit of 52 consecutive cases. *Ann Surg* 2003;**238**(5):720–727. doi:10.1097/01.sla.0000094437.68038.a3.

179. Miyazaki M, *et al.* Combined vascular resection in operative resection for hilar cholangiocarcinoma: does it work or not? *Surgery* 2007;**141**(5):581–588. doi:10.1016/j.surg.2006.09.016.

180. de Jong MC, *et al.* The impact of portal vein resection on outcomes for hilar cholangiocarcinoma: a multi-institutional analysis of 305 cases. *Cancer* 2012;**118**(19):4737–4747. doi:10.1002/cncr.27492.

181. Yu W, *et al.* Effect evaluation of vascular resection for patients with hilar cholangiocarcinoma: original data and meta-analysis. *Hepatogastroenterology* 2014;**61**(130):307–313.

182. Lee SE, *et al.* Systematic review on the surgical treatment for T1 gallbladder cancer. *World J Gastroenterol* 2011;**17**(2):174–180. doi:10.3748/wjg.v17.i2.174.

183. de Aretxabala XA, *et al.* Curative resection in potentially resectable tumours of the gallbladder. *Eur J Surg.* 1997;**163**(6):419–426.

184. You DD, *et al.* What is an adequate extent of resection for T1 gallbladder cancers? *Ann Surg* 2008;**247**(5):835–838. doi:10.1097/SLA.0b013e3181675842.

185. Jensen EH, *et al.* A critical analysis of the surgical management of early-stage gallbladder cancer in the United States. *J Gastrointest Surg* 2009;**13**(4):722-727. doi:10.1007/s11605-008-0772-8.

186. Goetze TO, Paolucci V. [Immediate Radical Re-Resection of Incidental T1b Gallbladder Cancer and the Problem of an Adequate Extent of Resection (Results of the German Registry "Incidental Gallbladder Cancer").]. *Zentralbl Chir.* March 2011. doi:10.1055/s-0030-1262698.

187. Cavallaro A, *et al.* Incidental gallbladder cancer during laparoscopic cholecystectomy: managing an unexpected finding. *World J Gastroenterol* 2012;**18**(30):4019-4027. doi:10.3748/wjg.v18.i30.4019.

188. Yildirim E, *et al.* The surgical management of incidental gallbladder carcinoma. *Eur J Surg Oncol* 2005;**31**(1):45–52. doi:10.1016/j.ejso.2004.09.006.

189. Jensen EH, *et al.* Lymph node evaluation is associated with improved survival after surgery for early stage gallbladder cancer. *Surgery* 2009;**146**(4):706–11–discussion711–3. doi:10.1016/j.surg.2009.06.056.

190. Agarwal AK, *et al.* The role of staging laparoscopy in primary gall bladder cancer--an analysis of 409 patients: A prospective study to evaluate the role of staging laparoscopy in the management of gallbladder cancer. *Ann Surg* 2013;**258**(2):318–323. doi:10.1097/SLA.0b013e318271497e.

191. Belghiti J, *et al.* Seven hundred forty-seven hepatectomies in the 1990s: An update to evaluate the actual risk of liver resection. *J Am Coll Surg* 2000;**191**(1):38–46. doi:10.1007/s00535-010-0298-1.

192. Cherqui D, *et al.* Major liver resection for carcinoma in jaundiced patients without preoperative biliary drainage. *Arch Surg* 2000;**135**(3):302–308.

193. Audisio RA, *et al.* The outcome of cholangitis after percutaneous biliary drainage in neoplastic jaundice. *HPB Surg.* 1993;**6**(4):287–293. doi:10.1155/1993/17078.

194. Nomura T, *et al.* Bacteribilia and cholangitis after percutaneous transhepatic biliary drainage for malignant biliary obstruction. *Dig Dis Sci.* 1999;**44**(3):542–546. doi:10.1023/A:1026653306735.

195. Al-Bahrani AZ, *et al.* Acute pancreatitis: an under-recognized risk of percutaneous transhepatic distal biliary intervention. *MHPB* 2006;**8**(6):446–450. doi:10.1080/13651820600917294.

196. Nimura Y. Preoperative biliary drainage before resection for cholangiocarcinoma (Pro). *MHPB* 2008;**10**(2):130–133. doi:10.1080/13651820801992666.

197. Hirano S, *et al.* Oncological benefit of preoperative endoscopic biliary drainage in patients with hilar cholangiocarcinoma. *J Hepatobiliary Pancreat Sci* 2014;**21**(8):533–540. doi:10.1002/jhbp.76.

198. Rocha FG, *et al.* Hilar cholangiocarcinoma: the Memorial Sloan-Kettering Cancer Center experience 2010;**17**(4):490–496. doi:10.1007/s00534-009-0205-4.

199. Higuchi R, Yamamoto M. Indications for portal vein embolization in perihilar cholangiocarcinoma. *J Hepatobiliary Pancreat Sci* 2014;**21**(8):542–549. doi:10.1002/jhbp.77.

200. Yi B, *et al.* Preoperative portal vein embolization for hilar cholangiocarcinoma--a comparative study. *Hepatogastroenterology* 2010;**57**(104):1341–1346.

201. Hong YK, *et al.* The efficacy of portal vein embolization prior to right extended hemihepatectomy for hilar cholangiocellular carcinoma: a retrospective cohort study. *Eur J Surg Oncol* 2011;**37**(3):237–244. doi:10.1016/j.ejso.2010.12.010.

202. Palavecino M, *et al.* Portal vein embolization in hilar cholangiocarcinoma. *Surg Oncol Clin N Am* 2009;**18**(2):257–67–viii. doi:10.1016/j.soc.2008.12.007.

203. Hemming AW, *et al.* Portal vein resection in management of hilar cholangiocarcinoma. *J Am Coll Surg* 2011;**212**(4):604–13–discussion613–6. doi:10.1016/j.jamcollsurg.2010.12.028.

204. Weber SM, *et al.* Intrahepatic cholangiocarcinoma: resectability, recurrence pattern, and outcomes. *J Am Coll Surg* 2001;**193**(4):384–391.

205. Hyder O, *et al.* Recurrence after operative management of intrahepatic cholangiocarcinoma. *Surgery* 2013;**153**(6):811–818. doi:10.1016/j.surg.2012.12.005.

206. National Comprehensive Cancer Network. Hepatobiliary Cancers (Version 2.2014) . http://www.nccn.org/professionals/physician_gls/pdf/hepatobiliary.pdf. Published April 1, 2014. Accessed August 25, 2014.

207. Eckel F, *et al.* ESMO Guidelines Working Group. Biliary cancer: ESMO Clinical Practice Guidelines for diagnosis, treatment and follow-up. *Ann Oncol* 2011;**22** Suppl 6(suppl 6):vi40-vi44. doi:10.1093/annonc/mdr375.

208. A Pitt H, *et al.* Adjuvant Therapy for Biliary Malignancies: International Trends and Possibilities. *Journal of Gastrointestinal Surgery* 2003;**7**(2):309. doi:10.1016/S1091-255X(02)00364-5.

209. Nakeeb A, Pitt HA. Radiation therapy, chemotherapy and chemoradiation in hilar cholangiocarcinoma. *MHPB* 2005;**7**(4):278-282. doi:10.1080/13651820500373028.

210. Schoenthaler R, *et al.* Carcinoma of the extrahepatic bile ducts. The University of California at San Francisco experience. *Ann Surg.* 1994;**219**(3):267–274.

211. Pitt HA, *et al.* Perihilar cholangiocarcinoma. Postoperative radiotherapy does not improve survival. *Ann Surg.* 1995;**221**(6):788-97-discussion 797–798.

212. Todoroki T, *et al.* Benefits of adjuvant radiotherapy after radical resection of locally advanced main hepatic duct carcinoma. *Int J Radiat Oncol Biol Phys* 2000;**46**(3): 581–587.

213. Serafini FM, *et al.* Location, not staging, of cholangiocarcinoma determines the role for adjuvant chemoradiation therapy. *Am Surg* 2001;**67**(9):839–43–discussion843–4.

214. Gerhards MF, *et al.* Results of postoperative radiotherapy for resectable hilar cholangiocarcinoma. *World J Surg* 2003;**27**(2):173–179. doi:10.1007/s00268-002-6434-1.

215. Takada T, *et al.* Is postoperative adjuvant chemotherapy useful for gallbladder carcinoma? A phase III multicenter prospective randomized controlled trial in patients with resected pancreaticobiliary carcinoma. *Cancer* 2002;**95**(8):1685–1695. doi:10.1002/cncr.10831.

216. Sagawa N, *et al.* Effectiveness of radiation therapy after surgery for hilar cholangiocarcinoma. *Surg Today* 2005;**35**(7):548–552. doi:10.1007/s00595-005-2989-4.
217. Balachandran P, *et al.* Predictors of long-term survival in patients with gallbladder cancer. *J Gastrointest Surg* 2006;**10**(6):848–854. doi:10.1016/j.gassur.2005.12.002.
218. Mojica P, *et al.* Adjuvant radiation therapy is associated with improved survival for gallbladder carcinoma with regional metastatic disease. *J Surg Oncol* 2007;**96**(1):8–13. doi:10.1002/jso.20831.
219. Wang SJ, *et al.* Prediction model for estimating the survival benefit of adjuvant radiotherapy for gallbladder cancer. *J Clin Oncol* 2008;**26**(13):2112–2117. doi:10.1200/JCO.2007.14.7934.
220. Borghero Y, *et al.* Extrahepatic bile duct adenocarcinoma: patients at high-risk for local recurrence treated with surgery and adjuvant chemoradiation have an equivalent overall survival to patients with standard-risk treated with surgery alone. *Ann Surg Oncol* 2008;**15**(11):3147–3156. doi:10.1245/s10434-008-9998-7.
221. Gold DG, *et al.* Adjuvant therapy for gallbladder carcinoma: the Mayo Clinic Experience. *Int J Radiat Oncol Biol Phys* 2009;**75**(1):150–155. doi:10.1016/j.ijrobp.2008.10.052.
222. Shinohara ET, *et al.* Radiotherapy is associated with improved survival in adjuvant and palliative treatment of extrahepatic cholangiocarcinomas. *Int J Radiat Oncol Biol Phys* 2009;**74**(4):1191–1198. doi:10.1016/j.ijrobp.2008.09.017.
223. Murakami Y, *et al.* Adjuvant gemcitabine plus S-1 chemotherapy improves survival after aggressive surgical resection for advanced biliary carcinoma. *Ann Surg* 2009; **250**(6):950–956.
224. Wirasorn K, *et al.* Adjuvant chemotherapy in resectable cholangiocarcinoma patients. *J Gastroenterol Hepatol* 2013;**28**(12):1885–1891. doi:10.1111/jgh.12321.
225. Horgan AM, *et al.* Adjuvant therapy in the treatment of biliary tract cancer: a systematic review and meta-analysis. *J Clin Oncol* 2012;**30**(16):1934–1940. doi:10.1200/JCO.2011.40.5381.
226. Casavilla FA, *et al.* Hepatic resection and transplantation for peripheral cholangiocarcinoma. *J Am Coll Surg.* 1997;**185**(5):429–436.
227. Iwatsuki S, *et al.* Treatment of hilar cholangiocarcinoma (Klatskin tumors) with hepatic resection or transplantation. *J Am Coll Surg.* 1998;**187**(4):358–364.
228. Meyer CG, *et al.* Liver transplantation for cholangiocarcinoma: results in 207 patients. *Transplantation* 2000;**69**(8):1633–1637.
229. Shimoda M, *et al.* Liver transplantation for cholangiocellular carcinoma: analysis of a single-center experience and review of the literature. *Liver Transpl* 2001;**7**(12): 1023–1033. doi:10.1053/jlts.2001.29419.
230. Brandsaeter B, *et al.* Liver transplantation for primary sclerosing cholangitis; Predictors and consequences of hepatobiliary malignancy. *J Hepatol* 2004;**40**(5): 815–822. doi:10.1016/j.jhep.2004.01.002.
231. Robles R, *et al.* Spanish experience in liver transplantation for hilar and peripheral cholangiocarcinoma. *Ann Surg* 2004;**239**(2):265–271. doi:10.1097/01.sla.0000108702.45715.81.

232. Sudan D, *et al.* Radiochemotherapy and transplantation allow long-term survival for nonresectable hilar cholangiocarcinoma. *Am J Transplant* 2002;**2**(8):774–779.

233. Rosen CB, *et al.* Surgery for cholangiocarcinoma: the role of liver transplantation. *HPB (Oxford)* 2008;**10**(3):186–189. doi:10.1080/13651820801992542.

234. Alden ME, Mohiuddin M. The impact of radiation dose in combined external beam and intraluminal Ir-192 brachytherapy for bile duct cancer. *Int J Radiat Oncol Biol Phys.* 1994;**28**(4):945–951.

235. Foo ML, *et al.* External radiation therapy and transcatheter iridium in the treatment of extrahepatic bile duct carcinoma. *Int J Radiat Oncol Biol Phys.* 1997;**39**(4):929–935.

236. Urego M, *et al.* Radiotherapy and multimodality management of cholangiocarcinoma. *Int J Radiat Oncol Biol Phys.* 1999;**44**(1):121–126. doi:10.1016/S0360-3016(98)00509-4.

237. Crane CH, *et al.* Limitations of conventional doses of chemoradiation for unresectable biliary cancer. *Int J Radiat Oncol Biol Phys* 2002;**53**(4):969–974.

238. Shin HS, *et al.* Combination of external beam irradiation and high-dose-rate intraluminal brachytherapy for inoperable carcinoma of the extrahepatic bile ducts. *Int J Radiat Oncol Biol Phys* 2003;**57**(1):105–112.

239. Park JY, *et al.* Concurrent chemoradiotherapy with doxifluridine and paclitaxel for extrahepatic bile duct cancer. *Am J Clin Oncol* 2006;**29**(3):240–245. doi:10.1097/01. coc.0000217829.77404.22.

240. Ben-David MA, *et al.* External-beam radiotherapy for localized extrahepatic cholangiocarcinoma. *Int J Radiat Oncol Biol Phys* 2006;**66**(3):772–779. doi:10.1016/j.ijrobp. 2006.05.061.

241. Deodato F, *et al.* Chemoradiation and brachytherapy in biliary tract carcinoma: long-term results. *Int J Radiat Oncol Biol Phys* 2006;**64**(2):483–488. doi:10.1016/j. ijrobp.2005.07.977.

242. Chen Y-X, *et al.* Determining the role of external beam radiotherapy in unresectable intrahepatic cholangiocarcinoma: a retrospective analysis of 84 patients. *BMC Cancer* 2010;**10**(1):492. doi:10.1186/1471-2407-10-492.

243. Kopek N, *et al.* Stereotactic body radiotherapy for unresectable cholangiocarcinoma. *Radiother Oncol* 2010;**94**(1):47-52. doi:10.1016/j.radonc.2009.11.004.

244. Park S-Y, *et al.* Transarterial chemoembolization versus supportive therapy in the palliative treatment of unresectable intrahepatic cholangiocarcinoma. *Clin Radiol* 2011;**66**(4):322–328. doi:10.1016/j.crad.2010.11.002.

245. Gusani NJ, *et al.* Treatment of unresectable cholangiocarcinoma with gemcitabine-based transcatheter arterial chemoembolization (TACE): a single-institution experience. *J Gastrointest Surg* 2008;**12**(1):129–137. doi:10.1007/s11605-007-0312-y.

246. Kiefer MV, *et al.* Chemoembolization of intrahepatic cholangiocarcinoma with cis-platinum, doxorubicin, mitomycin C, ethiodol, and polyvinyl alcohol: a 2-center study. *Cancer* 2011;**117**(7):1498–1505. doi:10.1002/cncr.25625.

247. Shen WF, *et al.* Adjuvant transcatheter arterial chemoembolization for intrahepatic cholangiocarcinoma after curative surgery: retrospective control study. *World J Surg* 2011;**35**(9):2083–2091. doi:10.1007/s00268-011-1171-y.

248. Wu ZF, *et al*. Postoperative adjuvant transcatheter arterial chemoembolisation improves survival of intrahepatic cholangiocarcinoma patients with poor prognostic factors: results of a large monocentric series. *Eur J Surg Oncol* 2012;**38**(7):602–610. doi:10.1016/j.ejso.2012.02.185.

249. Kim JH, *et al*. Radiofrequency ablation for the treatment of primary intrahepatic cholangiocarcinoma. *AJR Am J Roentgenol* 2011;**196**(2):W205-W209. doi:10.2214/AJR.10.4937.

250. Xu H-X, *et al*. Percutaneous ultrasound-guided thermal ablation for intrahepatic cholangiocarcinoma. *Br J Radiol* 2012;**85**(1016):1078–1084. doi:10.1259/bjr/2456 3774.

251. Ortner MEJ, *et al*. Successful photodynamic therapy for nonresectable cholangiocarcinoma: a randomized prospective study. *Gastroenterology* 2003;**125**(5):1355–1363.

252. Cheon YK, *et al*. Longterm outcome of photodynamic therapy compared with biliary stenting alone in patients with advanced hilar cholangiocarcinoma. *HPB (Oxford)* 2012;**14**(3):185–193. doi:10.1111/j.1477-2574.2011.00424.x.

253. Pereira S, *et al*. Photostent-02; porfimer sodium photodynamic therapy plus stenting versus stenting alone in patients (pts) with advanced or metastatic …. In: 2010.

254. Ellis PA, *et al*. Epirubicin, cisplatin and infusional 5-fluorouracil (5-FU) (ECF) in hepatobiliary tumours. *European Journal of Cancer*. 1995;**31**A(10):1594–1598.

255. Patt YZ, *et al*. Phase II trial of intravenous flourouracil and subcutaneous interferon alfa-2b for biliary tract cancer. *J Clin Oncol*. 1996;**14**(8):2311–2315.

256. Chen JS, *et al*. Weekly 24 h infusion of high-dose 5-fluorouracil and leucovorin in patients with biliary tract carcinomas. *Anticancer Drugs*. 1998;**9**(5):393–397.

257. Ducreux M, *et al*. Effective treatment of advanced biliary tract carcinoma using 5-fluorouracil continuous infusion with cisplatin. *Ann Oncol*. 1998;**9**(6):653–656.

258. Raderer M, *et al*. Two consecutive phase II studies of 5-fluorouracil/leucovorin/mitomycin C and of gemcitabine in patients with advanced biliary cancer. *Oncology*. 1999;**56**(3):177–180.

259. Choi CW, *et al*. Effects of 5-fluorouracil and leucovorin in the treatment of pancreatic-biliary tract adenocarcinomas. *Am J Clin Oncol* 2000;**23**(4):425–428.

260. Patt YZ, *et al*. Phase II trial of cisplatin, interferon alpha-2b, doxorubicin, and 5-fluorouracil for biliary tract cancer. *Clin Cancer Res* 2001;**7**(11):3375–3380.

261. Chen JS, *et al*. Mitomycin C with weekly 24-h infusion of high-dose 5-fluorouracil and leucovorin in patients with biliary tract and periampullar carcinomas. *Anticancer Drugs* 2001;**12**(4):339–343.

262. Kim TW, *et al*. Phase II study of capecitabine plus cisplatin as first-line chemotherapy in advanced biliary cancer. *Ann Oncol* 2003;**14**(7):1115–1120.

263. Kornek GV, *et al*. Mitomycin C in combination with capecitabine or biweekly high-dose gemcitabine in patients with advanced biliary tract cancer: a randomised phase II trial. *Ann Oncol* 2004;**15**(3):478–483.

264. Ueno H, *et al*. Phase II study of S-1 in patients with advanced biliary tract cancer. *Br J Cancer* 2004;**91**(10):1769–1774. doi:10.1038/sj.bjc.6602208.

265. Rao S, *et al.* Phase III study of 5FU, etoposide and leucovorin (FELV) compared to epirubicin, cisplatin and 5FU (ECF) in previously untreated patients with advanced biliary cancer. *Br J Cancer* 2005;**92**(9):1650–1654. doi:10.1038/sj.bjc.6602576.

266. Cho JY, *et al.* Capecitabine combined with gemcitabine (CapGem) as first-line treatment in patients with advanced/metastatic biliary tract carcinoma. *Cancer* 2005; **104**(12):2753–2758. doi:10.1002/cncr.21591.

267. Cho JY, *et al.* A Phase II study of capecitabine combined with gemcitabine in patients with advanced gallbladder carcinoma. *Yonsei Med J* 2005;**46**(4):526–531. doi:10.3349/ymj.2005.46.4.526.

268. Ducreux M, *et al.* A randomised phase II trial of weekly high-dose 5-fluorouracil with and without folinic acid and cisplatin in patients with advanced biliary tract carcinoma: results of the 40955 EORTC trial. *European Journal of Cancer* 2005;**41**(3):398–403. doi:10.1016/j.ejca.2004.10.026.

269. Park SH, *et al.* Phase II study of epirubicin, cisplatin, and capecitabine for advanced biliary tract adenocarcinoma. *Cancer* 2006;**106**(2):361–365. doi:10.1002/cncr.21621.

270. Hong YS, *et al.* Phase II study of capecitabine and cisplatin in previously untreated advanced biliary tract cancer. *Cancer Chemother Pharmacol* 2007;**60**(3):321–328. doi:10.1007/s00280-006-0380-9.

271. Feisthammel J, *et al.* Irinotecan with 5-FU/FA in advanced biliary tract adenocarcinomas: a multicenter phase II trial. *Am J Clin Oncol* 2007;**30**(3):319–324. doi:10.1097/01.coc.0000258124.72884.7a.

272. Furuse J, *et al.* A phase II study of uracil-tegafur plus doxorubicin and prognostic factors in patients with unresectable biliary tract cancer. *Cancer Chemother Pharmacol* 2009;**65**(1):113–120. doi:10.1007/s00280-009-1011-z.

273. Penz M, *et al.* Phase II trial of two-weekly gemcitabine in patients with advanced biliary tract cancer. *Ann Oncol* 2001;**12**(2):183–186.

274. Gebbia V, *et al.* Treatment of inoperable and/or metastatic biliary tree carcinomas with single-agent gemcitabine or in combination with levofolinic acid and infusional fluorouracil: results of a multicenter phase II study. *J Clin Oncol* 2001;**19**(20): 4089–4091.

275. Kuhn R, *et al.* Outpatient therapy with gemcitabine and docetaxel for gallbladder, biliary, and cholangio-carcinomas. *Invest New Drugs* 2002;**20**(3):351–356.

276. Bhargava P, *et al.* Gemcitabine and irinotecan in locally advanced or metastatic biliary cancer: preliminary report. *Oncology (Williston Park, NY)* 2003;**17**(9 Suppl 8):23–26.

277. André T, *et al.* Gemcitabine combined with oxaliplatin (GEMOX) in advanced biliary tract adenocarcinoma: a GERCOR study. *Ann Oncol* 2004;**15**(9):1339–1343. doi:10.1093/annonc/mdh351.

278. Knox JJ, *et al.* Gemcitabine concurrent with continuous infusional 5-fluorouracil in advanced biliary cancers: a review of the Princess Margaret Hospital experience. *Ann Oncol* 2004;**15**(5):770–774.

279. Alberts SR, *et al.* Gemcitabine, 5-fluorouracil, and leucovorin in advanced biliary tract and gallbladder carcinoma: a North Central Cancer Treatment Group phase II trial. *Cancer* 2005;**103**(1):111–118. doi:10.1002/cncr.20753.

280. Thongprasert S, *et al.* Phase II study of gemcitabine and cisplatin as first-line chemotherapy in inoperable biliary tract carcinoma. *Ann Oncol* 2005;**16**(2):279–281. doi:10.1093/annonc/mdi046.

281. Knox JJ, *et al.* Combining gemcitabine and capecitabine in patients with advanced biliary cancer: a phase II trial. *J Clin Oncol* 2005;**23**(10):2332–2338. doi:10.1200/JCO.2005.51.008.

282. Lee G-W, *et al.* Combination chemotherapy with gemcitabine and cisplatin as first-line treatment for immunohistochemically proven cholangiocarcinoma. *Am J Clin Oncol* 2006;**29**(2):127–131. doi:10.1097/01.coc.0000203742.22828.bb.

283. Kim ST, *et al.* A Phase II study of gemcitabine and cisplatin in advanced biliary tract cancer. *Cancer* 2006;**106**(6):1339–1346. doi:10.1002/cncr.21741.

284. Harder J, *et al.* Outpatient chemotherapy with gemcitabine and oxaliplatin in patients with biliary tract cancer. *Br J Cancer* 2006;**95**(7):848–852. doi:10.1038/sj.bjc.6603334.

285. Manzione L, *et al.* Chemotherapy with gemcitabine and oxaliplatin in patients with advanced biliary tract cancer: A single-institution experience. *Oncology* 2007;**73** (5–6):311–315. doi:10.1159/000134239.

286. Alberts SR, *et al.* Pemetrexed and gemcitabine for biliary tract and gallbladder carcinomas: a North Central Cancer Treatment Group (NCCTG) phase I and II Trial, N9943. *J Gastrointest Cancer* 2007;**38**(2–4):87–94. doi:10.1007/s12029-008-9037-8.

287. Riechelmann RP, *et al.* Expanded phase II trial of gemcitabine and capecitabine for advanced biliary cancer. *Cancer* 2007;**110**(6):1307-1312. doi:10.1002/cncr.22902.

288. Lee J, *et al.* Phase II trial of gemcitabine combined with cisplatin in patients with inoperable biliary tract carcinomas. *Cancer Chemother Pharmacol* 2008;**61**(1):47–52. doi:10.1007/s00280-007-0444-5.

289. André T, *et al.* Gemcitabine and oxaliplatin in advanced biliary tract carcinoma: a phase II study. *Br J Cancer* 2008;**99**(6):862–867. doi:10.1038/sj.bjc.6604628.

290. Meyerhardt JA, *et al.* Phase-II study of gemcitabine and cisplatin in patients with metastatic biliary and gallbladder cancer. *Dig Dis Sci* 2008;**53**(2):564–570. doi:10.1007/s10620-007-9885-2.

291. Kim HJ, *et al.* A phase II study of gemcitabine in combination with oxaliplatin as first-line chemotherapy in patients with inoperable biliary tract cancer. *Cancer Chemother Pharmacol* 2009;**64**(2):371–377. doi:10.1007/s00280-008-0883-7.

292. Jang J-S, *et al.* Gemcitabine and oxaliplatin in patients with unresectable biliary cancer including gall bladder cancer: a Korean Cancer Study Group phase II trial. *Cancer Chemother Pharmacol* 2010;**65**(4):641–647. doi:10.1007/s00280-009-1069-7.

293. Yonemoto N, *et al.* A multi-center retrospective analysis of survival benefits of chemotherapy for unresectable biliary tract cancer. *Jpn J Clin Oncol* 2007;**37**(11):843–851. doi:10.1093/jjco/hym116.

294. Eckel F, Schmid RM. Chemotherapy in advanced biliary tract carcinoma: a pooled analysis of clinical trials. *Br J Cancer* 2007;**96**(6):896–902. doi:10.1038/sj.bjc.6603648.

295. Valle J, *et al.* Cisplatin plus gemcitabine versus gemcitabine for biliary tract cancer 2010;**362**(14):1273–1281. doi:10.1056/NEJMoa0908721.

296. Malka D, *et al.* Gemcitabine and oxaliplatin with or without cetuximab in advanced biliary-tract cancer (BINGO): a randomised, open-label, non-comparative phase 2 trial. *Lancet Oncol* 2014;**15**(8):819–828. doi:10.1016/S1470-2045(14)70212-8.

297. Philip PA, *et al.* Phase II study of erlotinib in patients with advanced biliary cancer. *J Clin Oncol* 2006;**24**(19):3069–3074. doi:10.1200/JCO.2005.05.3579.

298. Chiorean EG, *et al.* Phase II trial of erlotinib and docetaxel in advanced and refractory hepatocellular and biliary cancers: Hoosier Oncology Group GI06-101. *The Oncologist* 2012;**17**(1):13. doi:10.1634/theoncologist.2011-0253.

299. Lee J, *et al.* Gemcitabine and oxaliplatin with or without erlotinib in advanced biliary-tract cancer: a multicentre, open-label, randomised, phase 3 study. *Lancet Oncol* 2012;**13**(2):181–188. doi:10.1016/S1470-2045(11)70301-1.

300. Paule B, *et al.* Cetuximab plus gemcitabine-oxaliplatin (GEMOX) in patients with refractory advanced intrahepatic cholangiocarcinomas. *Oncology* 2007;**72**(1–2): 105–110. doi:10.1159/111117.

301. Malka D, *et al.* Gemcitabine and oxaliplatin with or without cetuximab in advanced biliary-tract cancer (BINGO): a randomised, open-label, non-comparative phase 2 trial. *Lancet Oncol* 2014;**15**(8):819–828. doi:10.1016/S1470-2045(14)70212-8.

302. Jensen LH, *et al.* Phase II marker-driven trial of panitumumab and chemotherapy in KRAS wild-type biliary tract cancer. *Ann Oncol* 2012;**23**(9):2341–2346. doi:10.1093/annonc/mds008.

303. Sohal DPS, *et al.* A phase II trial of gemcitabine, irinotecan and panitumumab in advanced cholangiocarcinoma. *Ann Oncol* 2013;**24**(12):3061–3065. doi:10.1093/annonc/mdt416.

304. Zhu AX, *et al.* Efficacy and safety of gemcitabine, oxaliplatin, and bevacizumab in advanced biliary-tract cancers and correlation of changes in 18-fluorodeoxyglucose PET with clinical outcome: a phase 2 study. *Lancet Oncol* 2010;**11**(1):48–54. doi:10.1016/S1470-2045(09)70333-X.

305. Bengala C, *et al.* Sorafenib in patients with advanced biliary tract carcinoma: a phase II trial. *Br J Cancer* 2010;**102**(1):68–72. doi:10.1038/sj.bjc.6605458.

306. El-Khoueiry AB, *et al.* SWOG 0514: a phase II study of sorafenib in patients with unresectable or metastatic gallbladder carcinoma and cholangiocarcinoma. *Invest New Drugs* 2012;**30**(4):1646–1651. doi:10.1007/s10637-011-9719-0.

307. Yi JH, *et al.* A phase II study of sunitinib as a second-line treatment in advanced biliary tract carcinoma: a multicentre, multinational study. *Eur J Cancer* 2012;**48**(2):196–201. doi:10.1016/j.ejca.2011.11.017.

308. Valle JW, *et al.* ABC-03: A randomized phase II trial of cediranib (AZD2171) or placebo in combination with cisplatin/gemcitabine (CisGem) chemotherapy for patients (pts) with advanced biliary tract cancer (ABC). *J Clin Oncol* 2014;**32**(5s): (suppl–abstr4002).

309. Ramanathan RK, *et al.* A phase II study of lapatinib in patients with advanced biliary tree and hepatocellular cancer. *Cancer Chemother Pharmacol* 2009;**64**(4):777–783. doi:10.1007/s00280-009-0927-7.

310. Bekaii-Saab T, *et al.* Multi-institutional phase II study of selumetinib in patients with metastatic biliary cancers. *J Clin Oncol* 2011;**29**(17):2357–2363. doi:10.1200/JCO.2010.33.9473.

311. Lubner SJ, *et al.* Report of a multicenter phase II trial testing a combination of biweekly bevacizumab and daily erlotinib in patients with unresectable biliary cancer: a phase II Consortium study. *J Clin Oncol* 2010;**28**(21):3491–3497. doi:10.1200/JCO.2010.28.4075.

312. El-Khoueiry AB, *et al.* S0941: a phase 2 SWOG study of sorafenib and erlotinib in patients with advanced gallbladder carcinoma or cholangiocarcinoma. *Br J Cancer* 2014;**110**(4):882–887. doi:10.1038/bjc.2013.801.

Chapter 18

Neuroendocrine Tumors

Mauro Cives and Jonathan Strosberg

1 Introduction

Neuroendocrine tumors (NETs) are a heterogeneous group of malignancies originating in secretory cells of the diffuse neuroendocrine system. They are characterized by a relatively indolent rate of growth and the propensity to produce and secrete a variety of hormones and vasoactive peptides.[1,2] Gastroenteropancreatic-NETs (GEP-NETs) are subcategorized into two distinct biological entities: carcinoid tumors of the luminal gastrointestinal tract and pancreatic NETs (pNETs). The term 'carcinoid' was coined in 1907 by Siegfried Oberndorfer to describe a morphologically and clinically distinct type of intestinal neoplasm that was relatively benign.[1] However, it is now clear that most carcinoid tumors, even when biologically indolent, are malignant neoplasms. Nevertheless, the term 'carcinoid' still persists and is often used to describe well-differentiated NETs arising in the lung and digestive tract.

GEP-NETs have distinct clinical features depending on their site of origin. In 1963, Williams and Sandler categorized carcinoid tumors based on embryonic derivation, distinguishing between foregut (bronchial, gastric, duodenal), midgut (jejunal, ileal, cecal), and hindgut (distal colic and rectal) tumors.[3] Foregut and hindgut NETs are associated with a more aggressive clinical behavior and shorter life expectancy. Although gastrointestinal NETs originating in any site can produce hormones, metastatic midgut carcinoids are more strongly linked to the classical carcinoid syndrome, characterized by flushing, diarrhea, and right-sided valvular heart disease. Furthermore, midgut tumors are more prone to metastasize to liver, root of the mesentery, and locoregional lymph nodes, but once metastatic they often progress at an indolent pace.[4,5] Although of some utility, the embryological classification of gut NETs is somewhat oversimplified. For example, despite sharing the midgut origin, ileal carcinoids have a substantially higher metastatic potential when compared to appendiceal NETs. Similarly, colonic carcinoids are usually more aggressive than rectal NETs, despite the same embryological derivation.

NETs can present as hormonally functioning or nonfunctioning tumors. pNETs are usually hormonal silent, but can secrete a variety of peptide hormones including insulin, gastrin, glucagon, or vasoactive intestinal peptide (VIP).[6] Tumors should be described as functional only if they are associated with signs and symptoms consistent with excessive hormonal secretion, regardless of hormone staining on immunohistochemical testing.[7]

Although historically perceived as rare entities, GEP-NETs represent the second-most common digestive cancer in terms of prevalence.[5,8] The expanding role of somatostatin analogs (SSAs) and the availability of new systemic and liver-directed therapies have significantly improved the prognosis of patients with advanced carcinoid tumors in recent years.[5,9] In this context, a systematic multidisciplinary approach strongly impacts on GEP-NET patient care, maximizing the benefit of recent advancements in the field.[10]

2 Epidemiology

In the most updated series of 29,664 patients with GEP-NETs reported to the Surveillance, Epidemiology, and End Results (SEER) program of the National Cancer Institute, an incidence of 3.65 per 100,000 individuals per year was reported.[11] The age-adjusted incidence of GEP-NETs has steadily increased in the last four decades, with a 3.6-fold increase within the 1973–2007 time interval.[8] The expansion in diagnoses is likely related to the increased use of endoscopic and imaging studies as well as improved recognition of neuroendocrine histology. Small intestine (30.8%), rectum (26.3%), colon (17.6%), pancreas (12.1%), and appendix (5.7%) are the most common primary NET sites in the digestive tract.[12] While Caucasian patients seem more prone to develop small bowel carcinoid tumors, rectal NETs occur predominantly in African-American, Asian and Native American patients. Female patients are more likely to develop carcinoid tumors in the stomach, appendix or cecum, whereas male sex is associated with tumors in the jejunum–ileum, duodenum, and rectum.[5] Estimates of metastatic rates vary due to referral patterns, and even national databases such as SEER may underreport tumors that are not considered malignant. No environmental risk factors have been identified. Individuals with a family history of carcinoid tumor in a first-degree relative have a 3.6-fold increased risk of disease.[13]

3 The Cell of Origin

Gastrointestinal NETs arise from the malignant proliferation of neuroendocrine cells, which are located throughout the length of the gut and represent the largest group of hormone-producing cells in the body.[14] Historically regarded as originating from the neural crest, neuroendocrine cells have been shown to share the same endodermal origin with the other cell components of the intestinal mucosa and are currently thought to derive from local multipotent gastrointestinal stem cells.[15] Similarly, the islet-cell derivation of pNETs has been recently questioned and an alternative origin from precursors in the ductal epithelium has been postulated.[16] It is possible that tumorigenesis may originate in both islets of Langerhans and ductal epithelium.

Up to 14 distinct types of neuroendocrine cells have been identified in the digestive tract and pancreas, where they function to regulate hormone secretion and gastrointestinal motility (Table 1).[17] Discrepancies have been described between

Table 1 Gut neuroendocrine cells: distribution, function, and related hormonal syndrome.

Cell Type	Main Product	Localization	Related Hormonal Syndrome
A	Glucagon	Pancreas, fetal stomach	Glucagonoma
B	Insulin	Pancreas	Insulinoma
CCK	CCK	Duodenum, jejunum	
D	Somatostatin	Pancreas, stomach, duodenum	Somatostatinoma
D1	Ghrelin	Stomach	
EC	Serotonin	Stomach, small and large intestines, appendix	Carcinoid syndrome
ECL	Histamine	Stomach	Atypical carcinoid syndrome
G	Gastrin	Stomach antrum, duodenum	Zollinger–Ellison syndrome
GIP	GIP	Duodenum, jejunum	
L	GLI/PYY	Small and large intestines, appendix	
M	Motilin	Duodenum, jejunum	
N	Neurotensin	Small bowel	
PP	PP	Pancreas	
S	Secretin	Duodenum, jejunum	

Abbreviations: CCK, cholecystokinin; GIP, glucose-dependent insulin-releasing peptide; GLI, glicentin; PYY, peptide YY; PP, substance P.

the tissue distribution and prevalence of neuroendocrine cells and their malignant counterparts. For example, G cells are normally present in the antrum and, in minor extent, in the duodenum, whereas they are absent in the pancreas, apart from fetal life. Nevertheless, gastrinomas predominate in the duodenum and pancreas, within the so called "gastrinoma triangle," while being rare in the antrum. Similarly, although a plethora of endocrine cells populate the gastric mucosa, only enterochromaffin-like (ECL) cells account for the vast majority of gastric carcinoids.[18,19]

4 Tumor Biology

In recent years, whole exome sequencing has provided a more detailed picture of the genetic landscape of GEP-NETs, particularly for pNETs. In one study of 68 sporadic pNETs, mutations of *MEN1* and *DAXX/ATRX* were found in 44% and 43% of tumors, respectively, while 14% of specimens had mutations in genes associated with the mammalian target of rapamycin (mTOR) pathway including *PTEN*, *TSC2*, and *PIK3CA*.[20] In a cohort of 37 Chinese pNET patients, *MEN1*, *DAXX/ATRX*, and mTOR signaling genes were found to be mutated in 35%, 54%, and 54% of tumors. The same patient population showed also mutations of *KRAS*, *TP53*, and *VHL* in 11%, 13%, and 41% of specimens.[21] These mutations are not commonly detected in Caucasian patients. Mutations in *DAXX/ATRX* are strongly associated with the induction of the alternative lengthening of telomeres (ALT) pathway and chromosomal instability (CIN).[22] Conflicting data have been reported regarding the prognostic role of *DAXX/ATRX* in pNETs.[20–22]

The genetic underpinnings of small bowel carcinoid tumors are less understood. Massively parallel DNA sequencing of 48 small bowel carcinoids has shown a low mutational rate of 0.1 somatic single nucleotide variants (SSNVs) per 10^5 nucleotides. The discovery of mutations and deletions in *CDKN1B*, the cyclin-dependent kinase inhibitor gene encoding p27, has also raised the possibility that cell-cycle dysregulation may have a role in the pathogenesis of small bowel NETs.[23] Overexpression of mTOR and/or its downstream targets is observed with high frequency in small bowel NETs and is associated with higher proliferative activity and poorer clinical outcomes.[24]

The importance of the tumor microenvironment in GEP-NET pathogenesis has been recently recognized. GEP-NETs exhibit a high degree of vascularization and a consistent cross-talk exists between neuroendocrine cells and endothelial cells. In particular, NET cells overexpress proangiogenic factors including vascular endothelial growth factor (VEGF), fibroblast growth factor (FGF), and platelet-derived growth factor (PDGF).[25,26] Paradoxically, low-grade pNETs exhibit higher microvessel density than high-grade tumors.[27] The biological and clinical significance of this phenomenon needs to be further explored. Infiltration of inflammatory cells is a frequent event in NETs. In particular, the presence of CD3+ T cells has been associated with better survival in patients with intermediate-grade disease.[28] In midgut carcinoids, an increase of systemic FOXP3+ Treg cells drives energy by downregulating the T-cell proliferative capacity.[29] A rapid influx of mast cells has been described in animal models after development of *Myc*-driven pNETs, and inhibition of their degranulation is able to cause vasculature collapse and tumor regression.[30]

5 Pathology, Staging, and Prognosis

Tumor grade and differentiation are important prognostic and predictive factors in GEP-NETs. Despite often used interchangeably, grade and differentiation are not identical terms. In fact, while grade refers to the proliferative activity of the tumor, measured by ki-67 labeling index and/or mitotic rate, differentiation refers to the extent to which neoplastic cells resemble normal endocrine tissue. The most recent classification proposed by the World Health Organization (WHO) distinguishes between well-differentiated tumors (grade 1 or 2) and poorly differentiated tumors (grade 3). Well-differentiated tumors consist of small monomorphic cells arranged in islets or trabeculae with a "salt-and-pepper" chromatin pattern. By contrast, poorly differentiated tumors are often characterized as sheets of pleomorphic cells with extensive necrosis. Tumor grade is defined numerically, with grade 1 tumors having a mitotic rate of 0–1 per 10 high powered field (HPF) or ki-67 index of 0–2%; grade 2 tumors having mitotic rate of 2–20 per HPF or ki-67 index of 3–20%; and grade 3 tumors having higher mitotic rate or ki-67 index.[31] Tumor grade should always be measured in the most mitotically active areas of the pathology specimen. In this context, heterogeneity in mitotic activity between tumors within the same patient and even within a particular tumor should be always taken into account.[32] It should be emphasized that the expertise and experience of pathologists determines the accuracy of the diagnosis in this highly heterogeneous disease. The prognostic relevance of the 2010 WHO grading system has been confirmed by large series studies in both small bowel and pNETs. In one institutional study of midgut NETs, the five-year survival rates for low and intermediate grade tumors were 79% and 74%, respectively, whereas high grade NETs had a five-year survival rate of 40%. Similarly, in pNETs the five-year survival rates for low, intermediate and high grade tumors were 75%, 62%, and 7%, respectively.[9,33]

Formal TNM staging classifications have been only recently introduced for GEP-NETs. Both the European Neuroendocrine Tumor Society (ENETS) and the American Joint Committee on Cancer (AJCC) have adopted the same staging system for midgut and hindgut NETs, whereas slightly different classifications

Table 2   Five-year survival rates in midgut carcinoids and pNETs.

Stage	Midgut Carcinoids	pNETS	
	(ENETS/AJCC Classification)	ENETS Classification	AJCC Classification
Stage I	100%	100%	92%
Stage II	100%	88%	84%
Stage III	91%	85%	81%
Stage IV	72%	57%	57%

Data are taken from Refs. 9 and 37.

Table 3   Familial neuroendocrine syndromes: Genetic and clinical features.

Syndrome	Causative Gene	Gene Location	Protein	GEP-NET type (Penetrance)
MEN1	*MEN1*	11q13	Menin	Gastrinoma (40%)
				Non-functioning pNET (20%)
				Insulinoma (10%)
				Glucagonoma <1%
				VIPoma <1%
				Gastric carcinoid 10%
VHL syndrome	*VHL*	3p25	VHL	Non-functioning pNET (12–17%)
Tuberous sclerosis	*TSC1/TSC2*	9q34/16p13	Hamartin/tuberin	pNET (<5%)
NF1	*NF1*	17q11.2	Neurofibromin	Somatostatinoma (6%)

Data are taken from Refs. 22 and 139.

have been embraced for pNETs.[34,35] Validations of both staging systems have been performed on population and institutional databases[33,36] with some evidence suggesting a slightly higher prognostic relevance of the ENETS classification of pNETs.[37] Prognosis of patients with midgut carcinoid or pNET is summarized in Table 2.

6 Clinical Features

GEP-NETs are heterogeneous neoplasms in which diagnosis may arise from effects of tumor growth or hormone secretion. Increasingly, tumors are also detected incidentally, as a result of diagnostic evaluations for unrelated diseases or symptoms. The majority of GEP-NETs are sporadic, but they can also occur as part of inherited familial syndromes, such as multiple endocrine neoplasia type 1 (MEN-1), Von Hippel–Lindau syndrome, tuberous sclerosis, and neurofibromatosis type 1 (Table 3).

7 Familial Neuroendocrine Syndromes

MEN1 is a familial predisposition to tumors of the anterior pituitary, parathyroid glands and pancreaticoduodenal neuroendocrine cells. Carcinoid tumors, lipomas, and angiofibromas can also occur with increased frequency in this disorder. MEN1 is inherited as an autosomal-dominant syndrome and is caused by an inactivating mutation of the *MEN1* gene, located at 11q13. *MEN1* encodes for menin, a nuclear protein which has functions in cell division, genome stability, and transcription regulation via histone methylation. Up to 10% of patients with MEN1 syndrome may not harbor mutations in the coding regions of the *MEN1* gene, but in the gene promoter or untranslated regions, challenging the genetic diagnosis.[38,39] Parathyroid tumors, which typically develop during the third decade and result in primary hyper-parathyroidism, are the most common feature of MEN1, occurring in ~95% of MEN1 patients. Pituitary tumors, consisting of prolactinomas, somatotrophinomas, corticotrophinomas, and non-functioning adenomas, are observed in ~30% of patients. Pancreatic NETs, most commonly gastrinomas and nonfunctioning tumors, become clinically apparent in about one-third of patients, with a higher rate of subclinical disease. Although early resection can prevent the development of distant metastases, the invariably multifocal appearance of pNETs in patients with MEN1 limits the role of curative surgical therapy.[38,40] Most pNETs associated with MEN1 are exceptionally slow-growing and impact life expectancy very modestly.[41]

Von Hippel–Lindau (VHL) syndrome is an autosomal-dominant disorder caused by mutations in the *VHL* gene, mapping at 3p25. This gene encodes for a protein involved in the degradation of the α-subunits of hypoxia-inducible factor (HIF) in an oxygen-dependent manner.[42] Lack of degradation of HIF-1α results in uncontrolled production of hypoxia-associated cytokines including VEGF and PDGF. VHL may manifest with a variety of benign and malignant neoplasms, including clear renal cell carcinomas, pheochromocytomas (frequently bilateral), hemangioblastomas, retinal angiomas, paragangliomas, and pNETs, the latter developing in only 10% of cases.[43]

Tuberous sclerosis is an autosomal-dominant syndrome caused by mutations of either *TSC1* or *TSC2* genes, which map on 9q34 and 16p13 and encode for hamartin and tuberin respectively. Hamartin and tuberin form a complex that inhibits mTOR signaling. As consequence, when *TSC1* or *TSC2* are mutated, the mTOR pathway is constitutively upregulated. Clinically, the syndrome is characterized by widespread low-grade tumors and hamartomas in multiple organs, including the brain, heart, skin, eyes, kidney, lung, and liver. Pancreatic NETs are described in only 1–5% of cases.[44,45]

Neurofibromatosis type 1 (NF1) can rarely be associated with an increased risk of pNETs. NF1, formerly named von Recklinghausen's disease, is an autosomal dominant phakomatosis characterized by ubiquitous neurofibromas, multiple café-au-lait skin spots and susceptibility to gliomas, myeloid leukemia, and pheochromocytomas. It is caused by a deregulation of the Ras and mTOR pathways caused by the mutation of the GTPase protein neurofibromin.[46]

8 Sporadic GEP-NETs

8.1 *Small bowel NETs*

Most small bowel NETs originate within 60 cm of the ileocecal valve, where the concentration of enterochromaffin cells is highest. More than 25% of tumors are multifocal, often clustered in close proximity to each other. Abdominal pain, which can be crampy and intermittent, and/or bowel obstruction are common presenting manifestations of small intestinal NETs and can be related to both the mechanical effect of the intraluminal tumor and the desmoplastic response secondary to mesenteric lymph node involvement. Duodenal carcinoids may produce duodenal or biliary obstruction, but are usually detected incidentally. Although malignant potential of intestinal NETs strongly correlates with tumor size, even subcentimeter neoplasms can metastasize.[47] Liver, mesentery, and peritoneum are the most frequent sites of metastatic spread. Patients with liver metastases often present with carcinoid syndrome, a constellation of symptoms which can include diarrhea, flushing, bronchospasm, and right heart valvular disease caused by the excessive of serotonin and other vasoactive substances into the systemic circulation.

8.2 *Gastric NETs*

Gastric NETs are divided into three distinct types. Type 1 tumors account for about 75% of cases and are associated with atrophic gastritis, while type 2 tumors arise in the context of gastrinoma and Zollinger–Ellison syndrome. Both types I and II tumors are caused by hypergastrinemia, and tend to be small, multifocal, and clinically indolent. Management of types I and II gastric carcinoids is usually conservative, with endoscopic surveillance every 6–12 months. Sporadic gastric NETs (type III) occur in 15% of cases and are not associated with elevated gastrin levels. Their malignant potential is much higher than type I or II tumors and locally advanced forms are usually managed with radical gastrectomy.[48–50]

8.3 *Appendiceal and colorectal carcinoids*

NETs of the appendix are nearly always found incidentally during surgery for appendicitis.[49] The risk of malignant spread seems to correlate with tumor size and invasion of the mesoappendix. As rule of thumb, simple appendectomy can be considered sufficient for tumors <1 cm in size, whereas completion with right hemicolectomy is recommended for tumors larger than 2 cm. Hemicolectomy should be also considered in patients with tumors of intermediate size (1–2 cm) based on the depth of the mesoappendix invasion.[51,52]

Patients with colorectal NETs may present with rectal bleeding, pain, or change in bowel habits. However, at least half of rectal carcinoids are discovered incidentally during lower endoscopy.[53] Rectal tumors <1 cm in greatest diameter rarely metastasize, whereas neoplasms >2 cm metastasize in over 50% of cases.[54] Colonic NETs tend to be more aggressive than rectal ones and are often poorly differentiated. Once they have metastasized, both colonic and rectal tumors behave more aggressively than midgut NETs.[55]

8.4 *Pancreatic NETs*

In contemporary clinical series, fewer than 25% of pNETs are hormonally active.[6,33] Insulinomas and gastrinomas are the most common functional subtypes with an annual incidence of 1–4 cases per million. Less than 10% of insulinomas are considered malignant, although it is unclear whether the remainder are truly benign or of very low malignant potential. Clinical presentation of insulinomas is characterized by the classic "Whipple triad": consisting of symptomatic hypoglycemia, low blood glucose levels and relief of symptoms after glucose administration.[56] Gastrinomas originate in the duodenum and the pancreas, within the so-called 'gastrinoma triangle.' Tumors of pancreatic origin are more likely to metastasize than duodenal ones. Patients with gastrinoma usually present with the Zollinger–Ellison syndrome, although the use of high-dose proton pump inhibitors can delay the diagnosis.[57] Clinical manifestations of glucagonomas include hyperglycemia, weight loss, venous thromboses, glossitis, and an unusual rash called necrolytic migratory erythema. Causes of necrolytic migratory erythema are unclear, but amino-acid or zinc deficiencies are thought to play a role.[58] VIPomas usually originate in the tail of the pancreas and result in the Verner–Morrison syndrome, characterized by watery diarrhea, often exceeding 3 L a day, with consequent severe electrolyte imbalances.[59]

Nonfunctioning pNETs are usually detected as a result of tumor growth leading to symptoms such as weight loss, abdominal pain, and jaundice. Most patients are diagnosed in the metastatic setting with the liver being the most common site of distant spread, followed by retroperitoneum and bone.[60] An increasing proportion of pNETs is diagnosed incidentally and the optimal management of small (<2 cm), asymptomatic tumors is uncertain.[61]

9 Diagnosis

Diagnosis of GEP-NETs is based on clinical presentation and pathology. Due to their lack of specificity, tumor markers should be obtained only after pathologic diagnosis and not as part of routine initial assessment. Patients presenting with chronic diarrhea and/or flushing should undergo measurement of 24-h urinary excretion of 5-hydroxyindoleacetic acid (5-HIAA), the breakdown product of serotonin.[62] Although there is often no clear correlation between 5-HIAA levels and severity of carcinoid syndrome, patients with very high 5-HIAA (>100 mg/day) are particularly prone to develop carcinoid heart disease. False-positive elevations of 5-HIAA may be recorded in patients with malabsorptive syndromes such as celiac sprue. Measurement of 5-HIAA is rarely of benefit in foregut and hindgut tumors, due to their low propensity to produce serotonin.[63] In recent years, a plasma 5-HIAA assay has been described as equivalent in accuracy to 24-h urine 5-HIAA measurement, but its clinical use is still limited.[64] Markers common to well-differentiated NETs include chromogranin A (CgA), a glycoprotein stored within secretory vesicles and released with peptides and amines from neuroendocrine cells.[65] False-positive elevations of CgA are associated with a number of conditions including chronic atrophic gastritis, renal insufficiency, and inflammatory bowel disease are almost invariably observed in patients taking proton-pump inhibitors (PPIs).[66] The use of multiple different CgA assays limits reproducibility across treatment centers in the United States. Other secretory proteins can function as tumor markers in patients with GEP-NETs. These include pancreastatin, neuron specific enolase (NSE), substance P, and neurokinin A. Pancreastatin is a breakdown fragment of CgA and is not falsely elevated by chronic use of PPIs.[67] NSE is present in the cytoplasmic compartment of neuroendocrine cells but tends to be less sensitive and specific compared to CgA.[68] The National Comprehensive Cancer Network (NCCN) guidelines do not endorse routine measurement of any particular tumor marker.[48]

Assessment of the location and extent of GEP-NETs is crucial for their management. Imaging studies should focus on abdomen for pNETs and abdomen/pelvis for small bowel carcinoids. Since GEP-NETs are typically vascular and may enhance with iodinated contrast during early arterial phases with washout during the portal venous phase, three-phase computed tomography (CT) scans are recommended for optimal evaluation of liver metastases.[69] CT scans are also useful for detecting primary small intestinal carcinoids as well as pNETs. Carcinoid tumors often produce mesenteric masses with dense desmoplastic fibrosis, either due to direct extension of the primary tumors into the mesentery or due to mesenteric lymph node metastases. Radiographically, they often appear as infiltrative masses with a circumferential pattern of soft-tissue strands which tether surrounding bowel. pNETs often appear as homogeneous enhancing masses during arterial and pancreatic or portal venous phases of imaging. They can occasionally be cystic.[70] Magnetic resonance imaging (MRI) scans represent a valuable alternative to CT scans for the detection of liver metastases. The number of hepatic lesions visualized by MRI has been demonstrated to be higher as compared to CT scans or somatostatin receptor scintigraphy (SRS, OctreoScan®) in a series of 64 patients with metastatic gastrointestinal NETs. The optimal MRI sequences were T2-weighted images and arterial phase-enhanced T1-weighted images.[71] Eovist contrast may be used to optimize detection of sub-centimeter liver metastases.[72] Many NETs express somatostatin receptors (SSTRs) and can therefore be imaged with a radiolabeled form of the somatostatin analogue octreotide ([111]indium pentetreotide). SRS is the most established functional imaging for NET. It images the entire body, enabling detection of metastases outside of the abdominopelvic region. The sensitivity of SRS for small intestine carcinoids and pNETs is reported to be 86–95% and 60–90%, respectively.[73,74] Levels of radiotracer uptake can be also used to predict response to peptide–receptor radiotherapy (PRRT), whereas the predictive value for response to octreotide is still debated. The accuracy of SRS has improved with the addition of single photon emission computed tomography (SPECT) to planar imaging. In one report of 72 patients with NETs who were examined with SPECT/CT hybrid imaging, the combination improved localization in 23 of 44 cases, affecting clinical management in 10 patients.[75] Although in older studies the sensitivity of SRS compared favorably with other imaging techniques, recent advancements in CT and MRI technology have raised questions regarding the role of SRS in the staging workup of NETs. OctreoScan is particularly inadequate for detection of metastases <1.5 cm, with a sensitivity of <35%.[71] New SSTR targeting PET scans have recently emerged and offer higher spatial resolution and improved sensitivity for detection of small lesions. Innovative radiotracers include ^{18}F-dihydroxy-phenyl-alanine (^{18}F-DOPA), 11c-5-hydroxytryptophan (^{11}C-5-HTP), and ^{68}Ga-DOTATOC.[76] Conventional 18-fluorodeoxyglucose (FDG) PET scans are not useful for imaging patients with low-grade GEP-NETs which are relatively slow growing and metabolically inactive. However, due to their higher proliferative activity, FDG-PET scans are considered standard for imaging high-grade or poorly differentiated tumors.[77]

10 Follow-Up

GEP-NETs are typically slow-growing tumors. As a consequence, imaging studies and tumor markers measurements can often be obtained at relatively infrequent intervals (4–12 months). Post-operative surveillance of localized resected tumors can be performed twice yearly for the first 1–2 years, then annually with CT or MRI scans and tumor markers. Since recurrences can occur many years after the initial diagnosis, long-term follow-up (more than five years) is advisable. Patients with unresectable metastatic tumors should be imaged at a frequency that is based on rate of prior disease progression. Treatment decisions should typically not be based on tumor marker changes alone.[78]

11 Surgical Approach to GEP-NETs

Patients with localized GEP-NETs are usually treated surgically. The approach to surgery primarily depends on the primary tumor size and localization and can vary from conservative procedures to extended surgical resection. Surgery is recommended even for small, asymptomatic midgut NETs detected incidentally. Right hemicolectomy is usually performed for tumors arising in or near the ileocecal valve, whereas partial small bowel resection can be used for more proximal tumors. Resection of the involved small bowel mesentery is recommended for lymph node sampling. Since multifocality is a common feature of small bowel carcinoids, careful examination of the entire intestine is mandatory during the surgical procedure. There is some controversy regarding the necessity of resecting primary small bowel NETs in patients with distant metastases. While some non-randomized institutional studies suggest that resection of the primary tumor is associated with improved survival,[79] some experts advocate resection only in patients who are experiencing symptoms (pain, bleeding, intermittent bowel obstruction) or are likely to survive long enough to experience such symptoms in the future.[48] Rectal carcinoid tumors <1–2 cm can be managed with endoscopic resection or transanal excision. In a study of 115 patients with rectal carcinoids, endoscopic submucosal resection with a ligation device and endoscopic submucosal dissection showed superiority in terms of resection rate when compared with endoscopic mucosal resection.[80] Low anterior resection or abdominoperineal resection should be performed for larger rectal carcinoid tumors. Since most of colonic NETs are relatively large and invasive at diagnosis, a formal partial colectomy is usually indicated. Very little data guide the management of small duodenal NETs. Surgical options range from endoscopic resection for superficial, asymptomatic tumors, to duodenectomy or pancreaticoduodenectomy for more invasive neoplasms.[48] There is increasing awareness that a conservative or "watchful waiting" approach is indicated for small, incidentally discovered pNETs. In particular, based on the evidence that incidentally diagnosed pNETs <2 cm have a five-year overall survival (OS) of 100%,[81] the ENETS guidelines currently recommend a "wait-and-see" policy in selected patients with asymptomatic sporadic pNETs.[82] This approach should be considered only in the presence of low-grade tumors, thus rendering mandatory the fine-needle aspiration or biopsy. Patients with pNETs >2 cm and/or symptomatic should undergo pancreaticoduodenectomy or distal pancreatectomy for neoplasms involving the head or body/tail of the pancreas, respectively.

12 Systemic Treatment of Metastatic GEP-NETs

12.1 *Somatostatin analogs and peptide–receptor radiotherapy*

Native human somatostatin is a peptide hormone which interacts with five SSTR subtypes belonging to a family of G-protein coupled receptors (GPCRs) with seven transmembrane domains. Somatostatin has an inhibitory effect on gastrointestinal motility, secretion, and absorption. Also, it can reduce mesenteric blood flow and suppress the secretion of hormones including gastrin, cholecystokinin and serotonin.[83] The clinical use of native somatostatin is limited by its half-life of only 2 min. As consequence, SSAs were developed in the 1980s by eliminating enzymatic cleavage sites but conserving binding sites, thus prolonging half-life significantly. SSAs currently available in the clinical practice are octreotide and lanreotide. Both compounds bind avidly to $SSTR_2$ and moderately to $SSTR_5$.[84] The first trial of octreotide evaluated the drug in 25 patients with malignant carcinoid syndrome.[85] Major (>50%) improvement of flushing and diarrhea and significant urine 5-HIAA reductions were reported in 19 and 18 patients, respectively, leading to FDA approval of the compound for the management of the carcinoid syndrome. Similar efficacy was shown in subsequent studies of lanreotide.[86,87] Loss of response to SSAs in patients with carcinoid syndrome has been associated to tachyphylaxis, resulting from SSTR desensitization and/or SSTR gene mutations.[88] Both octreotide and lanreotide are particularly active at controlling the symptoms associated with VIPomas and glucagonomas, whereas poor efficacy has been documented in insulinoma syndrome, likely due to low expression of $SSTR_2$ by most insulinomas. Although active in the palliation of gastrinoma syndrome, SSAs seem less essential than PPIs in the management of gastric acid secretion.[89] Octreotide long-acting repeatable (LAR) has been found to be at least as effective as subcutaneous (SC) octreotide. A 20-mg starting dose of octreotide LAR is recommended for treatment of carcinoid syndrome with titration to 30 mg in patients with suboptimal symptom control.[90] Depot lanreotide is administered as a deep SC injection at doses ranging from 60 to 120 mg every four weeks. SSAs are exceptionally well-tolerated agents. Side effects are generally mild and include nausea, gas, steatorrhea, and bloating. These symptoms are related to suppression of the pancreatic exocrine activity and can be occasionally alleviated by supplementation with digestive enzymes.

Long-term administration of SSAs can result in an increased rate of biliary stone and sludge formation due to the inhibitory effects on gallbladder contractility. Escalation to above the standard dose of octreotide LAR of 30 mg every four weeks may result in improved control of carcinoid syndrome symptoms.[91] Patients experiencing exacerbation of symptoms toward the final week of each treatment cycle may benefit from an increased frequency of drug administration.

High-level evidence for the antiproliferative activity of SSAs has emerged only in recent years. Both direct and indirect mechanisms concur to this effect. Interaction of SSAs with SSTRs on tumor cells leads to activation of phosphotyrosine phosphatase and modulation of the MAP-kinase signaling pathway. This, in turn, inhibits both cell growth (direct effect) and release of cytokines including insulin-like growth factor (IGF) and VEGF (indirect effect).[92,93] The PROMID study,[94] a randomized phase III trial, was designed to test the hypothesis that SSAs inhibit tumor growth. The study compared octreotide LAR 30 mg versus placebo in 85 patients with advanced midgut NETs. It reported a statistically and clinically significant improvement in median time to progression (TTP) from six months on the placebo arm to 14.3 months on the experimental arm (hazard ratio, HR 0.34; $p = 0.0000072$). The small number of deaths in each treatment arm and the high rate of crossover precluded any analysis of difference in OS. On subset analysis, patients with low tumor burden (<10% hepatic involvement) and resected primary tumors benefitted most significantly from treatment with octreotide LAR versus placebo. Based on these results, octreotide LAR therapy is considered an appropriate first-line systemic treatment for patients with metastatic, unresectable midgut NETs. More recently, the CLARINET trial[95] has expanded the role of SSAs in NETs. This study randomized 204 patients with hormonally nonfunctioning GEP-NETs to receive depot lanreotide 120 mg every four weeks or placebo. Lanreotide was associated with significantly prolonged progression-free survival (PFS), with a median not reached versus a median of 18 months in the experimental and placebo arm respectively. The estimated rates of PFS at 24 months were 65.1% in the lanreotide group and 33% in the placebo group. The most common treatment-related adverse event was diarrhea. A population of patients with very indolent disease (96% of patients had no tumor progression in the 3–6 months before randomization) was enrolled on the trial, possibly explaining the unprecedented observed PFS. Comparison between the results of the PROMID study and the CLARINET trial is hindered by the use of different criteria for enrollment and tumor response assessment (WHO and RECIST 1.0, respectively). As a consequence, no specific recommendations can be formulated regarding the preferential use of octreotide or lanreotide in the daily clinical practice. Patient preference and drug cost should be taken into account.

Pasireotide is a novel multi-receptor targeted SSA with avid binding affinity to four of the five SSTR subtypes. It has been investigated as a salvage agent in single-arm trial of patients whose carcinoid syndrome was suboptimally controlled on octreotide, and demonstrated symptom improvement in a minority of patients.[96] In a phase III trial of patients with refractory carcinoid syndrome, pasireotide failed to demonstrate improvement in control of flushing or diarrhea.[97] The antiproliferative effects of pasireotide are being tested in several clinical studies. A high rate of hyperglycemia represent the major side effect of this drug.

The overexpression of SSTRs in NETs provides a useful target for radiolabeled SSA therapy, also known as PRRT. Radiopeptides bind $SSTR_2$ and are internalized, delivering radiation to the tumor cells. Selection criteria for PRRT include evidence of strong radiotracer uptake on SRS or ^{68}Ga-DOTATOC PET (positron emission tomography) scan. Three radionuclides (^{111}In, ^{177}Lu, ^{90}Y), somewhat differing in their physical characteristics, have been conjugated to SSAs. Early clinical trials of PRRT used octreotide labeled with ^{111}In, the Auger-electron emitting isotope used in SRS. However, Auger electrons have a short particle range, thus resulting in suboptimal treatment of large tumors. Although symptom relief was often observed, objective tumor responses were rare.[98] ^{90}Y is a high-energy β-particle emitter and was initially reported to cause objective radiographic responses in over 25% of patients.[99] A more recent multicenter trial of 90 patients with metastatic carcinoid tumors reported a 70% rate of disease stabilization, but an objective response rate of only 4%.[100] Due to the emission of both β- and γ-rays, ^{177}Lu-labeled peptides can be used for treatment as well as for dosimetry and monitoring of tumor response. A large, non-randomized trial recently reported a 30% radiographic response rate among 310 patients with GEP-NETs receiving the drug.[101] Toxicities of PRRT include myelosuppression and renal insufficiency, which is partially ameliorated by concurrent amino acids infusion. Acute gastrointestinal toxicities such as nausea and vomiting are primarily attributable to the amino acid infusion. Rare cases of leukemia or myelodysplastic syndrome have been reported in patients treated with PRRT.

12.2 *Interferon-α*

Interferons (IFNs) inhibit tumor growth through a variety of mechanisms including stimulation of T cells, inhibition of angiogenesis, and induction of cell-cycle arrest.[102] Seminal trials of IFN-α in hormonally functional NETs reported significant palliation of carcinoid syndrome as well as reduction of tumor markers in over 50% of patients.[103] The observed objective response rate was in the 5–10% range, with higher degree of disease stabilization. Since IFN-α *in vitro* upregulates SSTR expression in NET cells, several clinical trials have investigated the combination of IFN with SSAs. In one trial of patients with suboptimally controlled carcinoid syndrome, addition of IFN-α to octreotide was shown to improve symptoms in 49% of patients.[104] One multicenter study of 68 patients with metastatic midgut carcinoid tumors compared octreotide alone versus combination with IFN-α. A strong trend towards improvement of the five-year OS in the combination arm (57% *vs.* 37%; $p = 0.13$) was reported.[105] Another study has randomized 109 progressive metastatic GEP-NET patients to octreotide alone or in combination with IFN-α and showed prolongation of the median OS in the combination arm (54 months *vs.* 32 months). However, results did not achieve statistical significance ($p = 0.38$).[106] A three-arm trial of 80 therapy-naïve patients with advanced GEP-NETs compared subcutaneous lanreotide to IFN-α or in combination. Objective responses were rare ($\leq 7\%$) in all three arms and time to tumor progression was nearly identical.[107] The underpowered design of these randomized trials precludes any definitive conclusions regarding the impact of IFN-α on OS. Furthermore, no optimal dosing regimen has been established. Side effects of IFN treatment including flu-like symptoms, myelosuppression, myalgias, and depression limit its widespread use in clinical practice. Low doses of IFNα and weekly administration of PEGylated IFN-α have better tolerability, thus leading to improved patient compliance.[108] In clinical practice, the use of IFN-α is likely most appropriate in patients with symptomatically and/or radiographically progressive well-differentiated midgut NETs and carcinoid syndrome.

12.3 *mTOR inhibitors*

mTOR is a conserved serine/threonine kinase that is associated with the phosphatidylinositide 3-kinase (PI3K)/protein kinase B (AKT) pathway and regulates cell growth, metabolism, and proliferation in response to stimulation by growth factors and cytokines.[109] Everolimus is an oral mTOR inhibitor and is currently approved for treatment of patients with advanced pNETs. The phase II RADIANT 1 trial compared everolimus alone versus everolimus plus octreotide in a cohort of 160 patients with advanced, progressive pNET. Response rate and median PFS were 9% and 9.7 months in the monotherapy arm versus 4% and 16.7 months in the combined therapy arm, and patients with an early CgA and NSE response had a longer PFS.[110] A subsequent phase III trial (RADIANT 2) randomized 429 patients with hormonally active carcinoid tumors to treatment with everolimus plus octreotide versus placebo plus octreotide. On central radiographic review, median PFS increased from 11.3 months on the control arm to 16.4 months on the experimental arm ($p = 0.026$). Despite being clinically significant, the primary endpoint fell short of its prespecified statistical significance threshold ($p < 0.0246$). There was no trend toward improvement in OS in the experimental arm, possibly due to high rate of crossover to everolimus in the placebo arm.[111] The RADIANT 2 trial has generated some controversy regarding the role of everolimus in non-pancreatic NETs. A phase III study of everolimus in non-functional NETs (RADIANT 4) is currently ongoing and may settle the controversy, leading to a better understanding of the role of mTOR inhibition in non-pancreatic NETs. The phase III trial RADIANT 3 randomly assigned 410 patients with low- and intermediate-grade pNET to treatment with everolimus versus placebo. Concurrent SSA therapy was allowed. Everolimus was associated with an objective response rate of only 5%, but the study demonstrated a clinically and statistically significant improvement in PFS, which increased from 4.6 months on the placebo arm to 11 months on the everolimus arm ($p < 0.001$). OS differences were not observed, possibly due to crossover design.[112] These results granted FDA approval of the drug in advanced pNETs. Side effects of everolimus include hyperglycemia, cytopenias, aphtous oral ulcers, rash, diarrhea, and atypical infections. While most toxicities are mild, chronic adverse effects may negatively impact patient quality of life. The single-agent activity of temsirolimus, another analog of rapamycin, and an intravenous mTOR inhibitor, has been evaluated in a multicenter phase II study of 37 patients with advanced, progressive NETs. Median TTP was 10.6 months and six months in patients with pNET and carcinoid, respectively.[113] However, the small size of the study limits definite conclusions regarding the efficacy of temsirolimus in NETs.

12.4 *Angiogenesis inhibitors*

NETs are among the most vascularized cancers. As consequence, inhibition of angiogenesis has been envisaged as an attractive treatment target. Several tyrosine kinase inhibitors (TKIs) of VEGFR have been evaluated in advanced NETs. Sunitinib targets VEGFR-1, -2, and -3, PDGFR, and c-Kit. A phase II trial demonstrated that sunitinib was associated with objective response rates of 2.4% and 16.7% in carcinoid tumors and pNETs, respectively.[114] In a subsequent phase III study, sunitinib was evaluated versus placebo in 171 patients with low- and intermediate-grade pNET. A statistically significant improvement in PFS from 5.5 months on the placebo arm to 11.1 months on the sunitinib arm was reported. The objective response rate associated with sunitinib was 9.3%.[115] Based on these results, sunitinib is approved by the FDA for the treatment of pNETs. Side effects include diarrhea, nausea, fatigue, hypertension, palmar-plantar erythrodysesthesia, and cytopenias. Pazopanib, a TKI with target profile similar to sunitinib, was recently evaluated in a phase II study of 37 GEP-NET patients. The objective response rate was 24% on independent review and a median PFS of 9.1 months was observed.[116]

Bevacizumab is a mAb against VEGF-A. In a randomized phase II trial, 44 patients with metastatic carcinoid tumors were randomly assigned to receive bevacizumab or PEGylated IFN-α for 18 weeks, followed by both agents in combination. At the end of the single-agent administration period, the rate of PFS after 18 weeks of monotherapy was 95% on the bevacizumab arm versus 68% on the IFN-α arm. Bevacizumab was associated to a response rate of 18%.[117] Despite these encouraging results, a follow-up phase III study comparing bevacizumab to interferon did not meet its primary endpoint of improvement in PFS (personal communication to trial investigators; ClinicalTrials.gov identifier: NCT00569127).

12.5 Cytotoxic chemotherapy

Responses to chemotherapeutics are extremely heterogeneous in GEP-NETs and are influenced by tumor differentiation/grade and primary site location. Tumors with ki67 fractions above 55% are significantly more likely to respond to etoposide/cisplatin compared with high-grade tumors with lower rates of proliferative activity.[118] Several alkylating agents, alone or in combination with fluoropyrimidines such as 5-fluorouracil (5-FU) or capecitabine, have shown activity in pNETs. In a clinical trial of streptozocin monotherapy versus streptozocin plus 5-FU, a response rate of 36% and 63%, respectively, was reported.[119] In another study of streptozocin plus doxorubicin versus streptozocin plus 5-FU, the response rates were 69% and 45%.[120] However, these trials did not employ strict radiographic criteria for measurement of response rates, thus hindering definite conclusions on the efficacy of streptozocin. More recently, a retrospective study has investigated the combination of streptozocin, 5-FU and doxorubicin in 84 patients with pNET and reported a response rate of 39%, with median response duration of 9.3 months.[121] Myelosuppression, nausea and renal insufficiency limit the clinical use of streptozocin.

In recent years, the alkylating agent temozolomide has emerged as a promising agent in pNETs. Temozolomide induces DNA methylation in guanine residues of DNA and is counteracted by methyl-guanine-methyl-transferase (MGMT), a DNA repair enzyme. A phase II study investigated the combination of temozolomide and thalidomide, demonstrating an overall response rate (ORR) of 45% in the subset of 11 patients with pNET.[122] When combined to bevacizumab, temozolomide was associated with a response rate of 33% and a median PFS of 14.3 months.[123] Based on preclinical synergistic activity against NET cell lines, temozolomide has been investigated in several retrospective studies in combination with capecitabine. In one institutional series of 30 chemo-naïve patients with pNETs, the radiographic response rate was 70% and the median PFS was 18 months.[124] A response rate of

61% was also reported in another institutional series consisting primarily of pNET patients administered with the same combination of chemotherapeutics.[125] An ECOG-sponsored prospective randomized trial of temozolomide alone or in combination with capecitabine is currently running in the United States.

Midgut NETs are particularly chemoresistant, possibly due to their extremely low proliferative activity as well as their high expression of MGMT.[126] Clinical trials of cytotoxic chemotherapy in carcinoid tumors usually report response rates below 10%.[122,123,127] There are no studies comparing cytotoxic drugs to targeted agents. As a rule of thumb, chemotherapy may be more appropriate in patients with rapidly progressive, bulky, high-grade, and/or symptomatic tumors of pancreatic origin.

13 Management of Liver Metastases

The liver is the predominant site of metastases in patients with GEP-NETs. Patients with liver disease may experience symptoms such as anorexia, weight loss, and pain related to progressive tumor bulk, as well as flushing and/or diarrhea caused by hormonal secretion. Liver-directed therapies are designed to palliate or prevent both types of symptoms and include surgical resection or ablation, transarterial embolization (TAE) or chemoembolization (TACE), and liver transplantation.

Hepatic cytoreductive surgery has been advocated for patients with limited hepatic disease if greater than 90% of tumors can be successfully resected or ablated.[128] Different ablation techniques can be used, including cryoablation, alcohol ablation, and radiofrequency ablation (RFA).[129] Ablation methods are usually reserved for patients with unresectable oligometastases smaller than 5–7 cm in diameter. Although prolonged survival durations have been reported in institutional series,[130] no randomized trials have compared surgical versus non-surgical approaches in the management of GEP-NET liver metastases. As a consequence, the degree of survival benefit conferred by surgical therapy remains speculative.

Hepatic TAE or TACE are typically used in the context of diffuse or widely scattered liver metastases. The biologic rationale supporting the use of embolization strategies is that hepatic tumors are vascularized primarily by the arterial hepatic circulation, whereas normal parenchymal cells are supplied predominantly from the portal vein.[131] Moreover, the high vascularity of GEP-NETs renders them particularly sensitive to embolic therapies. Various particulate and occluding materials have been used including polyvinyl alcohol (PVA) and trisacryl gelatin microspheres. TACE is performed by infusing an emulsion of cytotoxic drugs, such as doxorubicin or cisplatin, with iodized oil until complete or near-complete stasis of flow.[132] Staged lobar embolizations may be necessary in the presence of bilobar metastases. Short term toxicities include nausea, fatigue, abdominal pain, and fevers, all caused by induction of ischaemic hepatitis. Severe complications are quite rare, but patients who have undergone prior Whipple surgery are particularly prone to develop liver abscesses after embolization. Data on angiographic liver-directed techniques have been drawn from retrospective institutional studies and the superiority of one technique has never been demonstrated. As a result, there is no consensus favoring a particular approach. Symptomatic and radiographic responses to embolization have been reported in 53–100% and 35–74% of patients, respectively. The median PFS has been estimated to be roughly 18 months.[133]

A novel liver-directed approach involves embolization of ^{90}Y embedded either in a resin microsphere (SirSphere) or a glass microsphere (TheraSphere). This technique, also called selective intrahepatic radiotherapy (SIRT), produces tumor necrosis through direct delivery of radiation. The ^{90}Y microspheres are not infused until stasis of blood flow, since radiotherapy requires normal oxygen tension. As result, patients with mild to moderate liver dysfunction or portal vein thrombosis who are ineligible for bland embolization or TACE may be able to tolerate SIRT. The procedure can be performed on an outpatient basis. Potentially serious but rare toxicities include chronic radiation hepatitis and radiation enteritis, which can occur if particles are accidentally infused into arteries supplying the gastrointestinal tract. In one retrospective multicenter trial of 148 patients treated with SirSpheres, the ORR was 63%.[134] In another study of 42 patients treated with either SirSpheres or TheraSpheres, the ORR was 51%, but only 29 patients were evaluable for response.[135] SIRT has never been compared prospectively to other embolic treatments and data from studies with long-term follow-up are lacking.

The role of liver transplantation for patients with metastatic GEP-NETs is still debated. In well-differentiated GEP-NETs, this procedure is associated with a five-year survival up to 90%, but long-term cures are rare.[136] According to ENETS guidelines, strict criteria should be used for selection of patients candidate to liver transplantation including low proliferative rate (ki67 <10%), age <55 years, absence of extrahepatic disease, pre-transplant primary tumor resection, limited (<50%) liver involvement, and stable disease for at least six months before transplantation.[137] Predictors of poor outcome include hepatomegaly, tumor dedifferentiation and major surgical resection in addition to the transplant procedure. In a retrospective study of 213 patients who underwent liver transplantation for NET metastases, 17% of the cohort died from early or late complications of the liver transplantation.[138]

14 Conclusions

Recent years have seen a significant expansion of our understanding of the pathobiology of NETs. Multiple studies have investigated targeted therapies, expanding the role of SSAs and placing new drugs such as everolimus and sunitinib within the therapeutic armamentarium of the practitioner. Radiolabeled SSAs show significant promise in the treatment of SSTR-expressing GEP-NETs, and results from large randomized trials are awaited. Alkylating agents such as streptozocin and temozolomide continue to play an important role in the management of pNETs, particularly tumors that are clinically aggressive.

With the availability of new and potentially toxic new treatment options, clinicians must be judicious in their choice of therapies. It is important to remember that (1) the heterogeneous nature of NETs including the extent and aggressiveness of disease, clinical presentation, and symptoms, plus the therapeutic options *vs.* goals; and (2) the clinically indolent behavior of many NETs, where some treatments may pose greater risk than benefit. Identification of prognostic and predictive biomarkers may enable a more rational and individualized approach to GEP-NET patient care.

References

1. Oberndorfer S. Karzinoide Tumoren des Dünndarms. *Frankf Z Pathol* 1907;**1**: 425–429.
2. Modlin IM, *et al.* Evolution of the diffuse neuroendocrine system — clear cells and cloudy origins. *Neuroendocrinology* 2006;**84**(2):69–82.
3. Williams ED, Sandler M. The classification of carcinoid tumours. *Lancet* 1963;**1**: 238–239.
4. Maggard MA, *et al.* Updated population-based review of carcinoid tumors. *Ann Surg* 2004;**240**(1):117–122.
5. Yao JC, *et al.* One hundred years after "carcinoid": Epidemiology of and prognostic factors for neuroendocrine tumors in 35,825 cases in the United States. *J Clin Oncol* 2008;**26**(18):3063–3072.
6. Halfdanarson TR, *et al.* Pancreatic endocrine neoplasms: Epidemiology and prognosis of pancreatic endocrine tumors. *Endocr Relat Cancer* 2008;**15**(2):409–427.
7. Klöppel G, *et al.* Pathology and nomenclature of human gastrointestinal neuroendocrine (carcinoid) tumors and related lesions. *World J Surg* 1996;**20**(2):132–141.
8. Fraenkel M, *et al.* Incidence of gastroenteropancreatic neuroendocrine tumours: A systematic review of the literature. *Endocr Relat Cancer* 2014;**21**(3):R153–R163.
9. Strosberg JR, *et al.* Prognostic validity of the American Joint Committee on Cancer staging classification for midgut neuroendocrine tumors. *J Clin Oncol* 2013;**31**(4): 420–425.
10. Tamagno G, *et al.* Initial impact of a systematic multidisciplinary approach on the management of patients with gastroenteropancreatic neuroendocrine tumor. *Endocrine* 2013;**44**(2):504–509.
11. Lawrence B, *et al.* The epidemiology of gastroenteropancreatic neuroendocrine tumors. *Endocrinol Metab Clin North Am* 2011;**40**(1):1–18.
12. Frilling A, *et al.* Neuroendocrine tumor disease: An evolving landscape. *Endocr Relat Cancer* 2012;**19**(5):R163–R185.

13. Hemminki K, Li X. Incidence trends and risk factors of carcinoid tumors: A nation-wide epidemiologic study from Sweden. *Cancer* 2001;**92**(8):2204–2210.

14. Rehfeld JF. The new biology of gastrointestinal hormones. *Physiol Rev* 1998;**78**(4): 1087–1108.

15. Rosai J. The origin of neuroendocrine tumors and the neural crest saga. *Mod Pathol* 2011;**24**(Suppl. 2):S53–S57.

16. Vortmeyer AO, *et al*. Non-islet origin of pancreatic islet cell tumors. *J Clin Endocrinol Metab* 2004;**89**(4):1934–1938.

17. Rindi G, *et al*. The "normal" endocrine cell of the gut: Changing concepts and new evidences. *Ann N Y Acad Sci* 2004;**1014**:1–12.

18. Solcia E, Vanoli A. Histogenesis and natural history of gut neuroendocrine tumors: Present status. *Endocr Pathol* 2014;**25**(2):165–170.

19. La Rosa S, *et al*. Histologic characterization and improved prognostic evaluation of 209 gastric neuroendocrine neoplasms. *Hum Pathol* 2011;**42**(10):1373–1384.

20. Jiao Y, *et al*. DAXX/ATRX, MEN1, and mTOR pathway genes are frequently altered in pancreatic neuroendocrine tumors. *Science* 2011;**331**(6021):1199–1203.

21. Yuan F, *et al*. *KRAS* and *DAXX/ATRX* gene mutations are correlated with the clinico-pathological features, advanced diseases, and poor prognosis in Chinese patients with pancreatic neuroendocrine tumors. *Int J Biol Sci* 2014;**10**(9):957–965.

22. Marinoni I, *et al*. Loss of DAXX and ATRX are associated with chromosome instability and reduced survival of patients with pancreatic neuroendocrine tumors. *Gastroenterology* 2014;**146**(2):453–460.

23. Francis JM, *et al*. Somatic mutation of *CDKN1B* in small intestine neuroendocrine tumors. *Nat Genet* 2013;**45**(12):1483–1486.

24. Qian ZR, *et al*. Prognostic significance of MTOR pathway component expression in neuroendocrine tumors. *J Clin Oncol* 2013;**31**(27):3418–3425.

25. Christofori G, *et al*. Vascular endothelial growth factor and its receptors, flt-1 and flk-1, are expressed in normal pancreatic islets and throughout islet cell tumorigenesis. *Mol Endocrinol* 1995;**9**(12):1760–1770.

26. Terris B, *et al*. Expression of vascular endothelial growth factor in digestive neuroendocrine tumours. *Histopathology* 1998;**32**(2):133–138.

27. Marion-Audibert AM, *et al*. Low microvessel density is an unfavorable histoprognostic factor in pancreatic endocrine tumors. *Gastroenterology* 2003;**125**(4):1094–1104.

28. Katz SC, *et al*. T cell infiltrate and outcome following resection of intermediate-grade primary neuroendocrine tumours and liver metastases. *HPB (Oxford)* 2010;**12**(10): 674–683.

29. Vikman S, *et al*. Midgut carcinoid patients display increased numbers of regulatory T cells in peripheral blood with infiltration into tumor tissue. *Acta Oncol* 2009; **48**(3):391–400.

30. Soucek L, *et al*. Modeling pharmacological inhibition of mast cell degranulation as a therapy for insulinoma. *Neoplasia* 2011;**13**(11):1093–1100.

31. Klimstra DS, *et al*. The pathologic classification of neuroendocrine tumors: A review of nomenclature, grading, and staging systems. *Pancreas* 2010;**39**(6):707–712.

32. Yang Z, *et al*. Effect of tumor heterogeneity on the assessment of Ki67 labeling index in well-differentiated neuroendocrine tumors metastatic to the liver: Implications for prognostic stratification. *Am J Surg Pathol* 2011;**35**:853–860.

33. Strosberg JR, *et al*. Prognostic validity of a novel American Joint Committee on Cancer Staging Classification for pancreatic neuroendocrine tumors. *J Clin Oncol* 2011;**29**(22):3044–3049.

34. Rindi G, *et al*. TNM staging of midgut and hindgut (neuro) endocrine tumors: A consensus proposal including a grading system. *Virchows Arch* 2007;**451**(4): 757–762.

35. Edge S, *et al* (eds.). *AJCC Cancer Staging Manual*, 7th ed. Chicago: Springer; 2010.

36. Rindi G, Wiedenmann B. Neuroendocrine neoplasms of the gut and pancreas: new insights. *Nat Rev Endocrinol* 2011;**8**(1):54–64.

37. Rindi G, *et al*. TNM staging of neoplasms of the endocrine pancreas: results from a large international cohort study. *J Natl Cancer Inst* 2012;**104**(10):764–777.

38. Thakker RV. Multiple endocrine neoplasia type 1 (MEN1) and type 4 (MEN4). *Mol Cell Endocrinol* 2014;**386**(1–2):2–15.

39. Lemos MC, Thakker RV. Multiple endocrine neoplasia type 1 (MEN1): Analysis of 1336 mutations reported in the first decade following identification of the gene. *Hum Mutat* 2008;**29**(1):22–32.

40. Lopez CL, *et al*. Long-term results of surgery for pancreatic neuroendocrine neoplasms in patients with MEN1. *Langenbecks Arch Surg* 2011;**396**(8):1187–1196.

41. Ebeling T, *et al*. Effect of multiple endocrine neoplasia type 1 (*MEN1*) gene mutations on premature mortality in familial MEN1 syndrome with founder mutations. *J Clin Endocrinol Metab* 2004;**89**:3392–3396.

42. Kaelin WG, Jr. The von Hippel–Lindau tumour suppressor protein: O_2 sensing and cancer. *Nat Rev Cancer* 2008;**8**(11):865–873.

43. Woodward ER, Maher ER. Von Hippel–Lindau disease and endocrine tumour susceptibility. *Endocr Relat Cancer* 2006;**13**:415–425.

44. Curatolo P, *et al*. Tuberous sclerosis. *Lancet* 2008;**372**(9639):657–668.

45. Dworakowska D, Grossman AB. Are neuroendocrine tumours a feature of tuberous sclerosis? A systematic review. *Endocr Relat Cancer* 2009;**16**(1):45–58.

46. McClatchey AI. Neurofibromatosis. *Annu Rev Pathol* 2007;**2**:191–216.

47. Moertel CG. Karnofsky memorial lecture. An odyssey in the land of small tumors. *J Clin Oncol* 1987;**5**(10):1502–1522.

48. Kulke MH, *et al*. Neuroendocrine tumors. *J Natl Compr Canc Netw* 2012;**10**(6): 724–764.

49. Kulke MH, Mayer RJ. Carcinoid tumors. *N Engl J Med* 1999;**340**(11):858–868.

50. Shah P, *et al*. Hypochlorhydria and achlorhydria are associated with false-positive secretin stimulation testing for Zollinger–Ellison syndrome. *Pancreas* 2013;**42**(6): 932–936.

51. Pape UF, *et al*. ENETS Consensus Guidelines for the management of patients with neuroendocrine neoplasms from the jejuno–ileum and the appendix including goblet cell carcinomas. *Neuroendocrinology* 2012;**95**(2):135–156.

52. Grozinsky-Glasberg S, *et al.* Current size criteria for the management of neuroendocrine tumors of the appendix: Are they valid? Clinical experience and review of the literature. *Neuroendocrinology* 2013;**98**(1):31–37.

53. Buitrago D, *et al.* The impact of incidental identification on the stage at presentation of lower gastrointestinal carcinoids. *J Am Coll Surg* 2011;**213**(5):652–656.

54. Fahy BN, *et al.* Carcinoid of the rectum risk stratification (CaRRs): A strategy for preoperative outcome assessment. *Ann Surg Oncol* 2007;**14**(5):1735–1743.

55. Anthony LB, *et al.* The NANETS consensus guidelines for the diagnosis and management of gastrointestinal neuroendocrine tumors (nets): Well-differentiated nets of the distal colon and rectum. *Pancreas* 2010;**39**(6):767–774.

56. Whipple Ao. Islet cell tumors of the pancreas. *Can Med Assoc J* 1952;**66**(4):334–342.

57. Wolfe MM, Jensen RT. Zollinger–Ellison syndrome. Current concepts in diagnosis and management. *N Engl J Med* 1987;**317**(19):1200–1209.

58. Van Beek AP, *et al.* The glucagonoma syndrome and necrolytic migratory erythema: a clinical review. *Eur J Endocrinol* 2004;**151**(5):531–537.

59. Verner JV, Morrison AB. Islet cell tumor and a syndrome of refractory watery diarrhea and hypokalemia. *Am J Med* 1958;**25**(3):374–380.

60. Strosberg J, *et al.* Survival and prognostic factor analysis in patients with metastatic pancreatic endocrine carcinomas. *Pancreas* 2009;**38**(3):255–258.

61. Cheema A, *et al.* Incidental detection of pancreatic neuroendocrine tumors: an analysis of incidence and outcomes. *Ann Surg Oncol* 2012;**19**(9):2932–2936.

62. Modlin IM, *et al.* Gastroenteropancreatic neuroendocrine tumours. *Lancet Oncol* 2008;**9**(1):61–72.

63. Caldarola VT, *et al.* Carcinoid tumors of the rectum. *Am J Surg* 1964;**107**:844–849.

64. Degg TJ, *et al.* Measurement of plasma 5-hydroxyindoleacetic acid in carcinoid disease: an alternative to 24-h urine collections? *Ann Clin Biochem* 2000;**37**: 724–726.

65. O'Connor DT, Deftos LJ. Secretion of chromogranin A by peptide-producing endocrine neoplasms. *N Engl J Med* 1986;**314**(18):1145–1151.

66. Conlon JM. Granin-derived peptides as diagnostic and prognostic markers for endocrine tumors. *Regul Pept* 2010;**165**(1):5–11.

67. Raines D, *et al.* A prospective evaluation of the effect of chronic proton pump inhibitor use on plasma biomarker levels in humans. *Pancreas* 2012;**41**(4):508–511.

68. Bajetta E, *et al.* Chromogranin A, neuron specific enolase, carcinoembryonic antigen, and hydroxyindole acetic acid evaluation in patients with neuroendocrine tumors. *Cancer* 1999;**86**(5):858–865.

69. Paulson EK, *et al.* Carcinoid metastases to the liver: Role of triple-phase helical CT. *Radiology* 1998;**206**:143–150.

70. Legmann P, *et al.* Pancreatic tumors: Comparison of dual-phase helical CT and endoscopic sonography. *AJR Am J Roentgenol* 1998;**170**:1315–1322.

71. Dromain C, *et al.* Detection of liver metastases from endocrine tumors: a prospective comparison of somatostatin receptor scintigraphy, computed tomography, and magnetic resonance imaging. *J Clin Oncol* 2005;**23**:70–78.

72. Kim YK, *et al*. Diagnostic accuracy and sensitivity of diffusion-weighted and of gadoxetic acid-enhanced 3-T MR imaging alone or in combination in the detection of small liver metastasis (≤1.5 cm in diameter). *Invest Radiol* 2012;**47**(3):159–166.

73. Sundin A, *et al*. Nuclear imaging of neuroendocrine tumours. *Best Pract Res Clin Endocrinol Metab* 2007;**21**(1):69–85.

74. Binderup T, *et al*. Functional imaging of neuroendocrine tumors: A head-to-head comparison of somatostatin receptor scintigraphy, 123I-MIBG scintigraphy, and 18F-FDG PET. *J Nucl Med* 2010;**51**(5):704–712.

75. Krausz Y, *et al*. SPECT/CT hybrid imaging with 111In-pentetreotide in assessment of neuroendocrine tumours. *Clin Endocrinol (Oxf)* 2003;**59**(5):565–573.

76. Toumpanakis C, *et al*. Combination of cross-sectional and molecular imaging studies in the localization of gastroenteropancreatic neuroendocrine tumors. *Neuroendocrinology* 2014;**99**(2):63–74.

77. Sundin A, *et al*. PET in the diagnosis of neuroendocrine tumors. *Ann N Y Acad Sci* 2004;**1014**:246–257.

78. Strosberg J. Neuroendocrine tumours of the small intestine. *Best Pract Res Clin Gastroenterol* 2012;**26**(6):755–773.

79. Capurso G, *et al*. Systematic review of resection of primary midgut carcinoid tumour in patients with unresectable liver metastases. *Br J Surg* 2012;**99**(11):1480–1486.

80. Kim KM, *et al*. Treatment outcomes according to endoscopic treatment modalities for rectal carcinoid tumors. *Clin Res Hepatol Gastroenterol* 2013;**37**(3):275–282.

81. Bettini R, *et al*. Tumor size correlates with malignancy in nonfunctioning pancreatic endocrine tumor. *Surgery* 2011;**150**(1):75–82.

82. Falconi M, *et al*. ENETS Consensus Guidelines for the management of patients with digestive neuroendocrine neoplasms of the digestive system: Well-differentiated pancreatic non-functioning tumors. *Neuroendocrinology* 2012;**95**(2):120–134.

83. Reichlin S. Somatostatin. *N Engl J Med* 1983;**309**(24):1495–1501.

84. Lamberts SW, *et al*. Octreotide. *N Engl J Med* 1996;**334**(4):246–254.

85. Kvols LK, *et al*. Treatment of the malignant carcinoid syndrome. Evaluation of a long-acting somatostatin analogue. *N Engl J Med* 1986;**315**:663–666.

86. Ruszniewski P, *et al*. Treatment of the carcinoid syndrome with the longacting somatostatin analogue lanreotide: A prospective study in 39 patients. *Gut* 1996;**39**(2):279–283.

87. O'Toole D, *et al*. Treatment of carcinoid syndrome: A prospective crossover evaluation of lanreotide versus octreotide in terms of efficacy, patient acceptability, and tolerance. *Cancer* 2000;**88**(4):770–776.

88. Hofland LJ, Lamberts SW. The pathophysiological consequences of somatostatin receptor internalization and resistance. *Endocr Rev* 2003;**24**(1):28–47.

89. Jensen RT. Gastrinomas: Advances in diagnosis and management. *Neuroendocrinology* 2004;**80**(Suppl. 1):23–27.

90. Rubin J, *et al*. Octreotide acetate long-acting formulation versus open-label subcutaneous octreotide acetate in malignant carcinoid syndrome. *J Clin Oncol* 1999;**17**:600–606.

91. Strosberg JR, *et al.* Clinical benefits of above-standard dose of octreotide LAR in patients with neuroendocrine tumors for control of carcinoid syndrome symptoms: A multicenter retrospective chart review study. *Oncologist* 2014;**19**(9):930–936.

92. Florio T, *et al.* Somatostatin activation of mitogen-activated protein kinase via somatostatin receptor 1 (SSTR1). *Mol Endocrinol* 1999;**13**(1):24–37.

93. Woltering EA, *et al.* Somatostatin analogs: Angiogenesis inhibitors with novel mechanisms of action. *Invest New Drugs* 1997;**15**(1):77–86.

94. Rinke A, *et al.* Placebo-controlled, double-blind, prospective, randomized study on the effect of octreotide LAR in the control of tumor growth in patients with metastatic neuroendocrine midgut tumors: A report from the PROMID Study Group. *J Clin Oncol* 2009;**27**(28):4656–4663.

95. Caplin ME, *et al.* Lanreotide in metastatic enteropancreatic neuroendocrine tumors. *N Engl J Med* 2014;**371**(3):224–233.

96. Kvols LK, *et al.* Pasireotide (SOM230) shows efficacy and tolerability in the treatment of patients with advanced neuroendocrine tumors refractory or resistant to octreotide LAR: Results from a phase II study. *Endocr Relat Cancer* 2012;**19**(5): 657–666.

97. Wolin EM, *et al.* A multicenter, randomized, blinded, phase III study of pasireotide LAR versus octreotide LAR in patients with metastatic neuroendocrine tumors (NET) with disease-related symptoms inadequately controlled by somatostatin analogs. *ASCO Annu Meet* (Abstr.); 2013.

98. Valkema R, *et al.* Phase I study of peptide receptor radionuclide therapy with [In-DTPA]octreotide: The Rotterdam experience. *Semin Nucl Med* 2002;**32**(2): 110–122.

99. Valkema R, *et al.* Survival and response after peptide receptor radionuclide therapy with [90Y-DOTA0,Tyr3]octreotide in patients with advanced gastroenteropancreatic neuroendocrine tumors. *Semin Nucl Med* 2006;**36**(2):147–156.

100. Bushnell DL Jr, *et al.* ^{90}Y-edotreotide for metastatic carcinoid refractory to octreotide. *J Clin Oncol* 2010;**28**(10):1652–1659.

101. Kwekkeboom DJ, *et al.* Treatment with the radiolabeled somatostatin analog [177 Lu-DOTA 0,Tyr3]octreotate: Toxicity, efficacy, and survival. *J Clin Oncol* 2008;**26**(13):2124–2130.

102. Detjen KM, *et al.* Molecular mechanism of interferon alfa-mediated growth inhibition in human neuroendocrine tumor cells. *Gastroenterology* 2000;**118**(4):735–748.

103. Oberg K, *et al.* Effects of leukocyte interferon on clinical symptoms and hormone levels in patients with mid-gut carcinoid tumors and carcinoid syndrome. *N Engl J Med* 1983;**309**(3):129–133.

104. Janson ET, Oberg K. Long-term management of the carcinoid syndrome. Treatment with octreotide alone and in combination with alpha-interferon. *Acta Oncol* 1993; **32**(2):225–229.

105. Kölby L, *et al.* Randomized clinical trial of the effect of interferon alpha on survival in patients with disseminated midgut carcinoid tumours. *Br J Surg* 2003;**90**(6): 687–693.

106. Arnold R, *et al.* Octreotide versus octreotide plus interferon-alpha in endocrine gastro-enteropancreatic tumors: A randomized trial. *Clin Gastroenterol Hepatol* 2005; **3**(8):761–771.

107. Faiss S, *et al.* Prospective, randomized, multicenter trial on the antiproliferative effect of lanreotide, interferon alfa, and their combination for therapy of metastatic neuroendocrine gastroenteropancreatic tumors — the International Lanreotide and Interferon Alfa Study Group. *J Clin Oncol* 2003;**21**(14):2689–2696.

108. Pavel ME, *et al.* Efficacy and tolerability of PEGylated IFN-alpha in patients with neuroendocrine gastroenteropancreatic carcinomas. *J Interferon Cytokine Res* 2006; **26**(1):8–13.

109. Laplante M, Sabatini DM. mTOR signaling in growth control and disease. *Cell* 2012;**149**(2):274–293.

110. Yao JC, *et al.* Daily oral everolimus activity in patients with metastatic pancreatic neuroendocrine tumors after failure of cytotoxic chemotherapy: A phase II trial. *J Clin Oncol* 2010;**28**(1):69–76.

111. Pavel ME, *et al.* Everolimus plus octreotide long-acting repeatable for the treatment of advanced neuroendocrine tumours associated with carcinoid syndrome (RADIANT-2): A randomised, placebo-controlled, phase 3 study. *Lancet* 2011;**378**(9808):2005–2012.

112. Yao JC, *et al.* Everolimus for advanced pancreatic neuroendocrine tumors. *N Engl J Med* 2011;**364**(6):514–523.

113. Duran I, *et al.* A phase II clinical and pharmacodynamic study of temsirolimus in advanced neuroendocrine carcinomas. *Br J Cancer* 2006;**95**(9):1148–1154.

114. Kulke MH, *et al.* Activity of sunitinib in patients with advanced neuroendocrine tumors. *J Clin Oncol* 2008;**26**(20):3403–3410.

115. Raymond E, *et al.* Sunitinib malate for the treatment of pancreatic neuroendocrine tumors. *N Engl J Med* 2011;**364**(6):501–513.

116. Ahn HK, *et al.* Phase II study of pazopanib monotherapy in metastatic gastroenteropancreatic neuroendocrine tumours. *Br J Cancer* 2013;**109**(6):1414–1419.

117. Yao JC, *et al.* Targeting vascular endothelial growth factor in advanced carcinoid tumor: A random assignment phase II study of depot octreotide with bevacizumab and PEGylated interferon alpha-2b. *J Clin Oncol* 2008;**26**(8):1316–1323.

118. Sorbye H, *et al.* Predictive and prognostic factors for treatment and survival in 305 patients with advanced gastrointestinal neuroendocrine carcinoma (WHO G3): The NORDIC NEC study. *Ann Oncol* 2013;**24**(1):152–160.

119. Moertel CG, *et al.* Streptozocin alone compared with streptozocin plus fluorouracil in the treatment of advanced islet-cell carcinoma. *N Engl J Med* 1980;**303**(21): 1189–1194.

120. Moertel CG, *et al.* Streptozocin-doxorubicin, streptozocin-fluorouracil or chlorozotocin in the treatment of advanced islet-cell carcinoma. *N Engl J Med* 1992;**326**(8): 519–523.

121. Kouvaraki MA, *et al.* Fluorouracil, doxorubicin, and streptozocin in the treatment of patients with locally advanced and metastatic pancreatic endocrine carcinomas. *J Clin Oncol* 2004;**22**(23):4762–4771.

122. Kulke MH, *et al.* Phase II study of temozolomide and thalidomide in patients with metastatic neuroendocrine tumors. *J Clin Oncol* 2006;**24**(3):401–406.

123. Chan JA, *et al.* Prospective study of bevacizumab plus temozolomide in patients with advanced neuroendocrine tumors. *J Clin Oncol* 2012;**30**(24):2963–2968.

124. Strosberg JR, *et al.* First-line chemotherapy with capecitabine and temozolomide in patients with metastatic pancreatic endocrine carcinomas. *Cancer* 2011;**117**(2): 268–275.

125. Fine RL, *et al.* Capecitabine and temozolomide (CAPTEM) for metastatic, well-differentiated neuroendocrine cancers: The Pancreas Center at Columbia University experience. *Cancer Chemother Pharmacol* 2013;**71**:663–670.

126. Kulke MH, *et al.* O6-methylguanine DNA methyltransferase deficiency and response to temozolomide-based therapy in patients with neuroendocrine tumors. *Clin Cancer Res* 2009;**15**(1):338–345.

127. Sun W, *et al.* Phase II/III study of doxorubicin with fluorouracil compared with streptozocin with fluorouracil or dacarbazine in the treatment of advanced carcinoid tumors: Eastern Cooperative Oncology Group Study E1281. *J Clin Oncol* 2005; **23**:4897–4904.

128. Sarmiento JM, *et al.* Surgical treatment of neuroendocrine metastases to the liver: a plea for resection to increase survival. *J Am Coll Surg* 2003;**197**:29–37.

129. Kvols LK, *et al.* Role of interventional radiology in the treatment of patients with neuroendocrine metastases in the liver. *J Natl Compr Canc Netw* 2009;**7**: 765–772.

130. Que FG, *et al.* Hepatic resection for metastatic neuroendocrine carcinomas. *Am J Surg* 1995;**169**(1):36–42.

131. Proye C. Natural history of liver metastasis of gastroenteropancreatic neuroendocrine tumors: Place for chemoembolization. *World J Surg* 2001;**25**(6):685–688.

132. Ruszniewski P, *et al.* Hepatic arterial chemoembolization in patients with liver metastases of endocrine tumors. A prospective phase II study in 24 patients. *Cancer* 1993;**71**: 2624–2630.

133. Frilling A, *et al.* Recommendations for management of patients with neuroendocrine liver metastases. *Lancet Oncol* 2014;**15**(1):e8–e21.

134. Kennedy AS, *et al.* Radioembolization for unresectable neuroendocrine hepatic metastases using resin 90Y-microspheres: Early results in 148 patients. *Am J Clin Oncol* 2008;**31**(3):271–279.

135. Rhee TK, *et al.* 90Y Radioembolization for metastatic neuroendocrine liver tumors: Preliminary results from a multi-institutional experience. *Ann Surg* 2008;**247**(6): 1029–1035.

136. Rossi RE, *et al.* Liver transplantation for unresectable neuroendocrine tumor liver metastases. *Ann Surg Oncol* 2014;**21**(7):2398–2405.

137. Pavel M, *et al.* ENETS Consensus Guidelines for the management of patients with liver and other distant metastases from neuroendocrine neoplasms of foregut, midgut, hindgut, and unknown primary. *Neuroendocrinology* 2012;**95**(2):157–176.

138. Le Treut YP, *et al*. Liver transplantation for neuroendocrine tumors in Europe-results and trends in patient selection: A 213-case European liver transplant registry study. *Ann Surg* 2013;**257**(5):807–815.

139. Chen M, *et al*. Molecular pathology of pancreatic neuroendocrine tumors. *J Gastrointest Oncol* 2012;**3**(3):182–188.

Chapter 19

Management of Gastrointestinal Stromal Tumors

Caroline Novak, Nisha A. Mohindra, Christina A. Minami,
Jeffrey D. Wayne and Mark Agulnik

1 Introduction

Gastrointestinal stromal tumor (GIST) is a rare malignancy representing 1% of gastrointestinal neoplasms. The national incidence of GIST is 4,000–6,000 cases annually.[1,2] GISTs were originally categorized as tumors of smooth muscle derivation. Despite histological similarities to leiomyomas, GISTs express membrane elements found on neural-derived interstitial cells of Cajal, the "pacemaker" cells of the gastrointestinal tract. It is from the stem cell precursors of this set of cells, that GIST is now known to originate.

GIST can be divided into two primary histologic subgroups; spindle cells and epithelioid variant.[3–5] GISTs can be identified by the overexpression of the c-KIT antigen (CD117), which occurs in 80–95% of GISTs. CD117 is a type III tyrosine kinase receptor for stem cell factor (SCF) that plays a role in cell cycle regulation.[3]

GISTs typically contain activating mutations in the *KIT* proto-oncogene (75–80%) or in the platelet-derived growth factor oncogene (*PDGFR-α*, 5–10%). For cases lacking an identifiable molecular phenotype, there is evidence that succinate dehydrogenase or BRAF mutations may be involved.[6] The majority of *KIT* mutations occur in exon 11 and less frequently in exons 9, 13, or 17. Exon 11 and 9 mutations lead to disruption in kinase regulation domains, whereas mutations on exons 13 and 17 are directly involved in kinase activity. For *PDGFR* mutations, the most common source of oncogenic behavior is a point mutation in the activation loop of the kinase

503

with a single amino acid substitution (translated to D842V) comprising almost half of PDGFR mutations.[4,5]

Under normal circumstances, binding of the ligand stem cell factor induces homodimerization of c-KIT and subsequent phosphorylation of downstream products that are involved in cell growth, differentiation, and proliferation. In GIST, however, mutations in the tyrosine kinase receptors cause functional changes that lead to constitutive activation and cell immortalization and neoplastic growth. The advent of molecular targeted therapy, specifically the development of tyrosine kinase inhibitors, rapidly revolutionized the treatment of GIST.

2 Clinical Presentation and Diagnosis:

2.1 *Clinical presentation*

GISTs may occur anywhere along the gastrointestinal (GI) tract. They are most commonly found in the stomach (60%), jejunum and ileum (30%), duodenum (4–5%), rectum (4%), colon and appendix (1–2%), and esophagus (<1%).[7] The peak age of diagnosis is in the sixth to seventh decade of life, with only 10% of patients presenting before ago 40.[7,8] GISTs are often asymptomatic and discovered incidentally on radiographic or endoscopic studies performed for other reasons. When they are symptomatic, however, patients may present with GI hemorrhage (30%) or vague GI pain or discomfort (40%). Some may also present with a palpable abdominal mass (38%) which, when present, is an ominous sign.[9,10] Also included in the constellation of symptomatology are more non-specific complaints, such as anorexia, weight loss, nausea, and fatigue. On rare occasions, GISTs may present with acute intraperitoneal bleeding or perforation.

2.2 *Diagnosis*

Because the majority of these signs and symptoms are common and non-specific, it is relatively rare to diagnose a GIST prior to histological examination of a biopsy specimen and/or surgery. Suspicion may be aroused by the appearance of an ulcerated intramural mass on esophagogastroduodenoscopy (EGD) or a heterogeneous mass with patchy enhancement on the contrast phase of a computed tomography (CT) (Figures 1 and 2].[11] If a GIST is suspected, these studies are followed by an endoscopic ultrasound with fine-needle aspiration (EUS-FNA). A gastric GIST on EUS will usually show up as a demarcated hypoechoic mass contiguous with the muscularis propria.[8] High-risk GIST features on EUS include a tumor size of >5

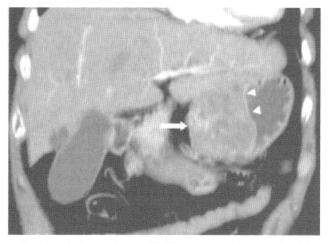

Figure 1 Gastrointestinal stromal tumor (GIST) on computed tomography (CT) imaging.[40]

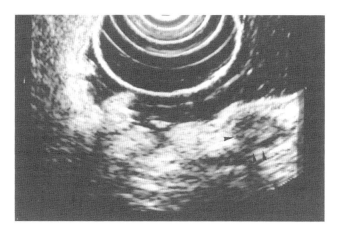

Figure 2 GIST on endoscopic ultrasound (EUS).[41]

cm, an irregular extraluminal border, local invasion, cystic spaces, ulceration, echogenic foci, and heterogeneity.[12] FNA biopsy will demonstrate spindle-cell predominance and the vast majority of GISTs will stain c-KIT positive on immunohistochemical (IHC) staining.[12] Staining for other markers are more variable, e.g. BCL-2, CD34, muscle-specific actin, smooth muscle actin, S-100, and desmin.[7] Mitotic index is rarely able to be gleaned from the FNA given the paucity of tissue.

2.3 *Staging and risk stratification*

A TNM (tumor–node–metastasis) staging system for GIST was developed by the American Joint Committee on Cancer (AJCC) and International Union Against Cancer (UICC), and published in the 2010 edition of the Cancer Staging Manual.[13] A commonly used approach is to classify GIST as either resectable or unresectable and subsequently risk-stratify resectable tumors based on the propensity of the tumor to recur after resection.

There have been three validated stratification schemas to assess risk of recurrence: the National Institutes of Health (NIH) consensus criteria, the Armed Forces Institute of Pathology (AFIP) Criteria, and the modified NIH criteria. Additionally, there are nomograms and prognostic contour heat maps available that measure risk as a continuous variable rather than into discrete categories.[14,15]

The first risk stratification system (Table 1) was developed from consensus criteria at the NIH GIST meeting in 2001. The "NIH criteria" identified size of the tumor and high mitotic count (number of mitoses per high-power field, HPF) as risk factors for recurrence based on data from historical series.[1,2,16] A second, AFIP, system, built upon the NIH criteria but also accounted for the tumor location in risk stratification (Table 1). The prognostic significance of tumor size and mitotic rate

Table 1   Stratification schemes for estimating risk of GIST recurrence after surgery

Risk group	Characteristics of operable GIST		10-year RFS (%) in pooled data from 10 population-based series[3]
	Diameter (cm)	Mitosis count (per 50 high power fields)	
NH consensus criteria[*]			
Very low risk	<2	<5	98.3
Low risk	2–5	<5	88.2
Intermediate risk	<5	6–10	79.8
	5–10	<5	
High risk	>5	>5	30.4
	>10	Any count	
	Any size	>10	
AFIP creteria for size and mitosis count[‡]			
Group 1	<2.0	≤5	95.0
Group 2	2.1–5.0	≤5	89.6
Group 3a	5.1–10.0	≤5	79.7

(Continued)

Table 1 (*Continued*)

Risk group	Characteristics of operable GIST		10-year RFS (%) in pooled data from 10 population-based series[3]
	Diameter (cm)	Mitosis count (per 50 high power fields)	
Group 3b	>10.0	≤5	64.9
Group 4	<2.0	>5	45.7
Group 5	2.1–5.0	>5	48.9
Group 6a	5.1–10.0	>5	25.1
Group 6b	>10.0	>5	9.4
Modified NIH criteria			
Very low risk[*]	<2.0	≤5	94.9
Low Risk[*]	2.1–5.0	≤5	89.7
Intermediate risk[§]	≤5.0	6–10	86.9
	5.1–10.0	≤5	
High risk	>10.0[*]	Any count[*]	36.2
	Any size[*]	>10[*]	
	>5.0[*]	>5*	
	≤5.0[‖]	>5[‖]	
	5.1–10.0[‖]	≤5[‖]	
	Any size[¶]	Any count[¶]	

[*]Criteria valid for any site. [‡]Risk stratification available for gastric,[27] duodenal,[41] ileal and jejunal,[28] and rectal[42] GISTs. [§]Gastric sites. [‖]Non-gastic sites. [¶]Any site, if tumor rupture present. Abbreviations: AFIP, Arrmed Forces Institute of Pathology; GIST, gastrointestinal stromal tumours; NIH, National Institutes of Health, RFS, recurrence-free survival.

Source: Joensuu H. Adjuvant treatment of GIST: Patient selection and treatment strategies. *Nat Rev Clin Oncol* 2012;**9**:351–358.

was confirmed in this cohort. In addition, tumor location was found to be an independent risk factor for recurrence and progression.[4,5]

Following the introduction of the AFIP stratification, the NIH introduced a modified system (Table 1) that took tumor site into account. Additionally, tumor rupture and peritoneal studding were considered high risk for recurrence regardless of size or mitotic count.[17] In addition to the risk factors incorporated into the conventional stratification systems above, there is increasing awareness of the impact of c-KIT mutational status on outcomes.

3 Treatment

3.1 *Surgical approach and principles*

In patients who are deemed reasonable candidates for resection, surgery remains the standard of care for non-metastatic GISTs. The patient's surgeon and oncologist may decide to administer preoperative imatinib, a tyrosine kinase inhibitor for c-KIT (see below), if a reduction in tumor size will improve surgical morbidity or enable a patient with unresectable or marginally resectable disease to become an operative candidate.[18]

The operation should always include a close inspection of the abdomen for metastases, especially the peritoneal surfaces and liver. Care should be taken during the procedure in handling the tumor and surrounding area. These masses may be fragile from intratumoral hemorrhage and necrosis, and any rupture of the tumoral pseudocapsule may lead to uncontrolled hemorrhage and peritoneal seeding. A formal anatomic resection is not usually necessary given that the exophytic growth pattern from the muscularis and the rare incidence of lymph node metastasis.[19] Lymphadenectomy is not warranted unless gross nodal involvement is present. Thus, an R0 resection of gastric GISTs can usually be achieved by a wedge or partial gastric resection. However, in the case of large pre-pyloric tumors, anything less than an anatomic gastrectomy may result in impedance of gastric emptying.[19] Though surgeons should strive for clear margins, the procurement of wide margins has not demonstrated any oncologic benefit[17]. One must be cognizant that GISTs can sometimes adhere to surrounding structure, necessitating the removal of adjacent tissue in order to achieve negative margins.[20]

Laparoscopy may be considered for small gastric GISTs; no evidence-based size limitation exists, and GISTs as large as 8 cm has been removed.[21] Using a size cut-off of 5 cm is likely a reasonable guideline when deciding between a laparoscopic and open procedure. The tumor should be placed in a protective bag in order to prevent port-site seeding and recurrence. It is highly encouraged to consult with a pathologist to ensure that negative margins have been achieved. Laparoscopic resection of gastric GISTs is not only feasible, it also offers a decreased length of hospital stay (three days *vs.* six days for open procedures) and a trend toward shorter operative times and decreased blood loss.[19]

3.2 *Adjuvant therapy*

Two multicenter, randomized phase III trials have explored the role of adjuvant imatinib.[22,23] Intergroup ACOSOG Z9001 enrolled from 2002–2007. Patients were included in this study if their tumors were ≥3 cm in size and if they were c-KIT positive by IHC. Thereafter, they were randomized to receive imatinib 400 mg daily for one year or placebo. In the initial analysis, a significant improvement was seen in one-year recurrence free survival (98% for imatinib *vs.* 83% for placebo) with an overall hazard ratio (HR) of 0.35 (0.22–0.53; *p* < 0.001) for recurrence favoring imatinib. Of note, patients were stratified by tumor size (3–6 cm, 6–10 cm, or greater than 10 cm) and the statistically significant improvement in recurrence-free survival persisted across all size subsets. Imatinib was well tolerated, with dermatitis, diarrhea, and abdominal pain representing the most common reported adverse events, all below 3%. This trial formed the basis for an expedited FDA approval for adjuvant imatinib therapy.

SSG XVIII/AIO, a large phase III multicenter randomized trial from the Scandinavian sarcoma group, randomized high risk, KIT-positive, postoperative patients to 12 or 36 months of adjuvant imatinib. High-risk tumors were defined as size >10 cm, mitotic count >10/50 hpf, size >5cm with mitotic count >5 hpf or by the presence of tumor rupture, in accordance with the modified consensus criteria. Patients were stratified by extent of resection (R0 *vs.* R1). At 54 months of follow-up, relapse-free survival was significantly improved in the group that received 36 months of therapy compared to those who were treated for 12 months (65.6% *vs.* 47.9%; *p* < 0.005). In this trial, an overall survival benefit was appreciated but the number of deaths was small and the survival benefit did not maintain statistical significant when limited to GIST-specific mortality. As in earlier studies, imatinib was well tolerated with few grade 3 or 4 toxicities. The most common serious side effects incurred were diarrhea in 4% and leukopenia in 3% of the patients on therapy for 36 months. A longer duration of therapy was associated with a statistically significant but small increased risk of treatment toxicity overall.[1]

As previously seen in earlier adjuvant and metastatic trials, the rate of tumor recurrence in both the ACOSOG Z9001 and SSGVXIII/ AIO, increased as therapy completed.[24] The PERSIST-5 trial is an ongoing single arm phase II trial of five years of imatinib following R0 resection with results anticipated in 2018 (NCT00867113).

3.3 *Neoadjuvant therapy*

The role of neoadjuvant therapy for GIST is limited to those tumors that are marginally resectable or where resection would be associated with significant organ dysfunction or morbidity due to the extent of the surgery. The Radiation Therapy Oncology Group (RTOG) 0132/American College of Radiology Imaging Network (ACRIN) 6665 trial was a prospective phase II trial evaluating neoadjuvant imatinib in 65 patients with a large (>5 cm) primary tumor or resectable metastatic disease.[25]

Patients received preoperative imatinib 600 mg daily for eight to 12 weeks, followed by surgical resection if possible. The majority (83%) of patients had stable disease on serial imaging and 2 patients had a demonstrable response to therapy by RECIST criteria. At a median follow-up of 5.1 years, disease free survival was 77% and 68% in patients with large primaries and resectable metastatic disease respectively; while progression free survival was 68% and 30%. Although these numbers compare favorably to historical controls, it is difficult to infer the amount of benefit due to neoadjuvant therapy because two-thirds of patients on trial received at least 18 months of adjuvant therapy following surgery.

The EORTC published a large retrospective series of patients who received neoadjuvant GIST for treatment of marginally resectable or initially unresectable disease with a goal of achieving an R0 resection. Patients received preoperative imatinib for a median of 40 weeks (range 6–190).[26] Prior to surgery, 80.1% of patients had a significant radiographic response and 83% went on to achieve an R0 resection. Only two patients experienced progression while on imatinib therapy. Five-year disease-free and disease-specific survival rates were 65% and 95%, respectively. As in the prospective trial, the majority of patients went on to adjuvant imatinib, with 56% of patients receiving therapy for at least one year postoperatively. The use of postoperative imatinib and tumor location were found to be independent prognostic indicators with improved disease-free survival in those patients who received adjuvant therapy as well as in those with gastric or rectal as oppose to small bowel primaries. This analysis highlights the safety of a neoadjuvant strategy even in the absence of randomized data in cases where physicians think an R0 resection would be feasible with minimal to moderate tumor shrinkage. In addition, it re-emphasizes the importance of adjuvant imatinib in patients with bulky disease at diagnosis regardless of extent of resection.

3.4 Recurrent and metastatic disease

In 2001, a paradigm-shifting case report was published which highlighted a dramatic response to imatinib 400 mg daily in a patient with metastatic GIST.[27] These results led to further investigation of imatinib in patients with unresectable or metastatic disease. The first phase II trial that evaluated imatinib in advanced GIST was B2222. This study randomized 147 patients to imatinib 400 mg daily or to imatinib 600 mg daily.[28] Patients receiving 400 mg daily were allowed to cross over to 600 mg at the time of progression. Ninety-eight percent of patients had undergone surgical resection and 51% had received prior cytotoxic chemotherapy. After a median follow-up of 288 days, 53.7% of patients had achieved a partial response and 27.9% of patients had stable disease. Survival at one year was 88%. At the end of this proof-of-concept period, the investigators revised the study to include a four-year extension trial. Median survival was 57 months, which was almost three times as long as that of historical controls (18 months). Patients who received 600 mg daily had a longer time to progression (20 months *vs.* 24 months; $p = 0.371$); however, this was not associated with a statistically significant difference in survival between the two dose groups. Further, there was no difference in overall survival between patients who experienced stable disease compared to those who had a partial response.[29]

Similar results were noted in larger phase III trials. The EORTC 62005 trial randomized 946 patients to imatinib 400mg daily or imatinib 400 mg BID,[30] with crossover to twice daily dosing of imatinib was allowed at time of progression. The primary endpoint was PFS. Patients treated with BID imatinib achieved a longer progression-free survival compared to the lower dose group (HR 0.82; 95% CI 0.69–0.98; $p = 0.026$). However, an increased risk of clinically significant toxicity was observed in the BID dose group compared to the daily dosing group (risk of grades 3–4 toxicity 50% *vs.* 41%).

Similarly, the SWOG S0033/CALGB 150105 randomized 694 patients to imatinib 400 mg daily (standard dose) or 800 mg daily (high dose), with cross over to higher dosing at progression. After a median follow-up of 4.5 years, no statistically significant differences in objective response rates, progression-free survival, or overall survival were detected between the two arms. However, more grade 3+ adverse events were noted in patients receiving high dose therapy.

Further analysis revealed that c- KIT mutation status plays a large role in treatment outcomes. There was a pronounced favorable outcome for patients with c- KIT exon 11 mutations relative to patients with exon 9, wild-type, or *PDGFR* mutations.[31] The patients with a c- KIT exon 11 mutation had a partial response rate of 83.5% compared to 47.8% of those with exon 9 mutations or wild type. Although there were a small population patients with *PDGFR* mutations, it was noted that patients with a *PDGFR D842V* mutations did not response to imatinib at all. Conformational changes of each receptor may provide an explanation for these results. As imatinib binds c-KIT or PDGFR in the inactive conformation, mutations that favor the active conformation of either receptor, such as the *PDGFR D842V* kinase domain mutation, may be primarily refractory to imatinib. This data suggests that for most patients, starting at a conventional dose of 400 mg daily and increasing the dose in the event of progression is a reasonable approach. A possible exception may be in those preselected patients with exon 9 mutations, in whom initiating therapy at a higher dose may lead to prolonged event free survival.

4 Resistance to Imatinib Treatment

4.1 Continue treatment vs. dose escalation

Resistance to imatinib can be classified in two categories: primary and secondary resistance. Primary resistance is defined as radiographic or clinical progression in previously imatinib-naïve patients during their first six months of treatment. Secondary resistance is progression after an initial response to imatinib therapy.[32] As described above, certain c-KIT mutations are associated with a higher incidence of primary imatinib resistance on a standard dose of 400 mg daily. In some circumstances, this initial resistance can be overwhelmed by dose escalation to 800 mg daily if tolerated. This effect was demonstrated both in the EORTC 62005 and SWOG S0033 trials as described above as well as a prospective single-arm dose escalation trial from China.

In all patients with metastatic disease, there is evidence to suggest that imatinib should be continued indefinitely, when tolerated, to avoid rapid progression after cessation of therapy. The prospective BFR14 phase III trial of 58 patients with metastatic or unresectable GIST on imatinib therapy (BFR14) randomized individuals to discontinuation or continued treatment after 12 months of treatment. All patients had initially achieved stable disease, partial response or complete response. At a median 24 months of follow-up, there was a substantial decrement in progression-free survival in the patients who had interrupted therapy, with a median progression free survival of only 6.1 months after imatinib discontinuation(95% CI 3.5–6.7) compared to 18 months (95% CI 15.0–23.6) in the group who continued imatinib therapy.[33] In patients who progressed, imatinib was reinstituted resulting in a disease control rate approaching 90%. No overall survival benefit was noted with continuous therapy.

Based on this documented ability to salvage progression and the knowledge that non-compliance with imatinib tends to increase over time, the investigators performed a second randomization in the patients who were originally assigned to continuous imatinib after three years of therapy, again either continuing imatinib or interrupting treatment. A significant benefit was seen with continuous imatinib, with a progression-free survival rate of 80% (95% CI 58–91) compared to 16% (95% CI 5–33) in patients who stopped therapy ($p < 0.0001$).[34] This data confirms that in patients who are able to tolerate imatinib, therapy should be continued indefinitely unless progression occurs.

Patients who progress on imatinib therapy, despite dose escalation and in the setting of good compliance, are said to have secondary, or acquired, resistance. A post-hoc analysis of the B222 provided significant information about the two distinct mechanisms by which imatinib resistance can arise; acquisition of a second mutation that confers resistance, or via genomic amplification of the original mutated receptor.[32] In the case of the former, the secondary acquired mutation is usually found in the kinase domain and creates a physical impediment to imatinib binding. A point mutation resulting in a V654A substitution is the most common example of this type of acquired resistance, and mirrors mechanisms of acquired resistance in chronic myelogenous leukemia (CML) patients treated with imatinib.[35]

4.2 *Other tyrosine kinase inhibitors*

In the event of acquired imatinib resistance, several other agents are available for treatment of metastatic GIST.

4.2.1 *Sunitinib*

Sunitinib is a second-generation tyrosine kinase inhibitor with activity against c-KIT. The results of a large phase III trial of sunitinib in patients who progressed on imatinib were dramatic enough to merit unblinding during an interim analysis so that patients on placebo could begin sunitinib immediately. Before unblinding, 7% of the patients showed objective response to sunitinib and an additional 58% demonstrated stable disease, with only 19% showing progressive disease. In the placebo group, comparable rates were 0%, 48%, and 37%. Overall, sunitinib conferred a significant benefit of at least an additional five months until disease progression.[36] Notably, response to sunitinib appeared to follow predictable patterns based on the KIT or *PDGFR* mutation implicated. GISTs with a primary mutation in exon 9 appeared to have a much more pronounced sunitinib response than those with an exon 11 mutation. It should be noted, however, that there is a possibility that this statistical relationship would be attenuated if the high rate of secondary mutations leading to imatinib resistance in exon 11 mutants were taken into account.

4.2.2 *Regorafenib*

A phase III placebo controlled trial of regorafenib for advanced gastrointestinal stromal tumors after failure of imatinib and sunitinib (GRID trial) revealed a significant progression-free survival benefit for regorafenib. Patients who received regorafenib experienced a mean progression-free survival of 4.8 months compared to 0.9 months for those receiving placebo, with a significantly reduced HR for progression (0.27; 95% CI 0·19–0·39; $p < 0.0001$).[37]

4.2.3. *Nilotinib*

Nilotinib is a tyrosine kinase inhibitor developed using advanced molecular modeling techniques for use in CML. *In vitro*, nilotinib exhibits binding ability and subsequent inhibitory capacity many times more potent than imatinib with activity against Bcr-Abl, c-KIT, and PDGFR. A single-arm phase II study evaluated nilotinib in 35 patients who progressed on sunitinib and imatinib. At 24 weeks of follow up, 29% (95% CI 16.4–43.6%) of patients had disease control, defined as complete response, partial response, or stable disease. Median progression-free survival was 113 days.[38] A phase III study of nilotinib compared to best supportive care failed to show a significant benefit in progression free or overall survival, although further investigation is needed to investigate any potential benefit in specific mutation subtypes.[39]

Several other kinase inhibitors are under investigation for the treatment of metastatic GIST and could be considered under the auspices of a clinical trial. Another avenue of treatment for progressive GIST is imatinib in combination with other agents. Although constitutive activation of kit kinase is the hallmark of GIST, it is hyperactivity of the various signaling pathways downstream from c-KIT that is directly responsible for the maladaptive cellular proliferation and tumor growth.

5 Conclusions

While classified as a sarcoma, GIST is a distinct oncogenic entity. Its tumorgenesis is derived by a distinct oncogenic mutation and its therapies beyond surgical resection are driven to specifically target this kinase mutation. While a complete surgical resection is necessary to cure patients with localized GIST, surgery in itself is inadequate for those patients with higher-risk features that derive benefit from tyrosine kinase inhibition of c-KIT and PDGFR. The optimal length of adjuvant therapy remains uncertain, but clinical judgment and expertise along with patient characteristics and preference will help individualize adjuvant therapy with the goal of establishing patients who will be treated for one year, three years, and beyond. For those unfortunate patients with metastatic disease, three molecularly targeted agents are approved and have substantially extended the survival for patients with this disease. As the multidisciplinary, dedicated field of GIST researchers continues to further understand the intricacies of this disease, the benefits to patients will likely transpire.

References

1. Tran T, *et al.* The epidemiology of malignant gastrointestinal stromal tumors: An analysis of 1,458 cases from 1992 to 2000. *Am J Gastroenterol* 2005;**100**(1):162–168.

2. Nilsson B, *et al.* Gastrointestinal stromal tumors: the incidence, prevalence, clinical course, and prognostication in the preimatinib mesylate era — a population-based study in western Sweden. *Cancer* 2005;**103**(4):821–829.

3. Kindblom LG, *et al.* Gastrointestinal pacemaker cell tumor (GIPACT): Gastrointestinal stromal tumors show phenotypic characteristics of the interstitial cells of Cajal. *Am J Pathol* 1998;**152**(5):1259–1269.

4. Miettinen M, Lasota J. Gastrointestinal stromal tumors — definition, clinical, histological, immunohistochemical, and molecular genetic features and differential diagnosis. *Virchows Arch* 2001;**438**(1):1–12.

5. Rubin BP, *et al.* Molecular insights into the histogenesis and pathogenesis of gastrointestinal stromal tumors. *Int J Surg Pathol* 2000;**8**(1):5–10.

6. Agaimy A, *et al.* V600E *BRAF* mutations are alternative early molecular events in a subset of KIT/PDGFRA wild-type gastrointestinal stromal tumours. *J Clin Pathol* 2009; **62**(7):613–616.

7. Corless CL, *et al.* Biology of gastrointestinal stromal tumors. *J Clin Oncol* 2004; **22**(18):3813–3825.

8. Novitsky YW, *et al.* Long-term outcomes of laparoscopic resection of gastric gastrointestinal stromal tumors. *Ann Surg* 2006;**243**(6):738–745; discussion 745–737.

9. Miettinen M, *et al.* Gastrointestinal stromal tumors: Recent advances in understanding of their biology. *Hum Pathol* 1999;**30**(10):1213–1220.

10. Nowain A, *et al.* Gastrointestinal stromal tumors: clinical profile, pathogenesis, treatment strategies and prognosis. *J Gastroenterol Hepatol* 2005;**20**(6):818–824.

11. King DM. The radiology of gastrointestinal stromal tumours (GIST). *Cancer Imaging* 2005;**5**:150–156.

12. Shah P, *et al.* Predicting malignant potential of gastrointestinal stromal tumors using endoscopic ultrasound. *Dig Dis Sci* 2009;**54**(6):1265–1269.

13. Edge S, *et al* (eds.). A*JCC Cancer Staging Manual*, 7th ed. Chicago: Springer; 2010.

14. Gold JS, *et al.* Development and validation of a prognostic nomogram for recurrence-free survival after complete surgical resection of localised primary gastrointestinal stromal tumour: A retrospective analysis. *Lancet Oncol* 2009;**10**(11):1045–1052.

15. Rossi S, *et al.* Natural history of imatinib-naïve GISTs: A retrospective analysis of 929 cases with long-term follow-up and development of a survival nomogram based on mitotic index and size as continuous variables. *Am J Surg Pathol* 2011;**35**(11): 1646–1656.

16. Miettinen M, *et al.* Gastrointestinal stromal tumors of the stomach: A clinicopathologic, immunohistochemical, and molecular genetic study of 1765 cases with long-term follow-up. *Am J Surg Pathol* 2005;**29**(1):52–68.

17. DeMatteo RP, *et al.* Two hundred gastrointestinal stromal tumors: Recurrence patterns and prognostic factors for survival. *Ann Surg* 2000;**231**(1):51–58.

18. National Cancer Comprehensive Network. Gastrointestinal Stromal Tumors (GIST). Retriebed from http://www.nccn.org/professionals/physician_gls/PDF/sarcoma.pdf. Accessed October 30, 2014.

19. Melstrom LG, *et al.* Laparoscopic versus open resection of gastric gastrointestinal stromal tumors. *Am J Clin Oncol* 2012;**35**(5):451–454.

20. Demetri G, DeMatteo RP. NCCN Task Force report: Gastrointestinal stromal tumor (GIST). *J Natl Compr Cancer Netw* 2004;**2**(Suppl. 3):S25–S28.

21. Raut CP, Ashley SW. How I do it: Surgical management of gastrointestinal stromal tumors. *J Gastrointest Surg* 2008;**1–2**(9):1592–1599.

22. Dematteo RP, *et al.* Adjuvant imatinib mesylate after resection of localised, primary gastrointestinal stromal tumour: A randomised, double-blind, placebo-controlled trial. *Lancet* 2009;**373**(9669):1097–1104.

23. Joensuu H, *et al.* One *vs* three years of adjuvant imatinib for operable gastrointestinal stromal tumor: A randomized trial. *JAMA* 2012;**307**(12):1265–1272.

24. Wang D, *et al.* Phase II trial of neoadjuvant/adjuvant imatinib mesylate for advanced primary and metastatic/recurrent operable gastrointestinal stromal tumors: Long-term follow-up results of Radiation Therapy Oncology Group 0132. *Ann Surg Oncol* 2012;**19**(4):1074–1080.

25. Eisenberg BL, *et al.* Phase II trial of neoadjuvant/adjuvant imatinib mesylate (IM) for advanced primary and metastatic/recurrent operable gastrointestinal stromal tumor (GIST): Early results of RTOG 0132/ACRIN 6665. *J Surg Oncol* 2009;**99**(1):42–47.

26. Rutkowski P, *et al.* Neoadjuvant imatinib in locally advanced gastrointestinal stromal tumors (GIST): The EORTC STBSG experience. *Ann Surg Oncol* 2013;**20**(9): 2937–2943.

27. Joensuu H, *et al.* Effect of the tyrosine kinase inhibitor STI571 in a patient with a metastatic gastrointestinal stromal tumor. *N Engl J Med* 2001;**344**(14):1052–1056.

28. Demetri GD, *et al.* Efficacy and safety of imatinib mesylate in advanced gastrointestinal stromal tumors. *N Engl J Med* 2002;**347**(7):472–480.

29. Blanke CD, *et al.* Long-term results from a randomized phase II trial of standard- versus higher-dose imatinib mesylate for patients with unresectable or metastatic gastrointestinal stromal tumors expressing KIT. *J Clin Oncol* 2008;**26**(4):620–625.

30. Verweij J, *et al.* Progression-free survival in gastrointestinal stromal tumours with high-dose imatinib: Randomised trial. *Lancet* 2004;**364**(9440):1127–1134.

31. Heinrich MC, *et al.* Correlation of kinase genotype and clinical outcome in the North American Intergroup Phase III Trial of imatinib mesylate for treatment of advanced gastrointestinal stromal tumor: CALGB 150105 Study by Cancer and Leukemia Group B and Southwest Oncology Group. *J Clin Oncol* 2008;**26**(33):5360–5367.

32. Agulnik M, Giel JL. Understanding rechallenge and resistance in the tyrosine kinase inhibitor era: Imatinib in gastrointestinal stromal tumor. *Am J Clin Oncol* 2014;**37**(4): 417–422.

33. Blay JY, *et al.* Prospective multicentric randomized phase III study of imatinib in patients with advanced gastrointestinal stromal tumors comparing interruption versus continuation of treatment beyond 1 year: The French Sarcoma Group. *J Clin Oncol* 2007; **25**(9):1107–1113.

34. Le Cesne A, *et al*. Discontinuation of imatinib in patients with advanced gastrointestinal stromal tumours after 3 years of treatment: An open-label multicentre randomised phase 3 trial. *Lancet Oncol* 2010;**11**(10):942–949.

35. Heinrich MC, *et al*. Molecular correlates of imatinib resistance in gastrointestinal stromal tumors. *J Clin Oncol* 2006;**24**(29):4764–4774.

36. Demetri GD, *et al*. Efficacy and safety of sunitinib in patients with advanced gastrointestinal stromal tumour after failure of imatinib: A randomised controlled trial. *Lancet* 2006;**368**(9544):1329–1338.

37. Demetri GD, *et al*. Efficacy and safety of regorafenib for advanced gastrointestinal stromal tumours after failure of imatinib and sunitinib (GRID): An international, multicentre, randomised, placebo-controlled, phase 3 trial. *Lancet* 2013;**381**(9863):295–302.

38. Sawaki A, *et al*. Phase 2 study of nilotinib as third-line therapy for patients with gastrointestinal stromal tumor. *Cancer* 2011;**117**(20):4633–4641.

39. Reichardt P, *et al*. Phase III study of nilotinib versus best supportive care with or without a TKI in patients with gastrointestinal stromal tumors resistant to or intolerant of imatinib and sunitinib. *Ann Oncol* 2012;**23**(7):1680–1687.

40. Gong J, *et al*. CT and MR imaging of gastrointestinal stromal tumor of stomach: A pictorial review. *Quant Imaging Med Surg* 2012;**2**(4):274–279.

41. Palazzo L, *et al*. Endosonographic features predictive of benign and malignant gastrointestinal stromal cell tumours. *Gut* 2000;**46**(1):88–92.

Chapter 20

Small Intestinal Cancers

Theofanis Floros

1 Introduction

Cancer of the small intestine is rare. Although comprising almost 75% of the gastrointestinal tract (GI), it accounts only for 2% of its malignancies. It includes the duodenum, jejunum, and ileum. Presenting symptoms are non-specific and variant, and late-stage diagnosis occurs frequently. The histology of these malignancies is diverse with the four most common types being carcinoid tumors, adenocarcinoma, lymphomas, and sarcomas (mainly GIST, GI stromal tumor).

2 Epidemiology

As mentioned, small intestine cancers (SICs) account for 2% of GI tract malignancies. The Surveillance, Epidemiology and End Results (SEER) database estimates 9,160 new cases in 2014 with 1,210 deaths from SIC (0.5% of all new cancer cases and 0.2% of cancer deaths, respectively). Incidence is rising through the last four decades, especially during the last one where a 0.5% annual increase was observed. Median age at diagnosis is 65. There is a slight predominance in males (for all races) and for African-Americans (both male/female).[1]

Incidence depends on the subsite with ileum being the most commonly affected, followed by duodenum and jejunum. In the past, adenocarcinoma was the predominant type, but this probably changed during the last decade where an increase in carcinoid tumors was observed. Histologic presentation varies considerably with

519

regard to the subsite involved. Thus, the four most common histologic types of SIC comprise carcinoid tumors (37%), adenocarcinomas (37%), lymphomas (17%), and sarcomas (10%). Adenocarcinomas are more common in the duodenum (including peri-ampullary carcinomas), whereas carcinoid tumors, lymphomas, and sarcomas occur predominantly in the ileum.[2–4]

With all histologic types combined, the average five-year survival has also risen from 33% in 1975 to an estimated 65% in 2014, reflecting the advances in diagnostic capabilities, surgical intervention, and systematic treatments (targeted therapies, chemotherapy, nuclear medicine) for these diverse diseases.[1]

2.1 Etiopathogenesis

Definitive large epidemiologic studies for SIC are lacking due to the rarity of this disease. Nevertheless, small studies have identified predisposing genetic and environmental factors that may explain why SIC is much less frequent than colorectal cancer (CRC) despite constituting 75% of the length of the GI tract and over 90% of its mucosal surface.

2.1.1 Lifestyle

Alcohol consumption, smoking, refined carbohydrates, smoked food, canned food and barbequed or grilled meat have been associated with a higher incidence of SIC (mainly adenocarcinomas[5,6]), whereas fruit, fish, and vegetable intake was inversely related.[7,8] A recent large Asian environmental study reviewing data from 12 smaller cohort studies failed to confirm a significant association between smoking and SIC, whereas elevated BMI (body–mass index) and alcohol (>400 g per week) showed a trend of a higher incidence of SIC.[9] Although these factors are also associated with CRC, the marked difference in incidence may suggest a different exposure. In the small intestine, the transient time is about six times shorter than the colon (5–8 h vs. 30–40 h for a full transit) which count for less time exposure.[10] The mucosa expresses high levels of benzopyrene hydroxylase, an enzyme that inactivates the carcinogen benzopyrene found in tobacco and smoked/canned/barbequed food.[10,11] The intestinal chime is alkaline, thus rendering most carcinogens less harmful.[12] The bacterial load (mainly anaerobic) is much less than in colon, although it increases as we move from the duodenum downwards. Bacteria produce xenobiotic transformation of bile salts to desoxycholic acid, a potential mutagen.[10–12] There is also a higher mucosal regeneration that leaves less time for mutations to accumulate and higher immune surveillance (Peyer's patches, high surface IgA secretion)[12].

2.1.2 *Crohn's disease*

Crohn's disease (CD) increases the risk for adenocarcinomas by approximately 30 times compared to the general population due to the chronic inflammation status,[10] and this risk augments with longstanding disease (estimated 2% at 10 years of active disease). In contrast to sporadic adenocarcinomas, it is more common in the ileum since CD affects the ileum more often. It also appears at a younger age (fourth decade). Systematic treatment and surgical management appear to reduce that risk.[13–16].

2.1.3 *Celiac disease*

Celiac disease, an autoimmune disorder caused by a reaction to gliadin, is characterized by excessive lymphocytic infiltration (predominantly T cells) and damage of the epithelial mucosal cells.[17,18] It is associated with an increased risk (39%) for lymphoma (enteropathy associated T-cell lymphoma, EATL) and to a lesser degree (8–13%) for adenocarcinomas as was shown in a British study.[19] Similar results were generated in a Swedish investigation.[20] Their main location is the jejunum, and prevention through gluten-free diet is feasible.

2.1.4 *Genetic predisposition*

2.1.4.1 Familial adenomatous polyposis

Familial adenomatous polyposis (FAP) is caused by a germline dominant mutation of the adenomatous polyposis coli (*APC*) gene, a tumor suppressor gene with a key role in the Wnt pathway. Patients not only develop hundreds to thousands of early adenomatous polyps in the colon, but also in the small bowel (mainly the duodenum and ampulla). These affected individuals undergo prophylactic proctocolectomy by the age of 30. Although SIC (adenocarcinomas) account for less than 5% of cancer in FAP patients, this is the leading cause of cancer related-death for those who have undergone a proctocolectomy.[21–23]

2.1.4.2 Hereditary non-polyposis colorectal cancer

Hereditary non-polyposis colorectal cancer (HNPCC), also called Lynch syndrome, is caused by a germline mutation in any of several genes that enable DNA mismatch repair (MMR) mechanism with *MLH1*, *MSH2*, and *MSH6* accounting for more than 90% of kindreds. The average risk for adenocarcinomas (in the duodenum and jejunum) is increased more than 100 times in average with a lifetime risk of 1–4%.

The MMR phenotype should be recommended in patients with small intestine adenocarcinomas since this may be the presenting tumor of Lynch syndrome.[24–26]

2.1.4.3 Peutz–Jeghers syndrome

Peutz–Jeghers syndrome (PJS) is caused by an autosomal dominant mutation of the *STK11* (*LKB1*) tumor suppressor gene and predisposes to hamartomatous GI polyposis. The relative risk for adenocarcinomas is reported to be 15 to 500 compared to the general population.[27,28]

2.1.4.4 Other genetic syndromes

Other genetic syndromes that have been reported to confer a relative increased risk for small intestine adenocarcinomas include Gardner syndrome, von Recklinghausen's disease, and cystic fibrosis.

3 Clinical Presentation

The symptomatology of SIC is non-specific. Patients (up to 45%) usually present with vague symptoms such as abdominal pain, nausea, vomiting, melena (dark stools), and weight loss. Another 50% present acutely manifesting bowel obstruction or perforation. Bowel obstruction is more common in jejunal and ileal carcinomas and less frequent in duodenal tumors (47% *vs.* 34%).[29] Adenocarcinomas tend to be associated more with pain and obstruction, while sarcomas and lymphomas frequently present with acute GI hemorrhage and perforation, respectively.[30,31] Carcinoid tumors may present (up to 10%) with a special constellation of symptoms including diarrhea, flushing and bronchospasm called carcinoid syndrome due to the secretion of various hormonal peptides (e.g. serotonin, histamine, dopamine, prostaglandins). Palpable abdominal masses are more often seen in sarcomas. In general, different cancer subtypes have predilection to different regions in the small intestine, generating diverse symptoms except for carcinoid syndrome which is a functional disorder.

4 Diagnosis

The non-specific symptomatology of SIC combined with the difficulty in visualizing these tumors with standard endoscopic techniques contribute to a delay in diagnosis in average 8–12 months. One also has to mention that the rarity of this disease renders doctors less susceptible.[32] Patients often present with acute symptomatology (obstruction, perforation) or with signs of advanced disease (e.g. jaundice, distant lymphadenopathy). It is not unusual to establish the diagnosis postoperatively following the pathology examination of a resected specimen.[33]

Diagnostic workup (especially in acute presentation) may commence with an abdominal X-ray. Unfortunately, it usually gives no further information except in case of bowel obstruction or perforation. The use of contrast either by the small bowel follow-through technique (SBFT) or enteroclysis (delivery of the contrast directly into the proximal jejunum via a nasopharynx tube) yields a greatest accuracy (33–60% *vs.* >90%, respectively) in identifying luminal disorder and mucosal morphology. The contrast consists of barium and a bowel distending substance as methylcellulose which does not affect its peristalsis.[34–37]

Computer tomography (CT) with intravenous and oral contrast is probably the most common radiographic modality used for both initial and late diagnosis. It has a reported accuracy of approximately 50%, but this varies among histologic type (adenocarcinoma 70–80%, lymphomas 58%, carcinoid 33%). More sensitive CT multi-detectors probably achieve a higher accuracy. CT is also helpful for the detection both intra-abdominal (peritoneal and liver) and distant metastases. In general, adenocarcinoma is shown as an annular lesion with irregular edges, eccentric thickening of the bowel wall or fixation with adjacent structures, lumen narrowing, and proximal bowel dilatation. Particularly, duodenal adenocarcinomas look polypoid (70%), ulcerated (20%), or infiltrative (10%). Depending on the lesion's size, a higher peripheral-to-central contrast attenuation can be observed. Lymphoma commonly demonstrates multiple luminal filling disruptions, more "flat" wall thickening that involves bigger bowel section, aneurysmal bowel dilatation with intermittent obstruction, and excessive mesenteric lymphadenopathy. Carcinoid tumors are usually small (0.5–2cm), submucosal–intramural lesions that due to local serotonin secretion produce hypertrophy of the muscularis propria and fibrosis. Fibrosis (or desmoplastic reaction) is responsible for the characteristic stellate pattern which comprises of fixation, kinking, and angulation of the bowel wall. Up to 70% of calcifications can be seen in the mesentery. Sarcomas usually present as well circumscribed, hypervascular, and a submucosal mass with a necrotic center (depending on the size) that are exoenteric and displace adjacent bowel loops. When they grow toward the lumen, sarcomas become polypoid and fungating and frequently have a central area of mucosal ulceration that causes a high incidence of intestinal bleeding. Metastatic lesions to the small intestine have been known to occur in cases of melanoma, carcinoma of cervix, lung, breast (mostly lobular carcinoma), and soft tissue tumors. Often, these metastases to the small intestine cause obstruction and bleeding. They tend to have a little stroma, and obstruction is rarely seen even in large tumors unless they cause intussusception. In a patient with a known history of malignancy, obstructive symptoms, or bleeding from the gastro-intestinal tract, a metastatic lesion must be considered.[38–43]

Enteroclysis can be combined with CT or MRI (magnetic resonance imaging) and yield better diagnostic accuracy. CT enteroclysis produces a sensitivity of 85% and a specificity of 97% with a positive predictive value of more than 90%.[36,44–47] On the other hand, MRI enteroclysis or MRI enterography (use of anti-peristaltic agents such as butyl bromide or glucagon for reducing motion artifacts) have achieved an accuracy of 98% and should be recommended as the initial diagnostic procedure in patients suspected to have SIC and in centers with adequate experience in this technique.[48–50]

Double balloon or push enteroscopy (DBE) is a technique in which two bal-loons at the distal ends of both an endoscope and an overtube are operated in com-bination. Although technically challenging, it allows visualization of the entire small bowel, the ability to biopsy any suspicious lesion, and also the performance of endoscopic procedures such as polypectomy, stent placement, etc. Its average diagnostic accuracy is about 80%.[51–57] These results are also reproducible by video capsule endoscopy (VCE) with the advantage of being more tolerable to patients than DBE and the disadvantages of not having the ability for tissue sampling and a retention rate that requires surgical removal of about 1%.[58–64]

Nuclear medicine can be helpful in distinguishing a carcinoid tumor and iden-tifying an active bleeding location. Octreoscan (Indium-111) detects somatostatin receptors (present almost always on carcinoid tumors) with a sensitivity of over 90% and is more accurate than CT in identifying both the location of the primary tumor and possible metastasis. It is also more sensitive in detecting early-stage disease.[65–67] Technetium-99 can be used in conjunction with angiography or SPECT/CT to locate a spot of active bowel bleeding, especially in hypervascular tumors like carcinoid or sarcomas.[68]

5 Adenocarcinoma

Small intestine adenocarcinoma (SIA) was the predominant histologic type in the past. Recent reports[4,10] indicate that carcinoid tumors have reached the same inci-dence. The median age of diagnosis is after the sixth decade of life for sporadic SIA with an earlier presentation occurring in patients with predisposing factors (genetic or autoimmune). Men are affected more than women (ratio 1:1.4) and African-Americans more than Caucasians (1.29:0.63).[69] These trends appear the same across North America, Europe, and Australia.[70,71]

SIA is more commonly observed in the duodenum (60–70%) in the elderly patients, followed by the jejunum (20%) and ileum (10%) in the younger patients.

This probably reflects the etiology and risk factors as adenomatous polyps are more common in the duodenum, whereas CD and celiac disease dominate the distant parts of the small intestine.[13–16,17–20]

5.1 *Genetics*

SIA and CRC share some common genetic alterations such as in *18qloss*, *TP53*, *KRAS*, and *SMAD4*, E-cadherin alterations, and marked differences such as low *APC* gene mutation, although the Wnt pathway appears to play a key role as several studies have reported abnormal nuclear expression of β-catenin.[72–77,84] The lack of *APC* mutations and the rarity of SIA compared to CRC may reflect different mechanisms in the onset of carcinogenesis and not the well-defined polyp-to-adenocarcinoma sequence for CRC. MMR deficiency with genetic or epigenetic (*MLH1*, *MSH2*, and *MSH6* mutations, gene promoter methylation) is reported to occur more frequently than CRC, in duodenal or jejunal (28%) rather than ileal cancers and in younger patients.[78–80] This might suggest a Lynch syndrome phenotype being more often in SIA than CRC or a consequence of the different risk factors like celiac disease. This particular subset of patients has been reported to bear up to 67% of gene *MLH-1* promoter methylation[81]. HER-2 expression has been assessed with negative results both in American and European studies.[77,8] In addition, it has been demonstrated recently that SIA has more similar genome copy alterations to CRC than gastric cancer by examining 85 microsatellite stable (MSS) tumors with comparative genomic hybridization (CGH) from these three sites.[83]

5.2 *Staging/prognosis*

The TNM staging system is used for SIA staging (Table 1). Usually, patients are diagnosed with advanced disease (32% stage IV, 27% stage III, 30% stage II, and 10% stage I) in contrast to CRC. This probably reflects the non-specific symptomatology, the absence of effective screening modalities, and the minor susceptibility from doctors due to the rarity of the disease. Five-year cancer specific survival has improved over the last years ranges at 65.3–80.3% for stage I, 55–69.9% for stage II, 40–45.1% for stage III, and less than 5% for stage IV when eight or more lymph nodes are removed as well.[85] Nevertheless, survival remains worse when compared stage to stage with CRC even after accounting for nodal sampling.[86] Older age, T4 tumors, number of infiltrated lymph nodes, duodenal or ileal primary tumors, grade 3 differentiation, <10 lymph nodes recovery, and positive margins are adverse prognostic factors.[4,87]

Table 1   TNM classification of small intestine adenocarcinomas (SIAs)

Primary Tumor (T)	Primary tumor cannot be assessed
T0	No evidence of primary tumor
Tis	Carcinoma in situ
T1	Tumor invades the lamina propria or submucosa
T2	Tumor invades the muscularis propria
T3	Tumor invades 2 cm or less into the subserosa or into the non-peritonealized perimuscular tissue (mesentery or retroperitoneum[*])
T4	Tumor perforates the visceral peritoneum or directly invades other organs or structures, including: • Other loops of the small intestine, mesentery or retroperitoneum by more than 2 cm • Through the serosa into the abdominal wall • The pancreas (only for tumors in the duodenum)
Regional lymph nodes (N)	
Nx	Regional lymph nodes cannot be assessed
N0	No regional lymph node metastasis
N1	Regional lymph node metastasis
Distant metastasis (M)	
M0	No distant metastasis
M1	Distant metastasis
Stage	
IA T1 N0 M0	
IB T2 N0 M0	
IIA T3 N0 M0	
IIB T4 N0 M0	
III Tany N1 M0	
IV Tany Nany M1	

[*]The non-peritonealized perimuscular tissue for the jejunum and ileum is part of the mesentery. For the duodenum, it is part of the retroperitoneum in areas where there is no serosa.

Updated from AJCC Cancer Staging Manual, 7th ed. (Ref. 121).

5.3 *Management*

5.3.1 *Localized disease*

Surgery remains the mainstay of treatment. The type of surgical resection depends on the location. For duodenal cancers, a Whipple procedure is many times required especially for second segment's lesions. For the jejunum or ileum, a segmental resection with 5-cm margins and adequate nodal removal is advocated. The number of retrieved lymph nodes usually varies with the affected part of the small intestine and duodenal adenocarcinoma is by far the most understaged.[85–87] Local relapse is more common in duodenal tumors although systemic recurrence predominate.[88] In the case of unresectable disease, options include palliative resection, diversion, and bypass. In the case of peritoneal carcinomatosis, cytoreductive surgery along with hyperthermic intraperitoneal chemotherapy (HIPEC) either with mitomycin-C or 5-fluorouracil (FU) remains an option.[89–92]

5.3.2 *Adjuvant therapy*

No randomized trials have been performed and clinical practice is guided by small retrospective and often single-institution studies. No clear advantage over surgery alone has been demonstrated so far, and the decision for administering is biased based on "high-risk features."[93–97] Physicians use adjuvant treatment more often during the last decades extrapolating results from its activity in the metastatic setting together with the proven benefit in CRC.[98] The most common regiment consists of a fluoropyrimidine analog plus or minus oxaliplatin depending on each patient's characteristics. For ampullary adenocarcinomas, gemcitabine/cisplatin is another option as many believe that this entity shares many similarities with biliary adenocarcinoma.[99] Recent report classify ampullary carcinomas into biliary-like (poor prognosis) and intestinal-like (better prognosis) using gene-expression profiling methods.[100,101] Currently, a large phase III trial termed BALLAD (Benefit of Adjuvant Chemotherapy for Small Bowel Adenocarcinoma) is ongoing to test observation *vs.* 24 weeks of chemotherapy (5-FU or capecitabine *vs.* 5-FU or capecitabine, plus oxaliplatin). Adjuvant radiation may have a role in duodenal tumors due to their retroperitoneal location and enhanced surgical difficulty for clear margins or adequate sampling.[102,103] Neoadjuvant chemoradiotherapy is reported to be a feasible and safe strategy in a try to downstage a locally advanced tumor.[103,104]

5.3.3 *Palliative chemotherapy*

There are no randomized trials that compare chemotherapy to best supportive care alone. All data come from retrospective studies that show a survival benefit with the use of chemotherapy. The most commonly used regimens mimic those in use for CRC. The combination of a fluoropyrimidine plus oxaliplatin has yielded response rates of 30–50% with median progression-free survival (PFS) and overall survival (OS) of 7.8–11.3 months and 10.5–20.4 months, respectively (Table 2). The role of targeted therapies is not established, yet there are reports of cetuximab activity in *KRAS* wild-type patients.[114] Clinical trials are ongoing (Table 3).[115]

Table 2   Newer studies of systemic chemotherapy for SIAs.

Author	Regimen	Patient N.	Study/Design	Year	RR%	PFS/OS (m)
Overman[105]	Cis-5-FU	29	Retrospective (1st L)	2008	46%	8.7/14.8
	5-FU	41			5-FU/Other	5F-U/Other
	other	10			16%	3.9/12
Overman[106]	CapeOx	30	Prospective (1st L)	2008	50%	11.3/20.4
Zaanan[107]	FOLFOX	48	Retrospective (1st L)	2010	34	6.9/17.8
	Cis-5-FU	16			31	4.8/9.3
	FOLFIRI	19			9	6.0/10.6
	5-FU/LV	10			0	7.7/13.5
Zaanan[108]	FOLFIRI	28	Retrospective (2nd L)	2010	20	3.2/10.5
Zhang[109]	FOLFOX/ CapOx	28	Retrospective (1st L)	2011	32.3	6.3/14.2
Koo[110]	5-FU based	40	Retrospective (1st L)	2011	11.1	5.7/11.8
Tsusima[111]	Fluor. mon	60	Retrospective (1st L)	2012	20	5.4/13.9
	Cis/Fluor.	17			38	3.8/12.6
	FOLFOX	22			42	8.2/22.2
	fluor/IRI	11			25	5.6/9.4
	other	22			21	3.8/8.1
Xiang[112]	FLOFOX	33	Prospective (1st L)	2012	48.5	7.8/15.2
McWilliams[113]	CAPOXIRI	28	Prospective (1st L)	2012	39	8.7/12.7

Abbreviations: Cis, cisplatin; CapeOx, capecitabine + oxaliplatin; FOLFOX, 5-FU + oxaliplatin; FOLFIRI, 5-FU + irinotecan; RR, response rate; PFS, progression-free survival; OS, overall survival.

Table 3   Clinical trials for advanced SIAs.

Agent	Phase	Tumor type	Tx Line	N	Identifier
CAPOX + Bevacizumab	II	SBA + ampullary	1st	30	NCT00354887
Capecitabine/oxaliplatin/irinotecan	II	SBA	1st	33	NCT00433550
CAPOX + panitumumab (KRAS wt)	II	SBA + ampullary	1st	20	NCT01202409
GEMOX + erlotinib	Ib	Duodenal + ampullary	1st	22	NCT00987766
Nab-paclitaxel	II	SBA	≥2nd	10	NCT01730586

Abbreviations: CAPOX, capecitabine + oxaliplatin; GEMOX, gemcitabine + oxaliplatin; N, number of patients; SBA, small bowel adenocarcinoma; Tx, treatment.

*Chemotherapy dosing determined based upon UGTA1 genotype.

6 Carcinoid Tumors

Carcinoid tumors arise from neuroendocrine cells throughout the body and synthesize bioactive amines and peptides. The small intestine is the most common location and Kultcitski cells are thought to be their origin. They are part of gastroenteropancreatic neuroendocrine tumors (GEP-NETs), mostly indolent tumors and may be numerous throughout the small intestine. The ileum is most frequently affected (70–87%), followed by the duodenum and jejunum.[116] Their incidence has markedly increased over the last decades.[2–4] Age at diagnosis is similar to that of adenocarcinoma; there is slight preponderance to men, and risk is higher for African-Americans and lower for Hispanics.[117] Carcinoid tumors are also often associated with other non-carcinoid neoplasms.

The tumor arises inside the bowel wall as a submucosal mass, creating a desmoplatic reaction (fibrosis) with a characteristic radiographic (under CT) appearance.[41] The gut or mesentery can be distorted and patients can present with obstruction or venous mesenteric infarction. Metastatic disease is frequently an issue with the liver, lung, and bone being the most commonly affected. Functional (or secreting) carcinoids may up to 10% present with carcinoid syndrome (flushing, diarrhea, bronchospasm, carcinoid heart disease), caused by the release of biologically active substances such as ACTH, somatostatin, tachykinins, histamine, and serotonin.[118] Patient diagnosis can be facilitated through 5-hydroxyindoloacetic acid (5-HIAA) urine levels or serum chromogranin-A (CgA), each with a different specificity and sensitivity.[119]

6.1 *Staging/prognosis*

Until recently, a well-defined staging and prognostic system has been absent. In 2007, the European Neuroendocrine Tumor Society (ENETS) proposed a staging system for NETs of the lower jejunum and ileum based on TNM features.[120] A pathologic grading variant (mitotic rate, Ki-67 expression) was also introduced to assess the aggressiveness of the neoplasm. The American Joint Committee on Cancer (AJCC) adopted this system for the seventh edition of its staging manual (2010).[121] The largest series to test the prognostic validity of this system was published in 2013 by Strosberg *et al.*[122] They proposed that stages I and II to be merged in a single early stage category, stage III tumors be separated into locally advanced resectable *vs.* unresectable categories, and the mitotic rate per 10 HPF cutoff be set at 5 instead of 2. Others have yielded similar results.[123] In general, node involvement or nonresectable disease (stage III) appears to be the critical survival endpoint since 95-999% of patients have well- or intermediate-grade tumors. Five-year OS was 100% for stages I-9II, 91% for stage III, and 72% for stage IV (Table 4).

Table 4   TNM staging of midgut NETS.

Primary Tumor (T)

T1	Tumor invades lamina propria or submucosa and is size 1 cm or less
T2	Tumor invades muscularis propria or is size > 1 cm
T3	Tumor invades through the muscularis propria into the subserosa or into the nonperitonealized tissue
T4	Tumor invades the visceral peritoneum (serosa) or any other organs or structures

Regional Lymph Nodes (N)

N0	No regional lymph node metastasis
N1	Regional lymph node metastasis

Distant Metastasis (M)

M0	No distant metastasis
M1	Distant metastasis

Stage

			Mitotic Count (10HPF)	Ki-67 Index (%)
I	T1N0M0	Differentiation/Grade		
IIA	T2N0M0	Well-differentiated/ low-grade	<2	≤2
IIB	T3N0M0	Intermediate differentiation/ intermediate-grade	2–20	3–20
IIIA	T4N0M0	Poorly differentiated/ high-grade	>20	>20
IIIB	TanyN1M0			
IV	TanyNanyM1			

6.2 *Management*

6.2.1 *Localized disease*

Segmental resection with regional node dissection is mandatory. A thorough full length inspection of the bowel should be performed due to the increased risk for synchronous tumors.[12]

6.2.2 *Advanced disease*

Surgical removal of the primary tumor and its lymph nodes maybe necessary to treat or prevent bowel hemorrhage or obstruction, and subsequent metastasizing.

It may improve both survival and symptom control.[124–127] The liver is the most common site for metastatic disease. If possible, liver resection with curative intent should be attempted. Surgical manipulations have the risk of provoking a carcinoid crisis, so pretreatment with octreotide is recommended.[119] If extensive bilobar disease is present, hepatic arterial embolization (HAE) with or without chemotherapy (TACE) can provide disease control. Radiofrequency ablation (RFA), radioembolization, or cryoamblation are also options.[128,129] Surgical debulking can sometimes palliate symptoms from carcinoid syndrome more efficiently than TACE or systemic therapy.[126,127] Liver transplantation has been performed with some long-lasting remissions observed but still remains investigational and not part of routine practice.[130,131]

6.2.3 *Systemic therapy*

For patients with low-burden disease and no symptoms, a watchful waiting is recommended. Treatment should start on evidence of progressive disease or symptom development.[120] Somatostatin analogs (SSAs) (short- or long-acting octreotide, lanreotide) are used primarily for symptom relief although there is evidence that they have anti-proliferative activity as well (octreotide LAR, the PROMID study).[132] Time for therapy initiation is debatable in low-burden, asymptomatic patients. The CLARINET study tested lanreotide *vs.* placebo only in patients with non-functioning GEP-NETs. Results indicate that antitumor activity is present (two-year PFS, 62% *vs.* 22%, respectively).[133] IFN-α can be added to SSAs for carcinoid syndrome control in cases where they alone are not effective. It has been shown to have anti-tumor effect by itself in non-randomized studies. Combination with octreotide or lanreotide has not showed survival benefit and is rarely used in this setting.[134–136]

Carcinoid tumors historically respond poorly to chemotherapy with median response rates (RR) of about 10–20%. Streptozocin (STZ), 5-FU, dacarbazine, and doxorubicin are the most frequently used agents. The combination of STZ/5-FU has yielded the best results, both in response rate and median survival. Newer agents such as temozolamide (TMZ) and capecitabine with or without oxaliplatin have failed to produce substantial results although the latter combination in a phase II study resulted in 23–30% response rate in poorly and well-differentiated tumors, respectively. A TMZ and capecitabine combination was tested in a phase II trial with an impressive response rate of 70% and a median PFS of 18 months — the best figures yet demonstrated.[120,136]

Carcinoid tumors are hypervascular tumors. Molecules targeting anti-angiogenesis pathways have been tested in small phase II trials. Bevacizumab (an anti-VEGFA antibody) has been compared to PEGylated (PEG)-IFN-α by Yao *et al.*, demonstrating a higher response rate and prolonged PFS.[137] It was also demonstrated in functional CT scans that bevacizumab decreases tumor blood flow. SWOG (formerly the Southwest Oncology Group) is currently conducting a phase III trial that compares octreotide combination with bevacizumab or IFN-α (NCT00569127). Other combinations with TMZ or sorafenib failed to show benefit in carcinoid tumors.[138,139] Sunitinib (a VEGFR/PDGFR inhibitor) was evaluated in a phase II study of advanced NETs and although it demonstrated antitumor activity against pancreatic NETs, its role against carcinoid is not clear.[140] Sorafenib (a VEGFR, PDGFR, c-KIT, and Raf inhibitor) has also yielded better results in pancreatic NETs than carcinoid with a response rate of 10% and a median six-month PFS of 40% for carcinoid tumors but with substantial toxicity (grade 3–4 in 43% of patients).[141] Vatalanib (a VEGFR/PDGFR inhibitor), thalidomide, and endostatin achieved no remissions.[136]

Imatinib achieved similar results with a median PFS of 24 weeks in a phase II trial.[142] Everolimus has also been tested in phases II and III trials.[143,144] RADIANT-2, an international phase III trial, randomized 429 patients with carcinoid syndrome to receive everolimus or placebo in addition to octreotide LAR. Median PFS was better in the everolimus arm (16.4 vs. 11.3 months for placebo) but did not meet the predefined threshold for statistical significance.

6.2.4 Peptide receptor radionuclide therapy

Peptide receptor radionuclide therapy (PRRT) presents another option. An SSA is linked with a radiolabeled particle (^{90}Y, ^{177}Lu). ^{90}Y-DOTATOC, ^{177}Lu-DOTATATE, annd ^{90}Y-edotreotide have been mostly used in studies. Objective responses are few but symptomatic disease control is often achieved. Median PFS is about 12–16 months. Toxicity is generally mild but cases of renal failure and severe bone marrow disease (myelodysplastic syndrome or acute myeloid leukemia) have been reported.[145]

7 Sarcomas

The majority of mesenchymal tumors (>90%) arising at the small intestine are gastrointestinal stromal tumor (GISTs). This entity was well defined during the 1990s when specific genetic alterations were identified to distinguish GISTs from other sarcomas. The small intestine is the second-most commonly affected site after the stomach with an occurrence of 30%. The jejunum is the most common site of origin followed by the ileum and duodenum.[146] It is estimated that there are

3,300–6,000 new cases in the United States each year with an incidence of 6.8 per million from 1992 to 2000, although this is probably underestimated because many tumors at that time (diagnosed as sarcomas) had not been tested for *KIT* or *PDGFR-A* mutations. The average age at diagnosis is during the seventh decade of life, with a female and Caucasian predominance.[147] Other rare entities include leiomyomas, leiomyosarcomas, and desmoid tumors.

7.1 *Genetics*

c-KIT oncogene mutations are found in about 80–85% of GISTs. The mutations can affect all parts of the KIT receptor (CD117). The juxtamembrane (exon 11) followed by the extracellular (exon 9) domains are the most commonly affected (70% *vs.* 16%, respectively). Alterations of the ATP-binding pocket (exon 13) or the activation loop (exon 17) are rare. Exon 11 mutations are the most common in all sites, whereas exon 9 mutations are specific for intestinal GISTs.[148,149] *PDGFR-A* mutations in the juxtamembrane domain (exon 12), the first tyrosine kinase domain (exon 14), and the activation loop (exon 18) are also associated with GIST pathogenesis in 5–10% of all cases.[150] These genes mutations are almost mutually exclusive in untreated GISTs. Developing resistance to imatinib treatment is usually correlated with acquired secondary *c-KIT* mutations in exons 13 and 17.[151,152] *PDGFR-A* secondary mutations in exons 14 and 18 have also been reported.[153]

For the rest of GISTs, no mutations are present and they are called 'wild-type GISTs.' The term 'SDH-deficient GIST' is preferred by many after the discovering that succinate dehydrogenase (SDH), a metabolic enzyme of the Krebs cycle, is often mutated in GISTs lacking *KIT/PDGFR-A* alterations.[154] *BRAF* (V600E) has also been identified in this subset of GISTs.[155]

7.2 *Prognosis*

GISTs arise from the submucosa. They are believed to originate from the interstitial calls of Cajal, the "pacemaker" of the GI system that coordinates its peristalsis.[156] They grow in an endophytic fashion and thus even very large tumors rarely cause bowel obstruction. They almost never spread to lymph nodes and metastasize primarily to the liver or the peritoneum. Prognosis depends on the resectability of the disease, tumor's size, mitotic index, and primary location (small intestine GISTs do worse than gastric ones).[148,157] The molecular profile is also important; exon 11 mutations are more sensitive to therapy with imatinib than exon 9 and variable mutations within exon 11 behave differently.[158,159]

7.3 Management

7.3.1 Limited disease

Complete surgical resection with clear margins is the mainstay of treatment. Usually a segmental resection with primary anastomosis and preservation of an intact capsule to avoid tumor rupture and spillage is the goal.[160] Lymph node dissection is generally not needed. In cases where preoperative treatment with imatinib has resulted in tumor stabilization and regression, metastasectomy with curative intent can be performed.[161,162] After an optimal resection, patients are classified having low to intermediate and high risk of recurrence according to the pathology report (Table 5).[163] Current guidelines indicate that imatinib at a dose of 400 mg daily (a TKI inhibitor of c-KIT, BCR-ABL, and PDGFR-A) should be administered for at least 36 months for intermediate- to high-risk patients after the results of the SSGXVIII/AIO phase III study. In this study, patients were randomized to receive imatinib for three years vs. one being the gold standard at the time (ACSOG Z9001 study).[165] PFS and OS were significantly improved (five-year PFS 66% vs. 48% and five-year OS 92% vs. 82%, respectively). Toxicities are manageable and include nausea, fatigue, abdominal pain, and a fluid retention syndrome that may rarely lead to congestive heart failure. However, benefit on PFS is evident during imatinib treatment and relapse occurs 6–12 months after imatinib discontinuation irrespective of the length of the treatment.[166] This raises the question for the optimal duration of treatment[166,167] with NCCN guidelines stating "that postoperative imatinib should be administered for at least 36 months for high-risk tumors." Imatinib dosage is another issue as seen for exon 9 bearers in advanced disease; oral absorption is not consistent across individuals though it impacts clinical benefit.[168]

7.3.2 Advanced disease

Imatinib was first tested in advanced disease and demonstrated durable responses and substantial clinical benefit in phase II and phase III trials with a response rate of 60–70%.[169–171] The dose approved by the FDA in 2002 was 400 mg once daily. Mutational status is predictor of response with patients bearing an exon 11 mutation achieving better results than exon 9 mutation-bearing tumors.[172] Responses, although shorter, occur even in c-KIT wild-type tumors while exons 13 and 17 tumors are insensitive.[173] Resistance develops within 2–3 years with exon 9 patients relapsing faster. Dose escalation from 400–800 mg can achieve disease control in 29% for these patients.[174] Later studies examined the increase the dose to 800 mg daily but failed to show any survival advantage except for the subset of exon 9-mutated tumors which was the single significant predictive factor.[170,172,175] This dose is currently recommended the initial treatment for exon 9 mutation-bearing patients. Imatinib

Table 5 Assessment of risk recurrence of small intestinal GIST.[*]

Tumor Parameters		Recurrence Risk	
Mitotic rate	Size	Duodenum	Jejunum/ileum
≤5 per 50 high-power fields (HPF)[**]	≤2cm	None (0%)	None (0%)
	>2 – ≤5 cm	Low (8.3%)	Low (4.3%)
	>5 – ≤10 cm	(Insufficient data)	Moderate (24%)
	>10cm	High (34%)	High (52%)
>5 per 50 high power fields (HPF)	≤2cm	(insufficient data)	High[***]
	>2 – ≤5 cm	High (50%)	High (73%)
	>5 – ≤10 cm	(insufficient data)	High (85%)
	>10cm	High (86%)	High (90%)

*Data based on long-term follow-up of 1,055 gastric, 629 small intestinal, 144 duodenal, and 111 rectal GISTs from the pre-imatinib era.

**CAP denotes that the required total count of mitoses is per 5 mm^2 on the glass slide section. With the use of older-model microscopes, 50 HPF is equivalent to 5 mm^2. Most modern microscopes with wider 40 × lenses/fields require only 20 HPF to embrace 5 mm^2.

***Small number of patients.

should be continued until disease progression since discontinuation results in early disease progression and poor PFS results after reintroduction.[176–178]

Imatinib can be used preoperatively in patients with potentially resectable primary or metastatic disease. Several prospective studies have demonstrated the efficacy and safety of "neoadjuvant" imatinib. Partial responses are variable, ranging from 7–60%, although a survival benefit could not be observed since all patients received imatinib postoperatively.[179,180] This approach should be made on an individual basis taking account that they included small or no number of small intestinal GISTs and that in exon 9 mutation-bearing patients, no response was seen (imatinib dose of 600 mg).

Sunitinib (a VEGFR/PDGFR inhibitor) is the first choice for imatinib-progressing or -intolerable patients. When tested against placebo in a randomized phase III trial, it resulted in significant improvement in PFS (27.3 *vs.* 6.4 weeks).[181] Sunitinib dose was 50 mg daily, four weeks on, two weeks off as in other malignancies. Toxicity is substantial in this dose, so George *et al.* tested the continuous 37.5 mg daily in a phase II trial.[182] Clinical benefit ratio, partial response, and stable disease (SD) were 53% with better tolerability and is an effective dosing alternative. Sunitinib appears to benefit more patients with exon 9-, exon 13-, and PDGFR-A-mutant tumors while activation loop mutations are cross-resistant with imatinib.[173]

Regorafenib (a c-KIT, PDGFR, VEGFR, RET, FGFR, and BRAF inhibitor) has been approved for third-line treatment. In a phase III study, patients with failure to both imatinib and Sunitinib were randomized to receive 160 mg of regorafenib daily or placebo (three weeks on, one week off). PFS at three and six months were 60% and 38%, respectively, compared to 11% and 0% for the placebo. No OS benefit was detected.[183]

Other targeted agents tested in GISTs include sorafenib,[184] nilotinib,[185] dasatinib,[186] pazopanib,[187] and masitinib.[188] Of these, masatinib has a greater affinity than imatinib for *KIT* exon 11-mutant tumors. It showed activity against wild-type tumors as well. After encouraging results in a phase II trial,[188] it is now tested against imatinib in a randomized phase III trial (NCT00812240).

8 Intestinal Lymphomas

The GI system is the most common site of extranodal lymphomas within the small intestine, accounting for 30%, second to gastric involvement (50–60%). For labeling a primary gastrointestinal lymphoma, Dawson's criteria are used: (1) absence of peripheral lymphadenopathy at the time of presentation; (2) lack of enlarged mediastinal lymph nodes; (3) normal total and differential white blood cell count; (4) predominance of bowel lesion at the time of laparotomy with only lymph nodes obviously affected in the immediate vicinity; and (5) no lymphomatous involvement of liver and spleen.[189] The ileum followed by the jejunum is most commonly affected. Their frequency in the United States according to the SEER database has risen from 0.22 to 0.35 between 1974 and 2003, reflecting perhaps the universal increasing trend in non-Hodgkin lymphoma (NHL) incidence.[190] This is maybe attributed to the increased number of immunosuppressed patients (transplantations, HIV, radiation, other malignancies, etc.), intestine specific diseases (e.g. CD and veliac disease), microbiota (*Campylobacter jejuni*), better diagnostic procedures (molecular discrimination from benign lymphoid hyperplasias), an aging population, or immigration from areas where primary intestinal lymphomas predominate extranodal NHL occurrence (Middle East, Pacific Islands).[191] The small intestine is extremely rich in lymphoid tissue (Peyer's patches) and diffuse lymphocyte infiltration, constantly exposed to antigens; the functional immune response is always active.[192] The age at diagnosis peaks during the seventh decade of life and slightly more men suffer from intestinal lymphomas than women do (60% *vs.* 40%, respectively).[190] Clinical presentation is non-specific with abdominal pain (71%), ileus (38%), weight loss (29%), bleeding (21%), perforation (16%), and palpable mass (12%) being the most common symptoms.[193]

8.1 *Histologic type/staging/prognosis*

Histologic classification is according to 2008 WHO classification for B and T cell lymphomas.[194] The majority of primary intestinal lymphomas are of B-cell (>90%)

Table 6 Most common primary intestinal lymphomas.[190,194]

NHL type	Incidence (%)	Grading
DLBCL	46,7	High-grade lymphoma
FL	17.7	Indolent lymphoma
		Grade 1: <5 centroblasts/HPF
		Grade 2: 6-15 centroblasts/HPF
		Grade 3:>15 centroblasts/HPF
		3A: centrocytes present (equals to high grade FL)
		3B: centrocytes not visible (equals to DLBCL)
BL	4.0	High-grade lymphoma
MZBCL	3.5	Indolent lymphoma
MCL	1.2	Intermediate Aggressive lymphoma
EATL	1.4	High-grade lymphoma

Abbreviations: DLBCL, diffuse large B-cell lymphoma; FL, follicular lymphoma; BL, Burkitt lymphoma; MZBCL, marginal zone B-cell lymphoma; MCL, mantle-cell lymphoma; EATL, enteropathy-associated T-cell lymphoma; HPF, high-power field.

Table 7a Ann Arbor staging system for NHL.[195]

Stage	Description
I (A, B)	Involvement of a single lymph node region or lymphoid structure (e.g. spleen, thymus, Waldeyer's ring).
II (A, B)	Involvement of two or more lymph node regions on the same side of the diaphragm
III (A, B)	Involvement of lymph regions or structures on both sides of the diaphragm.
IV (A, B)	Involvement of extranodal site(s) beyond that designated (E).

For all stages: (A) No symptoms, (B) fever (>38°C), drenching sweats, weight loss (10% body weight over six months)
For stages I to III: (E) Involvement of a single, extranodal site contiguous or proximal to known nodal site.

origin with the remaining being of T- or NK-cell lineage[189] (Table 6). Staging follows the Ann Arbor system (Table 7a),[195] which was developed initially for Hodgkin's disease and applies mostly on nodal lymphomas. However, this system is not fully applicable for primary lymphomas of the GI tract and the Lugano staging system was subsequently created[196] (Table 7b). The International Prognostic Index (IPI), a clinical tool for aggressive high-grade NHL prognosis assessment, has a higher prognostic value. Later, modifications for low- or intermediate-grade NHL were made to predict prognosis in follicular lymphoma (FL-IPI) and mantle-cell lymphoma (M-IPI)[197–199] (Table 8).

Table 7b   Lugano staging system for GI lymphomas.[196]

Stage I — The tumor is confined to the GI tract. It can be a single primary lesion or multiple, noncontiguous lesions.

Stage II — The tumor extends into the abdomen. This is further subdivided based upon the location of nodal involvement:

- Stage II: Involvement of local nodes (paragastric nodes for gastric lymphomas or para-intestinal nodes for intestinal lymphomas).
- Stage II: Involvement of distant nodes (para-aortic, para-caval, pelvic, or inguinal nodes for most tumors; mesenteric nodes in the case of intestinal lymphomas).
- Stage IIE: The tumor penetrates the serosa to involve adjacent organs or tissues.

Stage III — There is no stage III disease in this system.

Stage IV — There is disseminated extranodal involvement or concomitant supra-diaphragmatic nodal involvement.

Table 8   International Prognostic Index for NHL and modifications.

IPI[197]	FL-IPI[198]	M-IPI[199]
Age >60 years	Age >60 years	Age <50 years; <60 years; <70 years
Stage III/IV disease	Stage III/IV disease	Serum LDH <0.67; <1.0; <1.5 ULN
Elevated serum LDH	Elevated serum LDH	ECOG performance status >2
ECOG performance status >2	Serum Hemoglobin <12g/dl	WBC <6,700; <10,000; <15,000c/μL
>1 extranodal site	>4 lymph node group	
Each feature: 1 point	Each feature: 1 point	0 points: Age <50 years, ECOG 0-1, LDH <0.67 ULN, WBC <6,700/μl
		1 point: Ages 50– 59, LDH 0.67–0.99 ULN, WBC 6,700 to 9,999/μl
		2 points: Ages 60–69, ECOG 2–4, LDH 1–1.49 ULN, WBC 10,000–14,000/μl
		3 points: Ages >70, LDH >1.5 ULN, WBC > 15,000/μl
Low risk (0 points) — Five-year OS of 73%	Low risk (0-1 points) — Five- and 10-year OS of 91 and 71%	Low risk (0–3 points) — median survival not yet reached
Low–intermediate risk (1 point) — Five-year OS of 51%	Intermediate risk (2 points) — Five- and 10-year OS of 78 and 51%	Intermediate risk (4–5 points) — median survival of 51 months
High–intermediate risk (2 points) — Five-year OS of 43%	High risk (3-5 points) — Five- and 10-year OS of 53 and 36%	High risk (6–11 points) — median survival of 29 months
High risk (4-5 points) — Five-year OS of 26%		

Abbreviations: ECOG, Eastern Cooperative Oncology Group; ULN, upper limit of normal; WBC, white blood cells; OS, overall survival.

8.2 *Specific primary lymphoma subtypes and management*

8.2.1 *Diffuse large B-cell lymphoma*

Diffuse large B-cell lymphoma (DLBCL) presents usually as a unifocal ulcerated lesion commonly in the ileocecal area with complications, thus mandating surgical intervention. It comprises large cells (>double the size of a normal lymphocyte) with a diffuse growth pattern and a high proliferation (Ki-67) index.[193] Persisting β-type symptomatology (fever, sweats, body weight loss greater than 10%) is not unusual. Immunosuppression is a major risk factor.[193] Chemotherapy both in early or advanced disease is beneficial. The most commonly regimen consists of an anthracycline based combination (CHOP; Table 9) with the monoclonal anti-CD20 (commonly expressed surface marker on B-cell origin normal and neoplastic cells) antibody rituximab.[200,201] Radiotherapy is beneficial in bulky as well as in localized disease.[201]

8.2.2 *Follicular lymphoma*

An entity found exclusively in the small intestine (mainly duodenum) is the so-called 'follicular lymphoma (FL) of the small intestine.'[202] It shares common features with nodal FL like the formation of neoplastic follicles in the mucosa and submucosally. It is usually of a low-grade (Ki-67 <5%), affects the proximal part of the small intestine, and presents more often in younger or middle-aged women.[202] Transformation to high-grade lymphoma (DLBCL) can occur. Treatment depends on the stage and grading of the disease. Surgical excision[202] or watchful waiting[203] can provide cure in stage IE low to intermediate grade FL. For higher stage (≥IIE), additional radiotherapy is needed.[203] For grade 3 disease or higher-stage CHOP or CVP (Table 9), chemotherapy with the rituximab antibody is appropriate.[204,205] Rituximab can be used as maintenance therapy for up to two years since it has demonstrated an increase in PFS at three years (from 33% 68%) and a trend toward improved OS.[206]

Table 9 Common chemotherapy regimens used in small intestinal lymphomas.

CHOP: Cyclophosphamide, doxorubicin, vincristine, prednisone
CVP: Cyclophosphamide, vincristine, prednisone
HyperCyvad: Hyperfractionated cyclophosphamide, vincristine, doxorubicin, dexamethasone
CODOX-M/IVAC: Cyclophosphamide, etoposide, doxorubicin, high-dose methotrexate/ifosfamide, etoposide, high-dose cytarabine
FCR: Fludarabine, cyclophosphamide, rituximab

8.2.3 Burkitt lymphoma

Burkitt lymphoma (BL) is very highly aggressive lymphoma with endemic prevalence in some parts of the world (Africa, New Guinea).[194] In Western countries, it is sporadic and immunodeficiency related (HIV, medically induced). BL usually affects younger people except for the latter type. It has been linked to EBV (Epstein–Barr virus) infection (endemic variant) and the ileocecal area is the most common site to present (all variants).[194] It is highly curable (>80%) with intense but brief chemotherapy. Most commonly regimens used are CODOX-M/IVAC[207] or Hyper-CVAD[208] (Table 9). A recent study reported OS of 100% with low-intensity chemotherapy.[209] Rituximab has been added recently.[210] Prophylactic CNS (central nervous system) therapy is mandated due to the propensity for CNS infiltration.[211]

8.2.4 Marginal zone B-cell lymphoma

Previously designated as mucosal-associated lymphoid tissue lymphoma (MALT) or 'Western MALT,' marginal zone B-cell lymphoma (MZBCL) is correlated to chronic inflammation and *Campylobacter jejuni* has been implicated as a potential bacterial factor (similar to what is believed with *H. pylori* in gastric MZBCL). Patients are usually older adults.[194] Many have a history of autoimmune disease such as Sjögren syndrome or Hashimoto thyroiditis. Another variety of MZBCL known as immunoproliferative small intestinal disease (IPSID) is seen almost exclusively in Eastern Mediterranean region, affects younger patients, tends to be diffuse, and of the proximal small intestine. It is also associated with *Campylobacter jejuni* and characteristically secretes alpha heavy-chain immunoglobulins.[212] They can be multifocal. Treatment in IPSID can initially include antibiotics determined by culture results or in their absence, a combination of metronidazole plus ampicillin is a reasonable choice. For local non-IPSID disease, radiotherapy is an option.[213] For recurrent/non responsive/advanced disease, the mostly used regimen consists of chlorambucil[214] plus rituximab.[215]

8.2.5 Mantle-cell lymphoma

Mantle-cell lymphoma (MCL) is rare in the small intestine, and usually presents in older patients involving multiple sites throughout the GI tract (lymphomatous polyposis).[194] Surgery is for palliative purposes in cases of perforation, obstruction, and mass bleeding. If the disease is localized, chemotherapy with CHOP plus rituximab followed by radiation is the first choice although it has not showed superiority over CVP or MCP regimens but only to FCR.[216] However, most MCLs are diagnosed in stage IV; patients have a poor performance status and median survival is approximately three years. Rituximab maintenance until disease progression has been recently approved.[216]

8.2.6 *Enteropathy-associated T-cell intestinal lymphoma*

Enteropathy-associated T-cell intestinal lymphoma (EATL) is a rare, aggressive T-cell lymphoma. Type I is almost always for patients with celiac disease. Type II, equally aggressive, has no known premalignant condition. It is multifocal; the jejunum is the most commonly affected sited. It has the worst prognosis among all lymphomas. A gluten-free diet can most likely delay its appearance. Patients are often malnourished, have a poor performance status, and suffer from multiple infections due to perforation and fistula formation. Five-year survival with anthracycline-based chemotherapy (CHOP) is reported to be 10–20%.[217]

References

1. Surveillance, Epidemiology and End Results Program. SEER Stat Fact Sheets: Small Intestine Cancer. Retrieved from http://seer.cancer.gov/statfacts/html/smint.html; Accessed 1 November 2015.
2. Siegel R, *et al*. Cancer statistics 2013. *CA Cancer J Clin* 2013;**63**:11–30.
3. Hatzaras I, *et al*. Small-bowel tumors: Epidemiologic and clinical characteristics of 1260 cases from the Connecticut tumor registry. *Arch Surg* 2007;**142**(3):229.
4. Bilimoria KY, *et al*. Small bowel cancer in the United States: Changes in epidemiology, treatment, and survival over the last 20 years. *Ann Surg* 2009;**249**:63–71.
5. Wu AH, *et al*. Alcohol use, dietary factors and risk of small intestinal adenocarcinoma. *Int J Cancer* 1997;**70**:512–527.
6. Kaerlev L, *et al*. Is there an association between alcohol intake or smoking and small bowel adenocarcinoma? Results from a European multi-center case-control study. *Cancer Causes Control* 2000;**11**:791–797.
7. Chow WH, *et al*. Risk factors for small intestine cancer. *Cancer Causes Control* 1993;**4**:163–169.
8. Negri E, *et al*. Risk factors for adenocarcinoma of the small intestine. *Int J Cancer* 1999;**82**:171–174.
9. Boffetta , *et al*. Body mass, tobacco smoking, alcohol drinking and risk of cancer of the small intestine--a pooled analysis of over 500,000 subjects in the Asia Cohort Consortium. *Ann Oncol* 2012;**23**:1894–1898.
10. Schottenfeld D, *et al*. The epidemiology and pathogenesis of neoplasia in the small intestine. *Ann Epidemiol* 2009;**19**:58–69.
11. Delaunoit T, *et al*. Pathogenesis and risk factors of small bowel adenocarcinoma: A colorectal cancer sibling. *Am J Gastroenterol* 2005;**100**:703–10.

12. Zureikat A, *et al*. Cancer of the small intestine. In DeVita VT, Lawrence, TS, Rosenberg SA. *DeVita, Hellman and Rosenberg's Cancer Principles & Practice of Oncology*, 9th ed. Philadelphia: Wolters Kluwer, pp. 1048–1059.

13. Palascak-Juif V, *et al*. Small bowel adenocarcinoma inpatients with Crohn's disease compared with small bowel adenocarcinoma *de-novo*. *Inflamm Bowel Dis* 2005;**11**: 828–832.

14. Von Roon AC, *et al*. The risk of cancer in patients with Crohn's disease. *Dis Colon Rectum* 2007;**50**(6):839.

15. Piton G, *et al*. Risk factors associated with small bowel adenocarcinoma in Crohn's disease: a case-control study. *Am J Gastroenterol* 2008;**103**:1730–1736.

16. Osterman M. Big risk, small risk: Small bowel cancer in Crohn's disease. *Inflamm Bowel Dis* 2009;**9**:1434–1435.

17. Green PH, *et al*. Risk of malignancy in patients with celiac disease. *Am J Med* 2003;**115**(3):191.

18. Silano M, *et al*. Small bowel malignancy at diagnosis of coeliac disease. *Gut* 2005;**54**(4):565–566.

19. Howdle PD, *et al*. Primary small-bowel malignancy in the UK and its association with coeliac disease. *Quart J Med* 2003;**96**:345–353.

20. Askling J, *et al*. Cancer incidence in a population-based cohort of individuals hospitalized with celiac disease or dermatitis herpetiformis. *Gastroenterology* 2002;**123**:1428–1435.

21. Bjork J, *et al*. Periampullary adenomas and adenocarcinomas in familial adenomatous polyposis: Cumulative risks and *APC* gene mutations. *Gastroenterology* 2001;**121**(5):1127.

22. Belchetz LA, *et al*. Changing causes of mortality in patients with familial adenomatous polyposis. *Dis Colon Rectum* 1996;**39**(4):384.

23. Nugent KP, *et al*. Life expectancy after colectomy and ileorectal anastomosis for familial adenomatous polyposis. *Dis Colon Rectum* 1993;**36**(11):1059.

24. Schulmann K, *et al*. HNPCC-associated small bowel cancer: Clinical and molecular characteristics. *Gastroenterology* 2005;**128**:590–599.

25. Babba T, *et al*. Small bowel carcinoma revealing HNPCC syndrome. *Gastroentérol Clin Biol* 2010;**34**:325–328.

26. Bonadona V, *et al*. Cancer risks associated with germline mutations in *MLH1*, *MSH2*, and *MSH6* genes in Lynch syndrome. *J Am Med Assoc* 2011;**305**:2304–2310.

27. Hemminki A. The molecular basis and clinical aspects of Peutz–Jeghers syndrome. *Cell Mol Life Sci* 1999;**55**(5):735.

28. Giardiello FM, *et al*. Very high risk of cancer in familial Peutz–Jeghers syndrome. *Gastroenterology* 2000;**119**:1447–1453.

29. Dabaja BS, *et al*. Adenocarcinoma of the small bowel: Presentation, prognostic factors, and outcome of 217 patients. *Cancer* 2004;**101**:518–526.

30. Talamonti MS, *et al*. Primary cancers of the small bowel: Analysis of prognostic factors and results of surgical management. *Arch Surg* 2002;**137**(5):564–571.

31. Ciresi DL, *et al*. The continuing clinical dilemma of primary tumors of the small intestine. *Am Surg* 1995;**61**(8):698.

32. Maglinte DD, *et al.* The role of the physician in the late diagnosis of primary malignant tumors of the small intestine. *Am J Gastroenterol* 1991;**86**(3):304.

33. Broll R, *et al.* [Malignant tumors of the small intestine. Diagnostic problems and differentiated surgical therapy.] *Chirurg.* 1994;**65**(5):451–456.

34. Maglinte DD, *et al.* Current status of small bowel radiography. *Abdom Imaging* 1996;**21**(3):247–257.

35. Nolan DJ. The true yield of the small-intestinal barium study. *Endoscopy* 1997;**29**(6): 447–453.

36. Boudiaf M, *et al.* Small-bowel diseases: prospective evaluation of multi-detector row helical CT enteroclysis in 107 consecutive patients. *Radiology* 2004;**233**:338–344.

37. Levine MS, *et al.* Pattern approach for diseases of mesenteric small bowel on barium studies. *Radiology* 2008;**249**(2):445–460.

38. Buckley JA, *et al.* The accuracy of CT staging of small bowel adenocarcinoma: CT/ pathologic correlation. *J Comput Assist Tomogr* 1997;**21**(6):986–991.

39. Korman MU. Radiologic evaluation and staging of small intestine neoplasms. *Eur J Radiol* 2002;**42**(3):193–205.

40. Horton KM, *et al.* The current status of multi-detector row CT and three-dimensional imaging of the small bowel. *Radiol Clin North Am* 2003;**41**(2):199.

41. Horton KM, *et al.* Carcinoid tumors of the small bowel: A multitechnique imaging approach. *Am J Roentgenol* 2004;**182**:559–567.

42. Ramachandran I, *et al.* Multi-detector row CT of small bowel tumours. *Clin Radiol* 2007;**62**(7):607.

43. Fernandes DD, *et al.* Cross-sectional imaging of small bowel malignancies. *Can Assoc Radiol J.* 2012;**63**(3):215–221.

44. Pilleul F, *et al.* Possible small-bowel neoplasms: contrast-enhanced and water-enhanced multidetector CT enteroclysis. *Radiology* 2006;**241**(3):796–801.

45. Rajesh A, Maglinte DD. Multi-slice CT enteroclysis: Technique and clinical applications. *Clin Radiol* 2006;**61**(1):31–39.

46. Hristova L, *et al.* Small bowel tumors: spectrum of findings on 64-section CT entero-clysis with pathologic correlation. *Clin Imaging* 2012;**36**(2):104–112.

47. Soyer P, *et al.* Helical CT-enteroclysis in the detection of small-bowel tumours: A meta-analysis. *Eur Radiol* 2013;**23**(2):388–399.

48. Masselli G, *et al.* Small-bowel neoplasms: Prospective evaluation of MR enteroclysis. *Radiology* 2009;**251**(3):7437–7450.

49. Van Weyenberg SJ, *et al.* MR enteroclysis in the diagnosis of small-bowel neoplasms. *Radiology* 2010;**254**(3):765–773.

50. Masselli G, *et al.* Magnetic resonance imaging of small bowel neoplasms. *Cancer Imaging* 2013;**13**:92–99.

51. Kita H, *et al.* Double balloon endoscopy in two hundred fifty cases for the diagnosis and treatment of small intestinal disorders. *Inflammopharmacology* 2007;**15**(2):7–77.

52. Suzuki T, *et al.* Clinical utility of double-balloon enteroscopy for small intestinal bleeding. *Dig Dis Sci* 2007;**52**(8):1914–1918.

53. Zhong J, *et al*. A retrospective study of the application on double-balloon enteroscopy in 378 patients with suspected small-bowel diseases. *Endoscopy* 2007;**39**(3):208–215.

54. May A, *et al*. Endoscopic interventions in the small bowel using double balloon enteroscopy: Feasibility and limitations. *Am J Gastroenterol* 2007;**102**(3):527–535.

55. Imaoka H, *et al*. Characteristics of small bowel tumors detected by double balloon endoscopy. *Dig Dis Sci*. 2011;**56**(8):2366–2371.

56. Cangemi D, *et al*. Small bowel tumors discovered during double-balloon enteroscopy: Analysis of a large prospectively collected single-center database. *J Clin Gastroenterol*. 2013;**47**(9):769–772.

57. Islam S, *et al*. Evaluation and management of small-bowel tumors in the era of deep enteroscopy. *Gastrointest Endosc* 2014;**79**(5):732–740.

58. Pennazio M, *et al*. Outcome of patients with obscure gastrointestinal bleeding after capsule endoscopy: Report of 100 consecutive cases. *Gastroenterology* 2004; **126**(3):643–653.

59. Hartmann D, *et al*. A prospective two-center study comparing wireless capsule endoscopy with intraoperative enteroscopy in patients with obscure GI bleeding. *Gastrointest Endosc* 2005;**61**(7):826–832.

60. Hadithi M, *et al*. A prospective study comparing video capsule endoscopy with double-balloon enteroscopy in patients with obscure gastrointestinal bleeding. *Am J Gastroenterol* 2006;**101**(1):52–57.

61. Schwartz GD, Barkin JS. Small-bowel tumors detected by wireless capsule endoscopy. *Dig Dis Sci* 2007;**52**(4):1026–1030.

62. Ross A, *et al*. Double balloon enteroscopy detects small bowel mass lesions missed by capsule endoscopy. *Dig Dis Sci* 2008;**53**(8):2140–2143.

63. Liao Z, *et al*. Indications and detection, completion, and retention rates of small-bowel capsule endoscopy: A systematic review. *Gastrointest Endosc* 2010;**71**(2):280–286.

64. Gerson L. Capsule endoscopy and deep enteroscopy. *Gastrointest Endosc* 2013;**78**(3):439–443.

65. Oberg K, Eriksson B. Nuclear medicine in the detection, staging and treatment of gastrointestinal carcinoid tumours. *Best Pract Res Clin Endocrinol Metab* 2005; **19**(2):265–276.

66. Kocha W, *et al*. Consensus recommendations for the diagnosis and management of well-differentiated gastroenterohepatic neuroendocrine tumours: A revised statement from a Canadian National Expert Group. *Curr Oncol* 2010;**17**(3):49–64.

67. Teunissen JJ, *et al*. Nuclear medicine techniques for the imaging and treatment of neuroendocrine tumours. *Endocr Relat Cancer* 2011;**18**(Suppl. 1):S27–S51.

68. Allen TW, Tulchinsky M. Nuclear medicine tests for acute gastrointestinal conditions. *Semin Nucl Med* 2013;**43**(2):88–101.

69. Qubaiah O, *et al*. Small intestinal cancer: A population-based study of incidence and survival patterns in the United States, 1992 to 2006. *Cancer Epidemiol Biomarkers Prev* 2010;**19**:1908–1918.

70. Haselkorn T, *et al*. Incidence of small bowel cancer in the United States and worldwide: Geographic, temporal, and racial differences. *Cancer Causes Control* 2005;**16**:781–787.

71. Curado MP, *et al. Cancer Incidence in Five Continents*, Vol. IX. Lyon: IARC, IARC Scientific Publication, No. 160, 2007.

72. Wheeler JM, *et al.* An insight into the genetic pathway of adenocarcinoma of the small intestine. *Gut* 2002;**50**:218–223.

73. Blaker H, *et al.* Genetics of adenocarcinomas of the small intestine: Frequent deletions at chromosome 18q and mutations of the *SMAD4* gene. *Oncogene* 2002;**21**:158–164.

74. Svrcek M, *et al.* Immunohistochemical analysis of adenocarcinoma of the small intestine: A tissue microarray study. *J Clin Pathol* 2003;**56**:898–903.

75. Blaker H, *et al.* Mutational activation of the RAS-RAF-MAPK and the Wnt pathway in small intestinal adenocarcinomas. *Scand J Gastroenterol* 2004;**39**:748–753.

76. Breuhahn K, *et al.* Large-scale N-terminal deletions but not point mutations stabilize beta-catenin in small bowel carcinomas, suggesting divergent molecular pathways of small and large intestinal carcinogenesis. *J Pathol* 2008;**215**:300–307.

77. Aparicio T, *et al.* Small bowel adenocarcinoma phenotype according to the primary localisation. *Ann Oncol* 2012;**23**:ix234.

78. Planck M, *et al.* Microsatellite instability and expression of MLH1 and MSH2 in carcinomas of the small intestine. *Cancer* 2003;**97**:1551–1557.

79. Warth A, *et al.* Genetics and epigenetics of small bowel adenocarcinoma: The interactions of CIN, MSI, and CIMP. *Mod Pathol* 2011;**24**:564–570.

80. Fu T, *et al.* CpG island methylator phenotype-positive tumors in the absence of MLH1 methylation constitute a distinct subset of duodenal adenocarcinomas and are associated with poor prognosis. *Clin Cancer Res* 2012;**18**:4743–4752.

81. Diosdado B, *et al.* High-resolution array comparative genomic hybridization in sporadic and celiac disease-related small bowel adenocarcinomas. *Clin Cancer Res* 2010;**16**:1391–1401.

82. Overman MJ, *et al.* Immunophenotype and molecular characterization of adenocarcinoma of the small intestine. *Br J Cancer* 2010;**102**:144–150.

83. Haan JC, *et al.* Small bowel adenocarcinoma copy number profiles are more closely related to colorectal than to gastric cancers. *Ann Oncol* 2012;**23**:367–374.

84. Murphy J, *et al.* DNA mutation frequencies in metastatic small bowel adenocarcinoma (mSBA) in comparison to gastric (mGC), colon (mCC), and rectal cancer (mRC): Continuum or cutpoint? *J Clin Oncol* 2013;**31**(Suppl.):Abstr. e14636.

85. Overman MJ, *et al.* Prognostic value of lymph node evaluation in small bowel adenocarcinoma: Analysis of the surveillance, epidemiology, and end results database. *Cancer* 2010;**116**:5374–5382.

86. Overman MJ, *et al.* A population-based comparison of adenocarcinoma of the large and small intestine: Insights into a rare disease. *Ann Surg Oncol* 2012;**19**:1439–1445.

87. Nicholl MB, *et al.* Small bowel adenocarcinoma: understaged and undertreated? *Ann Surg Oncol* 2010;**17**:2728–2732.

88. Dabaja BS, *et al.* Adenocarcinoma of the small bowel: Presentation, prognostic factors, and outcome of 217 patients. *Cancer* 2004;**101**:518–526.

89. Marchettini P, *et al.* Mucinous adenocarcinoma of the small bowel with peritoneal seeding. *Eur J Surg Oncol* 2002;**28**(1):19–23.

90. Jacks SP, *et al*. Cytoreductive surgery and intraperitoneal hyperthermic chemotherapy for peritoneal carcinomatosis from small bowel adenocarcinoma. *J Surg Oncol* 2005;**91**:112.

91. Chua TC, *et al*. Cytoreductive surgery and perioperative intraperitoneal chemotherapy for peritoneal carcinomatosis from small bowel adenocarcinoma. *J Surg Oncol* 2009; **100**(2):139–143.

92. Sun Y, *et al*. Cytoreductive surgery and hyperthermic intraperitoneal chemotherapy for peritoneal carcinomatosis from small bowel adenocarcinoma. *Am Surg* 2013;**79**(6): 644–648.

93. Dabaja BS, *et al*. Adenocarcinoma of the small bowel: Presentation, prognostic factors, and outcome of 217 patients. *Cancer* 2004;**101**:518–526.

94. Halfdanarson TR, *et al*. A single-institution experience with 491 cases of small bowel adenocarcinoma. *Am J Surg* 2010;**199**:797–803.

95. Koo DH, *et al*. Adjuvant chemotherapy for small bowel adenocarcinoma after curative surgery. *Oncology* 2011;**80**(3–4):208–213.

96. Schwameis K, *et al*. Small bowel adenocarcinoma — terra incognita: A demand for cross-national pooling of data. *Oncol Lett* 2014;**7**(5):1613–1617.

97. Guo XC, *et al*. Retrospective analysis of 119 small bowel adenocarcinoma in Chinese patients. *Cancer Invest* 2014;**32**(5):178–183.

98. Raghav K, *et al*. Small bowel adenocarcinomas-existing evidence and evolving paradigms. *Nat Rev Clin Oncol* 2013;**10**:534–544.

99. Ynson ML, *et al*. What are the latest pharmacotherapy options for small bowel adenocarcinoma? *Expert Opin Pharmacother* 2014;**15**(6):745–748.

100. Overman MJ, *et al*. Gene expression profiling of ampullary carcinomas classifies ampullary carcinomas into biliary-like and intestinal-like subtypes that are prognostic of outcome. *PLoS ONE* 2013;**8**(6):e65144.

101. Chang DK, *et al*. Histomolecular phenotypes and outcome in adenocarcinoma of the ampulla of Vater. *J Clin Oncol* 2013;**31**:1348–1356.

102. Swartz MJ, *et al*. Adjuvant concurrent chemoradiation for node-positive adenocarcinoma of the duodenum. *Arch Surg* 2007;**142**(3):285–288.

103. Kelsey CR, *et al*. Duodenal adenocarcinoma: Patterns of failure after resection and the role of chemoradiotherapy. *Int J Radiat Oncol Biol Phys* 2007;**69**(5):1436–1441.

104. Onkendi EO, *et al*. Neoadjuvant treatment of duodenal adenocarcinoma: A rescue strategy. *J Gastrointest Surg* 2012;**16**:320–324.

105. Overman MJ, *et al*. Chemotherapy with 5-FU and a platinum compound improves outcomes in metastatic small bowel adenocarcinoma. *Cancer* 2008;**113**:2038–2045.

106. Overman MJ, *et al*. Phase II study of capecitabine and oxaliplatin for advanced adenocarcinoma of the small bowel and ampulla of Vater. *J Clin Oncol* 2009;**27**:2598–2603.

107. Zaanan A, *et al*. Chemotherapy of advanced small bowel adenocarcinoma: A multicenter AGEO study. *Ann Oncol* 2010;**21**:1786–1793.

108. Zaanan A, *et al*. Second line chemotherapy with fluorouracil, leucovorin and irinotecan (FOLFIRI Regimen) in patients with advanced small bowel adenocarcinoma after failure of first line platinum based chemotherapy a multicenter AGEO study. *Cancer* 2011;**117**:1422–1428.

109. Zhang L, *et al*. Efficacy of the FOLFOX/CAPOX regimen for advanced small bowel adenocarcinoma: A three-center study from China. *J BUON* 2011;**16**:689–696.

110. Koo DH, *et al*. Systemic chemotherapy for treatment of advanced small bowel adenocarcinoma with prognostic factor analysis: Retrospective study. *BMC Cancer* 2011;**11**:205.

111. Tsushima T, *et al*. Multicenter retrospective study of 132 patients with unresectable small bowel adenocarcinoma treated with chemotherapy. *Oncologist* 2012;**17**: 1163–1170.

112. Xiang XJ, *et al*. A phase II study of modified FOLFOX as first-line chemotherapy in advanced small bowel adenocarcinoma. *Anticancer Drugs* 2012;**23**:561–566.

113. McWilliams RR, *et al*. Pharmacogenetic dosing by UGT1A1 genotype as first-line therapy for advanced small-bowel adenocarcinoma: A North Central Cancer Treatment Group (NCCTG) trial. *J Clin Oncol* 2012;**30**:(Suppl. 4; Abstr. 314).

114. Santini D, *et al*. Cetuximab in small bowel adenocarcinoma: A new friend? *Br J Cancer* 2010;**103**:1305.

115. Overman MJ. Rare but real: Management of small bowel adenocarcinoma. *Am Soc Clin Oncol Educ Book* 2013;**33**:189–193.

116. Ferolla P, *et al*. The biological characterization of neuroendocrine tumors: The role of neuroendocrine markers. *J Endocrinol Invest* 2008;**31**(3):277–286.

117. Qubaiah O, *et al*. Small intestinal cancer: A population-based study of incidence and survival patterns in the United States, 1992 to 2006. *Cancer Epidemiol Biomarkers Prev* 2010;**19**(8):1908–1918.

118. Ramage JK, *et al*. Guidelines for the management of gastroenteropancreatic neuroendocrine (including carcinoid) tumours (NETs). *Gut* 2012;**61**(1):6–32.

119. Nandy N, *et al*. Management of advanced and/or metastatic carcinoid tumors: Historical perspectives and emerging therapies. *Expert Opin Pharmacother* 2013;**14**(12):1649–1658.

120. Rindi G, *et al*. TNM staging of midgut and hindgut (neuro) endocrine tumors: A consensus proposal including a grading system. *Virchows Arch* 2007;**451**:757–762.

121. Edge SB, *et al*. (eds.). *AJCC Cancer Staging Manual*, 7th ed. Chicago: Springer, 2010, p. 184.

122. Strosberg JR, *et al*. Prognostic Validity of the American Joint Committee on cancer staging classification for midgut neuroendocrine tumors. *J Clin Oncol* 2013;**31**(4): 420–425.

123. Jann H, *et al*. Neuroendocrine tumors of midgut and hindgut origin: Tumor-node-metastasis classification determines clinical outcome. *Cancer* 2011;**117**(15):3332–3341.

124. Hellman P, *et al*. Effect of surgery on the outcome of midgut carcinoid disease with lymph node and liver metastases. *World J Surg* 2002;**26**(8):991–997.

125. Givi B, *et al*. Operative resection of primary carcinoid neoplasms in patients with liver metastases yields significantly better survival. *Surgery* 2006;**140**(6):891–897.

126. Glazer ES, *et al*. Long-term survival after surgical management of neuroendocrine hepatic metastases. *HPB (Oxford)* 2010;**12**(6):427–433.

127. Capurso G, *et al*. Systematic review of resection of primary midgut carcinoid tumour in patients with unresectable liver metastases. *Br J Surg* 2012;**99**(11):1480–1486.

128. Taner T, *et al.* Adjunctive radiofrequency ablation of metastatic neuroendocrine cancer to the liver complements surgical resection. *HPB (Oxford)* 2013;**15**(3):190–195.

129. Johnston FM, *et al.* Local therapies for hepatic metastases. *J Natl Compr Canc Netw* 2013;**11**(2):153–160.

130. Gedaly R, *et al.* Liver transplantation for the treatment of liver metastases from neuroendocrine tumors: An analysis of the UNOS database. *Arch Surg* 2011;**146**: 953–958.

131. Le Treut YP, *et al.* Liver transplantation for neuroendocrine tumors in Europe-results and trends in patient selection: A 213-case European liver transplant registry study. *Ann Surg* 2013;**257**(5):807–815.

132. Rinke A, *et al.* Placebo-controlled, double-blind, prospective, randomized study on the effect of octreotide LAR in the control of tumor growth in patients with metastatic neuroendocrine midgut tumors: A report from the PROMID Study Group. *J Clin Oncol* 2009;**27**(28):4656–4663.

133. Ruszniewski P, *et al.* A randomized, double-blind, placebo-controlled study of lanreotide antiproliferative Response in patients with gastroenteropancreatic neuroendocrine tumors (CLARINET) [abstract]. *17th ECCO–38th ESMO–32nd ESTRO Eur Cancer Congr* 2013:E17–E7103.

134. Faiss S, *et al.* Prospective, randomized, multicenter trial on the antiproliferative effect of lanreotide, interferon alfa and their combination for therapy of metastatic neuroendocrine gastroenteropancreatic tumors-the International Lanreotide and Interferon Alfa Study Group. *J Clin Oncol* 2003;**21**:2689–2696.

135. Arnold R, *et al.* Octreotide *vs.* octreotide plus interferon alpha in endocrine gastroenteropancreatic tumors: A randomized trial. *Clin Gastroenterol Hepatol* 2005;**3**:761–171.

136. Pavel M, *et al.* Systemic therapeutic options for carcinoid. *Sem Oncol* 2013;**40**(1):84–99.

137. Yao JC, *et al.* Targeting vascular endothelial growth factor in advanced carcinoid tumor: A random assignment phase II study of depot octrotide with bevacizumab and PEGylated interferon alfa-2b. *J Clin Oncol* 2008;**26**(8):1316–1323.

138. Chan JA, *et al.* Prospective study of bevacizumab plus temozolamide in patients with advanced neuroendocrine tumors. *J Clin Oncol* 2012;**30**(24):2963–2968.

139. Castellano DE, *et al.* Sorafenib and Bevacizumab combination targeted therapy in advanced neuroendocrine tumor: A phase II study of the Spanish neuroendocrine tumor group (GETNE0801). *Eur J Cancer* 2013;**49**(18):3780–3787.

140. Kulke MH, *et al.* Activity of sunitinib in patients with advanced neuroendocrine tumors. *J Clin Oncol* 2008;**26**(20):3403–3410.

141. Hobday TJ, *et al.* MC044h, a phase II trial of sorafenib in patients (pts) with metastatic neuroendocrine tumors (NET): A Phase II Consortium (P2C) study. 2007 ASCO Annu Meeting. *J Clin Oncol* 2007;**25**(18S):4504.

142. Yao JC, *et al.* Clinical and *in vitro* studies of imatinib in advanced carcinoid tumors. *Clin Cancer Res* 2007;**13**:234–240.

143. Yao JC, *et al.* Efficacy of RAD001 (everolimus) and octreotide LAR in advanced low-to intermediated-grade neuroendocrine tumors: Results of a phase II study. *J Clin Oncol* 2008;**26**:4311–4318.

144. Pavel ME, *et al*. Everolimus plus octreotide long-acting repeatable for the treatment of advanced neuroendocrine tumors associated with carcinoid syndrome (RADIANT-2): A randomized, placebo-controlled, phase 3 study. *Lancet* 2011;**378**:2005–2012.

145. Gulenchyn KY, *et al*. Radionuclide therapy in neuroendocrine tumours: A systematic review. *Clin Oncol* 2012;**24**(4):294–308.

146. Fletcher CD, *et al*. Diagnosis of gastrointestinal stromal tumors: A consensus approach. *Hum Pathol* 2002;**33**:459.

147. Rubin JL, *et al*. Epidemiology, survival, and costs of localized gastrointestinal stromal tumors. *Int J Gen Med* 2011;**14**(4):121–130.

148. Miettinen M, *et al*. Gastronitestinal stromal tumors: Pathology and prognosis at different sites. *Semin Diagn Pathol* 2006;**23**:70–83.

149. Corless CL, *et al*. Gastrointestinal stromal tumors: origin and molecular oncology. *Nat Rev Cancer* 2011;**11**:865–878

150. Lasota J, *et al*. Clinical significance of oncogenic *KIT* and *PDGFR-A* mutations in gastrointestinal tumors. *Histopathology* 2008;**53**:245–266.

151. Antonescu CR, *et al*. Acquired resistance to imatinib in gastrointestinal stromal tumors occurs through secondary gene mutation. *Clin Cancer Res* 2005;**11**:4182–4190.

152. Wardelmann E, *et al*. Acquired resistance to imatinib in gastrointestinal stromal tumors caused by multiple *KIT* mutations. *Lancet Oncol* 2005;**6**:249–251.

153. Lim KH, *et al*. Molecular analysis of secondary kinase mutations in imatinib-resistant gastrointestinal stromal tumors. *Med Oncol* 2008;**25**:207–213.

154. Janeway KA, *et al*. Defects in succinate dehydrogenase in gastrointestinal stromal tumors lacking KIT and *PDGFR-A* mutations. *Proc Natl Acad Sci* 2011;**108**:314–318.

155. Agaimy A, *et al*. V600E *BRAF* mutations are alternative early molecular events in a subset of *KIT/PDGFR-A* wild-type gastrointestinal stromal tumors. *J Clin Pathol* 2009;**62**:613–616.

156. Sircar K, *et al*. Interstitial cells of Cajal as precursors of gastrointestinal stromal tumors. *Am J Surg Pathol* 1999;**23**(4):377–389.

157. Demetri GD, *et al*. NCCN task force report: Update on the management of patients with gastrointestinal stromal tumors. *J Natl Compr Canc Netw* 2010;**8**:S-1.

158. Martin J, *et al*. Deletions affecting codons 557–558 of the *c-KIT* gene indicate a poor prognosis in patients with completely resected gastrointestinal stromal tumors: A study by the Spanish Group for Sarcoma Research (GEIS). *J Clin Oncol* 2005;**23**(25): 6190–6198.

159. Corless CL, *et al*. Relation of tumor pathologic and molecular features to outcome after surgical resection of localized primary gastrointestinal stromal tumor (GIST): Results of the intergroup phase III trial ACOSOG Z9001. 2010 ASCO Annual Meeting. *J Clin Oncol* **28**:15s, 2010(Suppl.; Abstr. 10006).

160. Katrin S, *et al*. Surgical treatment of GISTuan institutional experience of a high volume center. *Int J Surg* 2013;**11**:801–806.

161. McAuliffe JC, *et al*. A randomized, phase II study of preoperative plus postoperative imatinib in GIST: Evidence of rapid radiographic response and temporal induction of tumor cell apoptosis. *Ann Surg Oncol* 2009;**16**(4):910–919.

162. Blesius A, *et al.* Neoadjuvant imatinib in patients with locally advanced non metastatic GIST in the prospective BFR14 trial. *BMC Cancer* 2011;**11**:72.

163. College of American Pathologists (CAP). Protocol for the Examination of Specimens from Patients with Gastrointestinal Stromal Tumor (GIST). Retrieved from http://www.cap.org/apps/docs/committees/cancer/cancer_protocols/2012/GIST_12protocol_3021.pdf; Accessed 1 November 2015.

164. Joensuu H, *et al.* One *vs.* three years of adjuvant imatinib for operable gastrointestinal stromal tumor: A randomized trial. *JAMA* 2012;**307**(12):1265–1272.

165. De Matteo RP, *et al.* Adjuvant imatinib mesylate after resection of localised, primary gastrointestinal stromal tumor: A randomised, doubleblind, placebo-controlled trial. *Lancet* 2009;**373**(9669):1097–1104.

166. Serrano C, *et al.* Recent advances in the treatment of gastrointestinal tumors. *Ther Adv Med Oncol* 2014;**6**(3):115–127.

167. Joensuu H. Adjuvant therapy for high-risk gastrointestinal stromal tumour, considerations for optimal management. *Drugs* 2012;**72**(15):1953–1963.

168. Yoo C, *et al.* Cross-sectional study of imatinib plasma trough levels in patients with advanced gastrointestinal stromal tumors: Impact of gastrointestinal resection on exposure to imatinib. *J Clin Oncol* 2010;**28**(9):1554–1559.

169. Demetri GD, *et al.* Efficacy and safety of imatinib mesylate in advanced gastrointestinal stromal tumors. *N Engl J Med* 2002;**347**(7):472–480.

170. Verweij J, *et al.* Progression-free survival in gastrointestinal stromal tumours with high-dose imatinib: Randomised trial. *Lancet* 2004;**364**(9440):1127–1134.

171. Blanke CD, *et al.* Long-term results from a randomized phase II trial of standard-versus higher-dose imatinib mesylate for patients with unresectable or metastatic gastrointestinal stromal tumors expressing KIT. *J Clin Oncol* 2008;**26**(4):620–625.

172. Heinrich MC, *et al.* Correlation of kinase genotype and clinical outcome in the North American Intergroup Phase III Trial of imatinib mesylate for treatment of advanced gastrointestinal stromal tumor: CALGB 150105 Study by Cancer and Leukemia Group B and Southwest Oncology Group. *J Clin Oncol* 2008;26(33):5360-67

173. Heinrich MC, *et al.* Primary and secondary kinase genotypes correlate with the biological and clinical activity of sunitinib in imatinib-resistant gastrointestinal stromal tumor. *J Clin Oncol* 2008;**26**(33):5352–5359.

174. Zalcberg JR, *et al.* Outcome of patients with advanced gastro-intestinal stromal tumours crossing over to a daily imatinib dose of 800 mg after progression on 400 mg. *Eur J Cancer* 2005;**41**(12):1751–1757.

175. Blanke CD, *et al.* Phase III randomized, intergroup trial assessing imatinib mesylate at two dose levels in patients with unresectable or metastatic gastrointestinal stromal tumors expressing the KIT receptor tyrosine kinase: S0033. *J Clin Oncol* 2008;**26**(4):626–632.

176. Blay JY, *et al.* Prospective multicentric randomized phase III study of imatinib in patients with advanced gastrointestinal stromal tumors comparing interruption versus continuation of treatment beyond 1 year: The French Sarcoma Group. *J Clin Oncol* 2007;**25**(9):1107–1113.

177. Le Cesne A, *et al.* Discontinuation of imatinib in patients with advanced gastrointestinal stromal tumours after 3 years of treatment: An open-label multicentre randomised phase 3 trial. *Lancet Oncol* 2010;**11**(10):942–949.

178. Patrikidou A, *et al.* Influence of imatinib interruption and rechallenge on the residual disease in patients with advanced GIST: Results of the BFR14 prospective French Sarcoma Group randomised, phase III trial. *Ann Oncol* 2013;**24**(4):1087–1093.

179. Eisenberg BL, *et al.* Phase II trial of neoadjuvant/adjuvant imatinib mesylate (IM) for advanced primary and metastatic/recurrent operable gastrointestinal stromal tumor (GIST): Early results of RTOG 0132/ACRIN 6665. *J Surg Oncol* 2009;**99**(1):42–47.

180. McAuliffe JC, *et al.* A randomized, phase II study of preoperative plus postoperative imatinib in GIST: Evidence of rapid radiographic response and temporal induction of tumor cell apoptosis. *Ann Surg Oncol* 2009;**16**(4):910–919.

181. Demetri GD, *et al.* Efficacy and safety of sunitinib in patients with advanced gastrointestinal stromal tumour after failure of imatinib: A randomised controlled trial. *Lancet* 2006;368(9544):1329–1338.

182. George S, *et al.* Clinical evaluation of continuous daily dosing of sunitinib malate in patients with advanced gastrointestinal stromal tumour after imatinib failure. *Eur J Cancer* 2009;**45**(11):1959–1968.

183. Demetri GD, *et al.* Efficacy and safety of regorafenib for advanced gastrointestinal stromal tumours after failure of imatinib and sunitinib (GRID): An international, multicentre, randomised, placebo-controlled, phase 3 trial. *Lancet* 2013;**381**(9863): 295–302.

184. Montemurro M, *et al.* Sorafenib as third- or fourth-line treatment of advanced gastrointestinal stromal tumour and pretreatment including both imatinib and sunitinib, and nilotinib: A retrospective analysis. *Eur J Cancer* 2013;**49**(5):1027–1031.

185. Reichardt P, *et al.* Phase III study of nilotinib versus best supportive care with or without a TKI in patients with gastrointestinal stromal tumors resistant to or intolerant of imatinib and sunitinib. *Ann Oncol* 2012;**23**(7):1680–1687.

186. Trent JC, *et al.* A phase II study of dasatinib for patients with imatinib-resistant gastrointestinal stromal tumor (GIST). *J Clin Oncol* 2011;**29**(15 Suppl.):Abstr. 10006.

187. Ganjoo KN, *et al.* A multicenter phase II study of pazopanib in patients with advanced gastrointestinal stromal tumors (GIST) following failure of at least imatinib and sunitinib. *Ann Oncol* 2014;**25**(1):236–240.

188. Le Cesne A, *et al.* Phase II study of oral masitinib mesilate in imatinib-naïve patients with locally advanced or metastatic gastro-intestinal stromal tumour (GIST). *Eur J Cancer* 2010;**46**(8):1344–1351.

189. Prasanna G, *et al.* Primary gastrointestinal lymphoma. *World J Gastroenterol* 2014; **17**(6):697–707.

190. Gustafsson BI, *et al.* Uncommon cancers of the small intestine, appendix and colon: An analysis of SEER 1973-2004 and current diagnosis and therapy. *Int J Oncol* 2008; **33**:1121–1131.

191. Müller A, *et al.* Epidemiology of non-Hodgkin's lymphoma (NHL): Trends, geographic distribution, and etiology. *Ann Hematol* 2004;**84**(1):1–12.

192. Carmack SW, *et al*. Lymphocytic disorders of the gastrointestinal tract: A review for the practicing pathologist. *Adv Anat Pathol* 2009;**16**(5):290–306.

193. Yin L, *et al*. Primary small-bowel non-Hodgkin's lymphoma: A study of clinical features, pathology, management and prognosis. *J Int Med Res* 2007;**35**(3):406–415.

194. Campo E, *et al*. The 2008 WHO classification of lymphoid neoplasms and beyond: evolving concepts and practical applications. *Blood* 2011;**117**(19):5019–5032.

195. Armitage JO. Staging non-Hodgkin lymphoma. *CA Cancer J Clin* 2009;**55**(6): 368–376.

196. Rohatiner A, *et al*. Report on a workshop convened to discuss the pathological and staging classifications of gastrointestinal tract lymphoma. *Ann Oncol* 1994;**5**(5): 397–400.

197. The International Non-Hodgkin's Lymphoma Prognostic Factors Project. A predictive model for aggressive non-Hodgkin's lymphoma. *N Engl J Med* 1993;**329**(14): 987–994.

198. Solal-Céligny P, *et al*. Follicular lymphoma international prognostic index. *Blood* 2004;**104**(5):1258–1265.

199. Hoster E, *et al*. A new prognostic index (MIPI) for patients with advanced-stage mantle cell lymphoma. *Blood* 2008;**111**(2):558–565.

200. Pfreundschuh M, *et al*. CHOP-like chemotherapy plus rituximab versus CHOP-like chemotherapy alone in young patients with good-prognosis diffuse large-B-cell lymphoma: a randomised controlled trial by the MabThera International Trial (MInT) Group. *Lancet Oncol* 2006;**7**(5):379–391.

201. Koniaris LG, *et al*. Management of gastrointestinal lymphoma. *J Am Coll Surg* 2003;**197**(1):127–141.

202. Misdraji J, *et al*. Primary follicular of the gastrointestinal tract. *Am J Surg Pathol* 2011;**35**:1255–1263.

203. Schmatz AI, *et al*. Primary follicular lymphoma of the duodenum is a distinct mucosal/submucosal variant of follicular lymphoma: A retrospective study of 63 cases. *J Clin Oncol* 2011;**29**(11):1445–1451.

204. Hiddemann W, *et al*. Frontline therapy with rituximab added to the combination of cyclophosphamide, doxorubicin, vincristine, and prednisone (CHOP) significantly improves the outcome for patients with advanced-stage follicular lymphoma compared with therapy with CHOP alone: Results of a prospective randomized study of the German Low-Grade Lymphoma Study Group. *Blood* 2005;**106**(12):3725–3732.

205. Marcus R, *et al*. Phase III study of R-CVP compared with cyclophosphamide, vincristine, and prednisone alone in patients with previously untreated advanced follicular lymphoma. *J Clin Oncol* 2008;**26**(28):4579–4586.

206. Van Oers MH, *et al*. Rituximab maintenance improves clinical outcome of relapsed/resistant follicular non-Hodgkin lymphoma in patients both with and without rituximab during induction: Results of a prospective randomized phase 3 intergroup trial. *Blood* 2006;**108**(10):3295–3301.

207. Magrath I, *et al*. Adults and children with small non-cleaved-cell lymphoma have a similar excellent outcome when treated with the same chemotherapy regimen. *J Clin Oncol* 1996;**14**(3):925–934.

208. Thomas DA, *et al*. Chemoimmunotherapy with hyper-CVAD plus rituximab for the treatment of adult Burkitt and Burkitt-type lymphoma or acute lymphoblastic leukemia. *Cancer* 2006;**106**(7):1569–1580.

209. Dunleavy K, *et al*. Low-intensity therapy in adults with Burkitt's lymphoma. *N Engl J Med* 2013;**369**(20):1915–1925.

210. Wildes T, *et al*. Rituximab is associated with improved survival in Burkitt lymphoma. *Ther Adv Hematol* 2014;**5**(1):3–12.

211. Hill QA. CNS prophylaxis in lymphoma: who to target and what therapy to use. Blood Rev. 2006;20(6):319–32

212. Lecuit M, *et al*. Immunoproliferative small intestinal disease associated with *Campylobacter jejuni. N Engl J Med*.2004;**350**(3):239–248.

213. Goda JS, *et al*. Long-term outcome in localized extranodal mucosa-associated lymphoid tissue lymphomas treated with radiotherapy. *Cancer* 2010;**116**(16): 3815–3824.

214. Zucca E, *et al*. Addition of rituximab to chlorambucil produces superior event-free survival in the treatment of patients with extranodal marginal-zone B-cell lymphoma: 5-year analysis of the IELSG-19 Randomized Study. *J Clin Oncol* 2013;**31**(5): 565–572.

215. Conconi A, *et al*. Clinical activity of rituximab in extranodal marginal zone B-cell lymphoma of MALT type. *Blood* 2003;**102**(8):2741–2745.

216. Kluin-Nelemans HC, *et al*. Treatment of older patients with mantle-cell lymphoma. *N Engl J Med* 2012;**367**(6):520–531.

217. Hawkes E, *et al*. Diagnosis and management of rare gastrointestinal lymphomas. *Leuk Lymphoma* 2012;**53**(12):2341–2350.

Chapter 21

Importance of Supportive and Palliative Care in Gastrointestinal Malignancies

Neha Jeurkar Darrah, Valaree Williams and Ursina R. Teitelbaum

1 Introduction

The European Organization for Research and Treatment of Cancer (EORTC) defines supportive care for cancer patients as "the multi professional attention to the individual's overall physical, psychosocial, spiritual, and culture needs" and states that it "should be available at all stages of the illness, for patients of all ages, and regardless of the current intention of any anti-cancer treatment."[1] This is particularly relevant for patients diagnosed with gastrointestinal (GI) malignancies who suffer from a wide range of symptoms. In this chapter, we will review general complications of GI malignancies, therapy related complications, and complications by cancer site.

2 General Complications of Gastrointestinal Cancers

2.1 *Psychosocial distress*

The National Comprehensive Cancer Network (NCCN) defines distress as "an emotionally unpleasant psychological, social, and/or spiritual existence that may interfere with a patient's ability to effectively cope with cancer, its physical symptoms and its treatment."[2] Psychosocial distress is common in patients with cancer but unfortunately often goes unrecognized and untreated.[3,4] Patients who are at particularly high risk for distress include those with a history of psychiatric disorder or substance use, cognitive impairment, communication barriers, uncontrolled symptoms, psychosocial factors, and spiritual and religious concerns.[2] Recognition and prompt treatment of psychosocial distress will help alleviate patient suffering and improve health outcomes.[5,6]

The NCCN recommends that patients should be screened for distress at their initial visit and at periods of increased vulnerability as clinically indicated.[2] These periods include the start of a new treatment modality, completion of therapy, and referral to hospice. Clinicians can screen for distress using either clinician-administered or patient-administered assessments. Regardless of which method is used, a standardized screening tool that adequately addresses the multi-faceted nature of distress should be utilized. Examples of validated screening tools for distress include the Hospital Anxiety and Depression Scale (HADS), Psychological Distress Inventory (PDI), Distress Thermometer (DT), Patient Health Questionnaire (PHQ-4), and the General Health Questionnaire (GHQ-12). The DT and PHQ-4 are the shortest tools. Patients with suspected mood disorder, anxiety disorder, or adjustment disorder should be referred for psychotherapy and initiated on medical treatment if appropriate.

2.2 *Fatigue*

Cancer-related fatigue (CRF) is the most common symptom encountered in patients with advanced cancer and consistently ranked as the most distressing symptom.[7–10] CRF is described as a persistent sense of diminished energy related to cancer and/or its treatment and is not relieved by rest. Multiple, interrelated factors contribute to CRF and include deconditioning, cancer therapy, cachexia/malnutrition, psychological factors, metabolic abnormalities, sedating medications, systemic infection or organ dysfunction anemia, and unmanaged symptoms such as pain.[11] A thorough history and physical examination with a specific focus on sleep patterns, depression, and anxiety can help elucidate the underlying cause. If a potential underlying cause for fatigue is identified, it should be treated. For patients without a treatable cause for fatigue, treatment with either psychostimulants or corticosteroids could be considered, although data for their use is limited. The most commonly used psychostimulant is methylphenidate. Dosing guidelines recommend starting at 2.5–5 mg daily and titrating as necessary to 15–30 mg at 8:00 am and noon. A recent systematic review found a suggested therapeutic benefit for methylphenidate in CRF but the absolute numbers were small.[12] Commonly reported side effects included vertigo, anxiety, anorexia, and nausea.[12] Another psychostimulant that is being evaluated is modafinil. Dosing guidelines recommend starting at 50 mg qAM and titrating as necessary to 200–400 mg PO qAM. Pilot studies have indicated efficacy in the treatment of fatigue associated with ALS and HIV.[13,14] A recent double blind RCT, however, found that modafinil has no effect in lung cancer patients suffering from CRF.[15] Research is needed to determine if this lack of efficacy is also applicable to gastrointestinal malignancies.

Another available option is steroids. Steroids provide modest benefit for a limited period of time (2–4 weeks) and are therefore most appropriate for patients with a limited life expectancy.[11] They decrease fatigue via unknown mechanisms.[16] Reported regimens include prednisone 7.5–10 mg daily, dexamethasone 2 mg daily, or methylprednisolone 32 mg daily. Long-term use may cause myopathy, increase risk of infection, and further contribute to fatigue.

All patients suffering from fatigue should be offered education and counseling about the options for management, expected outcomes, and potential for progressive debility and functional limitations if the disease progresses. This will help thepatient and family set realistic expectations and plan accordingly. For some patients, enrollment in exercise programs may be very beneficial. Several randomized controlled trials have shown that endurance exercise training improves fatigue and physical performance.[17,18] Low to moderate aerobic exercise for 20–30 min per day, 4–5 days per week is a reasonable goal.

2.3 *Anorexia/cachexia*

Many patients with advanced cancer suffer from a wasting syndrome known as the "cancer anorexia-cachexia syndrome" or CACS.[19] It is particularly common in patients with pancreatic ductal carcinoma and occurs in 80% of these patients.[20,21] CACS is characterized by weight loss (involuntary loss of more than 10% pre-diagnosis weight) accompanied by profound loss of skeletal muscle mass with or without loss of adipose tissue.[11] It negatively impacts quality of life, body image, and is an independent risk factor for early mortality.[11,22] The pathophysiology of CACS is complex and mediated by interactions between tumor by-products and host cytokines.[11] For patients with GI cancers, particularly upper GI, malignancy or treatment-related alterations to normal digestive or absorptive properties will also contribute to cachexia. For example, pancreatic adenocarcinoma is associated with severe cachexia and poor pancreatic function that leads to malabsorption.[23] In addition to the underlying malignancy, untreated symptoms such as pain, chronic nausea, depression, dysphagia, odynophagia, hypoguesia, hyposmia, taste alteration from chemotherapy and constipation may contribute to anorexia and should be addressed first.[11] A detailed evaluation conducted by the multidisciplinary oncology team should assess anorexia, decreased food intake, catabolic drivers, muscle mass and strength, and changes over time as well as symptoms and medications that may interfere with the ability to consume adequate intake. A plan to address nutrition-related contributors to cancer cachexia should include management of symptoms that impact intake. In order to promote adequate nutrition, patients need development of a plan to maximize nutrition and potentially consideration of pharmacologic interventions. Pharmacological options for treating anorexia include megestrol, corticosteroids, anti-depressants, and cannabinoids. No options exist for treating cachexia specifically and the aforementioned measures will not reverse cachexia in most patients. One of the most commonly prescribed appetite stimulants is megesterol. Megesterol exerts its effect by antagonizing the progesterone receptor. Megestrol is dosed once daily and is available as either tablets or liquid. Dosing guidelines recommend starting at 400 mg/day and titrating to 800 mg/day for effect.[24] Improvement in appetite generally occurs in under a week but weight gain may take 4–6 weeks of continuous medication use. Weight gain, however, is largely adipose tissue and water retention rather than lean muscle mass and no study has shown a survival benefit.[25] Notable side effects potentially include thromboembolic events, hypertension, hyperglycemia, and adrenal suppression if discontinued abruptly. A recent study demonstrated that 75% of patients with advanced gastrointestinal cancer achieve weight gain when prescribed megestrol.[26]

Another option is corticosteroids. Use of corticosteroids should be restricted to patients with a limited life expectancy (<6 months) because the risk of steroid-related side effects increases dramatically over time.[11] For patients with a longer life expectancy, megesterol should be used. An appropriate dose is prednisone 20 to 40 mg/day or its equivalent. For patients who cannot tolerate megestrol, dronabinol, a cannabinoid, may be an option. Some studies have found beneficial effects of dronabinol on appetite but the effect on cachexia seems to be limited.[27,28] Side effects include sedation, poor concentration, dysphoria, and hallucinations.

For patients with concomitant insomnia, low dose mirtazapine, a selective serotonin noradrenaline inhibitor that is more likely to cause somnolence than other anti-depressants, may be beneficial. Compared to other anti-depressants, it is more likely to cause weight gain and increased appetite.[29]

Fish oil supplementation continues to be explored as a method to preserve or improve lean body mass and body weight. The published Nutrition Practice Guideline from the Academy of Nutrition and Dietetics Evidence Analysis Library regarding dietary supplements containing fish oil for the adult oncology patient states, "If sub-optimal symptom control or inadequate dietary intake has been addressed and the adult oncology patient is still experiencing loss of weight and lean body mass (LBM), the registered dietitian nutritionist (RDN) may consider use of dietary supplements containing eicosapentaenoic acid (EPA) as a component of nutrition intervention. Research indicates that dietary supplements containing fish oil (actual consumption, 0.26 g to 6.0 g of EPA per day), resulted in a significant effect on preservation or improvement of weight and LBM in adult oncology patients with weight loss. Rating: Strong, Imperative".[30] Caution should be used in patients who are intolerant or allergic to fish and potential drug interactions should be evaluated prior to initiation of fish oil supplementation.

Anorexia and cachexia can be particularly difficult for families to watch and may lead to concerns about their loved one starving to death. Compassionate counseling is required to reframe the condition from starving to death to irreversible metabolic abnormalities from the underlying malignancy. Because food represents love and nurturing in many cultures, it is important to reassure families that they can continue to care for their loved one in other ways, even if they no longer can directly feed them.

2.4 *Early satiety*

Early satiety, the feeling of being full after eating or drinking a small amount, is a common issue and can lead to weight loss, nutrient insufficiencies and deficiencies, dehydration and malnutrition.[31] Delayed gastric emptying, gastroparesis, heartburn, certain medications, the gastrointestinal cancer itself, surgery and chemotherapy can contribute to early satiety. Evaluation of conditions and medications that may slow gastric emptying and influence GI function can assist with determining factors contributing to early satiety. Assisting the patient in adjusting eating and drinking patterns to decrease the impact of early satiety is necessary to promote adequate oral intake. Pharmacologic interventions include prokinetic agents such as metoclo-pramide. The following recommendations may also assist in maximizing oral intake despite the presence of early satiety:

- Choose calorie dense food or oral nutrition supplements
- Maximize intake when most hungry
- Transition to eating small, frequent meals
- Eat on a schedule rather than waiting for appetite or hunger cues
- Consume liquids between meals rather than at meals
- Engage in light physical activity to help move food through GI tract

2.5 *Role of nutrition support in gastrointestinal cancers*

Nutrition support, including enteral (EN) and parenteral nutrition (PN), is a neces-sary consideration when the oral feeding route is unavailable or not tolerated or oral nutritional intake is inadequate. Indicators for nutrition support in the oncology population include mechanical and functional dysfunctions such as dysphagia, gastrointestinal obstruction, inability to digest and/or absorb nutrients and inability to chew or swallow foods and liquids. The role for nutritional support in advanced GI malignancies in the absence of these indications is less clear. A small retrospective study of patients on home TPN identified 16 patients who survived a year or longer; most of these patients had carcinoid tumors.[32] A randomized prospective trial of patients with primarily gastrointestinal tumors showed a trend towards increased survival in patients who received TPN.[33] In contrast, a meta-analysis of cancer patients on TPN showed decreased survival and increased susceptibility to infection.[34] Decisions regarding the initiation of nutrition support should align with the overall plan of care and the individual patient's wishes.

2.5.1 *Enteral versus parenteral nutrition*

Once the need for nutrition support is identified, it is necessary to determine which route is most appropriate. If contraindications do not exist, the enteral route is preferred over the parenteral route. Enteral nutrition utilizes the gut and normal physiologic route of nutrition, which reduces the risk of bacterial translocation when compared to parenteral nutrition.[35] Compared to PN, EN has a lower prevalence of infectious complications and infectious morbidity and has been shown to reduce hospital length of stay and lower incidence of hyperglycemia.[36–38] In addition to improved outcomes, EN is less expensive as compared to PN.[36] Indications, risk, benefits and cost should be considered when deciding the method of nutrition support.

2.5.1.1 Enteral nutrition

Enteral nutrition provides nutrition directly into the GI system, bypassing the oral route. EN is most appropriate in patients receiving active anticancer treatment who are malnourished and who are anticipated to be unable to ingest and/or absorb adequate nutrients for greater than seven to 14 days.[39] According to the clinical guidelines of the American Society for Parenteral and Enteral Nutrition (ASPEN), patients undergoing major cancer-related surgeries do not benefit from routine use of EN.[40] Perioperative nutrition support may be beneficial in moderately or severely malnourished patients if administered for seven to 14 days preoperatively but the potential benefits must compared against potential risk and risk of delaying surgery. Contraindications of EN include bowel obstruction low in GI tract, hemodynamic instability, intractable diarrhea, severe active GI bleed, ischemic or perforated gut, high output fistula or ostomy, aggressive nutrition intervention not warranted, and extensive resection of small bowel.

Options for enteral access include short term nasogastric and nasoenteric tubes as well as longer term tubes inserted directly into the stomach or small intestine.

Nasogastric and nasoenteric tubes can be placed at the bedside or intraoperatively while gastrotomy and jejunostomy tubes are placed utilizing more invasive methods. Feedings into the stomach are typically well tolerated and provide flexibility in administration of feedings.[41] Post pyloric feedings are indicated in the presence of gastroparesis, gastric outlet or duodenal obstruction and fistula proximal to the feeding tube location.[42] Jejunal access is commonly utilized for patients requiring enteral access prior to anticipated esophagectomy, post-operatively after esophagectomy and in the post-operative stage after gastric or pancreatic resection.[43] Consideration of short and long term treatment plan is necessary in determining tube type and location. Once the feeding tube is placed, a Registered Dietitian-Nutritionist can assist with the selection of enteral formula and development of feeding schedule.

Enteral nutrition is not without potential complications. Complications include metabolic aberrations, gastrointestinal intolerance, enteral misconnections, mechanical/tube complications, microbial contamination and drug/nutrient interactions.[40]

2.5.1.2 Parenteral nutrition

Parenteral nutrition (PN) can be a life-saving modality for people with cancer but should not be a routine adjunct to chemotherapy or considered standard to cancer care.[39] PN is most often indicated in the setting of cancer for preoperative nutrition support in severely malnourished patients and for the following indications in GI cancer patients; non-functional or inaccessible GI tract, severe nausea with vomiting, severe diarrhea or malabsorption, GI fistula and severe acute necrotizing pancreatitis. Acute complications of PN include derangements in serum glucose and electrolytes, hypertriglyceridemia and volume/fluid management issues. Long-term complications include infection, metabolic derangements, nutrient deficiencies or toxicities, organ dysfunction and bone disease.[44] PN support is significantly more costly than EN and presents increased risks as compared to EN. Due to the risks and cost of PN, careful consideration of indications, risks, benefits and goals of care along with patient wishes is necessary to insure proper utilization of PN.

2.6 *Pain*

Chronic pain is common for patients with GI malignancies and unrelieved pain is one of the most feared and burdensome of symptoms, leading to decreased quality of life.[45] In two thirds of cancer patients, pain is directly related to the presence of primary or metastatic disease.[46] For the remaining third, pain is related to treatment or complications such as osteoporosis and infection.[46] Untreated pain may lead to other symptoms such as anorexia, chronic nausea, anxiety, and depression.

In 1986, the WHO developed a three-step "ladder" to guide management of cancer-related pain based on severity.[47] Non-opioids such as non-steroidal anti-inflammatories and acetaminophen are recommended for mild pain.[47] NSAIDs are not recommended for patients with a known history of gastrointestinal bleeding. Weak opioids such as codeine, hydrocodone, and tramadol are recommended for moderate pain.[47] Unfortunately, potential for dose escalation is low for these drugs because of unacceptable toxicities. For severe pain, strong opioids such as morphine, oxycodone, hydromorphone, fentanyl, and methadone are recommended.[47] Starting doses for opioid-naïve patients are given in Table 1.[48] Most patients can be managed using this algorithm. For the remaining patients, a multi-dimensional approach to pain management should be taken. A referral to a palliative care specialist should also be considered.

For patients with renal and liver failure, starting doses should be decreased and dosing intervals increased.[48] The safest opioids to use in renal failure are fentanyl and methadone and the safest opioids to use in liver failure are fentanyl and hydromorphone.[49,50] Morphine should be avoided in patients with renal and liver failure.[48,50] Once patients have achieved good pain control on short acting opioids, it is generally possible to convert them to long-acting opioids such as morphine every 8 to 24 h, oxycodone every 12 h, or transdermal fentanyl patch every 3 days.[51] Patients prescribed transdermal fentanyl patches should be cautioned that fever causes rapid absorption of the drug and may lead to toxicities.[52] Long-acting opioids should be used with extreme caution in patients with liver and renal failure. Patients should have a short acting opioid, generally 10 to 20% of total daily dose, available for breakthrough pain.[51]

Table 1   Starting doses for opioids.

Opioid	PO	IV/SC
Moderate Opioids		
Codeine	30–60 mg q3–4 h	15–30 mg IM/SC q4 h
		IV contradicted
Tramadol		
Hydrocodone	5 mg q3–4 h	Not available
Strong Opioids		
Morphine	5–15 mg q3–4 h	2.5–5 mg SC/IV q3–4 h
Oxycodone	5–10 mg q3–4 h	Not available
Hydromorphone	1–2 q3–4 h	0.2–0.6 SC/IV q2–3 h
Methadone	2.5–5 mg q8 h	1.25–2.5 mg q8 h
Fentanyl	Transdermal patch	25–50 mcg IM/IV q1–3 h
	12.5 mcg/h q72 h	

Common side effects include nausea, sedation, and constipation. Nausea and sedation will abate in three to seven days with the development of tolerance.[51,53] Scheduled metoclopramide can be helpful in managing opioid-related nausea.[54] Constipation, however, will not improve with time and all patients prescribed opioids should be given a standing bowel regimen with the goal of having one soft bowel movement per day.[51] All bowel regimens should contain senna, uptitrated to 6 tablets/day for effect.

In addition to traditional analgesics, some patients may benefit from an adjuvant agent. Adjuvants are drugs without intrinsic analgesic properties but that are capable of producing analgesia in certain situations. Commonly used adjuvants include anti-convulsants such as gabapentin, corticosteroids, and anti-depressants. Corticosteroids are especially helpful for reducing edema and therefore capsular stretch in patients with metastatic disease to the liver.[51] Medications such as gabapentin and nortryptiline may be helpful for patients with a neuropathic component to their pain such as those patients with chemotherapy-related peripheral neuropathy.[51] All of the neuropathic agents work centrally and can cause sedation.

For patients who continue to have severe pain despite multiple opioid trials and use of adjuvant drugs, referral to an interventional pain specialist may be appropriate. General interventions include spinal analgesics where opioids with or without anesthetics are delivered directly into the intrathecal or epidural space. Consideration of spinal analgesics is appropriate for patients with cancer pain resistant to high doses of systemic opioids or when side effects are intolerable.[55] Spinal analgesics in general are both safe and effective for most patients.[56]

Patients with severe, upper abdominal pain, particularly those with pancreatic cancer, should be considered for a celiac plexus block.[55] The celiac plexus is a retroperitoneal structure, comprised for sympathetic nerve fibers, that mediates painful sensations from viscera including the pancreas, stomach, distal esophagus, and liver. The block, which uses either alcohol or phenol or destroys nerve tissue, is typically performed as an outpatient procedure.[55] The most common complications are hypotension and chronic diarrhea.[57] Severe spinal cord injury is extremely rare.[58]

2.7 *Nausea/vomiting*

Nausea is defined as a sensation of unease or discomfort in the back of the throat or epigastrium that may culminate in vomiting. Despite improvements in pharmacological treatments, nausea and vomiting remain two of the most distressing side effects for patients and their families.[58,59] Nausea in this population is often multifactorial and requires a multi-pronged and chronic approach to treatment.

Nausea and vomiting is coordinated by the vomiting center, a group of loosely organized neuronal areas in the lateral reticular formulation of the medulla.[60,61] The vomiting center receives input from the following sources: (1) higher cortical pathways that respond to sensory stimuli and psychogenic stimuli; (2) vestibular pathways; (3) peripheral pathways from the GI tract, parietal serosal surfaces, and visceral capsules; and (4) chemoreceptor trigger zone.[62] The chemoreceptor trigger zone is located in the floor of the fourth ventricle, outside of the blood brain barrier. It is able to sample emetogenic toxins, metabolic derangements such as uremia or hypercalcemia, and drugs in the blood or spinal fluid.[63] The chemoreceptor trigger zone also receives input from the GI tract via vagus and splanchnic nerves.[62] Nausea and vomiting in GI malignancies are primarily coordinated via peripheral pathways from the GI tract and the chemoreceptor trigger zone. Dopamine and serotonin are the most important neurotransmitters involved in these pathways.

Nausea and vomiting in patients diagnosed with GI malignancies may be related to the cancer itself, side effects of the treatments, or certain medications. Common malignancy-related causes for nausea and vomiting include metabolic derangements, ascites, peritoneal carcinomatosis, hepatic metastases, obstruction (gastric outlet or bowel), and metastatic brain involvement.[62] Common medication offenders include chemotherapy, opioids, anti-inflammatories, anti-cholinergics, and antibiotics.[62]

A thorough history and physical can help elucidate the cause of nausea and vomiting. It is particularly important to ask about frequency and consistency of bowel movements since constipation can often contribute to nausea in this population. This should be accompanied by a rectal examination to rule out fecal impaction. Diagnostic tests include evaluation of renal and hepatic function and serum electrolytes, particularly calcium.[62] Abdominal imaging may reveal obstruction or fecal impaction.[62]

When treating nausea and vomiting, both pharmacological and non-pharmacological measures are important to consider. Eating is often problematic for patients suffering from nausea and vomiting. Strategies such as eating small, frequent meals and avoiding foods with strong odors or unpleasant tastes can be helpful. Relaxation techniques are also useful adjuncts to medication management.

There is a lack of large, adequately powered randomized controlled trials to guide treatment of nausea. Management of nausea is based more on expert opinion rather than evidence. Most palliative care specialists support a "mechanistic" approach to anti-emetic therapy.[62] This depends on identifying the most likely cause of nausea and basing treatment decisions on the probable mechanism and neuropharmacology of the emetic pathway.[62] Two prospective audits of current practice have shown response rates of 80–90% when following this approach.[64,65] Others have proposed using an empiric approach and in studies this has been found to be highly effective.[54,56,66,67]

Major classes of anti-emetics include prokinetic agents, antihistamines, dopamine antagonists, serotonin receptor antagonists, benzodiazepines, corticosteroids, and anti-cholinergics. Table 2 presents the major classes with dosing and side

Table 2 Anti-emetic dosing table.

Anti-emetic	Available Forms	Starting Dose	Side Effects/Monitoring
	5-HT3 Antagonist		
Ondansetron (Zofran)	IV, ODT, PO	0.15 mg/kg/dose every 6 h to a maximum 8 h IV = PO	Constipation, HA Prolongs QTc (rare)
	Dopamine Antagonist		
Prochlorperazine (Compazine)	IV, SC, PO, PR	5–10 mg q6–8 h 0.15 mg/kg/dose every 4 h to a max of 10 mg/dose	Prolongs QTc, sedation, EPS
Haldol	IV, SC, PO	0.5 to 5 mg/dose every 8 h up to 30 mg/day	
	Pro-kinetic		
Metoclopramide (Reglan)	IV, SC, PO	5–15 mg qAC and qHS PO = IV/SC	Prolongs Qtc, EPS
	Histamine Receptor Blockade		
Diphenhydramine (Benadryl)	PO, IV	1 mg/kg/dose PO every 4 h to max 100 mg/dose SC/IV = PO	Anti-cholinergic SE (confusion, constipation, xerostomia, urine retention)
Hydroxyzine	PO, IV	0.5 to 1 mg/kg/dose every 4 h to max 600 mg/day SC/IV = PO	
Promethazine (Phenergan)	PO, IV, PR	12.5–25 q4–6 hrs 0.25 to 1 mg/kg every 4 h	

(Continued)

Table 2   (*Continued*)

Anti-emetic	Available Forms	Starting Dose	Side Effects/Monitoring
Muscarinic Receptor Blockade			
Scopolamine	Patch	1 patch q72 h	Same as histamine receptor blockade
Meclizine	PO	25 TID	
Glycopyrolate	PO, IV		
Benzodiazepines			
Lorazepam	IV, PO, IM		Sedation, confusion, paradoxical reaction
Dexamethasone	IV, PO	2–4 mg two to four times/day	As with steroids (hyperglycemia, fat redistribution, psychosis, immunosuppression, etc.)

effects. It is important to remember that for many patients, a single anti-emetic is not enough to produce relief. In these cases, multiple anti-emetics from different classes should be prescribed and patients should be instructed to take anti-emetics at regular scheduled intervals rather than as needed.

Dopamine plays a significant role in mediating nausea from peripheral pathways and the chemoreceptor trigger zone. Therefore, initiating a dopamine antagonist such as haloperidol may be very beneficial for a variety of nauseating states.[68] Prochlorperazine, another dopamine antagonist, is often prescribed but may be too sedating for some patients because of its anti-histamine properties.[68] If nausea and vomiting persists despite treatment with a dopamine antagonist, NCCN guidelines suggest initiating treatment with a 5-HT3 antagonist such as ondansetron followed by an anti-cholinergic agent or an antihistamine.[68] If nausea persists despite scheduling multiple, traditional anti-emetics from different classes, non-traditional anti-emetics such as cannabinoids, steroids, or atypical antipsychotics, particularly olanzapine, may be beneficial.[68]

3 Metastatic Complications of Gastrointestinal Malignancies

3.1 *Malignant bowel obstruction*

Malignant bowel obstruction is a common oncologic complication of advanced gastrointestinal malignancies and may occur in up to 28% of patients with colorectal cancer.[69] Common causes of bowel obstruction include extrinsic compression of the bowel wall, endoluminal obstruction by a primary cancerous mass or functional obstruction.[70] Extrinsic compression may be caused by a primary cancerous mass or metastasis, radiation-induced fibrosis, or abdominal or pelvic adhesions.[70] Functional obstruction results from impaired intestinal motility. Potential causes include tumor infiltration of the mesentery or nerves involved in intestinal motility or drugs, such as opioids and anti-cholinergics that cause ileus.[70]

In patients with advanced gastrointestinal malignancies, bowel obstruction develops insidiously over several weeks and presents with episodes of abdominal pain, abdominal distension, nausea, and vomiting.[71] If malignant bowel obstruction is suspected, a computer tomography of the abdomen should be ordered to confirm the diagnosis and determine the cause of the obstruction.[70] Complications such as strangulation, volvulus, and perforation may necessitate emergency surgery.

After a surgical emergency has been ruled out, options for treatment include surgical correction, stent placement, and medical management. Treatment decisions should be made in a multi-disciplinary team with the patient's performance status and prognosis in mind. When possible, endoscopic procedures with stent placement are preferred to surgery because they have lower morbidity and mortality rates.[70] Clinical success rates vary from 88% for colorectal stents to 91% for gastroduodenal stents.[72–74] The most serious complication is perforation and occurs in 0.5 to 4% of patients.[70] Use of anti-angiogenic drugs, concurrent radiotherapy, and history of radiotherapy (esophagus) increase the risk of perforation.[72,74,75]

By comparison, palliative surgery for bowel obstruction has a clinical success rate of 32 to 100% but has a far higher complication rate.[76] Mortality is high (6–32%) and serious complications are common (7–44%).[76] Patients who choose surgery should be counseled about the realistic goals and limitations of surgery. It is also important to inform patients that malignant bowel obstruction can be palliated without surgery or endoscopic procedures.

For some advanced cancer patients, the invasive options are not possible because of poor functional status or limited prognosis and medical management is appropriate. Medical management of malignant bowel obstruction without surgery relies on the use of the following symptomatic medications: analgesics, anti-emetics, anti-secretory agents, and glucocorticoids. In general, patients will not be able to take oral medications and IV or SC preparations should be used. While medications are being titrated, patients may require temporary placement of a NGT for decompression.

Haloperidol is usually considered as a first-line treatment in medical management of malignant bowel obstruction although data about its efficacy is lacking.[77] For patients without IV access, sublingual haloperidol concentrate can be used. Metoclopramide can be used in patients with incomplete obstruction but should be promptly discontinued if patients develop worsening abdominal pain.[70] In patients with intractable vomiting, 5-HT3 receptor antagonists can be used as second-line treatment.[70] Glucocorticoids help reduce bowel wall edema and are recommended at the time of diagnosis.[70] They should be administered in short courses of 5 to 10 days to limit long-term side effects.[70] The mean dose is 1 to 4 mg/kg/24 h for methylprednisolone or equivalent.[70] Anti-secretory agents such as hyoscyamine or glycopyrolate are helpful to reduce secretions and colicky pain but may worsen delirium because of their anti-cholinergic properties. If symptoms persist, a somatostatin analogue such as octreotide can be considered. Recent studies have confirmed the efficacy of octretide in relieving obstruction-related symptoms. The high cost of these drugs, however, limits their use as first-line treatment, particularly when patients are enrolled in hospice. Major side effects include local skin irritation, headache and qTC prolongation.

For patients who continue to have obstructive symptoms resistant to medical treatment, a venting gastrostomy is indicated. Patients should be counseled that the role of the venting gastrostomy is not to provide nutrition. Most venting gastrostomies are placed endoscopically. Contraindications to endoscopic placement include parietal masses with advanced stage carcinomatosis and a history of gastrectomy or abdominal surgery with adherences that prevents clear gastric transillumination.[70] In these cases, the venting gastrostomy should be placed surgically. Complications of placement include gastric bleeding, skin infection, tube blockage, leakage around tube, and perotinitis.[79]

Depending on patient goals and prognosis, artificial nutrition may be beneficial. A recent prospective study demonstrated that patients with malignant bowel obstruction survived longer if TPN was initiated but was associated with an increased risk of infectious complications.[80] Patients who are in the last days to weeks of life, however, will unlikely benefit from parenteral nutrition.[81]

3.2 *Malignant ascites*

Malignant ascites is defined as the cancer-related accumulation of fluid in the peritoneal cavity. Mechanisms by which cancer causes malignant ascites include peritoneal carcinomatosis, malignant obstruction of draining lymphatics, portal vein thrombosis, and massive hepatic metastases.[82] The pathophysiology of malignant ascites is not well understood but thought to result from the complex interaction of a variety of factors. Contributing mechanisms include obstruction of lymphatic drainage, increased vascular permeability, activation of the RAS system, neoplastic fluid production, and production of enzymes that degrade the extracellular matrix.[82]

Patients with colon, stomach, and pancreatic cancers are most likely to develop malignant ascites.[83] Common symptoms associated with ascites include pain, dyspnea, anorexia, nausea, reduced mobility, and difficulty with body image. Appropriate management of malignant ascites is important to improve these patients' quality of life.

Most patients with suspected malignant ascites should undergo a diagnostic paracentesis because it will inform both prognosis and treatment approach.[84] Appropriate classification of ascites is based on calculating the serum-ascites albumin gradient (SAAG). This requires measuring ascitic fluid for albumin and protein as well as determining serum albumin and protein levels. The SAAG is calculated by subtracting ascetic fluid albumin concentration from serum albumin concentration. A SAAG > 1.1 g/dl indicates ascites secondary to portal hypertension and is most commonly seen in patients with CHF and cirrhosis. A SAAG < 1.1 g/dl indicates that the ascites is not caused by portal hypertension; common causes include peritoneal carcinomatosis, nephrotic syndrome, spontaneous bacterial peritonitis. Ascitic fluid should also be sent for cytology. Cytologic evaluation is 97% sensitive for patients with peritoneal carcinomatosis but will not detect malignancy if ascites is caused by massive hepatic metastases or obstruction of lymphatic drainage.[84]

A large volume paracentesis is generally the first step in managing malignant ascites. It can provide immediate relief of symptoms in up to 90% of patients and can be done safely and quickly in clinic, at home, or in the hospital.[82] Patients generally note significant symptomatic improvement with the removal of a few liters.[85] For patients who require frequent paracentesis, a peritoneal drainage catheter should be placed to avoid frequent needle sticks and increased risk for infection. Two types of catheters are available: pigtail catheter and tunneled catheter. A pigtail catheter is a simple drainage catheter that is prone to complications such as occlusion, accidental removal and leakage when used for a long period of time.[84] A tunneled catheter is tunneled under the skin and is less infection prone than the pigtail catheter.[84] At the site of entry, it has an antibiotic-impregnated Dacron cuff in subcutaneous tissue.[84] The Pleurex catheter is FDA approved for malignant ascites. Once placed, the patient, caregiver, or home nurse can manage drainage. How frequently drainage should occur is patient dependent and may change as the disease progresses.

Another option is diuretics although the evidence for the use of diuretics in malignant ascites is weak.[82] Malignant ascites generally does not respond well to diuretic treatments and may cause intravascular fluid depletion without affecting the ascites. Diuretics may also be troublesome for patients who are deconditioned or bed bound. Patients with portal hypertension are more likely to respond to diuretics than cancer patients.[82]

Less frequently used modalities include peritoneovenous shunts and dietary measures such as salt restriction.[86] Peritoneovenous shunts drain ascitic fluid from the perotineum into the superior vena cava. There are two types of shunt systems available: the Le Veen shunt and the Denver shunt.[82] Although there have not been any head to head randomized trials comparing the two systems, the Le Veen shunt seems to be associated with a lower risk of occlusion.[87] In general, peritovenous shunts should not be used in patients with gastrointestinal malignancies because of the low response rate (10–15%).[88]

Median survival after diagnosis of malignant ascites is one to four months.[84] Once diagnosed, it is important to discuss the implications of malignant ascites on the patient's prognosis and consider a referral to hospice.

3.3 *Pruritus 2/2 malignant obstructive jaundice*

Patients with advanced gastrointestinal malignancies are at risk for developing malignant obstructive jaundice, either from biliary obstruction or metastatic spread to the liver. Biliary obstruction occurs most frequently with pancreatic carcinoma but also may occur with ampullary cancer and cholangiocarcinoma.[89] Obstructive jaundice can cause a variety of symptoms, including anorexia, weight loss, and pruritus. Among these symptoms, pruritus is the most distressing and debilitating and markedly compromises quality of life for patients. The pathophysiology of pruritus is unknown but thought to be mediated by endogenous opioids.[90] Options for treating jaundice-related pruritus include local skin care, medications, and palliative interventions.

Local skin care includes avoiding heat and keeping skin moisturized.[91] Clothes and sheets should be washed in mild detergents and patients should be encouraged to wear loose fitting, cotton clothing. Topical corticosteroids are generally not indicated.

The mainstay of treating pruritus secondary to cholestasis is cholestyramine. Cholestyramine, a non-absorbable resin, increases fecal excretion of pruritus-causing agents.[90] Reported regimens include giving 4 g immediately before and after breakfast.[90] Additional doses may be given at lunch and dinnertime, not to exceed 16 g/day. Notable side effects include bloating, unpleasant taste, and interference with absorption of other drugs.

Other medications with possible benefit include anti-histamines, anti-depressants, ondansetron, rifampin, and opioid antagonists. Data for the use of all of these agents is limited and conflicting and no guidelines exist to direct treatment. Therefore, treatment recommendations should be made with known side effects in mind.

Patients who receive anti-histamines report some improvement of prutitus but it is unlikely that the reported relief is related to specific anti-pruritic effect from the anti-histamines.[90] Instead, patients may be responding to the sedating side effects of anti-histamines.

Anti-depressants such as paroxetine, sertraline, and mirtazapine have also been reported to relieve pruritus in small studies. For the SSRIs, it has been postulated that the drugs may inhibit conversion of endogenous substances, such as opioids, to a pruritus causing form of that substance.[90] Appropriate doses of the SSRIs include low dose paroxetine (5–10 mg) and 75 mg sertraline daily.[92,93] Mirtazapine is reported to relieve pruritis at doses ranging from 7.5 to 30 mg per day.[94]

Serotonin is thought to participate in nociception and therefore mediate pruritus. Based on this, ondansetron has been proposed as a potential treatment for pruritus. There is limited and conflicting evidence for the use of ondansetron in treating jaundice-related pruritus but may be appropriate for patients with concomitant nausea.[95,96]

Opioid antagonists such as naltrexone have also been reported to relieve pruritus. Because of the potential to develop opioid-withdrawal symptoms, these drugs must be introduced slowly and carefully and may initially require an infusion.[90] Naltrexone may be started at 6.25 to 12.5 mg per day and increased to a maximum of 100 mg per day.[90] As expected, treatment with chronic naltrexone makes pain management more complicated. In general, patients will require higher doses of opioids.

Rifampin has been used with some success in patients with pruritus secondary to cholestasis at doses ranging from 300 to 450 mg per day.[97] The mechanism by which rifampin exerts its anti-pruritic effect is unknown. Rifampin is a CYP450 inducer and therefore should be monitored closely for drug-drug interactions.

Novel therapies for pruritus include dronabinol and gabapentin. The efficacy of dronabinol in humans is limited to one case study with three patients.[98] In all three patients, dronabinol at 5 mg was associated with symptom relief. Gabapentin has been found to be effective in uremic pruritus, cancer/hematologic pruritus, opioid-induced itch, and pruritus of unknown origin.[99] It is unclear how either of these drugs mediates its anti-pruritic effects.

Surgical options also exist for palliation of obstructive jaundice but are not recommended for patients with poor performance status, intra-abdominal ascites, and/or expected survival of less than six months.[89] These options include surgical bypass or stent placement, either percutaneously or endoscopically. Decisions about which method to use should be made on a patient-by-patient basis using a multi-disciplinary approach. Refractory pruritus is an indication for biliary drainage by stent or percutaneously if feasible anatomically for patient comfort.

4. Treatment Related Complications of Gastrointestinal Malignancies

4.1 *Changes in taste and smell*

Changes in taste and smell may be caused by radiation or chemotherapy and can range from diminished taste or smell to heightened senses of taste or smell to metallic, bitter, salty or sweet tastes. These changes can take several months to a year to resolve after the end of treatment. Therefore intervention is necessary to prevent decreased oral food and fluid intake that may result from changes in taste and smell. The following recommendations may assist in coping with changes in taste and smell:

Taste changes

- Good oral hygiene including rinsing mouth or brushing teeth before eating
- Rinse mouth out with solution of baking soda, salt and water; 1 teaspoon each of salt and baking soda mixed in 1 quart of water
- Use sugar free lemon drops, gum or mints to improve mouth taste
- Increase the flavor of foods by choosing marinades for meats and using lemon, herbs and spices, pickles or condiments to season food
- Use of plastic silverware if metallic taste is reported
- If water has off taste, flavor water or try other beverage options

- If meats taste bitter or strange, add marinades and sauces or consider alternative protein sources such as eggs, tofu, dairy or beans
- Try different foods other than favorite foods

  Bothersome smells

- Avoid cooking areas during meal preparation
- Eat cold or room temperatures foods to lessen smells
- Use cup with lid and straw to mask food odors

4.2 *Chemotherapy-induced nausea/vomiting*

Patients starting chemotherapy consistently list chemotherapy-induced nausea and vomiting (CINV) as one of their greatest fears. Poorly controlled CINV leads to decreased quality of life, increased use of healthcare resources, and may lead to poor adherence to the treatment regimen. Prompt and informed treatment of CINV is therefore of the utmost importance.

Several factors have been identified that predispose to CINV and include sex and age with young, female patients being at the highest risk. Patients with a high pretreatment expectation for nausea are also at higher risk. Conversely, patients with a history of significant alcohol consumption are at lower risk. Treatment-related factors are also important. Of the known predictive factors, the intrinsic emetogenicity of the chemotherapy is the most relevant and should guide therapy. For patients with suspected chemotherapy induced nausea vomiting (CINV), 5-HT3 antagonists such as ondansetron, neurokinin-1 receptor antagonists such as aprepitant, or corticosteroids are the most effective.[100]

4.3 *Chemotherapy-induced neuropathy*

Chemotherapy induced peripheral neuropathy (CIPN) is a potentially significant complication of chemotherapies commonly given in gastrointestinal cancers, taxanes and platinum compounds, particularly oxaliplatin. Interestingly now that cytopenias and chemotherapy-induced nausea are better controlled with updated supportive agents, neuropathy can become the dose and even therapy limiting toxicity for an effective chemotherapy regimen. Sensory symptoms are the most common and may include pain, numbness, and tingling. Motor symptoms, such as weakness, autonomic neuropathy, and cranial involvement, may also be present.[101] CIPN can be clinically assessed with objective measurement and generally does not require electrophysiologic studies. There are multiple validated scales and neuropathy scoring tools, in addition to common toxicity criteria of NCI.[102]

Oxaliplatin-induced neuropathy is particularly vexing since this is a major agent in chemotherapy regimens for colorectal, gastroesophageal and pancreatic adenocarcinomas. Additionally oxaliplatin is the mainstay of therapy in the adjuvant setting for colorectal cancers and therefore the development of chronic neuropathies in potentially cured patients represents an additional burden. The mechanism for this neuropathy is not entirely elucidated but is thought to be caused by the accumulation of oxaliplatin in the dorsal root ganglia and associated axonal hyperexcitability and repetitive discharged due to alterations in voltage-dependent sodium (Na+) channels.[103,104] Oxalipatin is associated with two separate types of neuropathy: acute and chronic neuropathy. Acute neuropathy includes distal parasthesias, pain, and muscle contractions of hands, feet, and often perioral region ("first bite) and is generally cold triggered. Acute neuropathies occur in up to 90% of patients and typically reverse 7–10 days after drug administration.[105] Chronic neuropathy is cumulative and persists between and after treatment. CPIN typically is symmetric and affects the longest nerves in the body most significantly, impacting hands and feet in a "stocking and glove" distribution. Severe oxaliplatin-induced neuropathy resolves in approximate 13 weeks after cessation of treatment for most patients but a significant proportion of patients still experience significant neuropathy more than a year after. The degree of neuropathy is dependent on cumulative dose, duration of administration and dose intensity.[106] A recent study demonstrated persistent grade 2 and 3 neuropathy is more common in patients with cumulative dose of 900 mg/m2 or more of oxaliplatin.[107] Oxaliplatin-induced neuropathy may worsen for several months AFTER treatment is discontinued before stabilizing or improving. Given the widespread administration, it is frustrating that there are no well-established neuroprotective treatments to prevent the development of neuropathy and no effective agents to treat existing CIPN.

Patients with mild neuropathy can carefully continue on oxaliplatin therapy although dose modifications, such as increasing the duration of infusion to greater than two hours, may be required to prevent worsening.[108] Patients with more severe acute neuropathic symptoms may be at higher risk for development of chronic cumulative CIPN.[109] Because diabetic patients develop neuropathy at lower cumulative doses of oxaliplatin, treating providers need to be mindful of total dose and symptoms.[110] There is great interest in both the prevention and treatment of CIPN from oxaliplatin and the bulk of these efforts have been focused on dose modification, stop/start strategies and supplemental infusions and neuromodulating agents. When possible, "maintenance" therapies that omit oxaliplatin in the metastatic setting are useful. Studies of supplemental intravenous calcium and magnesium infusions given together with oxaliplatin did not confer benefit and are not recommended.[111] Drugs that are commonly used for neuropathic pain, such as duloxetine, gabapentin, pregabalin, may be tried but there is not great data to suggest benefit.

ASCO 2014 review of neuroprotectants concluded that no recommendations could be made for preventative agents currently being investigated, including oxycarbazepine or carbamazepine.[112]

4.4 *Chemotherapy-associated diarrhea*

Chemotherapy-induced diarrhea is most associated with fluoropyrimidines (infusional, bolus, and oral prodrug capecitabine) as well as irinotecan. Diarrhea induced by these chemotherapies can be very severe and associated with significant morbidity and may even lead to limiting of dosages. 5-fluorouracil and irinotecan both cause acute damage to intestinal mucosa and manifests as epithelial loss and increased loss of fluid from small bowel. This increased small bowel fluid loss is transmitted to the large bowel where it exceeds ability of colon to absorb and causes significant diarrhea. Initial diarrhea after irinotecan administration is thought to be cholinergically mediated and atropine is routinely administered prior to infusion in the chemotherapy suite to address this concern.[113] Delayed onset diarrhea with irinotecan is related to mucosal injury which is multifactorial but with significant contribution from accumulation of active metabolite of irinotecan, SN-38, in the intestinal mucosa.[114] Diarrhea can be very severe and can limit patient clinically but can also contribute to ED visits, hospitalizations due to dehydration and metabolic and electrolyte derangements. Diarrhea is also a common side effect of tyrosine kinase inhibitors, vascular endothelial growth factor inhibitors, and anti-EGFR monoclonal antibodies. 5-fluorouracil, irinotecan, and the targeted agents are commonly combined which can aggravate diarrhea and requires careful supervision and management.

Patients are generally taught how to assess their fluid intake and losses and to guide their use of anti-diarrheals accordingly. Loperamide (Imodium) and diphenoxylate/atropine (Lomotil) are recommended upfront in control of diarrhea and both are FDA-approved for chemotherapy-induced diarrhea. Both agents have rapid onset of action and can be combined to improve efficacy. Loperamide can be dosed with each loose stool and appears to be more effective and tolerated.[115] Patients with diarrhea from fluoropyrimidines or irinotecan that are refractory to loperamide or diphenoxylate/atropine can be treated with octreotide but this is generally considered second-line therapy due to cost and the fact that when properly dosed, loperamide is usually effective.

4.5 *Chemotherapy-associated alopecia*

While hair loss from chemotherapy is not life-threatening and is usually temporary, it can be very upsetting to patients and may even affect treatment decision-making. Since chemotherapy affects cells that are most rapidly dividing in the body, hair matrix cells are directly affected. GI chemotherapy regimens usually cause gradual hair loss over several weeks/cycles and depend on dose and schedule. Small molecule inhibitors and monoclonal antibodies also cause abnormal hair growth in addition to rash and itching. CTCAE (National Cancer Institute Common Terminology Criteria for Adverse Events) also provides mechanism for grading alopecia. There has also been a lot of interest in prevention of alopecia, both by direct physical maneuvers to decrease drug delivery to hair bulb and by pharmacologic agents. Scalp tourniquets and scalp hypothermia have been tried but the studies are small and variable and difficult to extrapolate to larger populations. Benefit is also affected by specific chemotherapy agents and has been better evaluated in hematologic malignancies. Topical minoxidil was ineffective in preventing hair loss.[116] Many other intravenous and topical preparations are under investigation.

4.6 *Rash secondary to epidermal growth factor receptor (EGFR) inhibitors*

EGFR inhibitors are frequently used in treatment of metastatic colorectal cancers and cutaneous adverse events are very common due to expression of EGFR in the skin. Side effects include acneiform rash, abnormal growth of hair and eyelashes, paronychia and dryness and itching of the skin. While reversible and not life-threatening, the rash associated with EGFR inhibitors is very upsetting to patients and can lead to discontinuation of the therapy. The acneiform rash generally localizes to sun-exposed area including face, chest and back/torso. There are various factors that mayhelp predict severity including age <70, male gender and prior significant experiences with acne.[117] Patients can develop red pustules or papules, generally on face and scalp and most prominently at nasolabial folds. Patients describe itching, pain and irritation associated. In addition to the disfiguring appearance, these pustules can become superinfected and lead to scarring and hyperpigmentation if not properly managed.

Clinical practice includes grading severity and treating aggressively, often in combination with Dermatology, so that the therapy can be continued. For mild rash, patients can try topical antibiotics and topical corticosteroids in additional to gentle soaps and moisturizers. For more severe rash, oral antibiotics can be added with close reassessment of response. If rash is severe or refractory to intervention, specific guidelines exist to adjust dosing and of EGFR inhibitor. Low dose isotretinoin can also be added to severe, refractory acneiform rash.[118] Patients are also counseled on lifestyle adjustments that can ameliorate the rash including wearing sunscreen and limiting sun exposure, use of heavy moisturizers, decreased temperature of bath/shower water, and avoidance of detergents and soaps with heavy scents. There has also been interest in using oral agents preventatively to limit development of rash and potentially improve satisfaction with and adherence to EGFR inhibitor regimens with some success in small Phase II studies.[119]

5 Supportive Care by Cancer Site

5.1 *Esophageal cancer complications*

5.1.1 *Malignant dysphagia*

Globally over 70% of patients diagnosed with esophageal cancer present with weight loss and dysphagia.[120] Dysphagia develops when the tumor either causes a fistula or a malignant stricture. Evaluation of the dysphagia and appropriate adjustment of nutritional intake is necessary to promote adequate food and fluid consumption. Referral to a Speech and Language Pathologist can be beneficial to evaluate the presence of aspiration and determine the safest diet consistency.[121] Recommendations include high calorie, high protein foods that are soft and moist to assist with cohesive bolus formation as well as the use of oral nutrition supplements as indicated to promote adequate intake and deter weight loss. In some cases, enteral access and enteral nutrition may be required to provide adequate nutrition. For patients with inoperable esophageal cancer, prognosis is often limited to less than six months and the goal of treatment is to relieve dysphagia as rapidly and as safely as possible. The most commonly used treatment is placement of a self-expanding metal stent.[122] Almost all patients experience rapid improvement in dysphagia within a few days. Unfortunately, post-procedural complications are high and include recurrent dysphagia from stent migration, tumor overgrowth or food impaction, transient retrosternal pain after placement, and possible increased risk of late hemorrhage.[122] Recurrent dysphagia occurs in 30–45% of all patients.[122] Patients should be counseled about recurrent symptoms prior to placement so that they can make an educated decision. Other options include laser therapy, single dose brachytherapy, and palliative chemotherapy. Although laser therapy is safer than stent placement, it is not as effective and more expensive.[123–125] Compared to stent placement, single dose brachytherapy resulted in better long-term relief of dysphagia with lower complication rates and therefore should be strongly recommended.[126] Patients with a good performance status may be candidates for palliative chemotherapy; although no survival benefit has been established.[122] If dysphagia cannot be palliated, initiation of artificial nutrition should be considered if a patient is not in his/her last days to weeks of life.

5.1.2 *Radiation complications*

Patients undergoing radiation therapy for esophagogastric cancer are at risk for developing both acute and late esophageal toxicities. Acute radiation esophagitis leads to esophageal inflammation, resulting in dysphagia, odynophagia, and dysmotility. Commonly used treatment modalities include topical anesthetics such as viscous lidocaine, systemic analgesics including opioids and NSAIDs, proton pump inhibitor for reflux, and calcium channel blocker for esophageal spasm.[127] Grade 1–2 toxicities can generally be managed with good pain control and modifications to the diet, including pureeing the diet and adhering to a bland diet. Grade 3 toxicity is characterized by severe dysphagia or odynophagia with dehydration or weight loss >15%. These patients will require supportive hydration and nutrition with IV fluids or TPN. Rarely, patients may develop obstruction, perforation, or fistulas. Late toxicity involves fibrosis that may lead to stenosis. Patients with moderate to severe stenosis may require dilation.

5.1.3 *Nutritional concerns in esophageal cancer*

Issues impacting nutritional status after esophagectomy surgery include gastroparesis and dysmotility, dumping syndrome, early satiety and dysphagia. The anatomy changes after an esophagectomy and resulting issues require long term adaptations in food choices and eating habits that often require frequent reinforcement from the care team.

5.1.3.1 Changes in eating patterns

Due to changes in anatomy after surgery, long-term changes in eating habits are necessary. Since eating patterns and habits are developed over decades, patients often struggle with the diet limitations after surgery. Necessary changes in eating patterns and habits after esophagectomy include small, frequent meals on a schedule, eating slowly and chewing well and avoiding poorly tolerated foods.

The decreased capacity of the now stretched stomach takes away the ability to consume large meals because the stomach is no longer able to serve as the reservoir for food waiting to be digested. Small, frequent meals are encouraged and it is important for patients to monitor for signals of satiety to avoid overeating at a meal. In addition to the need for small meals, a meal schedule including small meals every two to three hours can be helpful to promote adequate intake despite a decreased appetite and early satiety. After surgery, the remaining esophagus may not be able to move foods as easily from mouth to stomach resulting in foods sticking, regurgitation and midsternal pain. Changes in motility can be managed by chewing foods well, eating soft or chopped foods, avoiding tough, gummy or stringy foods and taking sips of fluids as needed. Often tolerance of specific foods may change after surgery. Experimentation is necessary to test the tolerance of specific foods after the healing process is complete and a patient should test new foods one at a time in small amounts. Reinforcement of the diet principles after esophagectomy is necessary to promote adequate nutritional intake and avoid unintended weight loss.

5.1.3.2 Dumping syndrome

After esophagectomy, digestion and absorption is affected and may result in dumping syndrome. The procedure can speed up gastric emptying, which allows incompletely digested and hyperosmolar chyme to enter the small intestine.[120,128] This leads to fluids rushing into the small intestine to normalize osmolarity. High fluid volume along with hormonal and vasomotor changes results in bloating, abdominal cramping, nausea and dumping. Dumping syndrome can be categorized as early or late. Early dumping syndrome occurs in 75% of dumping syndromes cases and onset is 10–30 min after eating. Symptoms of early dumping include epigastric fullness, nausea, vomiting, abdominal cramping, bloating, diarrhea, lightheadedness, diaphoresis, desire to lie down, pallor and palpitations. Late dumping syndrome occurs one to three hours after meals and is thought to be the result of reactive hypoglycemia. It occurs in 25% of cases. Symptoms of late dumping include hunger, perspiration, tremors and difficulty concentrating. Both early and late dumping syndrome can be improved with changes in eating habits and food choices. Management of dumping syndrome is necessary to improve quality of life and promote adequate nutritional intake. A detailed review of intake and associated symptoms can assist with identifying areas of change in order to help patient identify trends and improve symptoms. Recommendations for managing dumping syndrome are as follows:

- Small, frequent meals at least six times a day
- Avoid large portions and overeating
- Eat slowly and relax while eating
- Minimize activity after meals to promote transit time of food
- Chew food completely so that it becomes liquid before swallowing
- Separate food and fluid intake; do not consume fluids 30 min before or one hour after meals
- Consume a high protein food at each meal and snack
- Avoid high sugar foods such as sweetened beverages, fruit juices, and desserts
- If planning to consume high sugar food, eat as part of a meal and not separately

- Foods high in soluble fiber may reduce symptoms by slowing rate of sugar absorption into the blood
- Limit very cold or very hot foods

5.2 Gastric Cancer Complications

5.2.1 Nutrition concerns in gastric cancer

Early satiety, heartburn or indigestion, abdominal pain and discomfort, nausea, vomiting, anorexia and unintended weight loss are common symptoms of gastric cancer.[129] These symptoms often lead to reduced food intake, which may in part explain why malnutrition and weight loss occurs in greater than 70% of people diagnosed with gastric cancer. Each treatment modality can result in a unique set of side effects. Surgical resection of gastric tumors results in several potential nutrition-related issues including dietary intolerances, weight loss and vitamin and mineral malabsorption. These issues can lead to long-term consequences including anemia and bone disease. Often nutrient deficiencies develop months to years after gastric resection therefore ongoing monitoring and treatment of potential nutrition complications is necessary.

5.2.1.1 Nutrition after Gastric resection

Gastric resection typically results in weight loss with reported loss ranging from 10–30% of preoperative weight, which has been attributed to inadequate oral intake, malabsorption, rapid intestinal transit time and bacterial overgrowth.[130] Frequent nutrition follow-up in the early postoperative period is necessary to prevent a decline in nutrition status.

5.2.1.2 Dumping syndrome

Digestion and absorption is affected due to the altered anatomy of the gastrointestinal tract after resection. Symptoms of dumping syndrome are more prevalent after gastrectomy and often improve over time. Causes, symptoms and management of dumping syndrome are discussed in the esophagectomy section of this chapter.

5.2.1.3 Fat maldigestion

The etiology of fat malabsorption after gastrectomy is multifactorial. Increased transit time prevents adequate mixing of food with digestive enzymes and bile salts, decreased enzyme production reduces the ratio of enzymes to food and loss of the antrum and its sieving function allows for larger than normal food particles to empty into the jejunum resulting in a challenge for enzymes to attack.[131,132] Consideration of pancreatic enzyme replacement therapy may be necessary for patients exhibiting signs and symptoms of fat maldigestion. Dosing and administration of pancreatic enzyme replacement is discussed in detail in the pancreatic cancer section of this chapter. If fat maldigestion and malabsorption is present, it is necessary to monitor for fat soluble vitamin (vitamins A, D, E and K) deficiencies and consider supplementation with water soluble versions as needed.

5.2.1.4 Gastric stasis

Dysmotility is common following stomach resection and can present as delayed or accelerated gastric emptying. Symptoms of poor emptying may present as postprandial bloating, discomfort or fullness lasting for hours. Emesis of undigested food ingested hours to days before may also be present.[131] These patients are at higher risk for bezoar formation, bacterial overgrowth and intolerance to solid foods. Diet manipulation including small, frequent and easy to digest meals may be beneficial to assist with adequate nutrition in the setting of dysmotility.

5.2.1.5 Lactose intolerance

Lactose intolerance may occur after resection of the gastrointestinal tract. Patients complaining of abdominal cramping, gas, bloating, diarrhea and distention after consuming lactose containing foods may benefit from decreasing intake of these foods. Tolerance to lactose is typically dose dependent and may improve over time. Although diet therapy may be helpful, it is important to minimize diet restrictions as it can lead to patient frustration, decreased nutritional intake and weight loss. Lactase enzymes are available over the counter and can be helpful in allowing patients to consume dairy foods with decreased lactose intolerance symptoms.

5.2.2 *Nutrition related anemia*

Nutrition related anemias resulting from a vitamin B12, folate or iron deficiency are common in gastrectomy patients and often present as late complications of surgery. Baseline and periodic monitoring is necessary due to the potential severe consequences of anemia.

After gastric resection, malabsorption of vitamin B12 may occur due to reduction in intrinsic factor and reduced gastric acidity, which impairs cleavage of protein, bound B12.[133] Bacterial overgrowth and decreased oral intake of B12 rich foods may also contribute to the deficiency.[130] Although deficiency of vitamin B12 can develop as early as one year after surgery, it is more common in late post-operative states.[134] Once diagnosed, vitamin B12 supplementation should be initiated orally, intranasally, or intramuscularly. Ongoing periodic monitoring for vitamin B12 deficiency is necessary because of the long term risk of deficiency in this population. Folate deficiency may also develop after gastric surgery because of malabsorption and impaired digestion.[135] Serum red blood cell (RBC) folate should be evaluated when diagnosing folate deficiency because it is a better indicator of body folate stores than serum folate.[135] Finally, alterations in digestion and absorption are associated with iron deficiency.[131] Reduced dietary iron intake may also play a role. Patients should be encouraged to increase their intake of iron rich foods as well as vitamin C, which can help with iron absorption. Maximizing iron intake and absorption may not be adequate to prevent iron deficiency for some people. Periodic and ongoing monitoring of serum iron stores is necessary to identify deficiency and oral iron supplementation should be initiated as indicated.

5.2.3 Osteoporosis risk

The risk for osteoporosis is increased post-gastrectomy due to:[136]

- Altered oral nutritional intake
- Higher losses of calcium and vitamin D in the presence of malabsorption
- Lower rates of absorption with dumping syndrome, rapid transit times and bypass of absorptive region of duodenum and jejunum
- Absence of stomach acid in lowering pH of the proximal duodenum and lack of production of gastrocalcin in stomach mucosa
- Other primary risk factors and impact of inflammation on osteoclastic activity

Several measures including monitoring, diet adjustments, and lifestyle modifications can be taken to lessen the risk for osteoporosis in this population. DEXA scanning is recommended every two years for individuals with low body mass index, significant weight loss or other risk factors. A goal intake of 1,500 mg of calcium daily is encouraged and can be accomplished through intake of calcium rich foods as tolerated and supplementation with calcium citrate in divided doses with ≤500 mg per dose. Routine monitoring of serum vitamin D levels should be conducted with subsequent supplementation as needed. Recommendations for lifestyle modifications to decrease osteoporosis risk include smoking cessation, limiting alcoholic beverage intake and increasing weight bearing exercises. A proactive approach to osteoporosis prevention is necessary in the gastrectomy population due to increased risk.

5.3 Colorectal Cancer Complications

5.3.1 Sacral pain management

Uncontrolled colorectal and anal malignancies in the pelvis can directly invade the sacral nerve plexus and cause intractable pain. Tumor can grow directly along nerve roots and can also invade bony structures and pain is further compounded by lymphovascular obstruction. The sacral pain syndromes are very difficult to manage and often require multidisciplinary involvement. Palliative irradiation may be required to quickly address pain due to visceral or lymphovascular obstruction due to tumor but is less effective for neuropathic pain associated with involvement of sacral plexus. Patients will generally require analgesic management of neuropathic pain including opioids, steroids and neuroleptic agents. Sacral plexus involvement usually also requires interventional pain specialists to administer intrathecal analgesia. Palliative chemotherapy can contribute to long-term pain control strategy if indicated and effective.

5.3.2 Pelvic bleeding

Bleeding rectal and anal tumors can be both uncomfortable and life-threatening. Uncontrolled bleeding and resultant anemia may also impact ability to continue chemotherapies as well ability to deliver meaningful palliative care. Radiation therapy is an effective means of treatment and can stop active bleeding within 24–48 h of the first fraction. Should the bleeding be refractory to radiation, endoscopic techniques including laser ablation or surgical interventions may be performed.

5.3.3 Low anterior resection (LAR) syndrome

Increasing numbers of patients are surviving locally advanced rectal carcinomas with a combination of surgery, radiotherapy, and systemic chemotherapy with over 50% reaching 5 year mark disease free. Patients treated with sphincter-sparing low anterior resection comprise the majority of surgically cured patients and 50–90% are reported to experience some degree of bowel dysfunction.[137] LAR is performed with the assumption that the quality of life with bowel continuity is superior to life with a permanent stoma. LAR syndrome patients have variable bowel dysfunction including fecal incontinence, urgency, frequent bowel movements, and stool clustering. Scoring tools exist to evaluate degree of LAR syndrome and it is well documented in surgical literature with regard to effect on physical, emotional, and social functioning. Of note, urinary and sexual alterations can also occur, in addition to bowel effects. Risk factors for severity include radiotherapy and distance of the tumor to the anal verge.[138] Outcomes are better both in terms of disease control and post surgical quality of life based on surgeon's experience and volume of anorectal surgeries. There are currently no specific treatment options for LAR syndrome or fecal incontinence associated with LAR. Patients can try dietary modifications and anti-diarrheal agents with limited success. Pelvic floor rehabilitation, including pelvic floor muscle training, biofeedback, and rectal balloon training techniques are available. Pelvic floor rehabilitation is noninvasive and without adverse effects. Pelvic floor rehabilitation is generally first line recommendation for improving functional outcomes after LAR as symptomatic review show benefits in continence, stool frequency and quality of life.[138]

5.3.4 *Nutrition concerns in colorectal cancers*

The presence of colorectal cancer and its treatments, including surgery, chemotherapy, radiation and targeted therapies, can lead to nutrition impact symptoms. Often times combined modality treatment is utilized and can result in mucositis, diarrhea, nausea, vomiting and fatigue which can lead to changes in appetite and unintended weight loss. Surgical resection presents short term nutrition challenges and potentially long term issues. As treatment progresses, nutrition impact symptoms may evolve therefore adjustment in diet and symptom management may be necessary.

Effects of surgery on nutrition impact symptoms and diet tolerance may be short term and a majority of individuals are ultimately able to tolerate most foods. Initially after surgery, diet may need to be modified to allow the body time to adapt to its new anatomy. Dietary modifications after surgery commonly focus on measures to slow movement of chyme through the remaining colon and retain as much fluid and electrolytes as possible. Nutritional complications are listed in Table 3.

5.4 *Pancreatic and Bile Duct Cancer Complications*

5.4.1 *Nutrition concerns in pancreatic and bile duct cancers*

Nutrition issues often present prior to the diagnosis of pancreatic and bile duct cancers and include weight loss, poor appetite, malabsorption, delayed gastric emptying, and diabetes. Symptoms of pancreatic and bile duct cancers combined with common treatments increase the risk of malnutrition in this population.

5.4.1.1 Pancreatic exocrine insufficiency and malabsorption

Pancreatic exocrine insufficiency (PEI) may be observed in patients at diagnosis, during chemotherapy and/or radiation treatments and following surgery for pancreatic

Table 3 Possible nutrition-related complications with colorectal cancer (1–2).

Nutrition Related Complication	Nutrition Management Suggestions
Small bowel resection	• Encourage 5–6 small, frequent meals each day to improve tolerance • Fluid and electrolytes should be provided in small, frequent amounts • If terminal ileum resection, monitor serum vitamin B12 levels and need for supplementation of fat soluble vitamins, calcium, zinc and magnesium • Bile acid sequestrants may be indicated if diarrhea is present
Colectomy with reanastomosis	• Encourage 5–6 small, frequent meals each day to improve tolerance • Monitor fluid and electrolyte status • Initiate nutrition interventions to slow transit time if indicated
Colostomy and ileostomy	• Monitor fluid and electrolytes imbalances and utilize electrolyte-containing fluids as needed (e.g. sports drinks, broth, vegetable juice and electrolyte solutions) • Suggest intake of at least 1 L more than daily ostomy output • Provide dietary strategies for stool consistency and odor as needed
Ileal pouch	• Monitor for pouchitis and treat as indicated • Educate regarding nutrition interventions and stress adequate fluid and electrolyte intake due to increased losses • Reinforce use of anti-diarrheal medication
Possible vitamin and mineral malabsorption	• Monitor serum vitamin D levels and supplement if indicated • Encourage calcium rich diet, supplement as needed to promote meeting DRI • Supplemental vitamin B12 if ileum resected

and periampullary cancer.[139] Recent studies indicate 80–90% of patients with pancreatic cancer may have PEI and malabsorption.[140,141] Malabsorption is often recognized by the presence of frequent or loose foul-smelling bowel movements. Opioid use will slow gut motility and the characteristic loose, frequent bowel movements associated with malabsorption may not be present. Tests exist to diagnosis PEI but can be cumbersome, difficult to conduct in clinical practice and expensive. In clinical practice, directed questioning is commonly used to determine signs and symptoms of PEI and provide timely medication management.[142] Pancreatic enzyme replacement should be prescribed when PEI is present. Currently, all FDA approved pancrelipase formulations are porcine derived. Caution should be exercised in using pancrelipase in patients with history of porcine allergy and use of this medication should be discussed with patients who avoid porcine products due to religious beliefs or other reasons.

Dosing recommendations vary but generally suggest starting at 10,000–40,000 lipase units per meal and 5,000–25,000 lipase units per snack.[143,144] Enzyme doses should start conservatively with titration until signs and symptoms of malabsorption have improved. Supplemental pancreatic enzyme dosages should not exceed 10,000 lipase units per kilogram per day or 2,500 lipase units per kilogram per meal up to four times a day.[144] For optimal replacement, the enzyme dose should be divided and administered throughout the meal to ensure adequate enzyme coverage. A fat restricted diet of 75 g of fat a day can also be used for symptom management but will exacerbate weight loss in a population that is already at high risk for malnutrition and is therefore not recommended.[145] For some patients, malabsorptive symptoms will persist after the enzyme dose has been titrated. The following steps should be taken to attempt to improve malabsorption:[146,147]

- Evaluate compliance with dose and timing
- Adjust dose and timing
- Change brand of enzyme and consider change in dosage form
- Add H_2-receptor antagonist or proton-pump inhibitor (if not already prescribed) to promote physiologically basic environment
- Assess for bacterial overgrowth or other malabsorptive disorder

5.4.1.2 Potential micronutrient deficiencies

Nutrient deficiencies may result from lack of nutritional intake, malabsorption or maldigestion of nutrients. Malabsorption can lead to increased risk of fat soluble vitamins and vitamin B12 deficiencies. With bypass of the duodenum and upper jejunum, the digestive processes between the stomach, duodenum and pancreatobiliary system are disrupted. The duodenum and proximal jejunum are important sites for absorption of iron, folate, fatty acids, proteins and trace elements therefore bypass of this part of the small bowel may result in impaired absorption of iron, calcium, zinc, copper and selenium.[146] If supplementation of fat-soluble vitamins is necessary in the presence of malabsorption, water miscible forms of fat-soluble vitamins should be used. Due to elevated risk of micronutrient deficiencies, periodic monitoring and supplementation as indicated is necessary.

5.4.2 *Diabetes and glucose intolerance*

The role of nutrition in the management of diabetes varies depending on the stage of the cancer and side effects or symptoms the patient is experiencing. The degree of dietary restrictions should be aligned with plan of care and patient's nutritional status. Diet should also be liberalized with advanced disease.[147] In patients who have completed treatment and have no evidence of disease, carbohydrate counting can be utilized to aid in glycemic control.

5.4.3 *Nutrition intolerances after pancreatic resection*

Nutrition related issues after pancreatic resection include pancreatic exocrine insufficiency, dumping syndrome, delayed gastric emptying, lactose intolerance, and diabetes/glucose intolerance.[146] Presence of symptoms depends on the extent of the surgical procedure. Management of nutrition related issues after surgery is important to minimize weight loss and risk for malnutrition.

References

1. Ahmedzai SH, *et al.* Towards a European standard for supportive care of cancer patients. A coordinated activity funded by DGV, final report for EC on behalf of the EORTC pain and symptom control task force. 2001, pp. 1–25.
2. National comprehensive cancer network (NCCN). NCCN clinical practice guidelines in oncology: Distress management (version I. 2014). Retrieved from http://www.nccn. org/professionals/physician_gls/pdf/distress.pdf. Accessed June 1, 2014.
3. Carlson LE, *et al.* High levels of untreated distress and fatigue in cancer patients. *Br J Cancer* 2004;**90**(12):2297–2304.
4. Passik SD, *et al.* Oncologists' recognition of depression in their patients with cancer. *J Clin Oncol* 1998;**16**(4):1594–1600.
5. Andersen BL, *et al.* Biobehavioral, immune, and health benefits following recurrence for psychological intervention participants. *Clin Cancer Res* 2010;**16**(12):3270–3278.
6. Giese-Davis J, *et al.* Decrease in depression symptoms is associated with longer survival in patients with metastatic breast cancer: A secondary analysis. *J Clin Oncol.* 2011;**29**(4):413–420.
7. Curt GA, *et al.* Impact of cancer-related fatigue on the lives of patients: New findings from the fatigue coalition. *Oncologist.* 2000;**5**(5):353–360.
8. Jenkins CA, *et al.* Demographic, symptom, and medication profiles of cancer patients seen by a palliative care consult team in a tertiary referral hospital. *J Pain Symptom Manage.* 2000;**19**(3):174–184.
9. Portenoy RK. Cancer-related fatigue: An immense problem. *Oncologist.* 2000;**5**(5): 350–352.
10. Teunissen SC, *et al.* Symptom prevalence in patients with incurable cancer: A systematic review. *J Pain Symptom Manage.* 2007;**34**(1):94–104.
11. Del Fabbro E, *et al.* Symptom control in palliative care — part II: Cachexia/anorexia and fatigue. *J Palliat Med.* 2006;**9**(2):409–421.

12. Gong S, *et al.* Effect of methylphenidate in patients with cancer-related fatigue: A systematic review and meta-analysis. *PLoS One.* 2014;**9**(1):e84391.

13. Breitbart W, *et al.* A randomized, double-blind, placebo-controlled trial of psycho-stimulants for the treatment of fatigue in ambulatory patients with human immunodeficiency virus disease. *Arch Intern Med.* 2001;**161**(3):411–420.

14. Rabkin JG, *et al.* Modafinil treatment of fatigue in patients with ALS: A placebo-controlled study. *Muscle Nerve.* 2009;**39**(3):297–303.

15. Spathis A, *et al.* Modafinil for the treatment of fatigue in lung cancer: Results of a placebo-controlled, double-blind, randomized trial. *J Clin Oncol.* 2014.

16. Bruera E, *et al.* Action of oral methylprednisolone in terminal cancer patients: A prospective randomized double-blind study. *Cancer Treat Rep.* 1985;**69**(7–8):751–754.

17. Mock V. Evidence-based treatment for cancer-related fatigue. *J Natl Cancer Inst Monogr.* 2004;(**32**):112–118.

18. Stricker CT, *et al.* Evidence-based practice for fatigue management in adults with cancer: Exercise as an intervention. *Oncol Nurs Forum.* 2004;**31**(5):963–976.

19. Inui A. Cancer anorexia-cachexia syndrome: Current issues in research and management. *CA Cancer J Clin.* 2002;**52**(2):72–91.

20. Bachmann J, *et al.* Pancreatic cancer related cachexia: Influence on metabolism and correlation to weight loss and pulmonary function. *BMC Cancer.* 2009;**9**:255–2407-9–255.

21. Ronga I, *et al.* Anorexia-cachexia syndrome in pancreatic cancer: Recent advances and new pharmacological approach. *Adv Med Sci.* 2014;**59**(1):1–6.

22. Ramos EJ, *et al.* Cancer anorexia-cachexia syndrome: Cytokines and neuropeptides. *Curr Opin Clin Nutr Metab Care.* 2004;**7**(4):427–434.

23. Bruno MJ, *et al.* Placebo controlled trial of enteric coated pancreatin microsphere treatment in patients with unresectable cancer of the pancreatic head region. *Gut.* 1998;**42**(1):92–96.

24. Kornblith AB, *et al.* Effect of megestrol acetate on quality of life in a dose-response trial in women with advanced breast cancer. the cancer and leukemia group B. *J Clin Oncol.* 1993;**11**(11):2081–2089.

25. Salacz M. Megestrol acetate for cancer anorexia/cachexia. fast facts and concepts. http://www.eperc.mcw.edu/EPERC/FastFactsIndex/ff_100.htm. Updated 2003. Accessed June 1, 2014.

26. Deutsch J, Kolhouse JF. Assessment of gastrointestinal function and response to megesterol acetate in subjects with gastrointestinal cancers and weight loss. *Support Care Cancer.* 2004;**12**(7):503–510.

27. Lane M, *et al.* Dronabinol and prochlorperazine in combination for treatment of cancer chemotherapy-induced nausea and vomiting. *J Pain Symptom Manage.* 1991;**6**(6):352–359.

28. Walsh D, *et al.* Established and potential therapeutic applications of cannabinoids in oncology. *Support Care Cancer.* 2003;**11**(3):137–143.

29. Watanabe N, *et al.* Mirtazapine versus other antidepressive agents for depression. *Cochrane Database Syst Rev.* 2011;(12):CD006528. doi(12):CD006528.

30. Evidence-based nutrition practice guideline on fish oil, lean body mass and weight in oncology patients. http://andevidencelibrary.com/template.cfm?template=guide_summary&key=4162&reset=true and. Updated 2013. Accessed June 5, 2014.

31. Cancer and chemo-based lack of appetite and early satiety. http://chemocare.com/chemotherapy/side-effects/cancer-and-chemobased-lack-of.aspx#.U5Bj8PmwL9U. Accessed June 5, 2014.

32. Hoda D, *et al.* Should patients with advanced, incurable cancers ever be sent home with total parenteral nutrition? A single institution's 20-year experience. *Cancer.* 2005;**103**(4):863–868.

33. Lundholm K, *et al.* Palliative nutritional intervention in addition to cyclooxygenase and erythropoietin treatment for patients with malignant disease: Effects on survival, metabolism, and function. *Cancer.* 2004;**100**(9):1967–1977.

34. McGeer AJ, *et al.* Parenteral nutrition in cancer patients undergoing chemotherapy: A meta-analysis. *Nutrition.* 1990;**6**(3):233–240.

35. Jeejeebhoy KN. Enteral and parenteral nutrition: Evidence-based approach. *Proc Nutr Soc.* 2001;**60**(3):399–402.

36. Huhmann MB, August DA. Perioperative nutrition support in cancer patients. *Nutr Clin Pract.* 2012;**27**(5):586–592.

37. McClave SA, *et al.* Guidelines for the provision and assessment of nutrition support therapy in the adult critically ill patient: Society of critical care medicine (SCCM) and american society for parenteral and enteral nutrition (A.S.P.E.N.). *JPEN J Parenter Enteral Nutr.* 2009;**33**(3):277–316.

38. Peter JV, *et al.* A metaanalysis of treatment outcomes of early enteral versus early parenteral nutrition in hospitalized patients. *Crit Care Med.* 2005;**33**(1):213–20; discussion 260–1.

39. August DA, Huhmann MB, American Society for Parenteral and Enteral Nutrition (A.S.P.E.N.) Board of Directors. A.S.P.E.N. clinical guidelines: Nutrition support therapy during adult anticancer treatment and in hematopoietic cell transplantation. *JPEN J Parenter Enteral Nutr.* 2009;**33**(5):472–500.

40. Bankhead R, Boullata J, Brantley S, *et al.* Enteral nutrition practice recommendations. *JPEN J Parenter Enteral Nutr.* 2009;**33**(2):122–167.

41. Krenitsky J. Gastric versus jejunal feeding: Evidence or emotion? *Nutr Issues Practl Gastroenterology.* 2006:46–55.

42. Itkin M, *et al.* Multidisciplinary practical guidelines for gastrointestinal access for enteral nutrition and decompression from the society of interventional radiology and american gastroenterological association (AGA) institute, with endorsement by canadian interventional radiological association (CIRA) and cardiovascular and interventional radiological society of europe (CIRSE). *J Vasc Interv Radiol.* 2011;**22**(8):1089–1106.

43. Gupta V. Benefits versus risks: A prospective audit. feeding jejunostomy during esophagectomy. *World J Surg.* 2009;**33**(7):1432–1438.

44. Fessler TA. Trace element monitoring and therapy for adult patients receiving long-term total parenteral nutrition. *Nutrition Issues in Gastroenterology.* Series #25, Editor Parrish CR, Practical Gastroenterology, 2005; page 44–65; 2005.

45. Foley KM. Controlling cancer pain. *Hosp Pract (1995)*. 2000;**35**(4):101–8, 111–2.

46. Cherney IN. Cancer pain: Principle of assessment and syndromes. In: Berger AM, Portenoy RK, Weissman DE, eds. *Principle and practice of palliative care and supportive oncology.* 2nd ed. Principle and Practice of Palliative Care and Supportive Oncology: Lippincott William & Wilkins; 2002:3–52.

47. World health organization. traitement de la douleur cancéreuse
. 1987.; access 2015/11/01

48. Quill TE, *et al.*, eds. *Primer of Palliative Care*, 5th ed. Glenview, IL: American Academy of Hospice and Palliative Medicine; 2010, pp. 11–35.

49. Chandok N, Watt KD. Pain management in the cirrhotic patient: The clinical challenge. *Mayo Clin Proc*. 2010;**85**(5):451–458.

50. Dean M. Opioids in renal failure and dialysis patients. *J Pain Symptom Manage.* 2004;**28**(5):497–504.

51. Bruera E, Kim HN. Cancer pain. *JAMA*. 2003;**290**(18):2476–2479.

52. McPherson ML. *Demystifying opioid conversion calculations: A guide for effective dosing.* Bethesda, MD: American Society of Health-System Pharmacists; 2010.

53. Bruera E, Macmillan K, Hanson J, MacDonald RN. The cognitive effects of the administration of narcotic analgesics in patients with cancer pain. *Pain*. 1989;**39**(1):13–16.

54. Bruera E, *et al.* Chronic nausea in advanced cancer patients: A retrospective assessment of a metoclopramide-based antiemetic regimen. *J Pain Symptom Manage.* 1996;**11**(3):147–153.

55. Birthi P, Sloan P. Interventional treatment of refractory cancer pain. *Cancer J.* 2013;**19**(5):390–396.

56. Nitescu P, *et al.* Complications of intrathecal opioids and bupivacaine in the treatment of "refractory" cancer pain. *Clin J Pain*. 1995;**11**(1):45–62.

57. Davies DD. Incidence of major complications of neurolytic coeliac plexus block. *J R Soc Med*. 1993;**86**(5):264–266.

58. Kinghorn S. Palliative care. nausea and vomiting. *Nurs Times*. 1997;**93**(33):57–60.

59. Portenoy RK, *et al.* Symptom prevalence, characteristics and distress in a cancer population. *Qual Life Res*. 1994;**3**(3):183–189.

60. Carpenter DO. Neural mechanisms of emesis. *Can J Physiol Pharmacol*. 1990; **68**(2):230–236.

61. Miller AD, Wilson VJ. 'Vomiting center' reanalyzed: An electrical stimulation study. *Brain Res*. 1983;**270**(1):154–158.

62. Dalal S, *et al.* Symptom control in palliative care — part I: Oncology as a paradigmatic example. *J Palliat Med*. 2006;**9**(2):391–408.

63. Borison HL, Wang SC. Physiology and pharmacology of vomiting. *Pharmacol Rev*. 1953;**5**(2):193–230.

64. Bentley A, Boyd K. Use of clinical pictures in the management of nausea and vomiting: A prospective audit. *Palliat Med*. 2001;**15**(3):247–253.

65. Lichter I. Results of antiemetic management in terminal illness. *J Palliat Care*. 1993;**9**(2):19–21.

66. Bruera E, *et al*. A double-blind, crossover study of controlled-release metoclopramide and placebo for the chronic nausea and dyspepsia of advanced cancer. *J Pain Symptom Manage*. 2000;**19**(6):427–435.

67. Corli O, *et al*. Effectiveness of levosulpiride versus metoclopramide for nausea and vomiting in advanced cancer patients: A double-blind, randomized, crossover study. *J Pain Symptom Manage*. 1995;**10**(7):521–526.

68. National comprehensive cancer network (NCCN). NCCN clinical practice guidelines in oncology: Palliative care (version 1. 2014). http://www.nccn.org/professionals/ physician_gls/pdf/palliative.pdf. Updated 2014. Accessed June 1, 2014.

69. Ripamonti C, *et al*. Management of bowel obstruction in advanced and terminal cancer patients. *Ann Oncol*. 1993;**4**(1):15–21.

70. Laval G, *et al*. Recommendations for bowel obstruction with peritoneal carcinomatosis. *J Pain Symptom Manage*. 2014.

71. Baines MJ. Symptom control in advanced gastrointestinal cancer. *Eur J Gastroenterol Hepatol*. 2000;**12**(4):375–379.

72. Costamagna G, *et al*. Treatment of malignant gastroduodenal obstruction with a nitinol self-expanding metal stent: An international prospective multicentre registry. *Dig Liver Dis*. 2012;**44**(1):37–43.

73. Khot UP, *et al*. Systematic review of the efficacy and safety of colorectal stents. *Br J Surg*. 2002;**89**(9):1096–1102.

74. Datye A, Hersh J. Colonic perforation after stent placement for malignant colorectal obstruction — causes and contributing factors. *Minim Invasive Ther Allied Technol*. 2011;**20**(3):133–140.

75. Siersema PD, *et al*. Coated self-expanding metal stents versus latex prostheses for esophagogastric cancer with special reference to prior radiation and chemotherapy: A controlled, prospective study. *Gastrointest Endosc*. 1998;**47**(2):113–120.

76. Paul Olson TJ, *et al*. Palliative surgery for malignant bowel obstruction from carcinomatosis: A systematic review. *JAMA Surg*. 2014;**149**(4):383–392.

77. Perkins P, Dorman S. Haloperidol for the treatment of nausea and vomiting in palliative care patients. *Cochrane Database Syst Rev*. 2009;(2):CD006271. doi(2):CD006271.

78. Ripamonti C, *et al*. The role of somatostatin and octreotide in bowel obstruction: Pre-clinical and clinical results. *Tumori*. 2001;**87**(1):1–9.

79. Brooksbank MA, *et al*. Palliative venting gastrostomy in malignant intestinal obstruction. *Palliat Med*. 2002;**16**(6):520–526.

80. Chermesh I, *et al*. Home parenteral nutrition (HTPN) for incurable patients with cancer with gastrointestinal obstruction: Do the benefits outweigh the risks? *Med Oncol*. 2011;**28**(1):83–88.

81. Dev R, *et al*. Is there a role for parenteral nutrition or hydration at the end of life? *Curr Opin Support Palliat Care*. 2012;**6**(3):365–370.

82. Becker G, *et al*. Malignant ascites: Systematic review and guideline for treatment. *Eur J Cancer*. 2006;**42**(5):589–597.

83. Runyon BA. Care of patients with ascites. *N Engl J Med*. 1994;**330**(5):337–342.

84. LeBlanc K, Arnold R. Evaluation of malignant ascites. Retrieved from http://www.eperc. mcw.edu/EPERC/FastFactsIndex/ff_176.htm. Updated 2007. Accessed June 3, 2014.

85. McNamara P. Paracentesis — an effective method of symptom control in the palliative care setting? *Palliat Med.* 2000;**14**(1):62–64.

86. Lee CW, *et al.* A survey of practice in management of malignant ascites. *J Pain Symptom Manage.* 1998;**16**(2):96–101.

87. Souter RG, *et al.* Surgical and pathologic complications associated with peritoneovenous shunts in management of malignant ascites. *Cancer.* 1985;**55**(9):1973–1978.

88. Becker G, *et al.* Malignant ascites: Systematic review and guideline for treatment. *Eur J Cancer.* 2006;**42**(5):589–597.

89. Baron TH. Palliation of malignant obstructive jaundice. *Gastroenterol Clin North Am.* 2006;**35**(1):101–112.

90. Bergasa NV. Medical palliation of the jaundiced patient with pruritus. *Gastroenterol Clin North Am.* 2006;**35**(1):113–123.

91. Bosonnet L. Pruritus: Scratching the surface. *Eur J Cancer Care (Engl).* 2003; **12**(2):162–165.

92. Browning J, *et al.* Long-term efficacy of sertraline as a treatment for cholestatic pruritus in patients with primary biliary cirrhosis. *Am J Gastroenterol.* 2003;**98**(12):2736–2741.

93. Zylicz Z, *et al.* Paroxetine for pruritus in advanced cancer. *J Pain Symptom Manage.* 1998;**16**(2):121–124.

94. Davis MP, *et al.* Mirtazapine for pruritus. *J Pain Symptom Manage.* 2003;**25**(3): 288–291.

95. O'Donohue JW, *et al.* A controlled trial of ondansetron in the pruritus of cholestasis. *Aliment Pharmacol Ther.* 2005;**21**(8):1041–1045.

96. Raderer M, *et al.* Ondansetron for pruritus due to cholestasis. *N Engl J Med.* 1994; **330**(21):1540.

97. Ghent CN, Carruthers SG. Treatment of pruritus in primary biliary cirrhosis with rifampin. results of a double-blind, crossover, randomized trial. *Gastroenterology.* 1988;**94**(2):488–493.

98. Neff GW, *et al.* Preliminary observation with dronabinol in patients with intractable pruritus secondary to cholestatic liver disease. *Am J Gastroenterol.* 2002;**97**(8): 2117–2119.

99. Anand S. Gabapentin for pruritus in palliative care. *Am J Hosp Palliat Care.* 2013; **30**(2):192–196.

100. Hesketh PJ. Chemotherapy-induced nausea and vomiting. *N Engl J Med.* 2008; **358**(23):2482–2494.

101. Xiao WH, *et al.* Characterization of oxaliplatin-induced chronic painful peripheral neuropathy in the rat and comparison with the neuropathy induced by paclitaxel. *Neuroscience.* 2012;**203**:194–206.

102. Cavaletti G, *et al.* The chemotherapy-induced peripheral neuropathy outcome measures standardization study: From consensus to the first validity and reliability findings. *Ann Oncol.* 2013;**24**(2):454–462.

103. Pasetto LM, *et al.* Oxaliplatin-related neurotoxicity: How and why? *Crit Rev Oncol Hematol.* 2006;**59**(2):159–168.

104. Park SB, *et al*. Dose effects of oxaliplatin on persistent and transient na+ conductances and the development of neurotoxicity. *PLoS One*. 2011;**6**(4):e18469.

105. Grothey A. Oxaliplatin-safety profile: Neurotoxicity. *Semin Oncol*. 2003;**30**(4 Suppl 15):5–13.

106. Beijers AJ, *et al*. A systematic review on chronic oxaliplatin-induced peripheral neuropathy and the relation with oxaliplatin administration. *Support Care Cancer*. 2014;**22**(7):1999–2007.

107. Vatandoust S, *et al*. A descriptive study of persistent oxaliplatin-induced peripheral neuropathy in patients with colorectal cancer. *Support Care Cancer*. 2014;**22**(2): 513–518.

108. Petrioli R, *et al*. Neurotoxicity of FOLFOX-4 as adjuvant treatment for patients with colon and gastric cancer: A randomized study of two different schedules of oxaliplatin. *Cancer Chemother Pharmacol*. 2008;**61**(1):105–111.

109. Argyriou AA, *et al*. Clinical pattern and associations of oxaliplatin acute neurotoxicity: A prospective study in 170 patients with colorectal cancer. *Cancer*. 2013;**119**(2): 438–444.

110. Uwah AN, *et al*. The effect of diabetes on oxaliplatin-induced peripheral neuropathy. *Clin Colorectal Cancer*. 2012;**11**(4):275–279.

111. Grothey A, *et al*. Intravenous calcium and magnesium for oxaliplatin-induced sensory neurotoxicity in adjuvant colon cancer: NCCTG N04C7. *J Clin Oncol*. 2011;**29**(4): 421–427.

112. Hershman DL, *et al*. Prevention and management of chemotherapy-induced peripheral neuropathy in survivors of adult cancers: American society of clinical oncology clinical practice guideline. *J Clin Oncol*. 2014;**32**(18):1941–1967.

113. Abigerges D, *et al*. Phase I and pharmacologic studies of the camptothecin analog irinotecan administered every 3 weeks in cancer patients. *J Clin Oncol*. 1995;**13**(1): 210–221.

114. Kawato Y, *et al*. Intracellular roles of SN-38, a metabolite of the camptothecin derivative CPT-11, in the antitumor effect of CPT-11. *Cancer Res*. 1991;**51**(16): 4187–4191.

115. Benson AB, *et al*. Recommended guidelines for the treatment of cancer treatment-induced diarrhea. *J Clin Oncol*. 2004;**22**(14):2918–2926.

116. Duvic M, *et al*. A randomized trial of minoxidil in chemotherapy-induced alopecia. *J Am Acad Dermatol*. 1996;**35**(1):74–78.

117. Jatoi A, *et al*. Clinical predictors of severe cetuximab-induced rash: Observations from 933 patients enrolled in north central cancer treatment group study N0147. *Oncology*. 2009;**77**(2):120–123.

118. Lacouture ME, *et al*. Clinical practice guidelines for the prevention and treatment of EGFR inhibitor-associated dermatologic toxicities. *Support Care Cancer*. 2011; **19**(8):1079–1095.

119. Lacouture ME, *et al*. Skin toxicity evaluation protocol with panitumumab (STEPP), a phase II, open-label, randomized trial evaluating the impact of a pre-emptive skin treatment regimen on skin toxicities and quality of life in patients with metastatic colorectal cancer. *J Clin Oncol*. 2010;**28**(8):1351–1357.

120. Lopes AB, Fagundes RB. Esophageal squamous cell carcinoma — precursor lesions and early diagnosis. *World J Gastrointest Endosc.* 2012;**4**(1):9–16.

121. Elliott L, *et al. Complete resource kit for oncology nutrition.* Academy of Nutrition and Dietetics Publication; 2012.

122. Homs MY, *et al.* Palliative therapy. *J Surg Oncol.* 2005;**92**(3):246–256.

123. Adam A, *et al.* Palliation of inoperable esophageal carcinoma: A prospective randomized trial of laser therapy and stent placement. *Radiology.* 1997;**202**(2):344–348.

124. Gevers AM, *et al.* A comparison of laser therapy, plastic stents, and expandable metal stents for palliation of malignant dysphagia in patients without a fistula. *Gastrointest Endosc.* 1998;**48**(4):383–388.

125. Sihvo EI, *et al.* Inoperable adenocarcinoma of the oesophagogastric junction: A comparative clinical study of laser coagulation versus self-expanding metallic stents with special reference to cost analysis. *Eur J Surg Oncol.* 2002;**28**(7):711–715.

126. Homs MY, *et al.* Single-dose brachytherapy versus metal stent placement for the palliation of dysphagia from oesophageal cancer: Multicentre randomised trial. *Lancet.* 2004;**364**(9444):1497–1504.

127. Berkey FJ. Managing the adverse effects of radiation therapy. *Am Fam Physician.* 2010;**82**(4):381–8, 394.

128. Ligthart-Melis GC, *et al.* Dietician-delivered intensive nutritional support is associated with a decrease in severe postoperative complications after surgery in patients with esophageal cancer. *Dis Esophagus.* 2013;**26**(6):587–593.

129. Feig BW, *et al. The MD Anderson surgical oncology handbook.* 2nd ed. Philadelphia, PA: Lippincott Williams and Wilkins; 1999.

130. Radigan AE. Post-gastrectomy: Managing the nutrition fall-out. *Practical Gastroenterology.* June 2004:63–75.

131. Meyer J. Morbidity after ulcer surgery. In: Sleisinger MH, Fordtran JS, eds. *Gastrointestinal diseases.* 5th ed. Philadelphia, PA: Saunders; 1994:731–744.

132. Stael von Holstein C, *et al.* Nutritional status after total and partial gastrectomy with roux-en-Y reconstruction. *Br J Surg.* 1991;**78**(9):1084–1087.

133. Oh R, Brown DL. Vitamin B12 deficiency. *Am Fam Physician.* 2003;**67**(5):979–986.

134. Tovey FI, Godfrey JE, Lewin MR. A gastrectomy population: 25–30 years on. *Postgrad Med J.* 1990;**66**(776):450–456.

135. Krenitsky J, Decher N. Medical nutrition therapy for upper gastrointestinal disorders. In: Mahan LK, Escott-Stump S, Raymond JL, eds. *Krause's food in the nutrition care process.* 13th ed. St. Louis, MO: Elsevier Saunders; 2012:592–609.

136. Carey S. Bone health after major upper gastrointestional surgery. *Practical Gastroenterology.* 2013:46–55.

137. Juul T, *et al.* Low anterior resection syndrome and quality of life: An international multicenter study. *Dis Colon Rectum.* 2014;**57**(5):585–591.

138. Lange MM, *et al.* Faecal and urinary incontinence after multimodality treatment of rectal cancer. *PLoS Med.* 2008;**5**(10):e202.

139. Ottery F. Supportive nutritional management of the patient with pancreatic cancer. *Oncology (Williston Park).* 1996;**10**(9 Suppl):26–32.

140. Imrie CW, *et al.* Review article: Enzyme supplementation in cystic fibrosis, chronic pancreatitis, pancreatic and periampullary cancer. *Aliment Pharmacol Ther.* 2010;**32** (Suppl 1):1–25.

141. Wakasugi H, *et al.* A study of malabsorption in pancreatic cancer. *J Gastroenterol.* 1996;**31**(1):81–85.

142. Ellison NM, *et al.* Supportive care for patients with pancreatic adenocarcinoma: Symptom control and nutrition. *Hematol Oncol Clin North Am.* 2002;**16**(1):105–121.

143. Dominguez-Munoz JE. Pancreatic enzyme therapy for pancreatic exocrine insufficiency. *Gastroenterol Hepatol (N Y).* 2011;**7**(6):401–403.

144. Fieker A, *et al.* Enzyme replacement therapy for pancreatic insufficiency: Present and future. *Clin Exp Gastroenterol.* 2011;**4**:55–73.

145. Sarner M. Treatment of pancreatic exocrine deficiency. *World J Surg.* 2003;**27**(11): 1192–1195.

146. Decher N, Berry A. Post-whipple: A practical approach to nutrition management. *Practical Gastroenterology.* 2012:30–42.

147. Poulson J. The management of diabetes in patients with advanced cancer. *J Pain Symptom Manage.* 1997;**13**(6):339–346.

Index